Advanced Respiratory Critical Care

Oxford Specialist Handbooks published and forthcoming

Oxford Specialist Handbooks in Critical Care

Advanced Respiratory Critical Care

Edited by

Martin Hughes

Consultant in Intensive Care Medicine
Royal Infirmary, Glasgow, UK

Roland Black

Consultant in Intensive Care Medicine
Royal Devon and Exeter Hospital
Exeter, UK

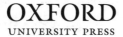

OXFORD
UNIVERSITY PRESS

OXFORD
UNIVERSITY PRESS

Great Clarendon Street, Oxford OX2 6DP

Oxford University Press is a department of the University of Oxford.
It furthers the University's objective of excellence in research, scholarship,
and education by publishing worldwide in

Oxford New York

Auckland Cape Town Dar es Salaam Hong Kong Karachi
Kuala Lumpur Madrid Melbourne Mexico City Nairobi
New Delhi Shanghai Taipei Toronto

With offices in

Argentina Austria Brazil Chile Czech Republic France Greece
Guatemala Hungary Italy Japan Poland Portugal Singapore
South Korea Switzerland Thailand Turkey Ukraine Vietnam

Oxford is a registered trade mark of Oxford University Press
in the UK and in certain other countries

Published in the United States
by Oxford University Press Inc., New York

© Oxford University Press 2011

British Library Cataloguing in Publication Data
Data available

Library of Congress Cataloging in Publication Data
Data available

Typeset by Cenveo, Bangalore, India
Printed in Great Britain on acid-free paper by
Ashford Colour Press Ltd, Gosport, Hampshire

ISBN 978–0–19–956928–1

10 9 8 7 6 5 4 3 2 1

Preface

Respiratory disease is the most common reason for admission to intensive care, and advanced respiratory support is one of the most frequently used interventions in critically ill patients. A clear understanding of respiratory disease is the cornerstone of high quality intensive care.

Although a plethora of literature is available, both in print and online, finding the necessary relevant information can be difficult and time consuming. This handbook provides comprehensive clinical detail in an easily readable format. It is written by practising clinicians and has both in-depth theoretical discussion and practical management advice.

The book is divided into sections
- Section 1 deals with the approach to the patient with respiratory failure – including pathophysiology, investigation, and diagnosis
- Section 2 covers non-invasive treatment modalities
- Sections 3 and 4 examine invasive ventilation in detail. Section 3 considers the principles of mechanical ventilation while section 4 deals with individual ventilator modes
- Section 5 discusses the management of the ventilated patient including sedation, monitoring, asynchrony, heart – lung interaction, hypercapnia and hypoxia, complications, weaning and extubation. It also has chapters on areas less frequently covered such as humidification, suction, tracheal tubes and principles of physiotherapy
- Section 6 is a comprehensive breakdown of each respiratory condition seen in ICU.

This book is designed to bridge the gap between Intensive Care starter texts and all-encompassing reference textbooks. It is aimed at consultants and senior trainees in Intensive Care Medicine, senior ICU nursing staff, consultants in other specialties and allied healthcare professionals who have an interest in advanced respiratory critical care.

Acknowledgements

The editors would like to acknowledge Dr Rajkumar Rajendram, Departments of General Medicine and Intensive Care, John Radcliffe Hospital, Oxford, UK, as a reviewer

Contents

Contributors

Rebecca Appelboam
Consultant in Intensive Care
Medicine
Derriford Hospital, Plymouth, UK

Hugh Bakere
Consultant in Respiratory
Medicine
Royal Devon and Exeter Hospital,
Exeter, UK

Steve Banham
Consultant in Respiratory
Medicine
Gartnavel General Hospital,
Glasgow, UK

Anthony Bateman
Consultant in Intensive Care and
Long Term Ventilation
Western General Hospital,
Edinburgh, UK

Catherine Bateman
Consultant Physician
United Bristol Hospitals NHS
Trust, Bristol, UK

Geoff Bellingan
Medical Director, Surgery and
Cancer Board
University College Hospital,
London, UK

Alexander Binning
Consultant in Intensive Care
Medicine
Western Infirmary, Glasgow, UK

Roland Black
Consultant in Intensive Care
Medicine
Royal Devon and Exeter Hospital,
Exeter, UK

Kevin Blyth
Consultant in Respiratory
Medicine
Southern General Hospital,
Glasgow, UK

Malcolm Booth
Consultant in Intensive Care
Medicine
Royal Infirmary, Glasgow, UK

Chris Cairns
Consultant in Intensive Care
Medicine
Royal Infirmary, Stirling, UK

Alyson Calder
Registrar in Anaesthesia
Royal Infirmary, Glasgow, UK

Luigi Camporota
Department of Adult
Critical Care Medicine
Guy's and St Thomas' NHS
Foundation Trust, London, UK

Colin Church
Research fellow in Respiratory
Medicine
Gartnavel General Hospital,
Glasgow, UK

Ian Colquhoun
Consultant Cardiothoracic
Surgeon
Golden Jubilee
National Hospital,
Clydebank, UK

Julius Cranshaw
Consultant in Intensive Care
Medicine and Anaesthesia
Royal Bournemouth Hospital,
Bournemouth, UK

Brian Cuthbertson
Professor and Chief of Department of Critical Care Medicine
Sunnybrook Health Sciences Centre, Toronto, UK

James Dale
Clinical Research Fellow
Institute of Infection, Inflammation and Immunity, University of Glasgow, UK

Dr Jonathan Dalzell
Clinical Research Fellow
British Heart Foundation Cardiovascular Research Centre, University of Glasgow, UK

Christopher Day
Consultant in Intensive Care Medicine,
Royal Devon and Exeter Hospital, Exeter, UK

Brian Digby
Consultant in Intensive Care Medicine and Anaesthesia
Royal Alexandria Hospital, Paisley, UK

Graham Douglas
Consultant Physician
Chest Clinic, Royal Infirmary, Aberdeen, UK

Dr Alasdair Dow
Consultant in Intensive Care Medicine
Royal Devon and Exeter Hospital, Exeter, UK

Tom Evans
Professor of Molecular Microbiology
Institute of Infection, Inflammation and Immunity, University of Glasgow, UK

Dawn Fabbroni
Consultant in Anaesthesia
Bradford Royal Infirmary, Bradford, UK

Timothy Felton
Clinical Research Training Fellow, Respiratory and Intensive Care Medicine
University of Manchester, UK

Andrew Foo
Registrar in Anaesthesia
North Bristol NHS Trust, Bristol, UK

Dimitris Georgopoulos
Professor of Medicine
Intensive Care Medicine Department, University Hospital of Heraklion, Crete, Greece

Dr Tim Gould
Consultant in Intensive Care Medicine and Anaesthesia
Royal Infirmary, Bristol, UK

Dr Duncan Gowans
Department of Haematology, Ninewells Hospital, Dundee, UK

Ian Grant
Consultant in Intensive Care Medicine and Long Term Ventilation
Western General Hospital, Edinburgh, UK

John Griffiths
Consultant and Honorary Senior Lecturer
Nuffield Department of Anaesthetics, John Radcliffe Hospital, Oxford, UK

Dr David Halpin
Consultant in Respiratory Medicine
Royal Devon and Exeter Hospital, Exeter, UK

Martyn Hawkins
Consultant in Intensive Care Medicine
Royal Infirmary, Stirling, UK

Nik Hirani
Senior Lecturer and Honorary
Consultant in Respiratory Medicine
Royal Infirmary, Edinburgh, UK

Martin Hughes
Consultant in Intensive Care
Medicine
Royal Infirmary, Glasgow, UK

Ben Ivory
Registrar in Anaesthesia
Royal Devon and Exeter Hospital,
Exeter, UK

Martin Johnson
Consultant in Respiratory Medicine
Scottish Pulmonary Vascular Unit,
Golden Jubilee National Hospital,
Clydebank, UK

Zuhal Karakurt
Sureyyepaşa Chest Disease and
Thoracic Surgery Training and
Research Hospital, Istanbul, Turkey

William Kinnear
Consultant in Respiratory Medicine
Nottingham University Hospitals
NHS Trust, Nottingham, UK

John Kinsella
Professor of Critical Care,
Anaesthesia and Pain Medicine
Royal Infirmary, Glasgow, UK

Maria Klimathianaki
Department of Intensive Care
Medicine
University Hospital of Heraklion,
Crete, Greece

Eumorfia Kondili
Department of Intensive Care
Medicine
University Hospital of Heraklion,
Crete, Greece

Nicola Lee
Pulmonary Vascular Fellow
Scottish Pulmonary Vascular Unit,
Golden Jubilee National Hospital,
Clydebank, UK

Andrew Lockwood
Team Leader in Critical Care
Physiotherapy
Royal Devon and Exeter Hospital,
Exeter, UK

Andrew Lumb
Consultant in Anaesthesia
St James's University Hospital,
Leeds, UK

Andrew MacDuff
Registrar in Respiratory and
Critical Care Medicine
Western General Hospital,
Edinburgh, UK

Peter MacNaughton
Consultant in Intensive Care
Derriford Hospital,
Plymouth, UK

Paul McConnell
Consultant in Intensive Care
Medicine
Crosshouse Hospital, Kilmarnock,
UK

Iain McInnes
Director and Professor of
Experimental Medicine and
Rheumatology
Institute of Infection, Inflammation
and Immunity, University of
Glasgow, UK

Elizabeth McGrady
Consultant in Anaesthesia
Royal Infirmary, Glasgow, UK

Stuart McLellan
Consultant in Intensive Care
Medicine
Western General Hospital,
Edinburgh, UK

Professor John McMurray
Professor of Medical Cardiology
British Heart Foundation
Cardiovascular Research Centre,
University of Glasgow, UK

Dr Nick Maskell
Senior Lecturer and Honorary
Consultant in Respiratory
Medicine
University of Bristol, UK

Dr Marina Morgan
Consultant in Medical
Microbiology
Royal Devon and Exeter Hospital,
Exeter, UK

David Mucuha Muigai
Assistant Professor, Department
Critical Care Medicine, University
of Pittsburgh; Medical Director,
Magee Womens Hospital of
UPMC, Adult ICU, Pittsburgh PA,
USA

Dr Julia Munn
Consultant in Intensive Care
Medicine
Royal Devon and Exeter Hospital,
Exeter, UK

Stephano Nava
Director of Respiratory and
Critical Care Unit
Sant'Orsola Malpighi University
Hospital, Bologna, Italy

Graham Nimmo
Consultant Physician in Intensive
Care Medicine and Clinical
Education,
Western General Hospital,
Edinburgh, UK

Dr Bipen Patel
Consultant in Respiratory
Medicine
Royal Devon and Exeter Hospital,
Exeter, UK

Ross Paterson
Consultant in Intensive Care
Medicine
Western General Hospital,
Edinburgh, UK

Derek Paul
Consultant in Cardiothoracic
Anaesthesia
Golden Jubilee National Hospital,
Clydebank, UK

Mr Giles Peek
Consultant in Cardiothoracic
Surgery and ECMO,
Glenfield Hospital, Leicester, UK

Michael Pinsky
Vice Chair, Academic Affairs
Professor of Critical Care
Medicine, Bioengineering,
Cardiovascular Disease and
Anesthesiology
University of Pittsburgh, PA, USA

Giles Roditi
Consultant in Radiology
Royal Infirmary, Glasgow, UK

Malcolm Sim
Consultant in Intensive Care
Medicine
Western Infirmary, Glasgow, UK

Christer Sinderby
Assistant Professor
Department of Medicine,
University of Toronto, Canada

Dr Lucy Smyth
Consultant in Renal Medicine
Royal Devon and Exeter Hospital,
Exeter, UK

Rosemary Snaith
Registrar in Anaesthesia
Royal Infirmary, Glasgow, UK

Dr Mike Spivey
Registrar in Anaesthesia
Royal Devon and Exeter Hospital,
Exeter, UK

David Swann
Consultant in Intensive Care
Medicine
Royal Infirmary, Edinburgh, UK

Anthony Todd
Consultant in Haematology
Royal Devon and Exeter Hospital,
Exeter, UK

Tim Walsh
Honorary Professor, Edinburgh
University and Consultant in
Critical Care
Royal Infirmary, Edinburgh, UK

Louise Watson
Clinical Lead in Critical Care
Physiotherapy
Royal Devon and Exeter Hospital,
Exeter, UK

Symbols and abbreviations

AAA	abdominal aortic aneurysm
AAFB	alcohol–acid fast bacilli
A-aO$_2$ gradient	alveolar-arterial oxygen gradient
ABG	arterial blood gas
ACBT	active cycle of breathing technique
ACE	angiotensin converting enzyme
ACh	acetylcholine
ACT	activated clotting time
ACV	assist control ventilation
AF	atrial fibrillation
AIDS	acquired immunodeficiency syndrome
AIP	acute interstitial pneumonia
AKI	acute kidney injury
ALI	acute lung injury
ANA	antinuclear antibody
ANCA	anti-neutrophil cytoplasmic antibody
AP	antero-posterior
APACHE	acute physiology and chronic health evaluation
APF	alveolo-pleural fistulae
APRV	airway pressure release ventilation
ARDS	acute respiratory distress syndrome
ARF	acute respiratory failure
AST	aspartamine transaminase
ASV	adaptive support ventilation
ATC	automatic tube compensation
ATLS	advanced trauma life support
AVCO$_2$R	artero-venous carbon dioxide removal
AVM	arteriovenous malformations
BAL	bronchoalveolar lavage
BCG	bacille Calmette-Guerin
BHL	bilateral hilar lymphadenopathy
BiPAP	bi-level positive airway pressure
BIPAP	biphasic positive airways pressure
BIS	bispectral index

BLS	basic life support
BMI	body mass index
BNP	brain natriuretic peptide
BOOP	bronchiolitis obliterans organizing pneumonia
BOS	bronchiolitis obliterans syndrome
BPF	broncho-pleural fistula
bpm	beats per minute
BTS	British Thoracic Society
BYCER	buffered yeast extract charcoal agar
CABG	coronary artery bypass graft
CAM-ICU	confusion assessment method for ICU
c-ANCA	antineutrophilic cytoplasmic antibody
CAP	community-acquired pneumonia
CAPS	COPD and asthma physiology score
CC	closing capacity
CCF	congestive cardiac failure
CDM	clinical decision making
CF	cystic fibrosis
CFA	cryptogenic fibrosing alveolitis
CHF	chronic heart failure
CI	cardiac index
CIM	critical illness myopathy
CIP	critical illness polyneuropathy
CIPM	critical illness polyneuromyopathy
CK	creatine kinase
CLED	cystine–lactose–electrolyte deficient
CMV	cytomegalovirus
CNS	central nervous system
CO	cardiac output
COP	cryptogenic organizing pneumonia
COPD	chronic obstructive pulmonary disease
CPAP	continuous positive airway pressure
CPB	cardiopulmonary bypass
CPG	central pattern generator
CPIS	clinical pulmonary infection score
CPO	cardiogenic pulmonary oedema
CPR	cardiopulmonary resuscitation
CROP	compliance respiratory rate oxygenation and pressure
CRP	C-reactive protein
CSF	cerebrospinal fluid

CSHT	context sensitive half times
CT	computerized tomography
CTPA	CT pulmonary angiography
CUS	compression ultrasonography
CVA	cerebrovascular accident
CVP	central venous pressure
CVS	cardiovascular system
CVVH	continuous veno-venous haemofiltration
CXR	chest X-ray
DAD	diffuse alveolar damage
DBP	diastolic blood pressure
DILD	drug-induced lung disease
DIP	desquamative interstitial pneumonia
DLCO	diffusing capacity of the lung for carbon monoxide
DMARD	disease-modifying antirheumatic drug
DMD	Duchenne muscular dystrophy
DTPA	diethylenetriaminepentaacetic acid
DVT	deep vein thrombosis
EAA	extrinsic allergic alveolitis
EAdi	electrical activity of the diaphragm
EBUS	endobronchial ultrasound
$ECCO_2R$	extra-corporeal CO_2 removal
ECG	electrocardiogram
ECMO	extracorporeal membrane oxygenation
ED	emergency department
EELV	end expiratory lung volume
EIT	electrical impedance tomography
ELISA	enzyme-linked immunosorbent assay
ELSO	extracorporeal life support registry
EMG	electromyogram
ENT	ear, nose and throat
EPAP	expiratory positive airways pressure
ESR	erythrocyte sedimentation rate
ET	endo-tracheal
ETT	endotracheal tube
ETS	expiratory trigger sensor
EVLW	extravascular lung water
FA	flow assist
FBC	full blood count
FEV	forced expiratory volume

FFP	fresh frozen plasma
FOB	fibreoptic bronchoscope
FRC	functional residual capacity
FSH	facioscapulohumeral
FVC	forced vital capacity
GABA	γ-amino butyrate
GBM	glomerular basement membrane
GCS	Glasgow Coma Score
GCSF	granulocyte macrophage colony-stimulating factor
GFR	glomerular filtration rate
GGO	ground glass opacity
GM-CSF	granulocyte-macrophage colony-stimulating factor
GTN	glyceryl trinitrate
HAART	highly active antiretroviral therapy
HAFOE	high air flow oxygen enrichment
HAP	hospital-acquired pneumonia
Hb	haemoglobin
HbA	haemoglobin A
HbF	foetal haemoglobin
HbO_2	oxyhaemoglobin
HbS	sickle cell haemoglobin
HDU	high-dependency unit
HELLP	syndrome of haemolysis, elevated liver enzymes, low platelets
HFOV	high frequency oscillatory ventilation
HH	heated humidifiers
HHb	deoxyhaemoglobin
HHT	hereditary haemorrhagic telangiectasia
HIV	human immunodeficiency virus
HME	heat and moisture exchanger
HPV	hypoxic pulmonary vasoconstriction
HR	heart rate
HRCT	high-resolution CT
HRQL	health-related quality of life
HRT	hormone replacement therapy
HSV	herpes simplex virus
HWH	heated water humidifier
IABP	intra-aortic balloon pumps
IBW	ideal body weight
ICMs	intercostal muscles

ICP	intracranial pressure
ICU	intensive care unit
I:E	inspiratory:expiratory
ILD	interstitial lung disease
IMV	intermittent mandatory ventilation
INR	international normalized ratio
IPAP	inspiratory positive airway pressure
IPF	idiopathic pulmonary fibrosis
IPPV	intermittent positive pressure ventilation
IRV	inverse ratio ventilation
ITP	intrathoracic pressure
IVC	inferior vena cava
IVIG	intravenous immunoglobulin
JVP	jugular venous pressure
KCO	transfer coefficient for carbon monoxide
LDH	lactate dehydrogenase
LFT	liver function tests
LMWH	low molecular weight heparin
LPS	lipopolysaccharide
LPV	lung protective ventilation
LR	likelihood ratio
LTV	long-term ventilation
LV	left ventricle
LVAD	left ventricular assist device
LVEDP	left ventricular end diastolic pressure
LVF	left ventricular failure
LVH	left ventricular hypertrophy
MAP	mean arterial pressure
MDR	multi-drug resistant
MDT	multidisciplinary team
MIC	minimum inhibitory concentration
met Hb	methaemoglobin
MH	malignant hyperpyrexia
MHI	manual hyperinflation
MI	myocardial infarction
MIGET	multiple inert gas elimination technique
MIP	maximal inspiratory pressure
MMF	mycophenolate mofetil
MND	motor neurone disease
MOF	multi organ failure

MPO	myeloperoxidase
MRC	medical research council
MRI	magnetic resonance imaging
MRSA	meticillin-resistant *Staphylococcus aureus*
MSSA	meticillin-sensitive *Staphylococcus aureus*
MV	minute volume
NAC	*N*-acetyl cysteine
NAECC	North American-European Consensus Conference
NAVA	neurally adjusted ventilatory assist
NGT	nasogastric tube
NICE	National Institute for Health and Clinical Excellence
NIV	non-invasive ventilation
NK	natural killer
NMBA	neuromuscular blockade agent
NNT	number needed to treat
NPV	negative pressure ventilation
NSAID	non-steroidal anti-inflammatory drug
NSIP	non-specific interstitial pneumonia
NSTEMI	non-ST-elevation myocardial infarction
nTe	neural expiratory time
NT-proBNP	N-terminal pro B type natriuretic peptide
NYHA	New York Heart Association
OHS	obesity hypoventilation syndrome
OLB	open-lung biopsy
OSA	obstructive sleep apnoea
PA	postero-anterior
PACS	picture archiving and communication systems
$PaCO_2$	arterial partial pressure of carbon dioxide
PAH	pulmonary artery hypertension
p-ANCA	antineutrophilic perinuclear antibody
PaO_2	arterial partial pressure of oxygen
PAO_2	alveolar partial pressure of oxygen
PAOP	pulmonary artery occlusion pressure
PAS	periodic acid-Schiff
PAV	proportional assist ventilation
PAVM	pulmonary arteriovenous malformations
PCI	percutaneous coronary intervention
PCP	*Pneumocystis jirovecii* pneumonia
PCR	polymerase chain reaction
PCV	pressure-controlled ventilation

PDE	phosphodiesterase
PDT	percutaneous dilational tracheostomy
PE	pulmonary thromboembolism
PEEP	positive end expiratory pressure
$PEEP_e$	extrinsic PEEP
$PEEP_i$	intrinsic PEEP
PEF	peak expiratory flow
PEFR	peak expiratory flow rate
P_{ES}	oesophageal pressure
PFT	pulmonary function tests
PGE1	prostaglandin E1
PH	pulmonary hypertension
PIFR	peak inspiratory flow rate
PIP	peak inspiratory pressure
pMDI	pressurized metered dose inhaler
PMP	polymethylpentene
PND	paroxysmal nocturnal dyspnoea
PO_2	partial pressure of oxygen
PS	pressure support
PSB	protected specimen brush
PSG	polysomnogram
PSI	Pneumonia Severity Index
PSV	pressure support ventilation
PTE	pulmonary thromboembolism
PTI	pressure time index
PTSD	post-traumatic stress disorder
PVL	Panton Valentine leukocidin
PVR	pulmonary vascular resistance
RA	right atrium
RACE	repetitive alveolar collapse expansion
RBC	red blood cell
RBILD	respiratory bronchiolitis-associated interstitial lung disease
RCT	randomized controlled trial
REM	rapid eye movement
RhF	rheumatoid factor
RIP	respiratory inductance plethysmography
RM	recruitment manoeuvres
ROS	reactive oxygen species
RQ	respiratory quotient

RR	relative risk
RSBI	rapid shallow breathing index
RSV	respiratory syncytial virus
rv	right ventricle
SAPS	simplified acute physiology score
SBD	sleep-disordered breathing
SBP	systolic blood pressure
SBT	spontaneous breathing trial
SDD	selective decontamination of the digestive tract
SIADH	syndrome of inappropriate anti-diuretic hormone
SIMV	synchronized intermittent mandatory ventilation
SIRS	systemic inflammatory response syndrome
SLB	surgical lung biopsy
SLE	systemic lupus erythematosis
SNIP	sniff nasal inspiratory pressure
SOD	selective oral decontamination
ST	surface tension
STEMI	ST elevation myocardial infarction
SV	stroke volume
SVR	systemic vascular resistance
TB	tuberculosis
TBLB	transbronchial lung biopsy
THAM	tris-hydroxymethyl aminomethane
TLC	total lung capacity
TPMT	thiopurine methyltransferase
TSST	toxic shock syndrome toxin
TTE	trans-thoracic echocardiography
TV	tidal volume
U+E	urea and electrolytes
UIP	usual interstitial pneumonia
VA	volume assist
VALI	ventilator associated lung injury
VAP	ventilator-associated pneumonia
VAS	visual analogue scale
VAT	ventilator-associated tracheobronchitis
VATS	video-assisted thoracic surgery
VC	vital capacity
VCV	volume controlled ventilation
VIDD	ventilator-induced diaphragmatic dysfunction
VILI	ventilator-induced lung injury

vTi	ventilator inspiratory time
VTE	venous thromboembolism
VZV	Varicella zoster virus
WCC	white cell count
WOB	work of breathing
ZA	zone of apposition
ZEEP	zero PEEP

Approach to the patient with respiratory failure

1.1 Respiratory physiology and pathophysiology

Control of breathing

Respiratory centre

The respiratory centre is located in the medulla. It generates the respiratory rhythm and co-ordinates voluntary and involuntary aspects of breathing. Functionally important components include the following.

Central pattern generator

The central pattern generator (CPG) is where the respiratory rhythm originates, with repetitive waves of activity in about six groups of interconnected neurones, thus allowing multiple patterns of respiratory activity to occur. A system which involves groups of neurones, rather than a single pacemaker cell, provides substantial physiological redundancy such that respiration in some form is preserved even under extreme physiological challenge. Unfortunately the large number of neurotransmitters involved in rhythm generation and modulation of the CPG also means that a wide variety of pathological situations and pharmacological agents will affect respiration.

Afferent inputs to the respiratory centre

Central:
- Pontine respiratory group—not essential for ventilation but influences fine control of respiration and co-ordinates the other central nervous system (CNS) connections to the CPG.
- Cerebral cortex—influences voluntary interruption in breathing required for speech, singing, sniffing, coughing etc.

Peripheral from the upper respiratory tract:
- Nasopharynx—water and irritants can cause apnoea, sneezing etc. Mechanoreceptors responding to negative pressure activate pharyngeal dilator muscles; abnormalities of this reflex are crucial in sleep-disordered breathing.
- Larynx—the supraglottic area receives sensory innervation from three groups: mechanoreceptors (as for the pharynx), cold receptors on the vocal folds that depress ventilation, and irritant receptors that cause cough, laryngeal closure, and bronchoconstriction.

From the lung:
- Slowly adapting stretch receptors are found in the airways and respond to sustained lung inflation.
- Rapidly adapting stretch receptors occur in the superficial mucosal layer and are stimulated by changes in tidal volume, respiratory rate, or lung compliance.
- C fibre endings are closely related to capillaries in the bronchial circulation and pulmonary microcirculation (J receptors). Stimulated by pathological conditions and by noxious substances, tissue damage, and accumulation of interstitial fluid, they may be responsible for dyspnoea associated with pulmonary vascular congestion or embolism.

Efferent output
Efferent pathways from the CPG go to separate inspiratory and expiratory motor neurone pools located in the brainstem. Arising from these are the motor nerves for the pharyngeal dilator muscles, intercostals, diaphragm, and expiratory muscles.

Influence of CO_2
Central chemoreceptors are located in the anterior medulla, separate from the respiratory centre. Carbon dioxide, but not H^+ ions, pass across the blood–brain barrier where carbonic anhydrase catalyses its hydration into H^+ and HCO_3^-. Central chemoreceptor neurones respond to a fall in pH with a linear increase in minute ventilation.

A compensatory shift in cerebrospinal fluid (CSF) bicarbonate concentration occurs with chronic hyper- and hypocapnia, and is seen in artificially ventilated patients. The speed of pH compensation by the bicarbonate shift depends on the extent of the arterial partial pressure ($PaCO_2$) change and can take hours. Artificially ventilated patients that have been hyperventilated may continue to hyperventilate after resuming spontaneous breathing because of this resetting of CSF pH by a compensatory decrease in CSF bicarbonate. Pathological states that directly lower the CSF bicarbonate concentration and pH can result in hyperventilation, for example following intracranial haemorrhage.

Influence of O_2 and peripheral chemoreceptors
Peripheral chemoreceptors are located close to the bifurcation of the common carotid artery and in the aortic bodies. They have a high perfusion rate, much greater than their metabolic rate, and a small arteriovenous PO_2 difference. The glomus cell is the site of oxygen sensing, a poorly understood process involving oxygen-sensitive voltage-gated potassium channels and a variety of neurotransmitters and modulators.

Features of the hypoxic ventilatory response include stimulation by:
- Decreased PaO_2, not oxygen content, therefore there is no response to anaemia, carboxyhaemoglobin. or methaemoglobin
- Decreased pH or increased $PaCO_2$—this response is only one-sixth of the central chemoreceptor response but occurs very rapidly; may also respond to cyclical oscillations in arterial $PaCO_2$ seen, for example, in time with respiration during the hyperventilation of exercise or altitude exposure
- Hypoperfusion (stagnant hypoxia) or raised temperature.

Stimulation results in an increase in depth and rate of breathing, bradycardia, hypertension, increased bronchiolar tone, and adrenal stimulation.

In response to sustained hypoxia, a series of ventilatory responses occur:

- Acute hypoxia produces a rapid increase in the ventilatory rate within a few seconds; with progressively severe hypoxia the increase in ventilation is not linear, and forms a rectangular hyperbola.
- The response curve is displaced upwards by hypercapnia and exercise, and displaced downwards by hypocapnia.
- After 5–10min of sustained hypoxia, hypoxic ventilatory decline occurs; there is a reduction in ventilation until a plateau is reached, which is still greater than the resting rate.
- Both the acute response and hypoxic ventilatory decline are less in poikilocapnic conditions when the hypocapnia induced by hyperventilation partly counteracts the ventilatory effects of hypoxia.
- With prolonged hypoxia there is a second slower rise in ventilation rate for about 8h.

Ventilation

Respiratory muscles

Numerous muscle groups are involved in changing lung volume. Their co-ordination by the medullary respiratory neurones and interaction with each other are complex.

- Upper airway muscles—pharyngeal dilator muscles contract both tonically and phasically (with respiration) to prevent upper airway collapse. Minor abnormalities of this system result in airway collapse by seemingly minor physiological challenges such as sleep or sedative drugs. Abduction and adduction of the posterior arytenoid muscles control vocal fold position to retard expiration and reduce lower airway collapse, in effect providing positive end expiratory pressure (PEEP).
- Diaphragm—the most important respiratory muscle. Contraction of the diaphragm causes reduction in the zone of apposition (the area around the outside of the diaphragm, which has direct contact with the inside of the ribcage), thus increasing lung volume in a 'piston-like' action. This is the most energy efficient way of converting diaphragm contraction into lung expansion, and is impaired either by hyperexpanded lung or by raised intra-abdominal pressure. Contraction of the diaphragm also increases thoracic volume by flattening of the diaphragm dome and expansion of the lower ribcage (Fig. 1.1).
- Ribcage muscles—three layers of intercostal muscles (ICMs) exist: external, internal, and intercostalis intima. Anteriorly the internal ICMs become thicker to form the parasternal ICMs. External ICMs are primarily inspiratory and internal ICMs are mainly expiratory, although these functions vary with posture. Elevation of the ribs by the ICMs results in a 'bucket handle' action to expand the chest wall while elevation of the sternum by the sternomastoid and scalene muscles results in a 'pump handle' action and opposes the upper ribs being pulled inward during inspiration. *In vivo*, these actions all occur together in a co-ordinated fashion and are significantly altered by posture (see below) and respiratory pattern.

- Abdominal muscles—rectus abdominis, external oblique, internal oblique, and transversalis muscle are mainly used in expiration. Contraction of these muscles increases intra-abdominal pressure, resulting in cephalad displacement of the diaphragm. Active expiration occurs during stimulated breathing if the minute volume is approximately >35L/min, or in the spontaneously breathing patient under general anaesthetic.
- Accessory muscles include the sternomastoids, pectoralis minor, trapezius, extensors of the spine, and serrati muscles. Inactive during normal ventilation, these are employed with increasing respiratory rate and tidal volume.

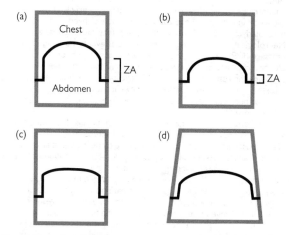

Fig. 1.1 Mechanisms of the respiratory actions of the diaphragm using a 'piston in a cylinder' analogy. (a) Resting end-expiratory position. (b) Inspiration showing 'piston-like' behaviour with shortening of the zone of apposition (ZA). (c) Inspiration with flattening of the diaphragm dome. (d) Combination of shortening of ZA, flattening of the dome, and expansion of the ribcage, which equates most closely with inspiration *in vivo*.

Effect of posture

- Upright—associated with greater expansion of the ribcage. Increased activity in scalene muscles, and parasternal and external ICMs.
- Supine—abdominal contents push the diaphragm cephalad, thus reducing functional residual capacity (FRC). The diaphragmatic zone of apposition (Fig. 1.1) is increased in this position so the diaphragm works efficiently.
- Lateral—the lower dome of the diaphragm is displaced cephalad so is more effective than the upper dome. Ventilation of the lower lung is twice that of the upper, which matches the preferential perfusion to the lower lung.

- Prone—as in the supine position the diaphragm moves cephalad into the chest. In anaesthetized patients movement of non-dependent areas of the diaphragm dominates. Upper chest and pelvis need support to allow free movement of the abdomen and chest.

Pathophysiology of ventilatory failure

Ventilatory failure occurs when a patient cannot achieve the required minute volume of alveolar ventilation. There are many causes, conveniently classified as shown in Fig. 1.2.

- Respiratory centre neurones: stimulated by hypoxia or high $PaCO_2$. The response to $PaCO_2$ is blunted by anaesthesia and some drugs. Apnoea occurs if $PaCO_2$ falls below the apnoeic threshold in an unconscious patient. Chronic respiratory diseases may lead to a reduction in the normal physiological response to hypercapnia. Drugs, particularly opioids and anaesthetic agents, may cause central apnoea. Neurological conditions, e.g. cerebrovascular events, raised intracranial pressure (ICP), or trauma may directly depress respiration.
- Upper motor neurones: cervical spine trauma may affect nerves supplying the respiratory muscles. Demyelination, tumours, and syringomyelia can involve upper motor neurones.
- Anterior horn cells: may be affected by various diseases, e.g. poliomyelitis.
- Lower motor neurones: may be affected by trauma and conditions such as advanced motor neurone disease or Guillain–Barré syndrome.
- Neuromuscular junction: routinely affected by neuromuscular blocking agents in anaesthesia or pathologically by botulism, organophosphate poisoning, nerve gas poisoning, or myasthenia gravis.
- Respiratory muscle pathology: may develop fatigue through increased work of breathing (WOB). Critical care patients commonly develop polyneuropathy and myopathy of respiratory muscles as a result of sepsis or prolonged disuse atrophy following a period of artificial ventilation. There is *in vitro* evidence indicating muscle fibre atrophy after only 18h of mechanical ventilation, and within days diaphragm strength is substantially reduced.
- Loss of lungs or chest wall elasticity: may occur within the lungs (pulmonary fibrosis or lung injury), the pleura (empyema), chest wall (kyphoscoliosis), or skin (contracted scars from burns).
- Loss of structural integrity of chest wall or pleural cavity: results from multiple fractured ribs producing a flail segment, or from a pneumothorax or pleural effusion.
- Small airway resistance: the most common cause of ventilatory failure, including asthma, chronic obstructive pulmonary disease (COPD), and cystic fibrosis.
- Upper airway obstruction: for example with airway and pharyngeal tumours, infections, inhaled foreign bodies, and tumour or bleeding in the neck.
- Increased dead space: caused by ventilation of large areas of unperfused lung, e.g. pulmonary embolism or pulmonary hypotension.

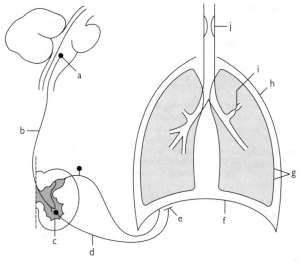

Fig. 1.2 Sites at which lesions, drug action, or malfunction may result in ventilatory failure. (a) Respiratory centre. (b) Upper motor neuron. (c) Anterior horn cell. (d) Lower motor neuron. (e) Neuromuscular junction. (f) Respiratory muscles. (g) Altered elasticity of lungs or chest wall. (h) Loss of structural integrity of chest wall or pleura. (i) Increased resistance of small airways. (j) Upper airway obstruction. Reproduced from *Nunn's Applied Respiratory Physiology* by permission of the author and publishers.

Respiratory system mechanics

Lung movements depend on external forces, caused either by the respiratory muscles in spontaneous breathing or a pressure gradient produced in artificial ventilation. The response of the lung to these forces is determined by the impedence of the respiratory system, which comprises:

- Elastic resistance of the lung tissue and chest wall, and resistance from the surface forces of the alveolar gas–liquid interface, which together are referred to as compliance
- Non-elastic resistance, which includes frictional resistance to gas flow through airways, deformation of thoracic tissue, and a negligible component from inertia associated with movement of gas and tissue. Together these are referred to as respiratory system resistance.

Compliance
- Definition: change in lung volume per unit change in transmural pressure gradient.
- Includes components from the lung and thoracic cage.
- Normal value for the whole respiratory system is 0.85L/kPa, for the lungs only the value is 1.5L/kPa.
- Elastance is the reciprocal of compliance.

Lung recoil

The tendency of the lung to collapse is balanced against the outward recoil of the thoracic cage. In expiration, when no air is flowing, the balance between these forces determines the FRC.

Recoil of the lung results from its inherent elasticity and surface tension (ST). ST, not inherent elasticity, accounts for most of the lung compliance. The ST of alveolar lining fluid is lower than that of water and changes according to the size of the alveolus because of the presence of surfactant.

Alveolar surfactant
- Structure—composed of 90% lipids, mostly dipalmitoyl phosphatidyl choline, and 10% proteins. In the alveolus hydrophobic fatty acids lie in parallel, projecting into the gas phase, with an opposite hydrophilic end extending into alveolar lining fluid.
- Synthesised in type II alveolar epithelial cells. Stored in lamellar bodies and released by exocytosis in response to high-volume inflation, increased ventilation rate, or endocrine stimulation.
- Alters the ST of alveoli as their size varies with inspiration and expiration. During expiration alveolar size decreases and surfactant molecules become more closely packed together, possibly forming multi-layered 'rafts', and exert a greater effect on ST. This action is controlled by the surfactant proteins, without which surfactant function is poor.
- Since the pulmonary capillary pressure in most of the lung is greater than alveolar pressure it encourages transudation, which is opposed by the oncotic pressure of plasma proteins. By decreasing the ST, surfactant reduces transudation.
- Immunological—surfactant proteins have a variety of roles in the defence of the lung from inhaled pathogens.

Altered surfactant function contributes to pathological states, e.g. acute lung injury (ALI). Surfactant is diluted by alveolar oedema and inactivated by inflammatory proteins, and cyclical closure of airways during expiration draws surfactant from the alveoli into small airways, contributing to atelectrauma.

Time dependence of pulmonary elasticity

If a lung is rapidly inflated and then held at that volume for a few seconds the inflation pressure quickly falls to a lower level. The extent to which this occurs affects measurements of lung compliance and can vary in different regions of lung, resulting in 'fast' and 'slow' alveoli and less than ideal V̇/Q̇ ratios (see below).

Causes of time dependency include:
- Changes in surfactant activity—the ST in alveoli is greater at larger lung volumes
- Stress relaxation—if any elastic material is stretched to a fixed length it produces maximal tension and then declines exponentially to a constant value
- Redistribution of gas—different parts of the lung have different time constants
- Recruitment of alveoli—some alveoli close at low lung volume; this is rare during normal breathing but occurs more easily in injured lungs. A much higher transmural pressure is needed to reopen them.

This time dependence may be assessed by the difference between static and dynamic compliance.

Static compliance is measured by inhalation of a range of known volumes of air from FRC and then allowing the patient to relax against a closed airway for a few seconds before the airway pressure is measured (relative to atmospheric). The volumes and pressures obtained are used to derive a compliance curve for the respiratory system (including lungs and thoracic cage).

Dynamic compliance is measured during rhythmical breathing, but calculated from measurements of pressure and volume made when there is no gas flowing, i.e. at end-inspiration and end-expiration. Many ventilators are able to produce pressure–volume loops and dynamic compliance can be displayed with each breath.

Factors affecting lung compliance:
- Lung volume: larger alveoli have higher compliance
- Posture: lung volume and therefore compliance changes with posture
- Pulmonary blood flow: venous congestion will decrease compliance
- Recent ventilation: hypoventilation may cause reduced compliance due to formation of atelectasis
- Bronchial smooth muscle tone: bronchoconstriction may enhance time dependence
- Disease: almost any lung disease will reduce lung compliance, either by affecting the elasticity of lung tissue or by impairing surfactant function.

Thoracic cage compliance
This includes compliance of the ribcage and diaphragm.
- Defined as change in lung volume per unit change in the pressure gradient between atmosphere and intrapleural space.
- Measured as described above but using intrapleural pressure (from an oesophageal balloon) rather than airway pressure.
- The diaphragm maintains some tone at end-expiration to prevent the abdominal contents pushing up into the thoracic cavity, which makes measurement difficult in a conscious patient.
- May be increased due to increased abdominal pressure, obesity, or from ossification of costal cartilages or chest wall scarring.

A reciprocal relationship exists between respiratory system compliance and its components:

$$\frac{1}{\text{total compliance}} = \frac{1}{\text{lung compliance}} = \frac{1}{\text{thoracic cage compliance}}$$

Respiratory system resistance
Respiratory system resistance has two components.

Tissue resistance
This is resistance caused by the deformation of lung and chest wall tissue during breathing. It includes the time-dependent element of elastance (see above): when the volume is changed there is initial resistance as tissue deformation occurs, but if inflation is held for a few seconds the elastance is reduced.

Airway resistance
This is the most important cause of respiratory system resistance in clinical practice and results from frictional resistance to gas flow within the airways. In healthy lungs the small airways contribute very little to total airway resistance because of their large combined cross-sectional area, so resistance is predominantly from larger airways. Gas flow within the lungs is a complex mixture of laminar and turbulent flow.

Turbulent flow occurs in conducting airways where gas velocity is high:
• Flow is therefore significantly influenced by the airway lining, e.g. mucus consistency.
• The turbulent flow increases the efficiency of humidification by mixing the inspired gas with the water vapour from the airway lining fluid.
• Helium gas mixtures (low Reynolds number, low viscosity) are of more benefit in overcoming resistance in large airways than small airways. Heliox has been used to treat acute asthmatic patients, perhaps because flow within narrowed, inflamed airways becomes turbulent.

Laminar flow normally occurs at around the 11th airway generation because:
• The velocity of gas flow decreases with successive airway generations
• In small airways the entrance length (distance required for laminar flow to become established) becomes short enough for laminar flow to develop before the next airway division.

Factors affecting respiratory resistance
Lung volume influences airway resistance. As lung volume is reduced all air containing components, including conducting airways, reduce in size and therefore resistance increases. At low lung volumes or during a rapid expiration airway collapse occurs and may result in gas becoming trapped distally. This causes an increase in FRC and residual volume. Use of continuous positive airway pressure (CPAP) or PEEP helps to prevent this by increasing the transmural pressure gradient, reducing airway resistance and preventing airway collapse and gas trapping.

Active physiological control of airway resistance occurs in the small airways where bronchial smooth muscle is under the influence of several systems:

- Neural:
  - Parasympathetic system via the vagus nerve—important in control of bronchomotor tone in humans. Afferent nerves respond to noxious stimuli or cytokines, and efferent nerves release acetylcholine (ACh) which acts on M3 muscarinic receptors to cause bronchoconstriction.
  - Sympathetic—minimal role in humans.
  - Non-adrenergic non-cholinergic system. Nerve fibres also in the vagus nerve. Neurotransmitter is vasoactive intestinal peptide that produces smooth muscle relaxation by production of NO.
- Humoral:
  - β2-adrenergic receptors responsive to circulating adrenaline.
- Local:
  - Mechanical stimulation by laryngoscopy, foreign bodies, or aerosols can cause bronchoconstriction.
  - Airway irritants, including air pollutants such as nitrogen dioxide and ozone, can produce bronchoconstriction.
  - Inflammatory mediators produce bronchoconstriction directly or by amplifying the physiological systems above.

Physiological response to increased resistance

- Inspiratory resistance: There is an immediate response detected by understretched muscle spindles, resulting in enhanced inspiratory muscle effort and little change in FRC. With prolonged and severe increased resistance a second compensation occurs over a few minutes, resulting from hypercapnia.
- Expiratory resistance: Expiration against a positive airway pressure of up to 10 cm H_2O does not cause any extra activation of expiratory muscles. Instead an increased respiratory force is produced to achieve a larger FRC with sufficient elastic recoil to overcome the expiratory resistance.

Intrinsic PEEP

If expiration is terminated early, before the lung volume has reached FRC, there will be residual alveolar pressure, termed intrinsic PEEP (PEEPi) or auto-PEEP. This is most commonly seen with artificial ventilation, increased expiratory flow resistance, or mucus retention. Alveolar pressures will rise with increased lung volumes and reduced lung compliance. Detrimental haemodynamic effects may also occur as a result of high alveolar pressure.

Pathophysiology of lung mechanics
Restrictive disease

These conditions result in reduced lung volumes (total lung capacity and vital capacity) because of either:

- Disease of lung parenchyma characterized by inflammation, scarring, and exudate-filled alveoli (e.g. pulmonary fibrosis)

- Disease of the chest wall or pleura, resulting in lung restriction, impaired ventilatory function, and respiratory failure (e.g. kyphoscoliosis) by reduction in the total compliance of the respiratory system.

Compensatory mechanisms include hyperventilation to maintain minute ventilation with smaller lung volumes.

Obstructive disease

In pathological states small airways obstruction is most important. In asthma, the increase in resistance is mostly due to airway mucosal inflammation and contraction of airway smooth muscle due to an exaggerated physiological response, both of which are quickly reversible. In COPD, damage to lung parenchyma, usually from smoking and repeated infections, causes a loss of lung elastin, so reducing the diameter of small airways that lack the intrinsic structural strength seen in larger airways. In either asthma or COPD long-term airway disease leads to remodelling of the airway smooth muscle and mucosal cells, resulting in a thickened mucosa and dense, incompliant musculature, giving rise to irreversible loss of lung function.

Pulmonary circulation

The lungs receive the entire blood volume but unlike the systemic circulation the pulmonary circulation is a low-pressure system because:

- Pulmonary arteries and arterioles contain only a small amount of smooth muscle compared with systemic vessels
- Pulmonary capillary networks surround alveoli to produce sheet-like blood flow to maximize the surface area for gas exchange
- With resting cardiac output pulmonary capillaries in non-dependent areas of the lung have little or no blood flow and can be 'recruited' if cardiac output increases
- Pulmonary capillaries are distensible vessels, easily doubling in diameter to accommodate large increases in flow with little change in driving pressure.

Pulmonary vascular resistance

pulmonary vascular resistance = pulmonary driving pressure/cardiac output

- The relationship is not linear due to flow being a mixture of laminar and turbulent forms.
- Increased blood flow only results in small increases in pulmonary arterial pressure due to the mechanisms described above.
- Changes in lung volume affect pulmonary vascular resistance, which is minimal at FRC. Alveolar capillaries lie between adjacent alveoli and so are compressed when lung volume increases. At low lung volumes capillaries may lose support from septal tissue and collapse. Extra-alveolar vessels may be compressed in dependent lung areas at low volumes.

Pulmonary blood flow

This is affected by:

- Posture—in the upright position pulmonary blood volume decreases by a third as a result of blood pooling in dependent regions of the systemic circulation. In the upright position hydrostatic pressure significantly affects blood flow as there may be a 20mmHg difference in vascular pressure between apex and lung bases
- Alveolar pressure—pulmonary capillary blood flow and vessel patency depend on both vascular and alveolar pressures, and lungs are traditionally divided into three zones:
  - Zone 1—$P_{alveolus} > P_{artery} > P_{venous}$: no blood flow and therefore alveolar dead space
  - Zone 2—$P_{artery} > P_{alveolus} > P_{venous}$: blood flow depends on the difference between arterial and alveolar pressure; venous pressure has no influence
  - Zone 3—$P_{artery} > P_{venous} > P_{alveolus}$: blood flow depends only on arterio-venous pressure difference
- Systemic vascular tone—the systemic vascular system has greater vasomotor activity so blood is diverted into the pulmonary circulation when vasoconstriction occurs and vice versa
- Left heart failure—pulmonary venous hypertension is likely to increase pulmonary blood volume and reduce flow in all three zones
- Positive pressure ventilation increases alveolar pressure, changing zone 3 areas into zone 2, and also reduces venous return, reducing global cardiac output.

Hypoxic pulmonary vasoconstriction

This reflex occurs in response to regional hypoxia in the lung, and is believed to optimize V̇/Q̇ matching by diverting pulmonary blood flow away from areas of low oxygen tension. Alveolar PO_2 has a greater influence than mixed venous (pulmonary arterial) PO_2, although both contribute. The reflex occurs within a few seconds of the onset of hypoxia, with constriction of small arterioles. With prolonged hypoxia the reflex is biphasic, with the initial rapid response being maximal after 5–10min and followed by a second phase of vasoconstriction, occurring gradually and reaching a plateau after 40min. Hypoxic pulmonary vasoconstriction is patchy in its onset even in healthy individuals exposed to global alveolar hypoxia. At high altitude the response also may be highly variable between individuals, explaining why some patients develop pulmonary hypertension with respiratory disease and some do not.

Mechanism of hypoxic pulmonary vasoconstriction

This is not fully elucidated. There is likely to be a direct action on smooth muscle and an indirect effect on endothelium-dependent systems. Proposed components include the following:

- Hypoxia may have a direct effect on pulmonary vascular smooth muscle by altering the membrane potential, affecting potassium channels, which in turn activate voltage-gated calcium channels to produce contraction.

- Inhibition of endothelial nitric oxide (NO) by hypoxia to produce vasoconstriction, although NO is more likely to modulate the response rather than initiate it.
- Cyclooxygenase activity is inhibited by hypoxia and promotes vasodilatory action by, for example, prostacyclin; this may also be a modulatory effect.
- Hypoxia promotes production of endothelin, a vasoconstrictor peptide, and this is accepted as being responsible for the second, slower phase of the response.

Pulmonary hypertension

This can be both primary and secondary. Secondary is more common. This is also discussed in 📖 Pulmonary vascular disease, p 541.

Primary pulmonary hypertension

This condition occurs in the absence of hypoxia and has a strong familial association and a poor prognosis. It is characterized by remodelling of the pulmonary arterioles (proliferation of endothelial cells and smooth muscle hypertrophy) and pulmonary vessel thrombosis. Treatments include pulmonary vasodilator drugs (oral or intravenous prostacyclin analogues or oral endothelin antagonists) and ultimately lung transplantation.

Secondary pulmonary hypertension

Chronic or intermittent hypoxic pulmonary vasoconstriction can lead to pulmonary hypertension by remodelling of the pulmonary vascular smooth muscle, producing irreversible increases in vascular resistance. The condition may occur with any disease that results in long-term hypoxia. It is also caused by several other conditions.

$\dot{V}/\dot{Q}$ relationships

Ventilation and perfusion are both preferentially distributed to dependent areas of the lung, partly as a result of gravity, and are therefore affected by posture.

Distribution of ventilation

The right lung is slightly larger so usually has 60% of total ventilation in either upright or supine positions. When lateral, the lower lung is always better ventilated but perfusion also preferentially goes to the lower lung and $\dot{V}/\dot{Q}$ matching is maintained.

Within each lung, regional ventilation is affected by gravity—lung tissue has weight, so alveoli in dependent areas become compressed. In the upright position alveoli at the lung apices will be almost fully inflated while those at the bases will be small. On inspiration the capacity of alveoli in non-dependent regions to expand is therefore limited, and regional ventilation increases with vertical distance down the lung. This variation in alveolar size causes regional differences in lung compliance. In a microgravity environment, where the lung has no weight, regional variation in ventilation disappears almost completely.

The ability of a lung region to ventilate may be quantified by considering its time constant. This is the product of compliance and airway resistance, and is a measure of the time that would be required for inflation of the lung region if the initial flow rate of gas were maintained throughout inflation.

Within the lung there are 'fast alveoli' with short time constants and 'slow alveoli' with long time constants. If the time constants are identical as the lung is inflated the pressure and volume changes will be identical so if inspiration stops there will be no redistribution of gas. The distribution is also independent of the rate, duration, or frequency of inspiration. However, if there are regions with different time constants within an area of the lung, gas distribution will be affected by the rate, duration, and frequency of inspiration. At the termination of gas flow there will be redistribution of gas because pressure and volume changes will be different between lung regions.

Distribution of perfusion

The pulmonary circulation is a low-pressure system and posture significantly alters blood distribution.

• Blood flow increases on descending down the lung, with minimal perfusion in non-dependent areas, particularly in the upright position.

• Lung perfusion *per alveolus* is reasonably uniform at normal tidal volumes. The dependent parts of the lung contain larger numbers of smaller alveoli than the apices at FRC, therefore perfusion per unit of lung volume is increased at the bases.

• When supine or prone the same perfusion differences occur between the anterior and posterior regions of the lung. Blood flow per unit lung volume increases by about 11% per centimetre of descent. Ventilation increases less so, resulting in a smaller $\dot{V}/\dot{Q}$ ratio in dependent areas.

It is now accepted that gravity is not the only factor affecting regional blood flow and may only account for 10–40% of regional blood flow variability. Pulmonary blood flow also varies in a radial fashion, with greater flow to central than peripheral lung regions in each horizontal slice. This results simply from the branching pattern of the pulmonary vasculature.

$\dot{V}/\dot{Q}$ ratios

For both lungs considered together $\dot{V}/\dot{Q}$ ratio = 0.8 (4L/min alveolar ventilation, 5L/min pulmonary blood flow). As already described, ventilation and perfusion are not uniform throughout the lung and within different lung regions there is a spectrum of $\dot{V}/\dot{Q}$ ratios from unventilated alveoli ($\dot{V}/\dot{Q}$ = 0) to unperfused alveoli ($\dot{V}/\dot{Q}$ = ∞) and all ratios in between.

The simplest way of understanding $\dot{V}/\dot{Q}$ ratios is the Riley three-compartment model, which considers the lungs as only having three regions (Fig. 1.3):

1 'Ideal' alveoli with a $\dot{V}/\dot{Q}$ ratio of 1—blood leaving these regions has PO_2 and PCO_2 values the same as for alveolar gas.

2 Alveoli with no ventilation ($\dot{V}/\dot{Q}$ ratio of 0), which constitutes an intrapulmonary shunt. PO_2 and PCO_2 values leaving these regions are the same as for mixed venous blood.

3 Alveoli with no perfusion ($\dot{V}/\dot{Q}$ ratio of ∞), which constitutes alveolar dead space. Gas leaving these alveoli has the same composition as inspired gas.

There are of course infinitely more compartments than this, but the three-compartment model is useful for understanding the clinically relevant concepts of shunt and dead space.

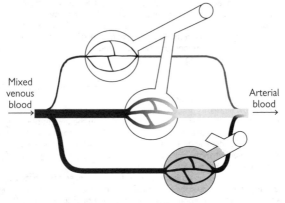

Mixed venous blood →

Arterial blood →

Fig. 1.3 Riley's three-compartment model of $\dot{V}/\dot{Q}$ relationships in the lung. The middle alveolus (1 in the text) has the 'ideal' ventilation and perfusion ($\dot{V}/\dot{Q} = 1$); the upper alveolus (3) is ventilated but not perfused ($\dot{V}/\dot{Q} = \infty$) so forms alveolar dead space; the lower alveolus (2) is perfused but not ventilated ($\dot{V}/\dot{Q} = 0$) and is an intrapulmonary shunt. In reality a wide range of $\dot{V}/\dot{Q}$ ratios exist.

Although not used in clinical practice, the multiple inert gas elimination technique (MIGET) allows assessment of the wide range of $\dot{V}/\dot{Q}$ ratios seen in the lungs. Several compounds of widely different solubility are administered intravenously and their elimination in exhaled air measured. This allows a graph to be drawn showing the distribution of $\dot{V}/\dot{Q}$ not by anatomical location but by a large number of compartments of different $\dot{V}/\dot{Q}$ ratio (Fig. 1.4), which gives a more realistic picture of $\dot{V}/\dot{Q}$ ratios *in vivo*.

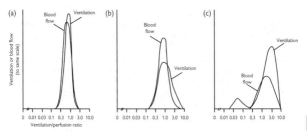

Fig. 1.4 Quantification of $\dot{V}/\dot{Q}$ ratios in the lungs using the multiple inert gas elimination technique. (a) Normal pattern from a healthy 22-year-old subject, with all lung regions having $\dot{V}/\dot{Q}$ ratios in the range 0.3–3.0. (b) Increased scatter of $\dot{V}/\dot{Q}$ ratios such as may occur in older subjects or in younger patients during general anaesthesia. Note that the overall $\dot{V}/\dot{Q}$ ratio remains normal at 0.8, but the areas of low and high $\dot{V}/\dot{Q}$ ratio will impair gas exchange. (c) patient with COPD with areas of low $\dot{V}/\dot{Q}$ ratio that will cause venous admixture and hypoxaemia.

Effect of $\dot{V}/\dot{Q}$ ratios on gas exchange

Areas of lung with high $\dot{V}/\dot{Q}$ ratios (between 1 and ∞) have more ventilation than is required for gas exchange with the blood perfusing that region. Gas in these alveoli will therefore have lower PCO_2 and higher PO_2 values than ideal alveolar gas, and these values will trend towards those of inspired gas as the $\dot{V}/\dot{Q}$ ratio increases. These regions contribute to alveolar dead space. CO_2 transfer from blood to alveolus will be increased because of the lower alveolar PCO_2, and the blood will be fully oxygenated.

Areas of lung with low $\dot{V}/\dot{Q}$ ratios (between 1 and 0) have less ventilation than is required for the blood flow. In these alveoli the PCO_2 will be higher and the PO_2 lower than in ideal alveolar gas, and these values will trend towards those of mixed venous blood with decreasing $\dot{V}/\dot{Q}$ ratio. CO_2 transfer between blood and alveolus will be reduced. Blood passing through these lung regions will not become fully oxygenated and when this mixes with blood from the rest of the lung arterial hypoxaemia occurs with an increase in the alveolar–arterial PO_2 gradient. In contrast to the compensation that occurs with increased CO_2 elimination elsewhere in the lung when dead space exists, there is no such mechanism for oxygenation as the lung regions with normal or high $\dot{V}/\dot{Q}$ ratios cannot carry extra oxygen because the haemoglobin is already fully saturated.

Shunt

Admixture of arterial blood with poorly oxygenated or mixed venous blood is the most important cause of arterial hypoxaemia.

Types of true shunt include:
- Intrapulmonary shunt: perfusion through lung regions with $\dot{V}/\dot{Q}$ ratio of 0, i.e. lung regions with non-ventilated alveoli such as atelectasis, pneumonia, or pulmonary oedema
- Anatomical (extrapulmonary) shunt: blood that passes from the right side of the circulation to the left without traversing the lung. May be physiological, including bronchial veins, Thebesian veins (small veins of the left side of the heart), or pathological, usually from cyanotic congenital heart disease.

Venous admixture, often loosely termed shunt, is the degree of admixture of mixed venous blood with pulmonary end-capillary blood that would be required to produce the observed difference between the arterial and pulmonary end-capillary PO_2. It is the calculated percentage of cardiac output required to result in the observed blood gases, and includes the effects of true shunt as described above along with a contribution from perfusion of lung regions with $\dot{V}/\dot{Q}$ ratio less than 1 but greater than 0 (see above). The amount of venous admixture seen in lung disease is variable and depends on the balance between hypoxic pulmonary vasoconstriction (HPV) and pathological pulmonary vasodilatation.

Effect of cardiac output on shunt

Within a few minutes a reduced cardiac output leads to a decrease in mixed venous oxygen content, so even if the shunt fraction remains unaltered there will be a greater reduction in arterial PO_2. However, a reduction in cardiac output is also believed to reduce the shunt fraction, possibly by activation of HPV due to the reduced mixed venous PO_2. As a result arterial PO_2 may be unaffected by reduced cardiac output. In an extrapulmonary shunt, such as seen in cyanotic congenital heart disease, this latter effect reduces shunt fraction, and arterial PO_2 becomes highly dependent on adequate cardiac output.

Dead space

This is the part of tidal volume that does not take part in gas exchange and is therefore exhaled unchanged. The part of the tidal volume involved in ventilation is the alveolar ventilation:

alveolar ventilation = respiratory frequency × (tidal volume − dead space)

It is alveolar ventilation that determines the arterial PCO_2, so in a hypercapnic patient all three terms on the right of this equation must be considered: dead space is often overlooked in the clinical setting.

Components of dead space include:
- Apparatus dead space, including face mask, breathing circuit connectors etc.
- Anatomical—the volume of air contained in the conducting airways (150mL approximately in normal subjects). Anatomical dead space is affected by subject size, age, posture, neck and jaw position, lung volume, presence of airway devices, endotracheal tubes or tracheostomy, bronchodilators, tidal volume, and respiratory rate
- Alveolar—this is the part of tidal volume that passes through the anatomical dead space to lung regions with $\dot{V}/\dot{Q}$ ratios greater

than 1 (see above). It is affected by decreased cardiac output, pulmonary embolism, and posture
- Physiological dead space is the sum of the anatomical and alveolar dead spaces.

Gas transport

O_2 cascade

The oxygen cascade describes the movement of oxygen down a partial pressure gradient from the inspired gas to its site of use in a mitochondrium. Various processes cause the drop in partial pressure:

- Humidification in the respiratory tract dilutes the inspired gas by a small amount (from 20.9 to 19.9kPa if breathing air). In quiet nasal breathing dry inspired gas is fully humidified in the pharynx, but in a mouth-breathing, hyperventilating subject the pharynx, larynx, and large airways are all required.
- On entering an alveolus inspired gas is further diluted by the CO_2 leaving the blood, the degree being determined by the alveolar gas equation (see below).
- Pulmonary alveolar to capillary diffusion barrier—this is very small even for the relatively poorly diffusible oxygen, although it may become important when breathing hypoxic mixtures such as at altitude or during exercise with a very high oxygen uptake.
- Venous admixture reduces the PO_2 of arterial blood below that of pulmonary venous blood, as described above. This component of the oxygen cascade is best represented by the alveolar to arterial PO_2 difference, which in healthy subjects is small (<2kPa). In patients with respiratory disease causing shunt or $\dot{V}/\dot{Q}$ mismatch this value can exceed 5kPa and is the most common cause of arterial hypoxaemia.
- Diffusion from the capillary into the mitochondria presents a highly variable barrier to oxygen transfer depending on the location of the cell concerned. Cells furthest away from the venous end of a capillary are said to be at a 'lethal corner' where tissue hypoxia will always occur first and probably work perfectly well under normal conditions at a PO_2 of less than 1kPa.

Alveolar gas equation

End-expired gas contains a variable mixture of gas from regions of alveolar dead space, from alveoli with $\dot{V}/\dot{Q}$ ratios > 1, and from 'ideal' alveoli. Ideal alveolar gas cannot therefore be measured and in order to quantify hypoxaemia by comparing alveolar and arterial PO_2 the alveolar air equation must be used to calculate the ideal alveolar PO_2. Many versions of this equation exist, but the most commonly used one is:

$$\text{alveolar } PO_2 = P_IO_2 - \frac{PaCO_2}{RQ}(1 - F_IO_2(1 - RQ))$$

Arterial PCO_2 is used because this is easy to measure and under most circumstances equals alveolar PCO_2, and the respiratory quotient (RQ) is included to account for differences in the relative amounts of oxygen uptake and CO_2 elimination in an alveolus. P_IO_2 is the partial pressure of inspired oxygen when fully humidified at body temperature:

$$P_IO_2 = F_IO_2 \times (PB - PH_2O)$$

where PB is barometric pressure and PH_2O is the saturated vapour pressure of water vapour at body temperature.

Oxygen carriage in the blood

Oxygen is carried in the blood in two forms: in combination with haemoglobin and in solution. The latter includes 0.0225mL/dL/kPa at 37°C or 0.3mL/dL when breathing air, compared with a total of about 20mL/dL.

Haemoglobin

The haemoglobin molecule consists of four subunits, each containing an iron-porphyrin group attached to a globin chain. Three normal forms of globin chain exist (α, β, and γ), with adult haemoglobin A (HbA) consisting of two α and two β chains.

Weak electrostatic bonds that determine the quaternary structure of haemoglobin are responsible for the features of the binding of oxygen by haemoglobin. In deoxyhaemoglobin (HHb) the electrostatic bonds are strong and the molecule is held in a tense (T) conformation which has low affinity for oxygen. In oxyhaemoglobin (HbO$_2$) the electrostatic bonds are weaker and haemoglobin assumes its relaxed (R) state. This allows an oxygen molecule better access to the haem group which lies at the bottom of a crevice in the globin chain, such that the affinity for oxygen increases by 500 times. One oxygen molecule binding to one globin chain alters the conformation, and therefore oxygen affinity, of the other three globins, an effect referred to as co-operativity that explains the well-known shape of the haemoglobin (Hb) dissociation curve. Conformational state, and therefore oxygen binding, is also altered by pH (the Bohr effect), CO_2, 2,3-diphosphoglycerate, and temperature by affecting the electrostatic bonds.

Abnormal haemoglobins

- *Fetal haemoglobin (HbF)*. This is made of two γ and two α globin chains. It has greater affinity for oxygen than HbA.
- *Sickle cell haemoglobin (HbS)*. A single amino acid substitution in the globin chain profoundly alters the function of the Hb molecule. In the deoxygenated state HbS becomes much less soluble and through its interaction with the red blood cell (RBC) cytoskeleton alters the shape and fragility of the red cell. The cell becomes sickle shaped and may cause obstruction to the microcirculation.
- *Thalassaemia*. Suppression of HbA production leads to a compensatory production of HbF, which shifts the oxyhaemoglobin dissociation curve to the left.

- *Methaemoglobin*. A small proportion of the iron in Hb exists as the ferric form (Fe^{3+}), and these molecules of methaemoglobin (metHb) are unable to carry oxygen. Some drugs (e.g. prilocaine, nitric oxide) or a deficiency of the red cell enzyme that converts Fe^{3+} to Fe^{2+} can increase the proportion of metHb.

CO_2 carriage in blood

Carbon dioxide is carried in the blood in three forms:

- In solution—although more soluble than oxygen, CO_2 in solution in blood again makes up only a small amount of the total. Its solubility is significantly affected by temperature, which makes interpretation of blood gases complex in hypothermic patients
- As carbamino compounds—amino groups in the uncharged $R-NH_2$ form can combine directly with CO_2 to form carbamic acid. Most is carried by haemoglobin and the capacity of HHb is 3.5 times that of HbO_2. The Haldane effect is the difference in the quantity of CO_2 carried, at constant $PaCO_2$, in oxygenated and deoxygenated blood, and is due to a combination of carbamino carriage and the altered buffering capacity of HHb and HbO_2
- As bicarbonate—most of the CO_2 carried in blood is in the form of bicarbonate. Carbon dioxide in solution hydrates to form carbonic acid, a reaction which is catalysed by the enzyme carbonic anhydrase, before the carbonic acid dissociates into bicarbonate and hydrogen ions.

Distribution of CO_2 within the blood

CO_2 can diffuse freely into RBCs, where the following occur:

- Rising intracellular PCO_2 increases carbamino carriage of CO_2 by Hb
- Hydration and dissociation of CO_2 to produce H^+ and bicarbonate ions. Intracellular accumulation of these ions is overcome by the following:
  - Buffering of H^+ ions by Hb, the capacity of which increases as oxygen is dissociated from the Hb
  - Hamburger or chloride shift—excess bicarbonate ions are actively transported out of the cell in exchange for chloride ions to maintain electrical neutrality. This process is facilitated by a RBC membrane-bound protein called band 3, which is attached to carbonic anhydrase, allowing the bicarbonate ions to be transferred directly between the proteins and transported out of the cell very rapidly.

The same processes occur in reverse in the pulmonary capillary.

Further reading

Boulet L-P and Sterk PJ (2007) Airway remodelling: the future. *Eur Respir J* **30**, 831–834.

Del Negro CA and Hayes JA (2008) A 'group pacemaker' mechanism for respiratory rhythm generation. *J Physiol* **586**, 2245–2246.

Galvin I, Drummond GB, and Nirmalan M (2007) Distribution of blood flow and ventilation in the lung: gravity is not the only factor. *Br J Anaesth* **98**, 420–428.

Lumb AB (2010) *Nunn's Applied Respiratory Physiology*, 7th edn. London: Elsevier.

Weir K, López-Barneo J, Buckler KJ, and Archer SL (2005) Acute oxygen-sensing mechanisms. *N Engl J Med* **353**, 2042–2055.

1.2 Diagnosis of respiratory failure

Definitions

Respiratory failure is defined as inadequate gas exchange. By convention respiratory failure is divided into:
- *Type 1 respiratory failure*—hypoxia (PaO_2 < 8kPa), $PaCO_2$ normal
- *Type 2 respiratory failure*—hypoxia with hypercapnia ($PaCO_2$ > 6.0kPa), plus accompanying acid–base changes.

This classification is in widespread use, but most diseases that traditionally cause Type 1 respiratory failure can also result in hypercapnia. It is therefore more useful to think in terms of:
- Failure of oxygenation
- Failure of CO_2 clearance.

The pathophysiological concepts responsible for the failure of gas exchange are fully dealt with in 📖 Respiratory physiology and pathophysiology, p 2, but for the purposes of diagnosis, the causes of hypoxia and hypercapnia can be simplified as follows.

Causes of hypoxia

- Regional mismatching of ventilation and perfusion ($\dot{V}/\dot{Q}$) in the lung.
- Right to left shunting—deoxygenated venous blood mixes with arterialized blood without participating in gas exchange. Usually intrapulmonary, but may be intracardiac.
- Reduced alveolar oxygen tension—hypoventilation, altitude, air travel.
- Impaired diffusion of oxygen across the alveolar capillary membrane.

Causes of hypercapnia

- Reduced minute ventilation.
  - Inadequate central ventilatory drive.
  - Disorders of motor neurons, neuromuscular junction, or respiratory muscles.
  - Reduced respiratory system compliance, including chest wall disease.
  - Increased airway resistance, including asthma, COPD, and cystic fibrosis.
  - Upper airway obstruction.
- Increased alveolar dead space, causing reduced alveolar ventilation.
  - Ventilation perfusion mismatch.
  - Pulmonary hypoperfusion (e.g. pulmonary embolism, cardiogenic shock, fibrotic acute respiratory distress syndrome (ARDS)).
  - Raised intra-alveolar pressures (e.g. dynamic hyperinflation, PEEP).
- Increased CO_2 production (e.g. malignant hyperpyrexia).

History

In intensive care, as in any other branch of medicine, the key to diagnosis is in the history and examination.

The history may be obtainable from the patient, but may have to be sought from the relatives, the notes, or other healthcare professionals.

Breathlessness

Breathlessness is the end result of complex signalling involving lungs, thorax, heart, and skeletal muscles, as well as the inputs and outputs of various CNS sites. Prognostically and diagnostically it is a poor discriminator.

Adaptive mechanisms may modify the perception of dyspnoea (e.g. some patients with severe COPD) and cortical inputs may cause hyperventilation without physiological stimulus.

Some types of severe hypoventilatory failure can develop with minimal breathlessness (particularly some chest bellows syndromes and muscular dystrophies). In these cases, worsening respiratory function is more likely to present as increasing lethargy and stupor.

Nevertheless, certain patterns of dyspnoea are helpful:
- Abrupt commanding dyspnoea suggests large airway narrowing (inhaled foreign body, anaphylactic laryngeal oedema), major pulmonary embolism (associated anterior chest tightness), or tension pneumothorax (often recall initial pleuritic pain when questioned).
- The acute breathlessness of severe pneumonia, pulmonary oedema, and ALI/ARDS tends to develop over hours to days.
- Breathlessness linked to time, place, or events, for example variation in breathlessness according to:
  - Time of year in farmer's lung.
  - Return to work or particular location in occupational lung disease (occupational asthma may lose this fluctuation as it progresses).
  - Exposure to precipitant in hypersensitivity pneumonitis (pigeon fancier's lung). This situational association may not always be present.
- Positional breathlessness:
  - Orthopnoea typifies cardiogenic pulmonary oedema, but may also be seen in diaphragmatic weakness and severe COPD.
  - Patients with expiratory muscle weakness (e.g. myotonic dystrophy) may prefer to lie flat.
  - Orthodeoxia (desaturation on sitting up) is associated with the intrapulmonary shunting seen in hepatopulmonary syndrome.
  - Choking and gasping episodes awakening patient from sleep (separate from orthopnoea) suggest sleep-related upper airway obstruction, which is a potential 'accelerating' factor for both pulmonary arterial hypertension and hypoventilatory respiratory failure.
- Sleep disturbance—poorly controlled asthmatics and bronchiectatics report nocturnal symptoms, disturbed sleep, and nocturnal inhaler use. Non-specific deterioration of sleep quality almost invariably characterizes extrapulmonary causes of hypoventilatory respiratory

failure, as sleep disordered breathing results in progressively more sleep fragmentation and altered sleep architecture.

Chest pain
- Central and restrictive chest pain—suggests myocardial ischaemia, but may be due to major pulmonary thromboembolism (PE) (RV ischaemia), and is sometimes described in advanced lung cancer with extensive mediastinal involvement.
- Pleuritic pain—occurs in primary pleural disease, inflammatory disease, pneumonia, lung abscess, vasculitis, or PE.

Cough
- Acute onset harsh cough—consider inhaled foreign body or tracheal injury.
- Dry cough:
  - Days to weeks—may herald any acute illness affecting lung parenchyma (pneumonia, pulmonary embolism, or pulmonary vasculitis).
  - Weeks to months—is often an early indicator of interstitial lung disease.
  - Exercise-induced and nocturnal exacerbations are often seen in asthma.
- Weak cough—raises suspicion of neuromuscular disease. It is also a risk factor for aspiration pneumonia.
- Productive cough—seen in bronchiectasis, COPD, pneumonia.

Sputum
- Amount—large volume suggests bronchiectasis.
- Character:
  - Serous in pulmonary oedema
  - Mucoid in COPD
  - Purulent in pneumonia.
- Viscosity—purulent sputum is less viscous.
- Taste/odour—offensive or fetid sputum suggests anaerobic or fungal infection.

Haemoptysis
Haemoptysis should be distinguished from haematemesis or epistaxis. Although always a worrying symptom for both patient and doctor, in many cases no underlying diagnosis is found.
- Frank haemoptysis—bronchiectasis, tuberculosis (TB), PE, aspergilloma, and vasculitis.
- Blood-stained sputum—lung abscess, bronchial carcinoma.
- Blood-streaked sputum—bronchial carcinoma, occasionally COPD.
- Rusty sputum—classically associated with pneumococcal pneumonia. The colour is due to haemoglobin degradation products.

Speed of onset of symptoms
  Acute
- Acute cardiogenic pulmonary oedema (ACPO).
- ARDS/ALI.
- Major pulmonary embolism.

- Community-acquired pneumonia (including viral).
- Pulmonary vasculitis/haemorrhage syndromes.
- Acute alveolitis (eosinophilic pneumonia, drug reactions).
- Upper airway closure (trauma, angio-oedema, foreign body).
- Loss of central drive (sedatives, stroke, encephalitis, myotonic dystrophy).
- Neuromuscular junction problems (botulism, acute poliomyelitis, tetanus, Guillain–Barre, acute myaesthenia gravis, organophosphate poisoning, transverse myelitis, and occasionally abrupt respiratory muscle failure in motor neurone disease).

Acute on chronic (or chronic)
- Interstitial lung disease (ILD).
- Granulomatous lung disease (sarcoidosis, berylliosis, hypersensitivity pneumonitis).
- Airflow obstruction (COPD, cystic fibrosis, bronchiectasis, asthma, bronchiolitis syndromes).
- Loss of central drive (congenital central hypoventilation, obesity hypoventilation).
- Chest wall disorders (congenital or acquired).
- Muscular dystrophies and myopathies (Duchenne, nemaline myopathy).

Past medical history
A past history of respiratory disease is clearly relevant but non-respiratory disease may also carry significance.
- Developmental and hereditary factors:
  - Alpha-1 antitrypsin deficiency in early-onset severe emphysema.
  - Kartegener's syndrome (primary ciliary dyskinesia) for unexplained severe bronchiectasis.
  - Common variable immune deficiency for repeated pneumonia (and possibly granulomatous lung disease).
  - Neurofibromatosis can result in pulmonary fibrosis, pneumothorax, and bullous emphysema.
  - Marfan's syndrome predisposes to apical fibrosis and pneumothorax.
  - Ehlers–Danlos syndrome can cause haemoptysis and pneumothorax.
- Family history, for example of cystic fibrosis (CF).
- Childhood illness:
  - Severe pneumonia, sinusitis, or dental caries may be a forerunner of severe non-CF bronchiectasis.
  - Pneumonia due to defective humoral immunity generally starts in the teenage years.
  - Paralytic polio may cause extrathoracic hypercarbic respiratory failure many years later (postpolio syndrome), especially where respiratory involvement had occurred originally.
- Sickle cell disease—crises can present as an acute chest syndrome, resulting in pleuritic chest pain, consolidation, and alveolar necrosis. Recurrent sickling results in pulmonary hypertension and a restrictive pattern of lung function.

- Rheumatoid arthritis—can cause pleural effusions, diffuse fibrosis, organizing and eosinophilic pneumonias, recurrent infections, pulmonary hypertension, and bronchiectasis.
- Connective tissue disease—many autoimmune conditions such as systemic sclerosis and systemic lupus erythematosus (SLE) have pulmonary manifestations.
- Organ transplantation—in addition to the increased infection risk due to immunosuppresion, organ transplantation is associated with a high risk of pulmonary damage:
  - Drug-induced lung disease.
  - Pulmonary malignancy (non-bronchogenic, e.g. lymphomas) in renal transplant patients.
  - Lymphoproliferative disorder in liver transplant.
  - Pleural effusions.
  - Alveolar haemorrhorage.
  - Bronchiolitis obliterans.
  - Idiopathic pneumonia syndrome associated with haemopoietic stem cells.

Travel

Air travel may predispose individuals to respiratory disease:
- Dehydration and immobility may increase the risk of deep vein thrombosis (DVT) and pulmonary embolus (PE).
- Altitude may expand bullae or pneumothoraces.
- Reduced oxygen tension can exacerbate pre-existing lung disease.
- Close proximity to 300 other passengers increases the airborne infective risk.
- Exposure to unusual infection, e.g. tropical disease or multi drug resistant tuberculosis.

Pets

The presence of pets can often give an indication to the potential underlying respiratory problem.
- Patients with asthma who may be unknowingly allergic to their cat or dog.
- Bird keepers can develop hypersensitivity pneumonitis from chronic antigen exposure, which can present in an acute form.
- Pigeon fanciers are also at risk of development of psittacosis.

Drug history

A history of prescribed and recreational drug use is important. Pulmonary reactions to prescribed drugs is dealt with in 📖 Drug-induced lung disease, p 438, but the following associations have been described with recreational drugs:
- Heroin use can cause ARDS, pneumonia, lung abscess, septic pulmonary emboli, and organizing pneumonia.
- Cannabis use has been associated with bullous lung disease.
- Crack cocaine use has been associated with interstitial pneumonitis, pulmonary fibrosis, alveolar haemorrhage, thermal airway injury, pulmonary hypertension, bullous emphysema, and eosinophilic lung disease.

- Amphetamine use can result in pulmonary fibrosis, right ventricular hypertrophy, and pulmonary hypertension.

Alcohol intake

Chronic alcohol ingestion is associated with an increased incidence of bacterial pneumonia and TB. This is partly explained by an increase in aspiration risk and impaired innate immunity (reduced macrophage phagocytic function and neutrophil chemotaxis). In addition, chronic alcohol ingestion renders patients four times more likely to develop ARDS when exposed to an inflammatory stimulus. This condition is now being described as 'alcoholic lung' and consists of:

- Reduced pulmonary glutathione levels.
- Impaired claudin protein production (a group of proteins responsible for maintaining a tight air–fluid barrier in the alveolus).
- Reduced granulocyte-macrophage colony stimulating factor (GM-CSF) receptors in the lung, leading to a blunted GM-CSF response.

The mortality of pneumonia in this group is much higher than the mortality predicted using physiological scoring systems.

Environmental history

- Work, home and hobbies.
  - Occupational asthma with plastics factories (isocyanates) and spray paints.
  - Hypersensitivity pneumonitis—over 300 antigens have been identified as triggers, many of which are found outwith the workplace.
- Lifestyle sexual exposures—HIV has numerous pulmonary complications. In addition to an increased susceptibility to bacterial pneumonia, these patients are also at risk of mycobacterial (typical and atypical), viral (cytomegalovirus (CMV)), fungal (histoplasmosis), and opportunistic (pneumocystis jiroveci) infections.
- Pregnancy (see 📖 Respiratory disease in pregnancy, p 515 for a full discussion of respiratory failure in pregnancy):
  - The cardiorespiratory demands of pregnancy may reveal previously undiagnosed disease and will worsen pre-existing respiratory disease.
  - Diagnoses specific to pregnancy include pre-eclampsia, haemolysis, elevated liver enzymes, low platelets (HELLP) syndrome, amniotic fluid embolism, peripartum cardiomyopathy, and tocolytic-induced pulmonary oedema.
  - There is a higher risk of pulmonary embolism, ARDS, and viral pneumonitis.
  - There are increased complications of bacterial pneumonias and viral infections.

Non-respiratory symptoms

- Loss of appetite, poor motivation, and fatigue are associated with gradually advancing hypoventilation in neuromuscular disorders.

- Systemic symptoms of fever, lethargy, malaise, myalgia, and diarrhoea are indicative of a significant inflammatory insult, including typical and atypical infection.
- Muscle weakness—the deterioration in neuromuscular function may be quite subtle ahead of precipitous acute respiratory failure in conditions such as acid maltase deficiency and motor neurone disease.
- Swallowing problems—result in aspiration risk and may be seen in:
  • Neuromuscular disorders (hypoventilation)
  • Connective tissue disease (associated with ILD)
  • Upper gastrointestinal disease.
- Skin rashes, joint problems, or neuropathies—important clues to interstitial and vasculitic lung disease.

Clinical setting
- Community—versus hospital-acquired disease.
- Post operative—nature of operation, adequacy of pain control, complication of surgery.
- Recent line insertion.
- Immobility.
- Intensive care unit (ICU)—lines, drains, ventilator induced lung injury (VILI), ventilator-associated pneumonia (VAP), ARDS.

Examination
Physical examination in the intensive care setting has constraints due to limited patient accessibility (intubation, invasive lines, monitoring equipment etc.). Nevertheless regular clinical examination should be conducted rather than relying solely on monitored physiological parameters, imaging, or laboratory results.

Initial observation
  Skin colour
- Central cyanosis due to deoxyhaemoglobin is readily detected in polycythaemia and easily missed in anaemia.
- The cherry red skin colour of carbon monoxide toxicity may mask tissue hypoxia in smoke inhalation.

  Skin perfusion
- Warm vasodilated extremities and bounding pulse associated with chronic hypercapnia, sepsis, or anaphylaxis.
- Cold, peripherally cyanosed extremities and rapid thready pulse associated with hypovolaemic, cardiogenic, or obstructive shock.

  Level of consciousness
- Somnolence in CO_2 retention, impending respiratory arrest, fatigue, or chronic hypoventilation.
- High respiratory drive in acute onset respiratory failure.

  Nutritional state
- Pickwickian habitus of chronic hypoventilation syndrome or obstructive sleep apnoea.
- Cachexia of malignancy or severe chronic disease.

Respiratory pattern
- Rate.
- Depth.
- Use of accessory muscles.
- Intercostal and subcostal recession.
- 'See-saw' respiration in airway obstruction.
- Purse-lipped breathing in obstructive airways disease.
- Asymmetrical chest movement in consolidation or pneumothorax.

Audible respiratory noises
- Wheeze.
- Stridor.
- Grunting.

Respiratory system assessment

The respiratory examination is well described elsewhere, and a detailed discussion is beyond the scope of this book. In summary it should include hands, head, neck, and chest.

- Signs suggesting sinus or orophayngeal sepsis—tenderness over facial bones, halitosis, or dental caries, which may indicate anaerobic bronchial sepsis.
- Signs suggesting malignancy—finger clubbing, Horner's syndrome, lymphadenopathy, non–pulsatile jugular venous distension, facial swelling, and distended superficial veins of superior vena cava obstruction.
- Wheeze.
  - Usual cause is bronchospasm.
  - Also seen in COPD, aspiration, pulmonary oedema, anaphylaxis, and even PE.
  - Cardiac asthma is often difficult to differentiate from bronchospasm, but the expiratory time is likely to be shorter in pulmonary oedema and longer in bronchospasm.
  - Localized or unilateral wheezing may indicate tumours, foreign bodies, or mucous plugging.
- Stridor is caused by upper airway disease and if associated with breathlessness, orthopnoea, voice changes, airway swelling, or obvious anatomical deformity should prompt urgent anaesthetic review. May be inspiratory or expiratory depending on whether the obstruction is extrathoracic or intrathoracic, respectively.
- Signs suggesting pleural involvement—asymmetry of chest movement, surgical emphysema, misplaced cardiac apex pleural rub, hyperresonant percussion note with absent breath sounds.
- Crepitations (now called 'crackles' by the American Thoracic Society).
  - Can be fine or coarse, early or late, inspiratory or expiratory.
  - Bibasal, late, fine, often described as 'velcro' sounding in ILD. Finger clubbing.
  - Bibasal, late, fine inspiratory ('wet') crackles of alveolar fluid. Third heart sound or associated effusion.

- Late coarse crackles in pneumonia. Evidence of infection.
- Coarse crackles in bronchiectasis are often asymmetric and improve after coughing.
- Early crackles occur in COPD and with consolidation.
- Often surprisingly few added sounds in ARDS.
- Expiratory crackles may represent upper airway noise or fluid in lower bronchi such as pulmonary oedema, bronchiectasis, or pneumonia.
- Signs suggesting non-aerated lung—dullness to percussion and reduced breath sounds similar in lobar collapse, pleural effusion, basal atelectasis, or consolidation.
- Bronchial breathing suggests breath sound conduction across 'solid' tissue through patent airways (consolidated lung), typically heard in lobar pneumonia and in the lung above effusions. Consolidation is also caused by fluid (pulmonary oedema), blood (pulmonary haemorrhage), and tumours.

General examination

The rheumatological system, CNS, and muscles are the systems most likely to reveal clues to a specific aetiology.

- Arthritis, arthralgia, and skin rashes or lesions may indicate connective tissue disease or vasculitis.
- Muscles.
  - Fasciculation in motor neurone disease.
  - Myotonia in myotonic dystrophy.
- Nervous system.
  - New, local weakness in post polio syndrome or cerebrovascular accident.
  - Bulbar dysfunction as a risk for aspiration syndrome or as an indicator of neuromuscular-related hypoventilation.
  - Encephalopathy of multi-organ failure—septic, hepatic, or renal.
  - Altered conscious level of encephalomyelitis.

Review of progress

Respiratory failure is a dynamic process that may alter during the course of the illness, and whilst therapy is directed where possible at restoring normal function, the underlying aetiology or the associated treatment (e.g. immunosuppressant drugs) may predispose the patient to complications which worsen or alter the existing pattern of respiratory failure. 'Secondary' alterations in the pattern of respiratory failure are more likely where prolonged and complex respiratory support is involved, such as intubation and mechanical ventilation. Vigilance for alterations in the pattern of respiratory failure and low threshold for diagnostic review is appropriate throughout but essential for patients in the critical care environment. If progress is unexpectedly slow, or deterioration takes place, consider:

- Is the diagnosis correct?
- New sepsis can cause ALI/ARDS. Consider all sources (brain, meninges, sinuses, pleura, lung, heart, biliary tree and liver, abdomen, bone, joints, vascular devices, drains, skin, urine, blood).

- Are the antibiotics likely to cover the organisms responsible?
- Is there any reason to suspect:
  - Interstitial lung disease, particularly acute interstitial pneumonitis (AIP) or cryptogenic organizing pneumonia (COP)
  - Pulmonary haemorrhage
  - Pulmonary embolus
  - Pneumothorax
  - Underlying malignancy.
- Cardiogenic or non-cardiogenic pulmonary oedema, worsened by administration of intravenous fluid or arrhythmias.
- Devices—occasionally movement or blockage of the endotracheal or tracheostomy tubes may cause airway compromise or secretion retention. Intercostal drains may cause lung damage and are a source of potential infection.

Whenever clinical concern is raised regarding worsening of respiratory failure, a complete reappraisal should be undertaken: reassess the history, examination, and investigations, and update the current examination and investigations. Was the diagnosis correct and has a new complication arisen?

Investigation of respiratory disease

Pulse oximetry

The amounts of red (660nm wavelength) and infra-red (940nm wavelength) light absorbed by blood varies with the proportion of oxygenated to deoxygenated haemoglobin. Pulse-oximetry uses this principle to measure the percentage oxygen saturation in arterial blood. It only measures pulsatile flow, so it is not affected by static signals (such as those from venous or capillary blood). It is accurate to 2% in healthy volunteers with oxygen saturations >90%. Readings are not affected by jaundice or anaemia, but there are some reports of inaccuracy in pigmented patients. Accuracy is also affected by:

- Haemodynamic instability
- Carboxyhaemoglobin (registers as SaO_2 90%)
- Methaemoglobinaemia (registers as SaO_2 85%)
- Low oxygen saturations (<80%)
- Pulsatile venous flow (e.g. tricuspid regurgitation, venous congestion, or arterio-venous fistulae)
- Intravenous dyes (e.g. methylene blue or indocyanine green)
- Motion artefact
- Blue, green, or black nail polish
- Fluorescent and xenon arc surgical lamps.

SaO_2 only allows assessment of hypoventilation when the patient is breathing air. The lowered alveolar PO_2 (PAO_2) and arterial PO_2 (PaO_2) produced by hypoventilation are easily corrected by a slight increase in FiO_2, so significant hypoventilation and increases in CO_2 may be overlooked if the patient is breathing oxygen.

Arterial blood gas analysis

Respiratory failure cannot be properly assessed without arterial blood gas sampling (ABGs). Repeated sampling is often appropriate. Capillary blood gas sampling offers an excellent but underutilized alternative to serial arterial puncture outside the high-dependency setting (allowing for an under-read of 0.5–1.0kPa for PaO_2).

PaO_2

PaO_2 alone is insufficient to fully evaluate the defect in oxygenation and a number of methods have been described to analyse it further:

- The PaO_2/FiO_2 ratio
- The A-aO_2 gradient.

PaO_2/FiO_2 ratio

PaO_2/FiO_2 attempts to quantify the severity of hypoxaemia, although gas exchange and ventilation are not analysed individually. The ratio in healthy lungs is >53kPa (e.g. 13kPa/0.21 = 62kPa). The American European Consensus Conference set the following PaO_2/FiO_2 ratio diagnostic criteria in 1994:

- Acute lung injury <40kPa (approx. 300mmHg)
- Adult respiratory distress syndrome <27kPa (approx. 200mmHg).

The PaO_2/FiO_2 ratio is simple to calculate and in widespread use, but both mathematical analyses and clinical studies have highlighted important shortcomings.

- As inspired O_2 is used in the calculation, if the disease is unresponsive to increased FiO_2 (mainly large shunts), simply increasing the FiO_2 will change the result.
- The calculation is affected by the applied airway pressures. The use of the oxygenation index allows for this:

   oxygenation index (OI) = mean airway pressure × FiO_2/PaO_2

The A-aO_2 gradient

The alveolar oxygen tension for a given inspired fraction of oxygen can be quickly calculated by making some approximations to the alveolar gas equation:

$$PAO_2 = FiO_2 (PB - PH_2O) - PaCO_2/RQ$$

$PB - PH_2O$ at sea level = 101.3kPa – 6.2kPa = 95kPa and assuming an RQ of 0.8, the equation above becomes

$$PAO_2 = FiO_2 × 0.95 - PaCO_2 × 1.2$$

The difference between the calculated PAO_2 and the measured PaO_2 is called the A-aO_2 gradient. The A-a gradient:

- Increases gradually with age ((0.044 × age) – 0.3kPa), and is a numerical value summating all the defects in gas exchange. These are most commonly due to $\dot{V}/\dot{Q}$ mismatch and shunt
- Allows assessment of the severity of the gas exchange defect
- Is a particularly useful tool in hypercarbic patients where hypoxaemia may occur in the absence of any gas exchange abnormality.

For example, a 50-year-old patient hypoventilating on air with a $PaCO_2$ of 9.5kPa has a PAO_2 of 8.6kPa. Even with a normal A-a gradient of 1.9kPa, their PaO_2 will be 6.7kPa.

- Helps to uncover gas exchange abnormalities masked by hyperventilation. Hyperventilation reduces $PaCO_2$ and $PACO_2$, increasing PAO_2. This may be sufficient to 'normalize' PaO_2 in the face of a gas exchange abnormality. For example, a hyperventilating 30-year-old patient has the following arterial blood gases: $PaCO_2$ 3.1kPa, PaO_2 12.1kPa. Even though the PaO_2 is within the normal range, the A-a gradient is elevated at 4.2kPa (should be 1kPa in 30-year-old)
- Allows us to spot aberrant results. For example, the A-a gradient tells us the following results are not possible on a patient breathing air: PaO_2 15kPa, $PaCO_2$ 5.5kPa.

Three important assumptions are made and should be kept in mind when using this analysis:
- Gas exchange is at a steady state.
- RQ is estimated rather than measured.
- Full equilibration of $PaCO_2$ and $PACO_2$ takes place. While this reliably happens in healthy lungs, in areas of high $\dot{V}/\dot{Q}$ there may not be full equilibration, and the A-a gradient will be underestimated.

$PaCO_2$
$PaCO_2$ depends on the balance between CO_2 production and CO_2 clearance in a relationship described by the equation

$$PaCO_2 = kVCO_2/VA$$

where VA is alveolar minute ventilation, VCO_2 is the rate of CO_2 production, k is a constant to equate the differing units of VCO_2 (mL/min) and $PaCO_2$ (kPa).

CO_2 production depends on metabolic rate and RQ, neither of which is easily manipulated, so the major determinant of $PaCO_2$ is alveolar minute ventilation. It can be seen that halving VA will double $PaCO_2$, therefore, in a normal metabolic state, hypercapnia results from reduced alveolar minute ventilation. There are only two causes:
- Reduced minute ventilation
- Increased dead space:
  - Anatomical as a result of equipment deadspace and rebreathing
  - Physiological as a result of alveolar dead space from $\dot{V}/\dot{Q}$ mismatch.

pH
The effects of $PaCO_2$ on pH are described by the Henderson–Hasselbalch equation:

$$pH = pKa + log (HCO_3/CO_2)$$

Any rise in $PaCO_2$ will result in a fall in pH. The relationship is non-linear as pH is a logarithmic measure, but for small changes of $PaCO_2$ and HCO_3 around normal values the following can be used as a rule of thumb:
- 0.13kPa rise in $PaCO_2$ causes a 0.01 decrease in pH
- 0.5mmol/L change in HCO_3 causes a 0.01 change pH.

Any acute changes are accompanied by physiological compensation (for example, respiratory acidosis promotes renal conservation of bicarbonate, with normalization of the pH). These compensatory mechanisms take days to weeks to occur, so the extent of compensation can be used as a measure of chronicity of the respiratory dysfunction.

Base excess represents the theoretical quantity of acid or alkali that needs to be added to the blood to return it to a normal pH (7.35–7.45) at a normal $PaCO_2$ (5.3kPa). First described by Astrup and Siggaard-Andersen in 1958, it is calculated using the pH and the $PaCO_2$. It is not a substitution for understanding of blood gas analysis, but it can be useful in detecting mixed respiratory and metabolic acidoses.

Standard base excess is the base excess calculated for anaemic blood (Hb 5g/dL). This reduces the haemoglobin buffering component and is thought to more closely represent whole body acid–base status.

Standard bicarbonate is the calculated bicarbonate level at standard conditions ($PaCO_2$ 5.3kPa, 37°C, full oxygen saturation).

Metabolic acidosis may also present as respiratory distress. The hyperventilation (Kussmaul respiration) is an attempt by the patient to reduce $PaCO_2$, creating a compensatory respiratory alkalosis.

It is important to recognize that these patients may not be in respiratory failure, and inappropriate mechanical ventilation may precipitate disaster. It would be impossible to mechanically match the minute ventilation spontaneously generated by the patient, worsening the acidaemia. A full discussion of metabolic acidosis (including Stewart's strong ion theory) is beyond the scope of this book, but a breakdown of causes using the traditional approach is shown in the text box below.

Metabolic acidosis

Anion gap quantifies unmeasured anions responsible for maintaining electroneutrality and is normally 8–16mEq/L. These are predominantly anionic groups on albumin and plasma proteins:

$$anion\ gap = (Na + K) - (HCO_3 + Cl)$$

The acidosis can be categorized into normal anion gap (bicarbonate wasting) or increased anion gap (increased non-volatile acids).

Albumin is the major unmeasured anion. Many critically ill patients are hypoalbuminaemic, and a high anion gap acidosis may appear to be a normal anion gap acidosis. The following formula corrects the anion gap:

$$observed\ anion\ gap + 0.25\ (normal\ albumin - measured\ albumin)$$

For example, Na 137, K 4, Cl 102, HCO_3 23, albumin 20g/L; anion gap 16mEq/L, adjusted to 16 + 0.25(44 − 20) = 22mEq/L.

Normal anion gap
Ureterostomy
Small bowel fistula
Excess chloride administration
Diarrhoea
Carbonic anhydrase inhibitors
Adrenal insufficiency
Renal tubular acidosis
Pancreatic fistula

Increased anion gap
Methanol
Uraemia
Diabetic keto-acidosis
Paraldehyde
Iron, izoniazid
Lactic acidosis
Ethanol, ethylene glycol
Salicylic acid

Pulmonary function tests
Pulmonary function tests (PFT) can be performed in the acute phase to aid diagnosis (although this is limited in ventilated patients), and examination of old PFT can give useful information about the nature and extent of any underlying lung disease.

Spirometry
This involves measurement of lung volumes as a function of time. The values are effort dependent and rely on patient co-operation. Tests are usually repeated to ensure reproducibility. Normal values are predicted from tables which take into account the patient's gender, height, and age.
- Forced expiratory volume in 1 second (FEV_1). Reduced in obstructive lung disease. There are significant limitations, even in COPD (see 📖 Chronic obstructive pulmonary disease, p 427), but the classification for severity of COPD is:

Table 1.1 Classification of severity of airflow obstruction

Severity	Post-bronchodilator FEV_1/FVC	Post-bronchodilator FEV_1 (% predicted)
Stage 1 – mild	<0.7	≥80%
Stage 2 – moderate	<0.7	50–79%
Stage 3 – severe	<0.7	30–49%
Stage 4 – very severe	<0.7	<30%

- Forced vital capacity (FVC).
  - Reduced in restrictive lung disease and neuromuscular disorders with respiratory muscle weakness.
  - Useful monitor of need for intervention in progressive neuromuscular disorders (e.g. Guilain–Barre). FVC <10mL/kg usually indicates a need for intervention.
  - Significant reduction when supine (>20%) suggests diaphragmatic weakness.

- FEV_1/FVC. Normal is 75–80%. The ratio is preserved or even increased in restrictive lung disease, and reduced significantly in obstructive lung disease.
- Peak expiratory flow rate (PEFR) is useful to monitor disease progression and response to therapy in obstructive diseases such as asthma.
- Flow volume loops provide a graphical representation of respiratory pattern. The loops have characteristic shapes in certain pathologies, but do not correspond to the loops produced by ventilators.

Plethysmography

This is a method of measuring FRC. The patient is sealed in an airtight box and breathes through a mouthpiece, which is closed at the end of inspiration. The resulting pressure changes within the mouthpiece and the airtight box allows the FRC to be calculated using Boyle's law. It is more accurate than gas dilution techniques, particularly where patients have air-spaces that do not communicate with the bronchial tree.

Diffusing capacity

Diffusing capacity of the lung for carbon monoxide (DLCO) measures the efficiency of gas exchange across the alveolar capillary interface. The patient holds a single breath of 0.3% CO and 10% helium for 10s. CO is used as it is rapidly taken up by haemoglobin, so the transfer is limited by diffusion rather than equilibration of partial pressures. Helium dilution allows measurement of total lung volume. Expired partial pressure of CO is measured. It is reduced in:
- Fibrosis
- Alveolitis
- Emphysema
- PE
- Low cardiac output states.

Elevated readings are found in:
- Alveolar haemorrhage
- Polycythaemia.

The diffusion coefficient for carbon monoxide (KCO) is DLCO indexed for lung volume.

Chest X-ray

Chest radiography remains the mainstay of imaging evaluation in respiratory failure, not only in primary diagnosis but also in monitoring of therapy and the day-to-day management of tubes and lines. The chest radiograph does, however, have limitations that must be borne in mind.
- Many of the patterns of abnormality are relatively non-specific in diagnostic terms.
- In ICU patients, positioning and exposure are often suboptimal and may well vary from examination to examination. Hence it is important to strive for radiographic continuity and recording of exposure factors for each patient to promote consistency and allow comparable follow-up examinations.

- ICU chest X-rays (CXRs) are usually performed anteroposterior (AP) and supine, resulting in magnification of the cardiac silhouette.
- Magnification also affects interpretation of mediastinal contours.
- Reduced achievable kilovoltage using mobile X-ray units may cause underexposure and motion blur due to the longer exposure times required.

Approach to chest radiograph interpretation
- Check patient demographics, date, and time.
- Check projection (AP or posteroanterior (PA)) and for any rotation— observe the relationship between medial ends of clavicles (anterior landmarks) and the spinous processes of the upper thoracic vertebrae (posterior midline landmarks). The upper spinous processes should be projected centrally between the medial ends of the clavicles.
- Assess penetration—vertebrae should be visible to T6, or halfway down cardiac shadow, and intervertebral disc spaces just visible through cardiac silhouette.
- Assess lung expansion—degree of inspiration/expiration. The anterior sixth rib should be visible above the diaphragm. The CXR is likely to have been taken in expiration if four anterior ribs or fewer are visible above diaphragm.
- Check positions and types of all tubes and lines methodically. Start with endotracheal tube (ETT) and nasogastric tube (NGT), then venous lines and surgical drains.
- Evaluate heart size—if the transverse diameter of the heart is <50% of the maximal internal thoracic diameter then it is not enlarged, especially with an AP film.
- Even with AP films, where a degree of magnification is inevitable, it is useful to check for serial changes in heart size, for example as a clue for developing pericardial effusion.
- Check mediastinum, particularly for aortic arch in trauma patients and for signs of pneumomedistinum in ventilated patients.
- Check for volume loss—compare sizes of hemithoraces, rib crowding, and deviation of trachea/mediastinum.
- Evaluate lungs, looking for regions of increased or decreased transradiancy, comparing side to side. Note that a general difference in transradiancy of the hemithoraces comparing right with left may be due to patient rotation (again check technical aspects of image).
- Localize and assess whether abnormalities of lung opacity are unilateral or bilateral, and predominantly upper or mid or lower zone. The zones of the lungs are a radiological definition to allow description and should not be confused with the lobes. The upper zones are defined as above the second anterior rib level, mid zones from second anterior to fourth anterior rib levels and lower zones below anterior fourth ribs.
- Are any areas of increased opacity discrete or general? Nodules are discrete opacities <3cm diameter while masses are >3cm.

Increased transradiancy (see also ▢ Pleural disease, p 481)

- Check for the presence of peripheral lung edge (pneumothorax) or whether lung markings are visible across areas of increased lucency or whether the lucency has defined borders.
- Pneumothorax—the main chest radiographic signs of pneumothorax are increased transradiancy, with a lung edge visible peripherally, demarcating the extent of the pneumothorax. With a tension pneumothorax the lung is usually extensively collapsed and the mediastinum plus heart deviated towards the opposite thorax. However, in the supine ICU patient a lung edge may not be visible and secondary signs of pneumothorax, such as a deep sulcus sign (the costophrenic angle is abnormally deepened) and/or abnormally well-demarcated mediastinum, should raise suspicion. Further clues are the development of abnormal air in other locations such as pneumomedistinum/pneumopericardium or surgical emphysema. Where pneumothorax develops on the background of an abnormal lung, tension may not be immediately apparent as the lung may not collapse.
- Emphysematous bullae may be manifest as very well-defined areas of lucency with imperceptibly thin margins. More often bullous lung disease is seen as areas of general increased transradiancy with sparse lung markings, commonly upper zone. Differentiation from pneumothorax is vital as introduction of an intercostal drain may be disastrous.
- Focal lucency within areas of increased opacity may be due to cavitation, e.g. cavitating pneumonia.
- Localized cavity with perceptible but thin wall is likely infectious in origin, e.g. TB.
- Cavities with thick walls are more likely to be neoplastic, e.g. squamous lung carcinoma.

Opacification

Categorize type:
- Dense with pulmonary vasculature obscured but air bronchograms visible (consolidation). The more common causes include pneumonia, aspiration pneumonitis, ARDS/ALI, pulmonary oedema, pulmonary haemorrhage, and pulmonary infarction. Rarer causes include alveolar proteinosis and some forms of malignancy, such as bronchoalveolar cell carcinoma.
- Opacity present but vasculature still visible ('ground glass'). Although the causes of consolidation and 'ground glass' opacity are essentially the same (alveolar air replacement by fluid, pus, haemorrhage, tumour etc.), the degree of opacity will give some indication of severity. One cause of a 'ground glass' type appearance on a CXR (as distinct from computerized tomography, CT) is the case of a small/moderate effusion on a supine radiograph where the combination of normally aerated lung anteriorly and dependent pleural fluid posteriorly results in increased density on which vascular structures are visible.

- Dense homogenous opacity without air bronchogram. The most common causes will be effusion (often combined with consolidation) or pulmonary collapse, but frank pulmonary masses will generally also be homogenous.

Intrathoracic fluid

Assessment of excess fluid within the thorax is of major importance in critical care patients. Predominantly the questions will be as to whether there is pleural fluid present fluid versus intrapulmonary fluid.

- Pleural effusions may not manifest the classic basal meniscus appearance familiar from erect films in the supine ICU patient, rather an effusion may appear as diffuse increase in the density of a lung. Clues may be apparent in the form of fluid tracking into the fissures and capping the lung apex.

Pulmonary oedema mainly manifests as consolidative shadowing and the main task in critical care patients is to try and differentiate cardiogenic oedema (fluid overload) from non-cardiogenic oedema (ARDS/ALI), although of course the two may coexist. Features favouring cardiogenic oedema/fluid overload are:

- Rapidity of onset or offset
- Changing appearances with time
- Associated effusions
- Septal lines (indicating interlobuar septal fluid)
- Peribronchial cuffing/perihailar haze (manifestaions of interstitial fluid in the loose peribronchial and perivascular spaces).

Review areas

Finally, for the lungs check the 'review areas'. These are the portions of the chest radiograph where research and experience have shown that pathology is most commonly missed. They are areas where interpretation may be hampered by superimposed structures and comprise:

- Lung apices (overlapping ribs + clavicles)
- Behind the heart
- Behind the diaphragm (posterior sulcus can be quite deep).

Final steps

- Check the skeleton of the thorax, particularly important in trauma patients, where flail rib fracture segments may be a missed contributory factor to respiratory failure.
- Review and compare to previous radiographs for serial changes and with premorbid images if available. This vital aspect of interpretation has been greatly improved with the widespread adoption of digital imaging systems (picture archiving and communication systems, PACS). The temporal evolution and change in a pattern on chest radiography may give the greatest information as to the likely cause of abnormality.

Integration of the above signs/patterns is required to aid formulation of a diagnosis. For example, homogenous opacification of a whole hemithorax will almost certainly be due to large pleural effusion where the volume of the hemithorax is maintained (the mediastinum may even be deviated away from the affected side due to space occupying effect) while it will denote complete lung collapse where the hemithorax is reduced and mediastinum deviated to that side.

Computerized tomography

Computerized tomography (CT) scanning is widely available and increasingly used for the investigation of respiratory disease in critically unwell patients. CT is useful where the CXR is non-diagnostic or complicated with both pleural and parenchymal involvement. CT defines mediastinal and vascular structures accurately, and gives more definitive information about the presence or absence of interstitial disease, fibrosis, atelectasis, consolidation, pneumothorax, pleural effusions, abscesses, cavitation, empyema, bronchial disease, and chest wall pathology. CT can be used to investigate known pathology, look for suspected pathology, or rule out the chest as a source of pathology (e.g. looking for a septic source).

With modern multidetector row CT scanners, image acquisition times have reduced markedly. This reduces movement and respiratory artefacts with resulting gains in image quality.

The thin 'high resolution' slices necessary for diagnosis of pulmonary parenchymal disease are now routinely available from volumetric studies performed in a single breath-hold.

Reconstruction of thin slice data from contrast media enhanced scans can provide angiographic images to rival conventional angiograms.

CT pulmonary angiography (CTPA) has revolutionized the investigation and diagnosis of PE in ICU patients. CTPA uses early phase scanning during contrast medium infusion for peak pulmonary arterial contrast enhancement.

A newer development in CT is the potential for the integration of electrocardiograph (ECG) gated scanning to allow cardiac assessment, particularly where cardiac pathology such as an intracardiac shunt is suspected. A controlled regular rhythm is preferable, and in patients who have COPD, or who are haemodynamically unstable, this may be achieved with esmolol or ivabradine.

While CT is undoubtedly more specific and better localizes disease in the thorax than CXR, many findings remain non-specific with wide differential diagnoses. There are also practical difficulties associated with implementing CT in critically ill patients:

- Patients must be moved to radiology, with the attendant risks such as disconnection of ventilators and monitoring equipment. Studies have shown that this can occur in a third of all transports outside the ICU with an even higher incidence in relation to CT transfers.
- Suspension of respiration must be co-ordinated with scan performance (preferably at full inspiration). With modern multidetector CT scanners image acquisition is <6s, making this somewhat less problematic, and with the most recent 'super premium' scanners whole thorax scanning in <1s may obviate the need for breath-holding.
- The administration of contrast media to these patients is not without risk (see below).

Contrast reactions

Idiosyncratic reactions to iodine-based contrast media are usually anaphylactoid (rather than anaphylactic) in nature (i.e. there is no prior sensitizing exposure). They are a 'toxic' reaction and not dose dependent. Treatment is as per anaphylaxis.

Non-idiosyncratic reactions are dose dependent and mediated by the following mechanisms:

- Vasomotor reactions, causing cardiovascular collapse
- Hyperosmolar effects, leading to endothelial damage and cardiac depression
- Chemotoxic effects, the most recognized of which is contrast-induced nephropathy (CIN), defined as a creatinine rise of >44.2µmol/L or >25% above baseline and occurs in 2% of general patients but in up to 50% of high-risk patients. In a study of 16,000 patients receiving contrast, mortality in those developing CIN was 34%, compared to 7% in those who did not. Risk factors for the development of CIN are:
  - Pre-existing renal impairment
  - Diabetes
  - Age >70
  - Dehydration
  - Nephrotoxic drugs
  - Respiratory failure
  - Sepsis.
- The avoidance of CIN entails refraining from unnecessary exposure to contrast in those at risk and ensuring adequate hydration while minimizing contrast dose when contrast administration is required. Other measures (e.g. mannitol, N-acetyl cysteine, calcium channel blockers, and ANP) have not been consistently shown to reduce the incidence of CIN.

Lung disease patterns on CT
  Alveolar opacity
- This refers simply to the replacement of 'alveolar' air spaces with material of increased density and ranges from ground glass opacity (GGO), where pulmonary vessels remain visible, through to consolidation, where vessels are obscured and air bronchograms are a hallmark. The material may be simple fluid (oedema), proteinaceous fluid, pus, haemorrhage etc. The pattern may give a clue to the aetiology.
- Ventrodorsal gradient is common in pulmonary haemorrhage (e.g. lupus pneumonia, Goodpastures syndrome) and also ARDS/diffuse alveolar damage associated with systemic inflammatory response syndrome (SIRS).
- Perihilar with gradient and subpleural sparing suggests cardiogenic oedema/fluid overload. Often with pleural effusions.
- No gradient with 'crazy paving' appearance (interlobular septal thickening with background GGO) suggests alveolar proteinosis.

  Interstitial opacites
- Interlobular septal thickening.
  - Smooth appearance is classically due to pulmonary oedema.
  - Nodular is suggestive of lymphangitis but also seen in sarcoid, among other conditions.

- Reticular opacities are seen in pulmonary fibrotic conditions.
  - Lower zone posterior distribution with subpleural honeycombing suggests usual interstitial pneumonitis.
  - Milder reticulation with GGO favours non-specific interstitial pneumonia (NSIP).
  - Presence of subpleural lines and bands along with pleural plaques is seen in asbestosis.
  - Upper zone predominance suggests chronic extrinsic allergic alveolitis (EAA).
- GGO.
  - Subacute EAA in non-smokers.
  - Respiratory bronchiolitis-associated interstitial lung disease (RBILD) in non-smokers is seen with coexistent emphysema.
  - Pneumocystis jirovecii pneumonia (PCP).

Nodular opacities
- 'Tree-in-bud' classically in TB.
- Ill-defined centrilobular nodules classically in subacute EAA, also seen with RBILD in smokers.
- PCP.

Reduced density
- Pneumothorax—peripheral pleural airspace outwith lung, may be loculated.
- Emphysema—air attenuation (increased lucency) without defined walls. Centrilobular, panacinar, and bullous types.
- Air trapping—reduced attenuation of lung parenchyma with small vessels. Usually seen as part of a mosaic pattern due to adjacent normal lung and small airways changes (bronchiolectasis and wall thickening), e.g. obliterative bronchiolitis.

Cysts
- Circumscribed low attenuation with defined walls.
- Uniform size in lymphangioleiomyomatosis.
- Bizarre shapes predominantly in upper and mid zones, with sparing of costophrenic recesses in histiocytosis.
- Combined with GGO in PCP.

Pulmonary thrombo-embolic disease
- CTPA specifically uses early phase scanning during contrast medium infusion for peak pulmonary arterial contrast enhancement.
- Pulmonary thromboembolism (PTE) is manifest as filling defects within the pulmonary arterial tree, contrasted against the high attenuation of enhanced blood. These filling defects may partially ('eyeball' and 'tram track' signs) or completely occlude the pulmonary arterial lumen (no contrast visible). Large emboli will obstruct central main pulmonary arteries; a more minor embolism may be limited to a few, or even one, subsegmental artery.
- Chronic PTE is more often eccentric/marginal, laminated, and smoothly contoured against the vessel wall.
- The severity of PTE is best determined by evaluation of its effect on right heart dynamics: in severe PTE the right heart chambers will be

dilated and the venae cavae engorged, often with reflux of contrast into the inferior vena cava and hepatic veins. Where the diameter of the RV exceeds that of the left (RV:LV > 1) this is a sign of severe haemodynamic compromise and poor prognosis without intervention.

Magnetic resonance imaging
- Magnetic resonance imaging (MRI) of the thorax has little role in the investigation of the critically ill patient with respiratory failure. It can be used for the evaluation of diaphragmatic integrity in cases of suspected rupture or as a dynamic method of assessing diaphragmatic movement.
- MRI of the brain and cervical cord may be required for investigation of central CNS causes of respiratory failure.
- Critically ill patients may require MRI evaluation for other reasons.
- MRI of the ventilated patient requires specialist equipment, free from ferromagnetic materials.
- Images are susceptible to movement artefact, so patients may require additional sedation.
- Image acquisition can take several minutes (rather than seconds for CT), with total room examination times for ventilated patients of up to an hour not unusual when including patient positioning and retrieval. This has implications for the patient and also for the staffing levels in the ICU.

Chest ultrasound
Ultrasound is becoming an integral part of the evaluation of patients with respiratory failure, and its use can both provide a prompt diagnostic service and facilitate therapeutic intervention. The most common use is in visualizing the pleural space but more recently ultrasound patterns of the lung parenchyma itself have been described.

In supine ventilated patients identification of fluid by physical examination is difficult and radiographic opacification on a supine x-ray can be difficult to interpret—effusions and consolidation can appear similar. Ultrasound can distinguish the two and allows marking for potential pleural drainage. Ultrasound also allows differentiation between simple effusion and loculated effusion, for which it is more accurate than CT.

Pneumothoraces in ICU can often be anterior in a supine patient and radio-occult on a plain film unless imaged by CT scan. Pleural ultrasound may help here, although the signs of a pneumothorax are more subtle than for an effusion. In normal pleural imaging with tidal breathing there is pleural sliding visualized as the visceral and parietal pleura move over each other. In the presence of air in the pleural space this is lost. Furthermore, the presence of a 'lung point' where the normal appearance returns adjacent to that of an area of air can delineate the extent of pneumothorax.

Lung sonography, in which the actual lung parenchyma is analysed, is being advocated in some ICUs to allow rapid bedside diagnosis. The analysis depends on the identification of certain patterns of appearance of the lung. For example, the loss of the normal lung sliding can also indicate the presence of pneumonia. Other conditions causing respiratory failure, such as cardiogenic pulmonary oedema and pulmonary embolism, can also be identified by means of lung ultrasound looking for the specific appearance of certain acoustic shadows and lines. The most characteristic features of increased interstitial lung water are lung comets or B-lines. These appearances reflect the presence of extravascular fluid in the lung and importantly the number seen correlates with the radiological extent of pulmonary oedema, wedge pressure, and New York Heart Association (NYHA) heart failure class. Ongoing work is suggestive that repeat imaging may also act as a method for assessing response to therapy, for example diuretics. The findings in pulmonary embolus (multiple, hypoechoic, wedge-shaped lesions with associated pleural fluid) are relatively non-specific.

A more minor role of ultrasound is to evaluate the function of the diaphragm, particularly in patients with ventilatory failure of unknown cause.

Microbiology

The investigation of a patient with ventilatory failure is not complete without adequate microbiological analysis. In patients with pulmonary infiltrates and ventilatory failure the exclusion of a microbiological cause is paramount, especially if the patient has risk factors such as immuno-suppression. The role of the microbiology laboratory is discussed fully in 📖 The microbiology laboratory, p 49.

Blood tests

Blood test results may direct and confirm diagnosis and assess the severity of the disease.

Haematology

- Elevated neutrophils can indicate infection or inflammation. In pneumonia white cell count (WCC) >20 or <4 × 10^9/ml indicates severe infection.
- If the neutrophil count is <1 × 10^9/ml, consider neutropaenic sepsis.
- Steroid therapy causes 'demargination'. Reduced adherence of neutrophils to the endothelium of blood vessels elevates circulating neutrophil levels, which are then less able to migrate to sites of infection, paradoxically resulting in immunosuppression.
- Viral infection may cause lymphocytosis or lymphopaenia.
- Causes of eosinophilia are numerous, but in the context of respiratory failure consider idiopathic eosinophilic pneumonia, connective tissue disease, vasculitis, and fungal disease.
- A drop in haemoglobin occurring in association with gas exchange deterioration may indicate diffuse alveolar haemorrhage. If the haemoglobin falls abruptly for no apparent reason, consider pulmonary haemorrhage or haemolysis.
- Coagulation abnormalities are seen in severe sepsis due to disseminated intravascular coagulation. The precise pattern is variable, but thrombocytopenia in the absence of even mild disturbance of clotting should lead to a search for other causes of low platelets.
- Thrombocytosis is associated with vasculitic disease and often missed.

Biochemistry
- Abnormal renal function may indicate severe disease or give clues to the origin, e.g. pulmonary-renal syndrome.
- C-reactive protein can be a better guide to infection than WCC, particularly if the patient is on immunosuppressant therapy. Furthermore, it can be used as serial measurements to assess response to treatment, with falling levels being a good indicator of sepsis resolution.
- Deranged liver function tests may be seen in any severe sepsis syndrome, but otherwise mild pneumonia is more common in atypical infections.
- Creatine kinase levels can be elevated in specific myopathies and in legionella infection.
- Hyponatraemia may suggest atypical pneumonia and associated syndrome of inappropriate anti-diuretic hormone.
- Thyroid function derangement is a potentially overlooked cause of failure to wean from ventilation.
- In the presence of renal failure, urine should be dipsticked and the presence of blood or protein should prompt a search for other signs or symptoms of glomerulonephritic/vasculitic disease:
  - Prolonged flu-like illness: malaise, arthralgia, myalgia, fatigue, night sweats, weight loss (median length of symptoms before diagnosis of Wegener's disease is 6 months).
  - Nasal discomfort and blockage together with ulceration, crusting, rhinorrhoea, and epistaxis (90% have upper airways disease).
  - SOB, cough, haemoptysis.
  - Late onset asthma.
  - Eosinophilia.
  - Thrombocytosis.

Immunology
- An urgent autoimmune screen should be sent in unexplained ventilatory failure with pulmonary infiltrates (antinuclear antibody, antineutrophilic cytoplasmic antibody, rheumatoid factor, and antiglomerular basement membrane), particularly in the presence of the symptoms, signs, or test results mentioned above.
- Anti-acetylcholinesterase antibodies can be useful if myasthenia gravis is suspected.

Serology
- Paired samples (within 7 days of onset of illness and repeated 7–10 days later) can be used to identify specific respiratory infections such as mycoplasma, chlamydia, and viral pathogens such as influenza or adenovirus. These depend on a rise in antibody titres at two separate time points. However, many laboratories are now using polymerase chain reaction (PCR) or enzyme-linked immunoassay to detect these organisms in respiratory secretions as the presence of organisms can be confirmed at an earlier stage.

- More specific serology can be used: legionella pneumophilia can be tested by PCR or serology, mycoplasma by complement fixation test.
- Often the results of these tests only become available after the patient has been treated and empirical cover is required.
- In immunocompromised patients, such as acquired immunodeficiency syndrome (AIDS) patients, consider sending serum for cryptococcal antigen.

Bronchoscopy

Bronchoscopy is an important investigation in the evaluation of a patient with respiratory failure. Broncoscopy in unintubated patients may precipitate a deterioration requiring intubation. For that reason, it is best performed in an ICU setting with the patient ventilated, or at least in a high-dependency environment where access to immediate intubation and ventilation is available.

Indications

- Diagnostic assessment:
  - Visualization of bronchial tree.
  - Collection of samples, e.g. bronchoalveolar lavage for microbiology and cytology.
  - Transbronchial biopsy (usually reserved for the post-transplant patient to exclude rejection).
- Relief of endobronchial obstruction.
- Localization and isolation of site of trauma or bleeding.
- Placement of percutaneous tracheostomy.

Technique

This is better demonstrated than described, but the following points are worthy of note:

- Patients should be preoxygenated with an appropriate FiO_2 (usually 100% in ventilated patients) and monitored with pulse oximetry and, if available, capnography throughout. Ideally patients should be ventilated and paralysed, which will reduce the risk of trauma to an agitated patient and damage to the fibreoptic bronchoscope (FOB).
- In intubated patients the FOB is introduced via a catheter mount, which has an airtight seal around it. Smallest size that can be used to accommodate an adult bronchoscope is an 8-mm ETT.
- There is a low incidence of complications (0.01–0.04% mortality in large series but may be higher in ventilated patients). The introduction of the FOB increases airway resistance and gas trapping; periodic removal of the bronchoscope allows exhalation.
- FOB can be performed in patients using non-invasive ventilation with a facemask interface. Air leaks can be a problem, causing further respiratory compromise.

Fluid/tissue sampling

- Sampling of the lower respiratory tract is usually through bronchoalveolar lavage; aliquots of 50–60mL (total volume 180–200mL) of sterile saline are introduced to a subsegment via a wedged bronchoscope and fluid is then aspirated and collected in a specimen pot attached to the FOB. The first lavage returned is usually discarded since it is most likely to be contaminated by organisms brought down by the scope on passage through the ETT. Lavage can cause hypoxia if too much fluid is instilled. This technique allows a wider area of lung parenchyma to be sampled.

- A protected specimen brush (PSB) is used to try and remove the risk of contamination from the upper airways. A brush is extended from a covering and used to collect distal tissue/fluid. It can be introduced blindly but is more commonly used under bronchoscopic guidance. This allows direct visualization of the area being sampled and reduces cross-contamination, although a much smaller area of lung is being sampled when compared to bronchoalveolar lavage (BAL). There are no differences in terms of sensitivity or specificity for microbiological analysis of either PSB or BAL.

- BAL can be used for cellular fluid analysis, which can be helpful in diagnosis and prognosis in terms of percentage of neutrophils, eosinophils, and lymphocytes present. For example, an elevated neutrophil count in the BAL in ARDS is associated with poorer outcome; elevated eosinophil count (>15%) is associated with only a limited number of conditions, namely Churg–Strauss, eosinophilic pneumonia, drug-induced reaction, helminthic infection, or AIDS-related infection.

- Cytological analysis of the fluid by an experienced pathologist is necessary; the detection of haemosiderin-laden macrophages or red blood corpuscles indicates recent alveolar haemorrhage, although the macrophages do not appear until 48h after the event. Foamy alveolar macrophages are associated with amiodarone-induced pulmonary toxicity.

- Biopsy of the lung in both ventilated and non-ventilated patients with respiratory failure can be very difficult with significant morbidity and mortality. Transbronchial lung biopsy (TBLB) and open lung biopsy have been used. TBLB is usually reserved for the post-transplant patient to exclude rejection. Pneumothorax is common (8–14% in TBLB in ventilated patients). Other complications include persistent air leaks and death.

- Endobronchial ultrasound (EBUS) allows visualization of structures within and adjacent to the airways. A common use is in the investigation of mediastinal lymphadenopathy of unknown cause. The ultrasound probe is integrated in the end of the bronchoscope and allows the simultaneous insertion of a 22-guage needle into the lymph node under real time.

Additional investigations
Pulmonary artery catheter
The use of the pulmonary artery catheter has diminished in recent years, but it still occasionally remains useful in the management of some respiratory diseases:

- Measurement of pulmonary artery pressures may help to distinguish RV dilatation secondary to PE from that due to RV infarct.
- Management of fluid balance in ARDS.
- 'Gold standard' for the measurement of cardiac output.

Pulmonary angiography

This can be used to exclude significant pulmonary emboli but dangers include contrast nephropathy. Its use has been largely superseded by CT angiography.

Neuromuscular investigations

The finding of ventilatory failure due to neuromuscular problems demands a full investigation.

- Spirometry and serum CK are useful screening investigations.
- Electromyography and neurophysiology can be used for diagnosis of motor neurone disease and myotonic dystrophy.
- MRI is the imaging modality of choice for the brainstem and spinal cord to exclude conditions such as syringomyelia or Arnold–Chiari malformation.
- Muscle biopsy may be required to look for rare myopathies such as Pompes' (acid maltase) disease and Duchenne's muscular dystrophy.

Sleep investigations

Sleep investigation can be complex and range from a simple screening test using overnight pulse oximetry to a full polysomnogram (PSG).

- In most patients the use of pulse oximetry and transcutaneous CO_2 can identify those who have obstructive sleep apnoea or obesity hypoventilation as a cause of their ventilatory failure. The appearance of large dips in nocturnal saturations associated with rises in transcutaneous CO_2 and heart rate can indicate sleep-disordered breathing.
- The role of the PSG in the ICU patient is limited. However, it can occasionally be useful if the patient has difficulty weaning, where a PSG may indicate sleep deprivation as a cause.

1.3 The microbiology laboratory

The services offered by the microbiology laboratory are invaluable in the management of respiratory disease in the ICU. This chapter covers the most commonly requested procedures carried out in the laboratory and should be read in conjunction with 📖 Diagnosis of respiratory failure, p 22.

Sputum

This is the most common sample sent to microbiology for the investigation of respiratory disease. Only 60% of patients with pneumonia produce sputum and neutropenic patients cannot produce purulent specimens.

Appearance
Colour
- Rusty sputum suggests old alveolar haemorrhage, especially in pneumococcal pneumonia.
- Frank haemoptysis suggests necrotizing pneumonias:
  - *Pseudomonas aeruginosa* or *Aspergillus* spp. in neutropenic patients
  - Panton Valentine leukocidin-associated staphylococcal pneumonia
  - *Mycobacterium tuberculosis*.
- Dark-red mucoid sputum ('redcurrant jelly') suggests *Klebsiella pneumoniae* (common in alcoholics following aspiration).

Volume
- Copious in bronchiectasis.
- Scant in viral, pneumocystis pneumonia (PCP), or atypical infection.

Consistency
- Mucopurulent—most commonly in bronchitis/pneumonia.
- Liquid—seen in neutropenic patients where there are no pus cells, or it may be saliva, which is usually not cultured.

Odour
- Foul smelling—often mixed anaerobes following aspiration, or may be due to anaerobic lung abscesses.

Microscopy
The utility of Gram staining in the diagnosis of pneumonia is disputed, since many organisms isolated may only be colonizing the airways rather than infecting lung parenchyma. In addition, >40% of bacteraemic patients with pneumococcal pneumonia will have negative sputum Gram films.

However, microscopy is a simple procedure that may reveal the identity of the infecting organism, and is helpful in determining the quality of the specimen. For example:
- An excess of epithelial cells present with few leukocytes indicate an upper respiratory tract sample and will grow mainly contaminants from the mouth.

- Lots of neutrophils with intracellular organisms indicate the sample is from the lower respiratory tract. Having been ingested by polymorphs, any isolated organisms are likely to be significant.

If TB is suspected, this must be stated on the request form otherwise only a Gram film will be done. Tuberculosis staining may be by the more old-fashioned alcohol acid fast bacilli (AAFB or Ziehl Neelsen) or the easier but less discriminatory auramine phenol techniques.

Sputum has to be treated before staining since organisms are not uniformly distributed though the specimen. This involves adding a mucous-disrupting solution followed by thorough mixing (vortexing). The process takes 15–20min and results in homogenization and decreased viscosity of the specimen.

Gram staining
After 'fixing' the specimen (usually by dry heat), Gram staining involves a four-stage procedure which takes about 5min.
- Add crystal violet (the blue stain).
- Add iodine to fix/mordant the stain.
- Decolourize with acetone.
- Counter-stain with carbol fuchsin or safranin (pink).

Classification
The retention of the different dyes differentiates the bacteria into:
- Gram positive (retain purple/blue stain) or
- Gram negative (retain pink stain).

They are classified by the appearance of individual organisms:
- Cocci—small and spherical (kokkos = berry)
- Bacilli—elongated or rod-shaped
- Cocco-bacilli—intermediate shape.

Gram-positive cocci are further classified by their arrangement:
- Staphylococci in clusters (staphyle = bunch of grapes)
- Streptococci in chains.

Limitations
- Cell wall deficient organisms not stained (eg mycoplasma).
- Acid fast bacilli not seen.

Ziehl Neelsen stain
This is a more involved process, taking more than 30min. It is more specific than auramine phenol so is often used for confirmation of species.
- Slide flooded with carbol fuchsin, heated gently, and left for 5min.
- Rinsed and decolorized with 3% acid alcohol solution for 2–3min.
- Rinsed and more acid alcohol solution added for 3–4min.
- Counter-stain with methylene blue or malachite green for 30s.

Limitations
- Preparation is time-consuming.
- Often few acid–alcohol fast bacilli (AAFB) present, which can be difficult to find, so slides need examining for 15–20min.
- A modification of this stain is also used for identifying *Nocardia* spp.

Auramine phenol
Auramine phenol (A-P) will show acid fast bacilli, but is not specific for mycobacteria. Processing time is approximately 20min.
- Pour freshly filtered A-P on the slide and leave for 10min.
- Wash with water and add acid-alcohol decolourizer for 3–5min.
- Wash and counter-stain with thiazine red or potassium permanganate. Slides are then examined under a fluorescent microscope.

Limitations
- Need fluorescent microscope.
- Not specific for mycobacterium.

Pneumocystis stains
Few hospitals in the UK routinely offer PCR or other molecular based tests for the diagnosis of *Pneumocystis jiroveci.*

Lower respiratory tract samples are needed. Induced sputum (provoked by hypertonic saline) can provide a suitable sample, but the high risk of transmitting infections such as TB during the deep coughing precludes its routine use. BAL specimens are best and easiest to deal with.

There are two commonly used methods:
- Immunofluorescent monoclonal antibody detection is the most sensitive test
- Variations of Wrights/Giemsa stains (Diff-Quik) and calco-fluor white are used in other countries.

Limitations
- May detect dead pneumocysts.
- Takes a minimum of 3h.

Culture
Conventional bacterial
Agar is a seaweed base of solidity with additives to encourage bacterial growth (for example sheep or horse blood). Other supplements can be added to encourage growth of unusual organisms. Most routine cultures are plated onto blood agar and cultured aerobically and anaerobically.
- Chocolate blood agar (lysed blood component) will encourage growth of delicate organisms such as Haemophilus spp.
- Selective agars with pH indicators (McConkey or cystine–lactose–electrolyte deficient (CLED)) are used for differentiating Gram-negative organisms, e.g. lactose-fermenting organisms (*E. coli,* Acinetobacter) from non-lactose fermenters (proteus, pseudomonas salmonellae).
- Legionella agar-buffered charcoal yeast.
- Burkholderia cepacia selective agar for cystic fibrosis patients.

Plates are incubated for 24h and then examined. Suspicious colonies are further examined for antibiotic sensitivities:

- Manually with antibiotic impregnated discs or
- Mechanically on an automated sensitivity machine (e.g. VITEK®).

Old-fashioned plating to culture and sensitivity results take >48h, longer if more sensitivity discs have to be added for a multi-resistant organism. Automated results may be available in 24–36h.

Mycobacterial culture
- 5mL early morning sputum, ideally three subsequent day specimens.
- Specimen decontaminated to remove organisms from the upper respiratory tract or, for example, pseudomonas in a cystic fibrosis patient.
- Inoculation of Lowenstein–Jensen medium (agar with potatoes and Dorset egg yolk), incubated for 3 months and examined weekly.

Rapid mycobacterial diagnosis
- BAL may be sent directly to reference laboratories for PCR, which will also detect rifampicin resistance genes.
- Liquid TB culture available in some centres; specially supplied bottles cultured on an automated machine.
- Speed of growth may be days rather than weeks.

Legionella culture
- Buffered yeast extract charcoal agar (BYCER) is used.
- Cultures may take 3–5 days to grow.

Blood cultures

Optimal timing of blood cultures is 15min before the temperature rise, as there is a delay in the hypothalamus generating pyrexia. Blood cultures are usually taken while the patient is febrile and hence the numbers of bacteria in the blood culture may be low or absent as circulating polymorphs have ingested them.

In patients where sepsis is suspected, blood cultures should be taken, even in the absence of pyrexia (25% of >65-year-olds with pneumococcal pneumonia are bacteremic but remain apyrexial). Continuing bacteraemia while on supposedly appropriate therapy may indicate an underlying intravascular focus (e.g. endocarditis). Low-level bacteremia may be present in line sepsis or translocation from an intrabdominal focus.

Generally one set suffices unless the patient has a central venous catheter or feeding line. In these circumstances a set of blood cultures should be taken from each lumen of every vascular device in addition to a peripheral set.

Several automated blood culture systems are in common use (e.g. Bac T Alert, Bactec). Some also contain a material to absorb antibiotics present in the patient's bloodstream that may otherwise inhibit growth. Systems usually consist of two bottles, one for aerobic and one for anaerobic culture. The manufacturer's instructions should be followed when adding blood as the amount differs between systems.

Once taken, the cultures should be sent directly to the laboratory for placing into the automated system. (If blood cultures cannot be placed in the system immediately then the bottles should at least be placed in an incubator rather than sitting on the ward or in a transit collection box, since delicate organisms such as Neisseria and some anaerobes will die at room temperature).

The activity within the bottles should be constantly monitored. More organisms in the initial inoculum results in a more rapid pH change and the bottle will 'flag' earlier (usually within 24h for septicaemic patients). Conversely, bottles showing growth after 2–3 days are either 'slow growing' or the result of a single organism harvested during aspiration of the blood, and are more likely to represent contaminants. Most pathogenic organisms, apart from brucella, cause the cultures to flag positive within 24–36h.

If many different pathogens are present within one blood culture set, then the results are suspicious of contamination, unless the blood was taken immediately peri-mortem or from a patient with intra-abdominal catastrophe.

Blood tests

Serology

Serology encompasses many different tests:

- Enzyme-linked immunosorbent assay (ELISA) tests for HIV and hepatitis B and C antibody detection.
- PCR (polymerase chain reaction) for viral loads (CMV, HIV) is now almost universally available in hospital laboratories, and same-day results are usually possible.
- Complement fixation tests. Some automated machine systems can detect mycoplasma IgM and other early evidence of respiratory infection, but usually most laboratories will offer the old-fashioned complement fixation tests. These rely on the production of antibody 7–10 days into the illness, and are most used for atypical infections (Mycoplasma, *C. psittaci* and *C. burnetii*). Antigen remaining free in the well after adding the patient's serum is indicative of low or no antibody formation, and the presence of free antigen is detected by an indicator system of red cells and complement. This is an overnight test, labour intensive and usually batched once or twice weekly.

Haematology

- Rapidly falling haemoglobin in the presence of a stable haematocrit may suggest intravascular hemolysis as found in streptococcal toxic shock or necrotizing fasciitis.
- The absolute neutrophil counts may be very high or very low in overwhelming bacterial sepsis.
- Infection with leukocytotoxin-producing organisms, e.g. Panton Valentine leukocidin (PVL) producing *S. aureus* and Group A beta haemolytic streptococci, often produces lymphopenia.
- While a lymphocytosis may indicate viral infection, the total white cell count is often unremarkable with viral infections other than infectious mononucleosis.

- Atypical lymphocytes in the presence of lymphadenopathy and a rash suggest Epstein–Barr virus, CMV or HIV acute seroconversion.
- A severe lymphopenia suggests Gram-positive sepsis (exotoxin driven) rather than Gram-negative (endotoxin). Exotoxins such as toxic shock syndrome toxin (TSST-1) and superantigens seem particularly associated with lymphopenia, and as the lymphocyte count rises to normal level the patient is usually improving.
- A neutrophilia indicates bacterial infection, a predominance of immature or band forms suggests increased cell turnover.
- Disseminated intravascular coagulation and thrombocytopenia are common in any severe sepsis. In community-acquired pneumonia, patients with platelet counts <100 have a worse outcome.
- Reactive thrombocythaemia is common in sepsis both as a reaction to the platelet consumption seen in Gram-negative sepsis, and also as a response to collection/abscess formation. A combination of relentlessly rising C-reactive protein (CRP), rising platelet count and swinging pyrexia almost invariably indicates a collection above or below the diaphragm.

Biochemistry

- Hyponatraemia is supposedly pathognomonic of Legionella infection, but in practice it can be seen in any severe pneumonia.
- Liver function tests are deranged in sepsis, and particularly so in streptococcal and staphylococcal sepsis. Some antibiotics are particularly hepatotoxic in high dosage (rifampicin and flucloxacillin). Intravenous fusidic acid should never be used.
- Renal failure often occurs in severe sepsis. Renal replacement therapy necessitates dosage adjustment of antimicrobials, particularly penicillins, and co-trimoxazole.
- High serum creatine kinase (CK) indicates myositis or myonecrosis, as well as the effects of circulating toxins or ischaemia.
- Hypocalcaemia due to calcium precipitation with fat necrosis is common in necrotizing fasciitis. Hypoalbuminaemia and hyponatraemia are common. Severe metabolic acidosis is the norm in streptococcal necrotizing fasciitis, and in this condition a high serum lactate combined with low sodium levels is predictive of mortality.

C-reactive protein

- CRP is one of many 'acute phase proteins' synthesized in the liver in response to inflammatory insults, usually bacterial infection.
- Other causes include surgery, venous thrombosis, and inflammatory or auto-immune disease.
- Levels of CRP correlate with the degree of inflammation; Crohn's disease, with transmural inflammation, will produce higher levels than relapses of ulcerative colitis with more superficial inflammation.
- CRP is rarely raised with malignancy, e.g. lymphomas.
- The CRP response to auto-immune disease rarely rises above 100mg/L. Levels above this should prompt investigation into the source of elevation.

- CRP is usually very high (300–400mg/L) with severe bacterial infection, and falls rapidly with effective treatment.
- Serial measurements over 48–72h are much more useful than a single level.
- In serious infections such as acute staphylococcal bacterial endocarditis, an initial response followed by a plateauing of the CRP at a high level may be the first indication of ring abscess.
- A high CRP combined with a high platelet count and a swinging pyrexia often indicates a collection somewhere.

Effects of corticosteroids on CRP

Although one would expect steroids to suppress CRP formation, there is in fact very little evidence to support this. Some blunting of CRP rises in those using inhaled steroids has been reported, and conversely anabolic steroids increase CRP. In practice, with the correct antimicrobial therapy, CRP will fall with or without steroids.

Other tests

Urinary antigens (Legionella and pneumococcal)

- Urine in a plain bottle (without preservative) should be sent.
- These tests are rapid (15–30min) and simple to perform.
- Negative results do not exclude the diagnosis. Commercial pneumococcal kits vary in performance, but most are around 50–80% sensitive and 90% specific.
- Tests remain positive up to 3 days into treatment.
- The Legionella antigen only detects limited serotypes, but remains positive for longer. Legionella serology takes weeks to become positive so antigen testing and specific culture techniques are preferred.

Polymerase chain reaction

- PCR tests for respiratory pathogens are really the domain of research establishments or regional reference laboratories rather than routine diagnostic laboratories.
- Local laboratories may refer specimens for PCR in certain circumstances, e.g. blood for aspergillus PCR in patients with suspected invasive aspergillosis.
- PCR is useful to detect the presence or absence of rifampicin resistance gene in cases where multiple drug resistant TB is suspected, and can confirm the species is M tuberculosis.

Experimental/less easily available tests

- Endotoxin detection in secretions or blood associated with Gram-negative infection is not commonly available.
- An exception is the exotoxin PVL test. Currently the gene is detected in isolates of staphylococci. However, kits have been developed to detect the PVL toxin in body fluids and sputum, using methodologies within the capabilities of routine diagnostic laboratories.

- A myriad of tests, including elastin fibre staining and antibody coating of bacteria, are, to date, not sensitive or specific enough for diagnosis.

Surveillance cultures

- Surveillance cultures of endotracheal aspirates may allow early identification of a causative organism of a subsequent VAP. Sensitivities would be expected to be available to guide therapy at an earlier stage.
- Tracheobronchial colonization, however, reflects a continually dynamic process, with complex interactions between colonizing flora.
- Tracheal colonization, even with organisms of low pathogenicity, poses a risk for downwards spread, but once established these organisms are likely to be difficult to treat and multiresistant. Hence, earlier detection of colonization with resistant organisms enables better antimicrobial stewardship and pre-emptive therapy where indicated.
- Colonization with meticillin-resistant *Staphylococcus aureus* (MRSA) increases the risk of VAP significantly. The positive predictive values are 62% for MRSA, 52% for *Pseudomonas aeruginosa*, and 24% for *Acinetobacter baumanii*.

Gram-positive organisms

Streptococcus pneumoniae (pneumococcus)

- This is one of the most common causes of pneumonia in fit healthy young people.
- It commonly colonizes the oro-pharynx; pulmonary infection can be due to aspiration or haematogenous spread.
- Isolation of *S. pneumoniae* in blood is now an indication for HIV testing (British Association of Sexual Heath and HIV guidelines).
- Vaccination protects the elderly, asplenic, and those with severe chronic disease from up to 23 serotypes, but not all strains of pneumococci.
- Pneumococcal pneumonia has a tendency to cause empyemas.
- Penicllin resistance is increasing and should be suspected in anyone recently returned from abroad, especially transfers from foreign intensive care units.
- Cephalosporins and vancomycin remain the recommended therapies. Some authorities prefer to change to penicillin once sensitivity is confirmed.

Staphylococcus aureus

- *S. aureus* is responsible for 2–5% of community acquired pneumonia.
- Historically it presents with dyspnoea out of proportion to the clinical findings of pneumonia, and dusky cyanosis of nail beds and lips.
- Staphylococcal pneumonia may present with classical lobar pneumonia, pneumatoceles, empyema, or septic emboli.
- When multilobar lung infiltrates are present, together with skin and soft tissue infection or osteomyelitis, staphylococcal infection is likely.

- Pleural effusions are common, especially in children.
- Nowadays primary staphylococcal pneumonias are rare, except in intravenous drug users or infections associated with PVL (see below).
- Secondary bacterial pneumonia with *S. aureus* is more frequent. Seen most commonly in two forms, post viral and hematogenous.

Post viral

Staphylococcal pneumonia is particularly common after influenza. Viral destruction of the cilia exposes raw collagen, to which staphylococci stick preferentially, allowing ingress into the lower airways.

Hematogenous

Blood-borne spread into the lungs is inevitable with tricuspid valve endocarditis in intravenous drug users. It is also particularly prevalent in patients with deep skin and soft tissue infections due to PVL producing *S. aureus*, and children with PVL *S. aureus* osteomyelitis.

Panton Valentine leukocidin staphylococcal infection

- Some 4% of staphylococci, whether MRSA or meticillin (flucloxacillin) sensitive, may produce PVL, a pore-forming toxin that kills leucocytes.
- Most patients suffer recurrent boils and abscesses, but some (especially younger adults and children) develop osteomyelitis with a high proportion of thromboses and necrotizing pneumonia.
- PVL-staphylococcal necrotizing pneumonia may rapidly progress to acute respiratory failure, and carries a high mortality (62–75%).
- Hypotension and haemoptysis make PVL more pneumonia likely.

The typical story is that of a previously fit, young patient, with a recent flu-like illness, now presenting with respiratory failure and haemoptysis. They are pyrexial (>39°C), tachycardic (>140bpm), tachypnoeic (respiratory rate >30/min), and hypotensive with a marked leucopoenia (due to PVL toxin), and very high CRP (~400g/L). Multilobular alveolar infiltrates are usual, and frequently cavitate. Pleural effusions are common.

An initially non-productive cough, low leucocyte count (due to toxins), and a normal CXR may falsely reassure the clinician. Hours later, as necrosis and consumption of platelets and neutrophils escalates, leukopenia occurs with septic shock.

There is much debate about the therapy of staphylococcal pneumonia, but with poor extracellular fluid concentrations and a mainly bacteriostatic mechanism of action, glycopeptides are not good choices for therapy. When sensitive, flucloxacillin is superior at killing staphylococci but has been shown to increase PVL toxin production, and should therefore not be used. In serious staphylococcal infections there are theoretical advantages of using exotoxin blocking agents such as clindamycin or linezolid. The former can be used in very high doses even with minimal renal function. Intravenous immunoglobulin 2g/kg has been recommended for neutralization of already formed toxin in the necrotic lung tissues.

Gram-negative organisms

These are responsible for 5–16% of pneumonia, and may be due to coliform bacteria such as *E. coli*, *Proteus*, *Klebsiellae* or *Pseudomonas aeruginosa*.

Gram-negative pneumonia is usually associated with bedridden elderly adults, hospital-acquired pneumonia, anaesthesia, or intubation.

Haemophilus influenzae

- This is a slim Gram-negative bacillus or cocco-bacillus.
- *H. influenzae* is most commonly found colonizing the airways of patients with chronic obstructive airways disease.
- Haemophilus infection is usually more insidious than pneumococcal or staphylococcal infection.
- In asplenic patients, both *H. influenzae* and *S. pneumoniae* can cause purpura fulminans similar to meningococcal septicaemia.
- Increasingly resistant to amoxicillin and occasionally to co-amoxiclav and tetracyclines, there are few options apart from macrolides and quinolones.
- Erythromycin minimum inhibitory concentration (MIC) for haemophilus cannot be achieved in the lungs *in vivo*, so it is completely ineffective even if the organism appears sensitive on a culture plate. Better penetration and intracellular concentration are achieved with azithromycin or clarithromycin.
- Vaccination against *H. influenzae* capsular type b has led to the relative increase of other capsular and non-typeable haemophili.

Legionella

- Legionella are environmental water-associated bacteria. They are small, fastidious, Gram-negative bacilli which grow best at 35°C.
- Nutritionally demanding, legionellae need enriched media containing L-cysteine for optimal culture.
- >50 species described, 20 of which infect humans.
- *L. pneumophila* is responsible for >90% of pneumonias due to Legionella. It has nearly 20 serogroups, not all of which are detectable with the urinary antigen test.
- Treatment is best with intracellular penetrating antimicrobials such as azithromycin, rifampicin, and quinolones.

Pseudomonas aeruginosa

- Typically a colonizer of watery habitats, pseudomonas is especially associated with bronchiectasis and cystic fibrosis.
- Extracellular proteases cause immense tissue destruction. It may be reduced by azithromycin therapy, which stops protease production but does not affect the pseudomonas itself.
- Generally, pseudomonas are among the more resistant of organisms— typically only ceftazidime, piperacillin-tazobactam, aminoglycosides, and the quinolones would cover pseudomonas. Resistance rapidly develops on therapy.

- Pseudomonas naturally produce pseudomonic acid (mupirocin), which is active against MRSA.

Acinetobacter

- Literally 'non-motile' or akinetic, this environmental Gram-negative cocco-bacillus is very uninteresting microbiologically and practically inert in most biochemical identification tests, but a nightmare for infection control.
- *A. baumanii* is inherently multiresistant, often necessitating therapy with toxic agents such as colistin. Some strains are resistant to all antibiotics.
- It is responsible for many outbreaks of invasive infection in intensive care units world wide, typically following construction work (Acinetobacter are easily transported in dust and room ventilation systems).

Fungi

Candida

- Candida is a common colonizer of the upper airways during ventilation and may cause superinfection, especially in the presence of escalating antibiotic therapy.
- Primary candida pneumonia is very rare. The most common cause of candidal empyema is anastomotic breakdown following oesophageal surgery.
- Candida are very large Gram-positive cocci. In the laboratory, a quick test for identification of likely *C. albicans* involves the proclivity for yeasts to produce 'germ tubes' in serum.
- *C. albicans* are almost always sensitive to fluconazole. 'Germ tube negative' Candida spp need further identification to ensure sensitivity to antifungal therapy.

Pneumocystis jiroveci pneumonia (pneumocystis pneumonia)

- Reclassified as a fungus, PJP still affects primarily immunosupressed patients and is a defining diagnosis for AIDS.
- Prophylactic co-trimoxazole has prevented many infections in transplant patients and neutropaenics.
- Diagnosis is mainly clinical, with extreme shortness of breath at rest.
- There is usually a ground glass appearance on CXR, although lobar presentations have been seen.
- Confirmation of diagnosis usually involves BAL and immunofluorescent antibody staining. Other tests (see above) may be used at specialist centres.

Viruses

- Almost any viral agent can cause pneumonia. The most common is influenza, although respiratory syncytial virus (RSV) and adenovirus can be responsible for pneumonia in children or the immunosupressed.
- Diagnosis usually involves PCR of secretions or a throat swab, and is usually a reference laboratory test.

- Viral cultures are expensive and cumbersome so now are rarely performed.
- Viral-induced death of the respiratory lining epithelium predisposes to *S. aureus* and especially PVL pneumonia ('secondary' pneumonia).

Mycobacteria

- Mycobacterial infections usually present in an indolent fashion with malaise, sweats, chronic cough, and constitutional symptoms, although in patients with chronic respiratory disease the symptomatology of the atypical infections may be obscured by the underlying disease process.
- CXR in *M. tuberculosis* often shows focal infiltrates, cavitation (especially in upper lobes), and hilar lymphadenopathy.
- In cases of confirmed TB, antimicrobial therapy has tended to remain the remit of respiratory physicians.
- The local health protection unit/public health department need to be notified so efforts to trace contacts are co-ordinated.
- Aggressive infection-control protocols are usually instituted, with staff wearing special 'fit tested masks' for invasive cough-inducing procedures such as suctioning.
- Respiratory isolation is essential, usually with a negative pressure room. It is mandatory for suspected multidrug resistant TB, pending PCR testing for rifampicin resistance.

Staining

- With a thick mycolic acid wall, mycobacteria are not Gram stainable and so are typically stained with Ziehl–Neelsen (red organisms against a blue background) or auramine phenol (yellow fluorescence).
- Atypical organisms (e.g. *M. fortuitum, xenopii*) may look more beaded or longer than conventional TB, but identification depends on isolation and biochemical testing, which may take weeks for the slow-growing mycobacteria.

Culture

- Liquid culture medium is not available at all laboratories.
- Specimens have to be sent in special bottles to reference laboratories for culture.
- Isolates are usually sent to reference laboratories for identification and sensitivity testing.
- Usually atypical mycobacteria are quicker growing (weeks rather than months).

Quantiferon-TB gold

- This has replaced the Mantoux test and is used to assist in diagnosis of TB infection, including latent disease.
- Whole blood is mixed in a special tube with antigens and controls and sent to a reference laboratory.
- Blood must be processed within 12h of collection.
- After incubation the level of interferon gamma is measured (released by white blood cells in response to contact with TB antigens).

- Results can be available within 24h. They are unaffected by prior bacillus Calmette–Guérin (BCG).
- Quantiferon assay may be prone to error. In addition, there are limited data for interpretation of results in HIV infection, in haematological malignancies in patients with chronic renal failure, and in children.

Antibiotic therapy

Antibiotic prescription should be made with knowledge of the local microbiological environment as well as the likely underlying diagnosis. Some general guidelines are presented in Figs 1.5, 1.6, 1.7, 1.8, and 1.9.

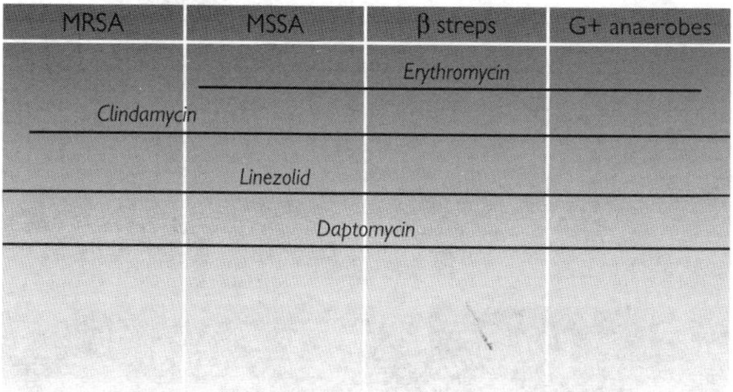

MRSA	MSSA	β streps	G+ anaerobes
		Erythromycin	
Clindamycin			
	Linezolid		
	Daptomycin		

Fig. 1.5 Exotoxin disease. MSSA, meticillin-sensitive *S. aureus*; β streps, β haemolytic streptococci; G+ anaerobes, Gram-positive anaerobes. © Marina Morgan 2009.

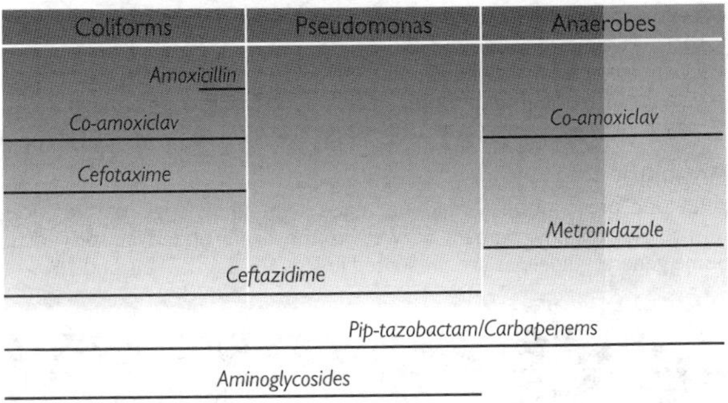

Fig. 1.6 Gram-negative sepsis. © Marina Morgan 2009.

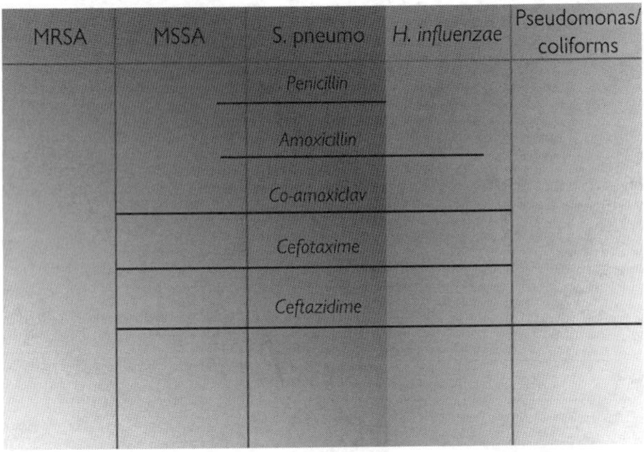

Fig. 1.7 Respiratory tract infections. © Marina Morgan 2009.

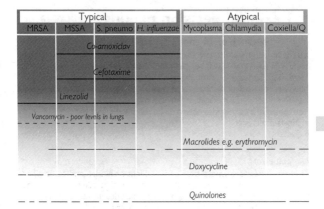

Typical				Atypical		
MRSA	MSSA	S. pneumo	H. influenzae	Mycoplasma	Chlamydia	Coxiella/Q

Co-amoxiclav

Cefotaxime

Linezolid

Vancomycin – poor levels in lungs

Macrolides e.g. erythromycin

Doxycycline

Quinolones

Fig. 1.8 Respiratory tract infections. © Marina Morgan 2009.

MRSA	MSSA	β streps	Anaerobes	GNB	
				Coliforms	Pseudomonas

Penicillin

Co-amoxiclav

Cefotaxime

Metronidazole

Carbapenems

Macrolides

Lincosamides (clindamycin)

Linezolid

Fig. 1.9 Skin and soft tissue infections. © Marina Morgan 2009.

1.4 Clinical decision making

The importance of diagnosis

This chapter is a short introduction to a vital, fascinating, and expanding branch of medicine. It will hopefully stimulate the interest of the reader to learn more about one of the most important aspects of being a clinician—how we make diagnoses. Failure to make a correct diagnosis is the second biggest cause (after medication errors) of preventable error in medicine. The causes of incorrect diagnosis may be subdivided into:

- No-fault errors
- System errors
- Cognitive errors.

No-fault errors

These include cases where the illness is silent or hidden and cases where the illness presents in such an atypical fashion that diagnosis could not have been expected. This category also includes instances where the history given by the patient is misleading or inaccurate.

These instances will probably reduce with time as medical knowledge and technology improve.

System errors

System errors are well documented and include:

- Fatigue
- Inadequate staffing
- Failure of senior input
- Poor working conditions
- Lack of diagnostic facilities
- Poor information technology and reference facilities
- Deficient lines of communication
- Context.

System error reduction has been the subject of much debate. Morbidity and mortality meetings, root cause analyses, clinical incident reporting systems, and an emphasis on clinical governance are part of the medical community's response.

Addressing system errors is not straightforward. Initial improvements often degrade over time and new sources of error may be inadvertently introduced with any fix. For example, a reduction in working hours means less continuity of care and results in less experiential learning.

Cognitive errors

It is important to understand how we think when making decisions, and to understand those factors which influence decision making. We might then be able to work out why things go wrong and employ strategies to improve clinical decision making (CDM). A system that explains how and why we make decisions, and why we get them wrong, will help clinicians improve their thinking processes and diagnostic skills.

Croskerry[1] has developed a Universal Theory of clinical decision making that incorporates the available psychological theory as well as other factors that affect decision making. This Universal Theory includes system 1 and system 2 processes.

System 1 processes
System 1 is a vital component of problem solving and uses mental short-cuts (heuristics). It is rapid, intuitive, context sensitive, and depends on pattern recognition. It allows experts to come to quick and often correct conclusions with a minimum of effort, usually when time is short and information is incomplete. It 'plays the odds'.

However, there may be conscious or subconscious influences magnifying potential sources of error, for example patient characteristics, illness characteristics, clinical workload, distractions, interruptions, and resource issues. This system is hardwired and will therefore also be used by inexperienced clinicians. These clinicians have a greater potential for error as they do not have the experience and wisdom to calibrate rapid decision making.

System 2 processes
System 2 reasoning is analytical and systematic. It takes more time and requires more effort. It permits abstract reasoning and hypothetical thinking, and is less likely to be erroneous. With experience, system 2 processes may devolve to system 1 processes, although during clinical encounters the clinician usually toggles between one and the other, calibrating and checking as more information becomes available.

System 1 reasoning is more prone to error than system 2 reasoning.

If the presentation is classical and clear, system 1 heuristics will allow a diagnosis to be made rapidly. If it is unrecognized or complex, or has atypical features, system 2 needs to be engaged. One danger is the application of system 1 to this latter situation. It is also possible that habit, training, and/or personality favour the use of either system 1 or system 2 processes by an individual clinician. Encouraging awareness of this personal tendency may allow the development of critical thinking and improved diagnostic skills.

Cognitive failure
Cognitive failures account for a significant proportion of diagnostic errors. A full discussion is beyond the scope of this chapter but it is important that doctors are aware of the ways their predispositions to a variety of flawed methods of reasoning may contribute to missed diagnoses.[2]
Examples include:
- Anchoring—focusing on some important features of the initial presentation, and failing to modify this impression in the face of subsequent contradictory information.

- Confirmation bias—accepting confirmatory evidence for the initial diagnosis and ignoring or rejecting evidence refuting the diagnosis, even when the latter is more persuasive.
- Premature closure—'when the diagnosis is made, the thinking stops'. Accepting a diagnosis before it has been fully verified. More information is needed.
- Search satisfying—calling off the search once something has been found. Co-morbidities and other pathologies may be missed. The information is there, but ignored. May exacerbate anchoring and confirmation bias.
- Gambler's error—the four previous patients with chest pain have had acute coronary syndrome, so the fifth can't also be acute coronary syndrome.
- Posterior probability error—confusion and agitation have been caused by alcohol withdrawal on the last four admissions, so this time it is also alcohol withdrawal and not, for example, hypoxia.
- Availability—the more recently a diagnosis has been seen, the more likely the physician is to make the diagnosis again. The patient with hypertension, cold peripheries, and pulmonary oedema is more likely to have serum catecholamine levels checked when the physician has seen a phaeochromocytoma present in this fashion.
- Sutton's slip—when bank robber Willie Sutton was asked by a judge why he robbed banks, he said, 'Because that's where the money is.' Sutton's law is going for the obvious; Sutton's slip is when other possibilities are given inadequate consideration.
- Sunk costs—the more that is invested in a diagnosis (time, thought, and personal reputation), the less likely the clinician is to consider another diagnosis.
- Investment bias—attaching more importance to information that we actively request or seek out than to information that was already available.

There are at least 30 of these cognitive errors and biases, and most diagnosticians have made most of the errors at some time.

There has been a general reluctance to address cognitive errors, possibly because of a belief that these errors are simply part of the human condition—we are programmed to think in these ways and there is nothing we can do about it. Part of the issue may be that these errors go unrecognized. In order to address these errors, we have to accept that they exist, look for them, and develop a reflective approach to diagnosis and clinical decision making, including metacognition—thinking about how we think.

Reducing cognitive errors
There are strategies available to reduce cognitive errors:[3]
- Teach doctors about cognitive errors, and make reflection on our reasoning skills and deficiencies (metacognition) routine. We should strive to be actively open minded.
- Reduce reliance on memory with cognitive aids (mnemonics, computer-aided diagnosis). Make important information available in a

clear and understandable format (e.g. automatically highlight abnormal results, present results in daily flow charts).
• Be familiar with proper data interpretation: what is the pretest probability and how does the investigation I am using alter the post test odds?

In ICU we need to constantly question ourselves:
• What else could it be—what is the differential diagnosis? Hypothesis generation is one of the earliest stages of diagnosis, and system 1 reasoning is often used to produce this first judgment. Central chest pain and cardiovascular instability are more likely to be caused by a myocardial infarction, but unless aortic dissection is contemplated, it is likely to be missed on those few occasions it presents. Differential diagnoses should be routinely considered (and listed) so that other less common or atypically presenting diseases processes are picked up.
• What new information (history, examination, and investigation) is there and does it fit with the current diagnosis?
• Is there more than one diagnosis? A unifying diagnosis is what doctors usually search for and it is more likely on average than multiple explanations. Occasionally, there will be more than one source for the problem.
• Is the information we have correct and have I personally checked it? Was it actually haemoptysis? What sort of pain was it? What was the time course of the interweaving events? What did the X-ray and ECG really show? Examine the raw evidence for the diagnosis.
• Have I taken into account the potential biases of the clinician reporting information to me? It is sometimes difficult to challenge the established thinking of a colleague, but it is necessary if previous errors are not to be amplified. Diagnoses once made gain a momentum of their own as the patient moves through the system: they become stickier. Stop, examine the evidence, and ask 'Does this all fit together?'
• Am I using predominantly system 1 (heuristic, intuitive) or system 2 (systematic, analytical) processes and is this method best for this diagnostic problem?
• Am I bored or depressed or annoyed by this patient and is that stopping me reassessing all the information?
• Are the direction and rate of progress as expected? If the patient is not improving on specific treatment reconsider the evidence.
  • Is the diagnosis correct but advanced or aggressive disease is preventing improvement?
  • Is the diagnosis incomplete?
  • Is it one of several diagnoses?
  • Is it wrong?
  • Has a complication or a new diagnosis arisen?

Final thought

Decision making pervades all of clinical activity. In intensive care we make multiple decisions every day. Many of these decisions involve the institution of supportive measures such as ventilation or, in an improving patient, the weaning of that support. However, the perfect application of multiple organ support is for naught if the underlying clinical condition(s) have not been diagnosed and if definitive treatment (as opposed to support) has not been instituted. We must constantly ask, 'Is this the correct diagnosis?'

1 Croskerry P (2009) A Universal Model of Diagnostic Reasoning. *Acad Med* **84**(8), 1022–8.
2 Croskerry P (2003) The Importance of Cognitive Errors in Diagnosis and Strategies to Minimize Them. *Acad Med* **78**, 775–80.
3 Graber M, Gordon R, and Franklin N (2002) Reducing Diagnostic Errors in Medicine: What's the Goal? *Acad Med* **77**, 981–92.

1.5 Indications for ventilatory support

Deciding when and whether to provide ventilatory support can be difficult. Careful assessment of each patient is essential and should involve consideration of pre-existing co-morbidities as well as the nature of the primary illness. The mode of support offered (CPAP, non-invasive ventilation (NIV) or intermittent positive airway pressure (IPPV)) must be appropriate and the following factors should be considered:
- Type of pathology and usual disease course
- Reversibility of pathology
- Appropriateness of non-invasive support
- Patients' wishes and previous treatment limitations.

Other considerations
- When the underlying diagnosis is unclear, respiratory support may be offered in order to 'buy time' whilst a diagnosis is made, and may facilitate investigations such as broncho-alveolar lavage or open lung biopsy.
- In chronic progressive pulmonary disease (e.g. pulmonary fibrosis, COPD), respiratory support may be appropriate whilst clarification between simple disease progression and an acute reversible deterioration (e.g. infection) is made.
- In patients with acute respiratory failure (e.g. pneumonia, ARDS) as opposed to acute-on chronic respiratory failure or cardiogenic pulmonary oedema, delaying invasive ventilation with a trial of NIV worsens outcome.
- If invasive ventilation is not appropriate, NIV can still be considered:
  - NIV reduces mortality in patients with COPD, and should be considered for all of those patients in whom a respiratory acidosis persists after an hour of standard medical therapy.
  - CPAP in acute cardiogenic pulmonary oedema has been shown to improve mortality, and improves dyspnoea scores and patient comfort. It should be considered as an adjunct to standard medical care.
- Prognostication in individual cases is extremely difficult, and there is evidence that clinicians are poor at predicting which patients will survive or wean successfully from the ventilator. However, being ventilated and treated in ICU is unpleasant for many patients. The SUPPORT trials demonstrated a range of disagreeable emotions and symptoms suffered by ICU patients.[1] Before placing this considerable burden on a patient, there should be a reasonable chance of benefit to that patient.

Indications
Patients are intubated for one of the following reasons:
- Hypoxaemia
- Hypercapnia
- Exhaustion

- To reduce oxygen consumption
- To protect airway
- To treat or prevent an obstructed airway
- To facilitate investigations
- To facilitate treatment of other conditions
- For transfer.

Hypoxaemia

Isolated hypoxaemia is a relatively infrequent indication for mechanical ventilation. More usually it is associated with hypercapnia or exhaustion and it is the combination, or speed of the deterioration, that dictates intubation. Isolated hypoxaemia may be relatively well tolerated, especially when associated with a normal or increased cardiac output. However, isolated hypoxaemia in critically ill patients will often lead to a fall in cardiac output and a dramatic deterioration in oxygen delivery.

Before intubation, consider an oxygen delivery device that will provide a high FiO_2.

Consider the underlying reason for respiratory failure and the likely response to positive pressure ventilation. Hypoxaemia due to shunts caused by unilateral lobar consolidation is not easily corrected by positive pressure. Indeed, blood may be diverted from the relatively compliant normal lung to the non-compliant consolidated lung, and there is often a period of profound and long-lasting hypoxaemia post intubation.

If the hypoxaemia is due to diffuse disease, improvement in gas exchange is more likely. Cardiogenic or early non-cardiogenic pulmonary oedema is likely to respond well to positive pressure ventilation. Patients with interstitial lung disease who require intubation have a poor prognosis and only those with a reversible component to the disease should have mechanical ventilation instituted.

Hypercapnia

Hypercapnia is discussed in detail in 📖 Hypercapnia while on a ventilator, p 296.

The physiological effects of hypercapnia, in particular neurological deterioration, are more important than precise figures for $PaCO_2$. However, at levels above 12kPa, unless the disease is quickly correctable (e.g. opiate overdose), NIV will not succeed and the patient should be intubated.

If hypercapnia is due to muscle fatigue and exhaustion (see below), then the reduction in oxygen consumption by removing the WOB may also be beneficial.

Exhaustion

This is probably the most common indication for mechanical ventilation. An experienced clinician will often know almost immediately that a patient requires intervention. Clues that the patient will not survive without intervention are:

- Confusion and somnolence
- Sweating

- Very high respiratory rate, use of accessory muscles, tracheal tug
- Very low respiratory rate
- Unable to complete sentences
- Marked sinus tachycardia, especially if associated with hypertension
- Hypotension.

Reducing oxygen consumption

The WOB may account for up to 30% of oxygen consumption in respiratory failure. If there is evidence of oxygen supply demand imbalance (acidosis and low SvO_2) and respiratory work is high, removal of, or reduction in, the WOB will reduce oxygen consumption and may improve oxygen delivery to other organ systems.

Airway protection

Critical care physicians are commonly asked to assess patients for intubation and ventilation in the case of a threatened airway associated with a decreased level of consciousness. Patients with a Glasgow Coma Score (GCS) <8 are at risk of airway obstruction attributable to the tongue falling back against the posterior pharyngeal wall, as well as obstruction by the soft palate and epiglottis due to a reduction in local muscular activity. Patients with impaired laryngeal reflexes are also at risk from aspiration of stomach contents, blood, or saliva. Assessment of patients with a decreased level of consciousness therefore requires assessment of airway patency and protection. An effective gag and cough indicates that laryngeal reflexes are likely to be adequate. Gag reflex is absent in a significant percentage of the normal population, and its absence is therefore difficult to interpret. If there is doubt about whether a patient is protecting their airway, it is usually better to proceed to intubation unless the risks of such a procedure are significant (for example difficult airway or co morbid respiratory disease).

Consider the cause of the reduced GCS and its likely time course. For example, a patient with a reduced GCS post-ictally or due to alcohol intoxication may be managed in a high-dependency area with the patient in the recovery position, as the time course is likely to be short, whereas a patient with a GCS 8 secondary to a head injury is better managed in a critical care environment with intubation and ventilation to prevent secondary brain injury.

Airway obstruction

Airway obstruction may present as an emergency requiring immediate intervention. It frequently presents in a more insidious fashion, with stridor, increased WOB, and agitation or somnolence. There may be more subtle signs, for example hoarse voice or difficulty swallowing. In patients with an ominous history (for example burns, neck trauma) a high index of suspicion is advisable and the airway should be secured (with awake fibreoptic intubation if necessary) at an early stage.

To facilitate investigations

A number of patients present to critical care with respiratory failure in whom the underlying diagnosis is unclear, but who are too unwell to tolerate investigation without respiratory support. Intubation and ventilation may be considered for these people to facilitate making a definitive diagnosis, for example radiological imaging or performing a bronchoscopy, BAL, or open-lung biopsy.

To assist in the treatment of other conditions

Controlled ventilation may be necessary to facilitate the treatment of other, non-respiratory conditions. Examples include therapeutic hypothermia post cardiac arrest and in preventing secondary brain injury in neurological intensive care. A common reason for ventilating patients post operatively who have undergone elective major surgery is to allow warming to normothermia, correction of peri-operative metabolic disturbance and fluid shifts, and ensure good analgesia and smooth emergence prior to extubation.

For transfer

In the UK, up to 10,000 critically ill patients are transported between hospitals for specialist care, repatriation, or due to a lack of local ICU resources. It is well established that patients should be stabilized prior to transfer to avoid potential difficulties *en route* in the event of a clinical deterioration, and intubation and ventilation are often considered part of this stabilization. While this is true in many situations, intubation inevitably delays transfer, and the sedation and paralysis necessary to allow ventilation removes the ability to assess neurological function and detect neurological deterioration. Therefore, the risks and benefits of intubation prior to transfer should be considered carefully in each individual case. Bear in mind the reason for transfer and clinical status, logistics of transfer (geography and length of journey, mode (air versus road), and accessibility of patient in transport vehicle), and skill of the transfer personnel.

1 SUPPORT Principal Investigators (1995) A controlled trial to improve care for seriously ill hospitalized patients: a study to understand prognosis and preferences for outcomes and risks of treatments. *JAMA* **274**, 1591–8. [Published correction appears in *JAMA* 1996, **275**, 1232.]

Non-invasive treatment modalities

2.1 Oxygen therapy

Joseph Priestley is credited with the first published description of oxygen. In 1774 he discovered that heating mercuric oxide released a gas which was 'five or six times better than common air for the purpose of respiration and inflammation', describing the gas as 'dephlogisticated[a] air'. It was renamed oxygen by Antoine Lavoisier in 1775 from the Greek word meaning 'acid former'. Although Priestly was credited with the discovery, a Swedish chemist, Carl Wilhelm Scheele, had independently made a similar discovery in 1772, but did not publish his findings until 1777. One hundred and seventy years before that, a Polish philosopher, Michał Sędziwój, discovered that heating saltpeter released a gas which he described as 'the elixir of life'. He was distracted from this discovery by his search for the philosopher's stone.

Oxygen (O_2) is the most commonly administered drug in hospital. It is widely used to help prevent tissue hypoxia and forms the cornerstone of resuscitation in the patient with respiratory distress. The administration of oxygen is often (wrongly) perceived as being a risk-free intervention, and it is incorrectly thought that it is not possible to give too much. In other circumstances (e.g. COPD) the administration of oxygen is thought to be detrimental to all, and patients are denied appropriate treatment.

This chapter will discuss when oxygen is indicated and when it is not, the side effects of administration and the mode of oxygen delivery.

Indications for oxygen therapy

Oxygen delivery to tissues is described by the equation

$$DO_2 = CO \text{ (L/min)} \times 10 \, [(Hb \times 1.34 \times SaO_2 \times 0.01) + (0.023 \times PaO_2)]$$

The characters within square brackets represent the oxygen content, which has been traditionally been expressed per 100mL of blood. In this equation Hb is measured in g/100mL. The equation does not take into account regional differences in perfusion. Nevertheless the major determinants of oxygen delivery are cardiac output, haemoglobin concentration, and oxygen saturation.

Administration of supplemental oxygen therefore achieves maximum benefit in conditions where there is arterial hypoxaemia and haemoglobin desaturation.

Conditions leading to arterial hypoxaemia

- Ventilation/perfusion ($\dot{V}/\dot{Q}$) mismatch. As the shunt fraction increases, supplemental O_2 becomes less effective. Examples include:
  - Pneumonia
  - Atelectasis
  - Asthma (small airway occlusion)
  - Pulmonary oedema.
- Gas diffusion abnormalities.

---

[a] Fire was postulated to be the visible escape of 'phlogiston' from a substance. Some gases encouraged combustion, so it was hypothesized that these gases were deficient in phlogiston (thereby encouraging the flame). One particular gas encouraged combustion to such an extent that it was assumed it had no phlogiston, or had been 'dephlogisticated'.

- Alveolar hypoventilation. Hypoxaemia caused by alveolar hypoventilation is easily corrected by low concentrations of additional oxygen.
  - Opiate overdose.
  - Neuromuscular disorders, e.g. motor neurone disease.

Conditions leading to normoxaemic hypoxia

The administration of supplemental oxygen may be useful in some conditions where there is no arterial hypoxaemia. Increasing the dissolved oxygen content of the blood may be critical in certain circumstances.

- Acute anaemia. It should be used only to temporize until appropriate red cell transfusion.
- Carbon monoxide (CO) poisoning. CO binds to haemoglobin with 200–250 times the affinity of O_2, rendering it unavailable for oxygen carriage. Morbidity and mortality correlate with the exposure COHb level. High inspired O_2 therapy decreases the half-life of carboxyhaemoglobin from 320min to 80min in healthy volunteers. In addition it increases the dissolved O_2 content of the blood. The use of hyperbaric oxygen therapy has been described where there is cardiovascular or neurological compromise, but there is no trial evidence to support its use.
- Cyanide poisoning inactivates mitochondrial cytochrome c oxidase in the electron transport chain and uncouples oxidative phosphorylation. Tissues and organs highly dependent on aerobic metabolism are very susceptible, e.g. the brain. Symptoms and signs include general weakness, confusion, arrhythmias, hypotension, apnoea, acidosis, and coma. Treatment includes sodium nitrite (to release the cytochrome oxidase enzyme) and sodium thiosulphate (which converts cyanide to the renally excreted thiocyanate). There is no logical reason why supplemental oxygen therapy should help, but anecdotal reports of clinical improvement with high-flow O_2 have led to oxygen being recommended in cyanide toxicity.

Oxygen toxicity

Absorption atelectasis

In normal subjects breathing 100% O_2, pulmonary shunts of up to 10% have been demonstrated after 10min. Other studies have demonstrated atelectasis radiologically under similar conditions. This atelectasis happens in alveolar units with a low $\dot{V}/\dot{Q}$ ratio, where the rate of absorption is greater than the rate of fresh gas replenishment. It is affected by breathing pattern (many studies did not allow patients to yawn, sigh, or breathe deeply), the duration of O_2 therapy, and the stability of the lung units (which may be affected by the toxic effects of high oxygen concentrations on type II pneumocytes).

Acute tracheobronchitis

Normal subjects breathing high (>90%) inspired oxygen concentrations complain of cough, retrosternal discomfort, inspiratory pain, and sore throat. The symptoms start in as little as 4h and ease with discontinuation of therapy, although full resolution may take days. The symptoms correspond to bronchoscopic findings of redness, oedema, and mucosal injection. These effects have not been demonstrated consistently.

Pulmonary oxygen toxicity
Prolonged administration (days to weeks) of 100% oxygen results in inflammatory changes in the lungs of experimental animals. The response to oxygen is species specific and humans appear to be less sensitive. The pathological findings (described as diffuse alveolar damage) are non-specific and are similar to those seen in any cause of pulmonary inflammation. The initial changes are exudative (vascular endothelial damage, alveolar epithelial cell destruction, oedema, fibrin deposition) followed by a proliferative phase after 1 week. These changes are often seen in patient post-mortem specimens, but due to their non-specific nature it is difficult to differentiate the contributions of the initial pathology from those potentially related to O_2 therapy.

Other effects
- Cardiovascular—hyperoxia causes ↓ heart rate (HR), ↑ systemic vascular resistance (SVR) and ↓ cardiac index (CI). The effects do not reverse immediately on restoring normoxia.
- Control of breathing—hyperoxia causes initial hypoventilation followed by a relative hyperventilation in normal subjects.
- CNS—hyperbaric oxygen toxicity can manifest as anxiety, visual and auditory disturbances, dizziness, twitching, seizures, and coma.

Mechanism
Oxygen toxicity is due to the excess formation of oxygen free radicals (e.g. O_2^-, H_2O_2, OH). These reactive oxygen species (ROS) are formed at a basal rate in the process of normal cellular metabolism and their damage is limited by antioxidant defenses such as glutathione, superoxide dismutase, and catalase. Under conditions of oxidant stress, such as inflammation or hyperoxia, the capacity of these defences is overwhelmed and the ROS accumulate. The ROS pull electrons from any available source, resulting in lipid peroxidation, enzyme inhibition, and DNA damage, leading to necrotic and apoptotic cell death.

FiO_2 should be kept to 0.5 or less if possible.
An exposure to FiO_2 >0.6 for >48h represents toxic exposure.

Detrimental clinical effects of oxygen therapy

Acute coronary syndrome
- Most patients with acute coronary syndromes are not hypoxaemic.
- Supplemental oxygen may increase infarct size and possibly increases mortality in uncomplicated myocardial infarction.

Congestive cardiac failure
- Supplemental oxygen impairs cardiac relaxation and increases left ventricular filling pressures.
- There is some evidence that hyperoxia should be avoided in normoxic patients with congestive cardiac failure.

Stroke
- Most stroke patients are not hypoxaemic.
- Supplemental oxygen may be harmful to non-hypoxaemic patients with mild to moderate strokes.

Pregnancy and obstetric emergencies
- Supplemental oxygen causes increased lipid peroxidation in the fetoplacental unit with caesarian section performed under regional anaesthesia.[1]
- There is little increase in umbilical oxygenation.

Bleomycin and paraquat poisining
- Bleomycin-injured lung tissue is less able to scavenge free oxygen radicals and may be further harmed by supplemental oxygen. This is also the case in paraquat poisoning.
- Avoid oxygen unless hypoxaemic.
- Aim for saturations of 88–92%.

Oxygen therapy in COPD
Many medical students are taught that patients with COPD have lost their chemoreceptor response to CO_2 and are dependent on their hypoxic drive to breathe.

This, it is explained, is why you should never give uncontrolled oxygen therapy to a patient with COPD. While this is true for a subset of COPD exacerbations, it is not applicable to all patients and is worth a more detailed discussion.

Mechanisms of hypercapnia in COPD
The causes of hypercapnia in patients with COPD are complex, multiple, and controversial. There are three main areas to consider.[2]

Magnitude of airflow obstruction
An FEV_1 of >1L tends not to be associated with significant hypercapnia. In patients with a very low FEV_1 there is wide variability in the degree of hypercapnia.

Inspiratory muscle function
Muscle weakness may be caused by increased lung volumes together with shortening and flattening of the diaphragm.

Individual ventilatory response to $PaCO_2$
Some individuals have a large ventilatory response to increasing $PaCO_2$, thus preserving their alveolar ventilation. Other individuals have a lower ventilatory response to increasing $PaCO_2$, tolerate higher values, hypoventilate, and develop a respiratory acidosis. The response to $PaCO_2$ levels is thought to be genetically determined.

Mechanisms of hypercapnia with oxygen administration in COPD
Some CO_2 retainers develop a life-threatening respiratory acidosis when oxygen is administered. Proposed mechanisms include the following:[3]

Depression of hypoxic respiratory drive
Ventilatory stimulus in individuals with a blunted ventilatory response to increasing $PaCO_2$ is generally attributed to hypoxic drive. Supplemental oxygen may attenuate this response with a subsequent decrease in minute ventilation.

The evidence for this is weak. Studies of COPD patients with acute respiratory failure have shown that the changes in $PaCO_2$ with supplemental oxygen do not correlate with changes in ventilation.

Ventilation-perfusion misdistribution
- Areas of local alveolar hypoxia result in hypoxic pulmonary vasoconstriction in breathing room air even in healthy patients.
- CO_2-rich blood is diverted to better ventilated regions of the lung.
- If local hypoxaemia is abolished with supplemental oxygen then hypoxic pulmonary vasoconstriction is abolished and poorly ventilated lung areas are perfused.
- Dead space increases and $PaCO_2$ rises.

Development of Haldane dead space
- Deoxygenated haemoglobin has a greater affinity for CO_2 than oxyhaemoglobin.
- Haldane effect enhances CO_2 excretion in health.
- Requires normal $\dot{V}/\dot{Q}$ ratios.
- Increased dead space will develop with supplemental oxygen (Haldane dead space).

Spotting individuals who may be at risk of severe hypercapnia
This is a subset of individuals who have advanced disease. There are no absolute rules but risk factors include:
- Hypercapnia on previous admissions
- Obesity
- Recurrent chest infections
- Periods of profound oxygen desaturations
- Clinical evidence of $\uparrow CO_2$ (vasodilation, warm peripheries, CO_2 flap, reduced conscious level)
- Signs of right heart failure, arrhythmias, hypertension
- Laboratory evidence of chronic respiratory disease ($\uparrow HCO_3$ levels, $\uparrow$haematocrit)
- Increased lung markings at lung bases on CXR.

It is important to identify these patients early. Hypercapnia decreases AO_2 (as described by the alveolar gas equation). Subsequently reducing the FiO_2 will cause a further drop in AO_2 and may precipitate life-threatening hypoxaemia.

The development of hypercapnia in patients at risk may not be accompanied by changes in the respiratory pattern or conscious level. The Standards of Care Committee of the British Thoracic Society have published a comprehensive set of guidelines[4] on the emergency use of oxygen in adults based on the best evidence available (see box).

It is important to distinguish chronically hypercapnic patients from patients who have acute type II respiratory failure. This second group is encountered in three main situations:
- Post operative: a mixture of hypoventilation from fatigue, opiates, diaphragmatic splinting, and pleural effusions, with $\dot{V}/\dot{Q}$ mismatch from infection, oedema, or atelectasis. O_2 therapy does not cause hypercapnia.
- Severe left ventricular failure (LVF) or ARDS. Profound $\dot{V}/\dot{Q}$ mismatch with increased dead space. O_2 therapy does not cause hypercapnia.

- Exhaustion following respiratory failure of any cause. O_2 therapy does not cause hypercapnia.

British Thoracic Society guidelines for the use of emergency oxygen

- Before blood gas results are available use a 28% Venturi mask at 4L/min and aim for a saturation of 88–92% for patients with risk factors for hypercapnia but no prior history of respiratory acidosis.
- Adjust target saturation to 94–98% if the $PaCO_2$ is normal (unless there is a history of previous NIV or IPPV) and recheck blood gases after 30–60min.
- If the $PaCO_2$ is raised, but the H^+ is lower than expected and associated with a raised bicarbonate, then the patient is likely to have longstanding hypercapnia. Maintain saturation at 88–92% and recheck blood gases at 30–60min, looking for hypercapnia or acidosis.
- If the patient is hypercapnic or acidotic consider NIV, especially if the patient has been acidotic for >30min despite appropriate therapy.

Patients with COPD and respiratory rate >30 should have the flow rate increased by 50% above the minimum flow rate specified for the Venturi mask (this increases the total gas flow from the mask but not the concentration of oxygen delivered).

Oxygen delivery devices

In the patient with respiratory failure the FiO_2 administered by the caregiver is often not that which reaches the distal airways or alveoli. Factors such as respiratory rate and pattern, expiratory pause, mask fit and position, and the presence or absence of a reservoir bag all have an influence on the final concentration of oxygen delivered to a patient's lungs. Of particular importance is the patient's peak inspiratory flow rate (PIFR). In health this is approximately 30L/min. In severe respiratory failure this can exceed 200L/min. When the PIFR exceeds the flow rate being administered from an oxygen delivery device, additional gas must be entrained. This additional gas will be air round the mask or may be oxygen from a reservoir bag, if present. The effective oxygen concentration is often diluted. In order to deliver a fixed or high concentration of oxygen, the delivery flow rate is as important as the set FiO_2.

Most oxygen flow meters are calibrated up to 15L/min, but in an emergency situation they can deliver up to 100L/min if the spindle valve is fully opened.

Fixed performance devices

High air flow oxygen enrichment (HAFOE) or Venturi masks deliver a constant FiO_2 using a combination of relatively high gas delivery rates and a fairly large mask reservoir. They use the Bernouille principle to entrain a fixed proportion of air. This entrainment ratio varies according to the mask and determines both the final oxygen concentration and gas delivery rates. The final flow rates are greater at low O_2 concentrations (Table 2.1). As the FiO_2 increases, the final gas delivery rate approaches PIFR and the performance may no longer be 'fixed'. This should be considered when interpreting blood gas results.

Table 2.1 Colour codes and FiO_2 delivered from Venturi-type masks

Valve colour	FiO_2	Flow meter setting (L/min)	Final gas delivery rate (L/min)
Blue	0.24	4	103
White	0.28	8	67
Yellow	0.35	10	56
Red	0.4	12	50
Green	0.6	15	30

Variable performance devices

Variable performance devices do not entrain additional gas in a calibrated fashion. As the maximum recommended flow rate is 15L/min, they are unlikely to match the patient's PIFR and are therefore particularly susceptible to the variability in final oxygen concentration described above.

They are useful where the final oxygen concentration is not critical. The variability in performance should be borne in mind when interpreting blood gas results.

High flow oxygen delivery
Devices with an oxygen reservoir

Often called trauma masks or non-rebreathing masks, these devices increase the final delivered oxygen concentration by incorporating a reservoir bag filled with oxygen. If the mask is tight fitting, entrainment of extra gas comes from the reservoir. FiO_2 concentrations of >0.8 have been described.

True non-rebreathing masks are fitted with both an inhalation valve and an exhalation valve so that all exhaled gas is vented to the atmosphere and inhaled gas comes only from a reservoir connected to the mask. Most 'non'-rebreathing masks are really partial rebreathing masks where intake of some exhaled and outside air is inevitable.

In a correctly fitting mask, the oxygen reservoir should be seen to collapse with inspiration.

Combination of devices

Devices can be combined to increase the final gas delivery rate. This may increase the final inspired O_2 concentration by reducing the entrainment of room air. Examples include:
• Nasal cannulae and face mask
• 'Double jet'—oxygen from two flow meters can be combined via a Y-connector. Increases FiO_2 to >0.7.

CPAP circuit manipulation

CPAP circuits are designed to deliver oxygen-enriched gas at high flow rates. When the CPAP valve is removed, the tubing can often be configured to deliver this high flow rate to a standard Hudson mask. This should only be performed by someone who has full understanding of the principles of the circuits.

Table 2.2 summarizes the advantages and disadvantages of some of the major devices used in modern clinical practice.

Table 2.2 Advantages and disadvantages of oxygen delivery devices

Device	Advantages	Disadvantages
Nasal cannulae	Well tolerated	Dry nasal secretions
	Patient able to eat and drink	Useful only in mild hypoxia
	Nasopharynx acts as O_2 reservoir	Septal erosion
Hudson mask	Range of flows/titratable	Patient unable to eat or drink
	Mask acts as reservoir	Potential for rebreathing of CO_2 at low flows
	Higher FiO_2 possible (0.6)	
Non-re-breathing mask	High FiO_2 possible (0.8)	Secretions rapidly dried
	Useful as first-line therapy during initial assessment	Reservoir bag has to be filled for maximum efficiency

With high flow or prolonged use of oxygen always use humidification. Failure to do so results in a rapid drying of secretions, which become tenacious and difficult to expectorate. There are commercially available devices that combine high flow oxygen with humidification (e.g. Vapotherm™).

FiO_2 delivered from different oxygen delivery devices
It is not possible to accurately predict the precise FiO_2 that will be delivered by a particular oxygen delivery device. There is also considerable variation in the literature. Table 2.3 gives an approximation of the ranges of FiO_2 that may be obtained from different devices.

Table 2.3 FiO_2 ranges that may be delivered by oxygen-delivery devices

Oxygen-delivery device	FiO_2 delivered
Nasal cannulae	0.24–0.28
Hudson mask	0.35–0.6
Venturi mask	0.24–0.6
Non-rebreathing mask	0.65–0.9
Combination devices, e.g. oxygen from two flow meters	0.7–0.8
High flow humidified O_2 via nasal prongs, e.g. Vapotherm™	up to 0.9

Capacity of oxygen cylinders
Transfer of the critically ill patient requires portable oxygen and high flow devices consume this quickly. A Whisperflow® valve uses a surprising 140L/min and will exhaust a size E cylinder in less than 5min. The capacity of common cylinders is shown in Table 2.4.

Table 2.4 The capacity of common cylinders

Size	C	D	E	F	G	J
Height (cm)	36	46	79	86	125	145
Capcity (L)	170	340	680	1360	3400	6800

Failure to respond to therapy

- Refractory hypoxia in critical illness is usually as a result of shunt rather than a diffusion abnormality or hypoventilation.
- With shunt fractions greater than 20% (e.g. in a severe pneumonia) increasing FiO_2 will not produce significant increases in SaO_2. In this situation the normally small proportion of oxygen dissolved in blood becomes more important and increasing supplemental oxygen is reasonable.
- On the ward, escalating FiO_2 may or may not be real. Patients often do not keep oxygen masks on. Entrainment of air, because of the unpredictable peak inspiratory flow rate seen in critical illness, can be highly variable. At the ward level it is almost impossible to say with any degree of accuracy what the actual FiO_2 is.
- Most patients who require invasive mechanical ventilation do so because of exhaustion rather than failure to oxygenate.

Summary

There are many firmly held, opposing views amongst the medical profession regarding oxygen administration. Few are backed up by robust evidence.
- Oxygen should be titrated to SaO_2 rather than PaO_2.
- Avoid hyperoxia unless specifically indicated.
- The majority of non-hypoxaemic breathless patients do not benefit from oxygen therapy.
- Initial oxygen therapy for critically ill patients should be a mask with a reservoir bag at 15L/min. In the absence of oximetry, continue to use a mask with a reservoir bag until definitive treatment is available.
- Aim for normal or near-normal oxygen saturation (SaO_2 94–98%) for all acutely ill patients except those at risk of hypercapnic respiratory failure.
- If at risk of hypercapnic respiratory failure aim for SaO_2 88–92%.
- Critically ill patients who also have COPD should have the same initial target saturation as other critically ill patients pending blood gas results, after which they may need controlled oxygen or ventilation.
- Once stabilized in ICU, SaO_2 92–94% is suitable for the majority of patients.

1 Khaw KS, Wang CC, Ngan Kee WD, Pang CP, and Rogers MS (2002) Effects of high inspired oxygen fraction during elective caesarean section under spinal anaesthesia on maternal and fetal oxygenation and lipid peroxidation. *Br J Anaesth* **88**, 18–23.
2 Caruana-Montaldo B, Gleeson K, and Zwillich C (2000) The control of breathing in clinical practice. *Chest* **117**(1), 205–25.
3 Hanson WC, Marshall BE, Frasch FH, and Marshall C (1996) Causes of hypercapnia with oxygen therapy in patients with chronic obstructive pulmonary disease. *Crit Care Med* **24**(1), 23–8.
4 O'Driscoll BR, Howard LS, and Davison AG on behalf of the British Thoracic Society (2008) BTS Guidelines for Emergency Oxygen Use in Adult Patients. *Thorax* **63** (S6), vi 1–68.

2.2 **Non-invasive respiratory support**

Effective mechanical ventilation can be provided non-invasively (i.e. without an endotracheal or tracheostomy tube) by applying negative extrathoracic pressure or positive airway pressure. Many other methods of NIV have been tried over the years, but most are of historical interest only.

Non-invasive ventilation

CPAP using a mask as the interface has been in use for many years as a way of improving oxygenation. The improvement in FRC associated with CPAP can improve pulmonary compliance and reduce WOB to a level that is sustainable by the patient (see 📖 Physiology and pathophysiology, p 2). This chapter will focus on NIV, i.e. circuit pressure alternating between two levels to achieve ventilation.

Basics

Inspiratory pressure
- NIV works by applying positive pressure to the airways during inspiration (inspiratory positive airway pressure, IPAP).
- The tidal volume generated depends on the respiratory compliance, patient effort, and magnitude of leaks.
- NIV is usually pressure-targeted, mainly because it is a 'leaky' system. Volume can be estimated by integrating the flow delivered by the ventilator, making adjustments for the intentional and unintentional leaks. Some newer modes of NIV will adjust the IPAP to maintain a set tidal volume, but there is no evidence that this is better than using a set pressure.
- IPAP is expressed as an absolute pressure (i.e. not relative to expiratory positive airways pressure (EPAP), see below). This can cause confusion in an ICU setting where inspiratory pressures are often expressed relative to the PEEP. Always double check that the patient is getting the pressures you want.

IPAP is titrated to clinical parameters starting at 10–15cmH$_2$O, aiming for 20–30cmH$_2$O. Increase the IPAP every few minutes using the following end points or until the patient finds the pressure or the mask leak too uncomfortable:
- Adequate chest expansion on inspection
- Less WOB indicated by reduced:
  - Use of accessory muscles.
  - Sweating.
  - Tracheal tug.
  - Intercostal recession.
- Improved respiratory comfort reported by patient.

An IPAP >30cmH$_2$O may be necessary (there is little risk of barotrauma with NIV). Problems associated with increasing IPAP include:
- Increased leaks.
- Delayed cycling to expiration.
- Non-voluntary glottic narrowing.
- Reduced patient tolerance.

Rise time

The time taken to reach the target IPAP is called the rise time (See Fig. 2.1). Patients with COPD usually prefer a shorter rise time (around 0.3s). In comparison, patients with neuromuscular problems, obesity-hypoventilation, or scoliosis may be more comfortable with a longer rise time (0.5s or longer). Patients are usually able to report which setting suits them best.

Consider shortening the rise time if the patient continues to use their accessory muscles on NIV, or they appear to be sucking against the ventilator.

Sometimes the rise time is so long that the target IPAP is not achieved. This usually indicates that there is a lot of leakage around the mask, with a ventilator that does not have the flow capacity to compensate.

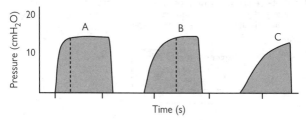

Fig. 2.1 This graph demonstrates short (A) and long (B) pressure rise times during NIV (dotted line indicates when target pressure of 14cmH$_2$O has been reached). Curve C shows target pressure failure, probably due to leaks.

Expiratory pressure

The EPAP is analogous to PEEP in invasive ventilation. EPAP has the following effects:
- Increases end-expiratory lung volume (and hence oxygenation).
- Overcomes intrinsic PEEP (see 📖 Pressure support ventilation, p 144, and Positive end expiratory pressure, p 119).
- Flushes exhaled gas out of the circuit.
- Reduces ventilation if IPAP not increased.

As IPAP and EPAP are absolute pressures, increases in EPAP will reduce the inspiratory pressure (and hence tidal volume) for a given IPAP.

Nomenclature

The nomenclature can be confusing. NIV is sometimes called bi-level positive airway pressure (BiPAP) outside an ICU environment. The clinician must be clear what BIPAP means for that patient.
- BIPAP is used as a generic term for a synchronized pressure-controlled time-cycled mode of ventilation (biphasic positive airway pressure). Alternative names are DuoPAP, Bi-Vent, BiLevel, and BiPhasic.
- BIPAP® is a ventilation mode trademarked by Drager with features of APRV, but more conventional I and E. inspiratory:expiratory (I:E) ratios.
- BiPAP® is a non invasive ventilator made by Respironics.

Triggering and cycling

In NIV inspiration is usually patient and flow triggered, with a backup time trigger (see 📖 Triggering and cycling, p 109). Failure to activate the flow trigger may be due to lack of patient effort, ineffective triggering, or excessive leaks.

Breaths are usually flow cycled, when inspiratory flow falls to a set percentage (around 50%) of the peak flow (expiratory trigger sensor, ETS). NIV can also be time-cycled. This is used as a backup to prevent failure of cycling because of excess leaks and is useful in neuromuscular conditions (see below).

Expiratory time should be sufficient to allow complete emptying and avoid breath stacking and dynamic hyperinflation (Fig. 2.2). Watch the patient's respiratory pattern or look at the ventilator flow/time trace to ensure that the ventilator settings allow the patient to spend adequate time in each phase of the respiratory cycle.

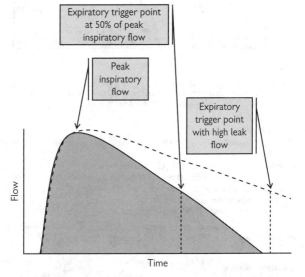

Fig. 2.2 Expiratory cycling in NIV with minimal leaks (solid line) and in a system with excessive leaks (dotted line). Excessive leaks will delay cycling and lengthen inspiration.

Indications

NIV works best in type 2 (hypercapnic) respiratory failure, although there is increasing evidence for its use in ICU in some patients with type 1 failure (Table 2.5).

Table 2.5 Indications for NIV

Condition	Strength of evidence	Comments
Acute exacerbations of COPD	+++	Not pneumonia, underweight
LV failure	++	Recent multicentre randomized controlled trials (RCTs) suggest more rapid improvement in physiology, but mortality unchanged by NIV
		Meta-analysis suggests mortality improvement for CPAP
Pneumonia	+	
Acute asthma	+	Small studies suggest more rapid improvement in peak flow with NIV, better delivery of nebulized drug
Acute neurological syndromes, e.g. Guillan–Barre	+/–	Anecdotal reports of NIV use
		By the time the respiratory muscles are involved, invasive ventilation is usually safer
Slowly progressive neurological conditions, e.g. muscular dystrophy	++	Extensive series of long-term NIV, in many instances started acutely
Obesity-hypoventilation	++	Increasing evidence of efficacy
Scoliosis	++	Long history of successful use
Fibrotic lung disease	–	The British Thoracic Society suggest worth trying, but seldom successful and no convincing evidence

The advantages of NIV over invasive ventilation include:
- Sedation usually not required.
- Complications of intubation are avoided (particularly ventilator-associated pneumonia).
- It can be alternated with periods of spontaneous breathing.
- The patient can eat and drink (and talk) during breaks from NIV.
- It can be used outside ICU.

Experience has shown that NIV is unlikely to work in the presence of:
• Significant metabolic acidosis.
• Hypotension.
• Severe hypoxia.

If the patient is unable to protect their airway then intubation is safer, although NIV may be tried if this is to be the ceiling of treatment. As a general rule, patients who are not for escalation to intubation (for example severe COPD, fibrotic lung disease, or patients with multiple co-morbidities) do not tend to do well on NIV either.

▶▶ *Do not persevere if NIV is clearly not working*

Weaning
NIV can be used to wean patients from invasive ventilation (for example, in patients with neuromuscular disease or chronic lung disease).
• Prior to extubation, the NIV ventilator should be used for invasive support, to ensure it is capable of providing effective ventilation.
• Immediately after extubation, make sure the pharynx is clear of secretions and start NIV—it is much less likely to work if you wait until the patient is exhausted.

NIV and tracheostomy
If the patient is being weaned with a tracheostomy and only overnight ventilation is required, NIV might be attractive as an alternative way of providing assisted ventilation at night and separating the patient from invasive respiratory support.
• The patient should ideally have an uncuffed fenestrated tracheostomy tube; failing that, the smallest tube practicable.
• Ensure adequate airflow by occluding the tracheostomy and seeing if the patient can breathe in.
• Occlude the stoma when you ultimately remove the tracheostomy by taping a pad of gauze tightly over the hole with an 'X' of elastic dressing. A simple occlusive dressing will simply blow off when you start NIV.

Pressure-control NIV
For patients with neuromuscular problems, scoliosis, and obesity-hypoventilation it is often best to provide mandatory pressure-control NIV rather than assisted ventilation. Home NIV ventilators are much better than most ICU ventilators for this purpose.

This will allow complete respiratory muscle rest. During nocturnal ventilation, this may lead to better quality sleep and falling bicarbonate levels (with improved daytime respiratory drive).

As this is a mandatory mode, patient compliance is needed. Encouragement, reassurance, and explanation are required.

Setting up pressure-control NIV:
• Select a mask.
• Set the respiratory rate to the patient's spontaneous rate.

- Set the inspiratory time to correspond to the patient's spontaneous breathing pattern.
- Set the IPAP to 20cmH$_2$O.
- Start NIV, holding the mask in place for the patient.
- Encourage the patient to relax and let the ventilator breathe for them.
- Strap the mask in place.
- Add supplemental oxygen if necessary.
- Increase the IPAP if the patient will tolerate it.

NIV outside the ICU

NIV is used extensively in clinical areas other than ICU. This is perfectly reasonable when intervening earlier in the natural history of respiratory failure, in an attempt to help prevent further deterioration to a stage where invasive ventilation will be needed. There is a danger that the availability of NIV on the wards means that patients who should be on ICU will not be transferred.

Training

Maintaining competency in NIV is not easy. Each clinical area will have its own solution to ensuring that a safe and effective NIV service is available around the clock.

- Choose a simple and robust ventilator for all areas (on the wards, the main adjustment you will need to make is to IPAP).
- Use only one model of ventilator.
- Mount it securely on a trolley (to prevent it getting lost or hidden away in a cupboard).
- Set up a simple training programme.

Problems

Leaks

Leaks are inevitable with NIV, through exhalation ports or around the mask. The ventilators are designed to generate sufficient flow to compensate for these leaks. Excessive leaks may:

- Prevent the target IPAP from being reached.
- Make inspiratory triggering less sensitive.
- Delay cycling from inspiration to expiration.
- Reduce the effect of supplemental oxygen on FiO$_2$.
- Interfere with the quality of sleep.

Adjusting the mask straps may be sufficient, but often it will be necessary to try a different style of mask (see below).

Nasal bridge pressure sores

Interface problems are one of the most frequent causes of failure of NIV. The skin over the bridge of the nose is particularly vulnerable to ulceration.

- If the skin is just reddened try loosening the straps a little, or using a mask with a strut that takes more pressure onto the forehead.

- Use a different mask, a smaller version that just fits over the tip of the nose or nasal pillows.
- Once the skin has started to break down, you must change to something that has no contact with the skin area under threat. Putting a dressing over the area and persevering with the same mask seldom works.

Rhinitis

Cooling and drying of the nasal mucosa causes rhinitis resulting in sneezing or rhinorrhoea. Intranasal steroid sprays or drops are sometimes effective.

Gastric dilatation

When patients first start NIV, they may complain of excessive belching and a bloated feeling. This usually settles, for reasons that are unclear, and is an infrequent problem in long-term users of NIV. The only solution is to reduce the IPAP.

Hypotension

Hypotension is much less common with positive airway pressure NIV than in external negative pressure ventilation or invasive ventilation. It tends to occur only in patients with poor cardiac function. Reduction of IPAP, EPAP, or both may be necessary.

Practicalities

Ventilators

On ICU the pressure driving the NIV ventilator is likely to be generated by the compressed gas supply. Outside ICU most NIV devices utilize a fan or turbine, although some home ventilators are still based on a simple bellows.

ICU ventilators designed to deliver invasive ventilation will sometimes struggle to cope with the inherent leaks of NIV. On certain ICU ventilators there are specific 'NIV' modes and some alterations of ventilator settings are required:

- Increase the expiratory trigger sensitivity to 50% so that cycling is more likely to take place despite ongoing leaks.
- Set a fallback time cycling (e.g. inspiratory time 2s) in case expiratory flows do not reach even the raised expiratory trigger.

Interfaces

The main choice for NIV is between a mask that covers the nose or one that covers the nose and mouth. The advantages and disadvantages of different interfaces are compared in Table 2.6.

Table 2.6 Interfaces for NIV

Interface	Comments
Nasal mask	Most commonly used interface for long-term NIV
	Good for alert patients
	Easier to obtain good seal than with oro-nasal mask
	Smaller is better
	Tendency to erode nasal bridge
Oro-nasal mask	Good for ill patients
	Widely available
	Leaks often a problem
Nasal pillows	Useful when nasal bridge pressure sores develop
Hybrid mask with pillows	Nasal pillows inside a mask
	Worth trying if problems obtaining a good seal
Nasal prongs	Large, soft prongs which fit inside the nose are an alternative to nasal pillows
Helmet	Encloses the whole face
	Patients may tolerate this mask better than smaller interfaces
	Large volume may dampen pressure waveform
Hood	Well tolerated and less claustrophobic
	Noisy
	Some ventilators struggle with the volumes required
Mouthpiece	Experienced NIV users sometimes use a simple mouthpiece in the daytime

Circuits

Simple NIV ventilators use a single tube circuit, with an exhalation port near the patient. On the high dependency unit (HDU) or ICU there may be separate expiratory and inspiratory tubes. Home NIV ventilators often employ an exhalation valve.

Humidification

The nose is an excellent humidifier. Most of the time additional humidification is not required. Heat/moisture exchangers can be used, but they may interfere with triggering. If the patient has a lot of thick secretions, or is severely troubled by the sensation of dryness when on NIV, a heated humidifier in the circuit may be used. Triggering may become more difficult because of the additional circuit volume.

Bacterial filters
A bacterial filter on the outlet of the ventilator will stop contamination of the machine if any secretions run back down the tubing. Use a thin bacterial filter, not a heat and moisture exchanger (HME) device (which will interfere with triggering).

Setting up NIV
When you are setting up NIV acutely, the mode will usually be pressure-support: the timing will be determined by the patient's own respiratory pattern.
- Choose a mask.
- Set IPAP 12cmH$_2$O and EPAP 5cmH$_2$O.
- Strap the mask in place.
- Titrate IPAP to clinical indicators (above) and as tolerated by patient.
- Observe patient to ensure patient's respiratory effort triggers ventilator (see 'Troubleshooting').

There will almost always be a back-up rate, for which you may need to set the timings, but the patient will dictate the respiratory pattern most of the time.

Oxygen
With an ICU or HDU ventilator, you may be able to set FiO$_2$, but on simpler ventilators you can add supplementary oxygen by adding a connector with a side-port into the circuit. The position of the connector makes little difference. Increase the oxygen flow rate until you achieve satisfactory oxygenation. A target range of 88–92% is reasonable for most patients.

Troubleshooting
Look at the patient first before you look at the numbers on the ventilator.

Asynchrony
The most common cause of asynchrony is mask leaks. This interferes with triggering (wasted efforts) and may cause failed cycling.
  Try adjusting the mask or consider a different interface.
  After an hour of NIV, arterial blood gases should be improving. If this is the case but the patient is not synchronizing with the ventilator, then they are getting better despite the impediment of NIV and you should leave them to breathe spontaneously.

Inadequate support
Many studies of NIV use an IPAP of 20 or 30cmH$_2$O. Provided you have a decent mask fit, titrate IPAP upward to clinical effect until leaks become excessive or the patient finds the pressure too much.
  Adjust the rise time to patient comfort.

Dynamic hyperinflation
In diseases with expiratory flow limitation (eg COPD), full expiration may not have occurred before the following inspiration. This leads to breath stacking and dynamic hyperinflation.

Although less problematic than in invasive ventilation (see 📖 Positive end expiratory pressure, p 119, and Pressure support ventilation, p 144), it is important to be aware of its existence and recognize it early. Measures to counteract dynamic hyperinflation include:

- Shortened rise time (allowing more time in expiration)
- Carefully increasing EPAP (may overcome some of effects of PEEPi)
- Removing NIV for a period.

> *If the arterial blood gases (particularly the pH or H⁺) are not improving after an hour of NIV, there is seldom any point in persevering.*

External negative pressure ventilation

Negative pressure ventilation can be delivered by 'iron lungs', used in the polio epidemics in the middle of the last century. (See 📖 Development of invasive ventilation, p 102). These devices, or smaller cuirass or jacket versions that only enclose the chest, are still used in some centres.

Iron lungs

Iron lungs are very effective at producing ventilation but they require a patent airway. Their use has declined since the 1960s, but they are still sometimes used in patients intolerant of facemasks (the cyclical pressure changes within the tank will still produce ventilation).

Iron lungs can generate negative pressures of $-40cmH_2O$. This can cause pooling of blood in the abdomen and limbs, with a concomitant fall in venous return and cardiac output ('tank shock').

They are large and cumbersome, patient access is limited, nursing care is restricted, and transport almost impossible.

Triggering

External negative pressure ventilation is time triggered, time cycled, and pressure targeted. Patient triggering has been reported using nasal pressure sensors, diaphragmatic electromyogram (EMG) or strain gauges around the chest. However, due to leaks and the volume gas pressurization required, there is considerable delay before the pumps are able to meet target pressure. This renders patient triggering of little value.

Upper airway obstruction

If a patient is able to co-ordinate their own respiratory cycle with the ventilator, then they 'prime' or open their upper airway before inspiration. If the patient cannot co-ordinate, or becomes apnoeic, this 'priming' is lost and upper airway obstruction can occur, usually at the level of the larynx or pharynx. Pharyngeal obstruction is particularly problematic because the patient has to lie on their back, with a tight collar around their neck where the seal is produced.

Cuirass ventilators

In a cuirass ventilator, negative pressure is applied only to the ribcage, which reduces the cardiovascular side-effects, but also the efficacy of ventilation. In addition, the rigid edges of the cuirass jacket restrict expansion of the lower abdomen and upper thorax. The Hayek oscillator uses a cuirass shell to deliver high-frequency negative pressure ventilation. It is the external equivalent of high-frequency oscillatory ventilation.

The decline of external negative pressure ventilation

In the poliomyelitis epidemic in Copenhagen in 1952, the limited supplies of negative pressure ventilators precipitated the use of positive pressure ventilation. The demonstration of a good outcome with 'long-term' invasive ventilation caused a swing away from negative pressure ventilation. The development of nasal masks in the 1980s allowed the easier application of traditional NIV and a further drift away from negative pressure ventilation. They are now little used, but units that still have an iron lung find that for a patient who cannot use a mask it can be a very effective way of assisting ventilation. Patients may require persuading to get into the iron lung first time, but they will often find the experience relaxing.

Rocking beds

These use the principle that when beds rock up and down, the abdomen acts as a piston, moving the diaphragm. It is quite an effective method of ventilating patients with isolated diaphragmatic paralysis. Surprisingly, motion sickness is not an issue, perhaps because the motion is only in one plane.

With the advent of nasal and facial masks, rocking beds have been largely superseded.

2.3 Continuous positive airway pressure

CPAP is the application of constant positive airway pressure throughout the respiratory cycle in the spontaneously breathing patient. A high flow oxygen/air mixture provides the positive pressure during inspiration with an expiratory valve creating PEEP. CPAP's uses can be broadly divided between the treatment of obstructive sleep apnoea (OSA, not discussed here) and acute respiratory compromise.

Physiology

CPAP causes many physiological changes, particularly in the respiratory and cardiovascular systems. These changes are fully discussed in 📖 Positive end expiratory pressure, p 119, and Heart–lung interaction, p 275.

Respiratory effects

CPAP is associated with the following beneficial effects:

- CPAP increases lung volumes and FRC. At low pressure levels, CPAP increases FRC by increasing the volume of already patent alveoli, while at higher pressure levels previously collapsed alveoli may be inflated (recruitment) with a reduction in intra-pulmonary shunting.
- CPAP may also lead to changes in the relative compliance of the upper and lower parts of the lung, improving ventilation to the well-perfused lower portion of the lung, and V̇/Q̇ matching.
- Improvements in compliance result in a decrease in WOB.
- Reduction in the threshold load from intrinsic PEEP (PEEPi).

However, inappropriate use of CPAP can worsen gas exchange and WOB.

- In unilateral or lobar disease, CPAP may increase shunt fraction by diverting blood away from healthy compliant lungs.
- In lungs which are already maximally recruited, the application of CPAP may increase alveolar deadspace.
- High levels of CPAP may actually increase WOB by:
  - Flattening the diaphragm
  - Increasing the need for an active expiratory phase.

Cardiovascular effects

In the healthy individual, CPAP may result in the following changes:

- Reduction in right atrial filling
- Reduced intra-abdominal vascular capacitance due to diaphragmatic descent
- Increase in sympathetic activity caused by reduced cardiac output
- Increase in pulmonary vascular resistance.

Despite these changes, in the healthy individual the reduction in cardiac output on application of CPAP at levels of less than $10cmH_2O$ is unlikely to be clinically detrimental.

In the failing heart, CPAP may have a number of advantageous clinical effects:

- Reduces the cardiac preload (see 📖 Heart-lung interaction, p 275)
- Reduces LV afterload by decreasing transmural pressure[1]

- Reduced heart rate (probably from pulmonary mediated vagal activity)
- Reduces alveolar oedema.

Miscellaneous effects
- Raised intracranial pressure (secondary to increased CVP).
- Reduced cerebral perfusion pressure.
- Hepatic venous congestion (raised CVP).
- Reduced cardiac output may compromise blood supply to other organs.

Indications

CPAP predominantly improves oxygenation. Its effects on WOB are more variable and depend on the underlying pathology. Its use in OSA is well described.

   When considering the use of CPAP it is important to address the natural history of the underlying condition. This includes an assessment of both the pathology (some diseases respond better than others) and time course (even the most compliant patient is unlikely to tolerate CPAP for more than 96h).

Cardiogenic pulmonary oedema
CPAP is associated with rapid symptom improvement in acute CPO.[2] This benefit has not been consistently shown in clinical trials, but meta-analyses have demonstrated a mortality reduction (relative risk 0.64, 95% confidence interval 0.44–0.92).[3]

   It is often useful as a 'therapeutic trial' to aid diagnosis, with many clinicians considering a rapid improvement in the patient's clinical state as supportive of a diagnosis of acute CPO.

Hypoxaemic respiratory failure
The evidence for the use of CPAP in unselected patients with respiratory failure is poor,[4] but initial response to treatment has been shown to be a good predictor of eventual outcome.[5]
- Patients with predominantly atelectasis/collapse respond better than those with consolidation.
- Its use in hypoxic respiratory failure must have a defined exit strategy. The use of CPAP should not hinder the decision to intubate.
- It may be used as a bridge to invasive respiratory support.
- There is evidence suggesting improved outcome when used for post-operative respiratory insufficiency after abdominal surgery.
- It may be used where therapy-limiting decisions are in place.

Prophylactic post-operative CPAP
- Lower rates of pneumonia and intubation have been demonstrated following oesophageal surgery and major abdominal surgery when CPAP is administered for approximately 24h post operatively.

Contraindications

Absolute contraindications
- Pneumothorax.
- Reduced conscious level (inability to protect airway).
- Ongoing upper gastrointestinal bleeding.
- Epistaxis.

- Severe facial trauma.
- Patient refusal.

Relative contraindications
- Asthma.
- Recent upper gastrointestinal or airway surgery.
- Cardiovascular instability.
- Non-respiratory organ failure.
- Active tuberculosis.
- Haemoptysis.
- Any condition where raised intracranial pressure is undesirable.
- Hypercapnia (but this may be improved in atelectasis causing ↑WOB).
- COPD or severe lung hyperinflation.
- Excessive secretions.
- Need for invasive procedures (central venous access, intercostal drains etc.).

Equipment
A CPAP circuit requires a flow generator, a CPAP valve, and a patient interface. The clinician setting up the circuit must understand the principles of CPAP and be familiar with the set up. Incorrectly set systems are dangerous and are the subject of a National Patient Safety Alert.

Flow generation
In order to provide positive pressure throughout the respiratory cycle, the CPAP system gas flow must be > peak inspiratory flow rate.
- Portable CPAP machines (commonly used in the treatment of OSA) provide flows of <30L/min. They are unable to deliver high FiO_2 levels and are therefore not usually used in the acute setting.
- CPAP bellows consist of an oxygen/air mixer and a pressurized gas reservoir storing at least three times the patient's minute volume to prevent a loss of inspiratory pressure. It will provide reliable flows/pressures with a high maximum FiO_2 and is suitable for use in the ICU.
- Venturi devices such as Whisperflow® and Vital Signs® using pressurized oxygen to entrain air can deliver gas flows of >150L/min. Circuit flow and FiO_2 are adjustable.

Valves
- Classically, CPAP/PEEP valves are either threshold resistors (CPAP/PEEP level not dependent on flow) or flow resistors (CPAP/PEEP level dependent on flow).
- In all new-generation ventilators, CPAP/PEEP is adjusted by microprocessors.
- Portable/interchangeable CPAP/PEEP valves are either spring loaded or magnetic.
  - All are combined threshold/flow resistors, with greater or lesser flow dependence.
  - Expiratory pressure during CPAP will increase by 2–3cmH$_2$O.
  - The actual CPAP level may vary from the indicated CPAP level by 3–4cmH$_2$O. It is preferable to measure the actual system pressure when using these devices.
  - These valves may impose extra WOB, (inspiratory as well as expiratory).

- Anti-asphyxia valves are necessary on facemasks should there be a failure in the gas supply.
- There should be a safety valve in the inspiratory limb, set at 5cmH$_2$O above the CPAP level. This prevents excessively high circuit pressure should the PEEP valve become occluded.

Patient interface

This discussion focuses on non-invasive provision of CPAP.

The patient interface is extremely important, as a significant number of late failures of CPAP therapy are due to mask intolerance, rather than failure of gas exchange.

No data exist for the superiority of one device over another, but anecdotally offering the patient a choice may improve compliance. Interface devices include the following.

Nasal masks

These are predominantly used in the treatment of OSA, although they may have a role following extubation of the obese patient and during the provision of mouth care.

Facemasks

- Some masks cover just the mouth and nose, while others cover the whole face. They are usually held in position by an elasticated harness.
- Patient comfort and the quality of the seal depend on proper sizing, positioning, cuff inflation, and tensioning of the restraining straps.
- If masks are not properly applied, patient tolerance will be poor (as well as discomfort, inadequately fitted masks may cause nasal bridge ulceration and corneal abrasions).
- Strapping the mask on more forcefully is not an adequate substitute for fitting the mask properly in the first place.
- Seal may be compromised by beards or atypical facial shape.

Helmets

CPAP helmets create a seal around the patient's neck rather than face. The helmet is kept in place by straps passed under the axillae.

- Sometimes better tolerated than facemask for prolonged periods.
- Provides protection from pressure damage around the face.
- May provide a better seal.
- Noise levels of up to 100dB have been recorded inside the helmet. Use of an HME filter on the inlet line significantly reduces the subjective perception of this noise.
- Humidification steams the mask up, reducing visibility.
- Increased device dead space:
  - Higher flows required.
  - Patient's minute ventilation may have to increase by up to 20%.

Other equipment

- Humidification is required for anything other than a brief trial of CPAP.
- Oxygen analyser.
- Manometer or pressure measurement.

Management

Setting up CPAP

Before commencing CPAP confirm the following:

- No contraindications to CPAP.
- Adequate explanation given to patient.
- Adequate monitoring *in situ*.
- Suitably trained staff available (nursing, physiotherapy etc.).
- 'Plan B' (e.g. intubation and IPPV) available or alternative plans made.

Initially, CPAP should be commenced at the maximal FiO_2 the system will allow at a pressure of $5cmH_2O$, or $10cmH_2O$ for acute CPO.
Common issues include:

- Leaks around facemasks or helmets:
  - Ensure mask properly sized and fitted.
  - Mask cuff appropriately filled.
  - Adequate tension on straps.
- Drop of pressure during inspiration:
  - Seen as an oscillating circuit pressure or a pressure dip during inspiration.
  - Increase flow rates to exceed peak inspiratory flow or to adequately fill bellows.
- Patient agitation/distress:
  - Attempt to reassure.
  - Address potential sources.
  - Consider sedation such as low dose remifentanil infusion.
  - Recognize as failure of CPAP.

Ongoing care

- After the initiation of CPAP therapy, many patients will require higher pressures. These should be provided in $2cmH_2O$ increments at 5-min intervals, with reassessment of patient comfort and physiological parameters.
- In acute CPO, the level of CPAP required needs to be sufficient to abolish negative intrathoracic pressure swings; this will reduce the left ventricular afterload and myocardial ischaemia without significantly reducing venous return and cardiac output. Higher levels of CPAP may therefore be required.
- CPAP is uncomfortable for the majority of patients and it may be necessary to provide breaks in therapy to increase the likelihood of ongoing compliance, as well as to allow for oral drug administration and nursing care. If the patient is unable to tolerate the levels of CPAP required to produce a physiological response it may be necessary to convert to IPPV.
- It is important to recognize early if you are not winning, and institute invasive ventilation.

1 Naughton MT, Rahman MA, Hara K, Floras JS, and Bradley TD (1995) Effect of continuous positive airway pressure on intrathoracic and left ventricular transmural pressures in patients with congestive heart failure. *Circulation* **91**, 1725–31.

2 Gray A, Goodacre S, Newby DE, Masson M, Sampson F, and Nicholl J on behalf of the 3CPO trialists (2008) Non-invasive ventilation in acute cardiogenic pulmonary edema. *N Engl J Med* **359**, 142–51.

3 Weng C, Zhao T, Liu Q, *et al.* (2010) Meta-analysis: Non-invasive ventilation in acute cardiogenic pulmonary edema. *Ann Int Med* **152**(9), 590–600.

4 Hill NS, Brennan J, Garpestad E, and Nava S (2007) Noninvasive ventilation in acute respiratory failure. *Crit Care Med* **35**(10), 2402–7.

5 Antonelli M, Conti G, Moro ML, *et al.* (2001). Predictors of failure of noninvasive positive pressure ventilation in patients with acute hypoxemic respiratory failure: a multicenter study. *Intensive Care Med* **27**, 1718–28.

Invasive ventilation basics

3.1 Development of invasive ventilation

Ancient history

- Tracheostomy was mentioned in the text of Hindu medicine, *Rig Veda*, as early as 2000BC, and in ancient Egyptian writings.
- It is reputed that elective tracheostomy was undertaken in Greece and Rome, 100BC–300AD, but there is little further mention of the technique until the middle ages.
- Hippocrates (460–380BC) wrote the first description of endotracheal intubation in man in *Treatise on Air*—'One should introduce a cannula into the trachea along the jaw bone so that air can be drawn into the lungs'.

Early modern history

- The first case of ventilatory assistance, rather than the provision of a patent airway alone, is credited to Andreas Vesalius (1514–64), the Belgian anatomist and Professor of Surgery and Anatomy at Padua, Italy. He wrote:

    'But that life may in manner of speaking be restored to the animal, an opening must be attempted in the trunk of the trachea into which a tube of reed or cane should be put; you will then blow into this, so that the lung may rise again and the animal take in air.......and the heart becomes strong and exhibits a wondrous variety of motions'.

    Vesalius' *de Humani Corporis Fabrica*, 1555, contains an illustrated letter 'Q' in which cherubs perform a tracheostomy on a pig (Fig. 3.1).
- In 1664 Robert Hooke (London) reported the first case of mechanical ventilation, as opposed to using expired air, when he ventilated a dog with a pair of fireside bellows via a tracheostomy.

Unfortunately the principles of ventilation demonstrated in early animal models were not put into routine use for resuscitation in humans for another 100 years. However, a large variety of alarming methods were employed, e.g. loud bells, bright lights, burning with red-hot irons, and rectal insufflation with tobacco smoke.

- 1744—John Fothergill described a case of successful mouth-to-mouth resuscitation.
- 1752—Joseph Black discovered carbon dioxide and showed its presence in exhaled air.
- 1774—Joseph Priestley discovered 'dephlogisticated' air, later named oxygen by Antoine Lavoisier, who described the relationship of these gases to metabolism.
- 1767—the Humane Society was founded in Amsterdam to aid victims of drowning in the city's waterways and the society spread to other European cities. Mouth-to-mouth respiration and fireside bellows were used for ventilation, as well as chest and abdominal compressions.
- 1776—John Hunter used a double bellows to provide positive pressure for inspiration and negative pressure to aid expiration. He also advised using oxygen and compressing the larynx against the oesophagus to prevent air entering stomach.

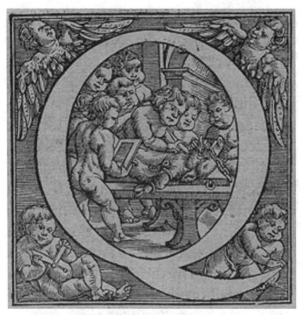

Fig. 3.1 Illustrated letter Q from Vesalius' de Humani Corporis Fabrica.

- In Scotland financial rewards were offered to members of the public who attempted resuscitation, with the tariff depending on the effort involved and the outcome.

By the early 1800s resuscitation of victims of drowning was abandoned when it was recognized that excessive pressure from the bellows could cause pneumothorax and the overall success rate was poor. Subsequently, the principles of resuscitation were largely forgotten for another century.

Negative pressure ventilation

From the mid 1800s to the early 1900s a large number of negative pressure 'tank ventilators' or 'iron lungs' were designed. In these devices the entire patient was encased in a rigid box in which negative pressure was created. Only the head protruded and the machine was sealed around the neck (Fig. 3.2). The energy source was usually a hand or foot pump operated by attendant. One paediatric ventilator was operated by the doctor breathing in and out of the box and in another the patient himself had to stand inside the box and generate pressure change by pumping giant bellows. There were few, if any, successful outcomes.

- 1929—Phillip Drinker (Harvard) designed the first electrically powered iron lung, which was used to ventilate a polio victim, who survived.

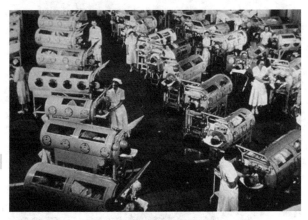

Fig. 3.2 Iron lung ward, Rancho Los Amigos Hospital, California, 1953.

It cost over $2000 (i.e. twice the price of a car—roughly the same price comparison exists today), which severely limited its availability during the 1937–38 UK polio epidemic.

- Edward and Donald Both (Adelaide) designed a less expensive model of the Drinker ventilator.
- 1938—Lord Nuffield (William Morris of the Morris car company, Oxford) was so shocked by news of a polio patient who died for lack of a ventilator that he manufactured over 1600 Both ventilators at his car plant. These were donated to hospitals throughout the commonwealth.
- Cuirass ventilators were developed during the same period. These consisted of a rigid shell covering the chest, under which a negative pressure was generated. They overcame the problems of claustrophobia, isolation, and inaccessibility for nursing care. The other advantages were cost and portability, which facilitated the advent of domiciliary ventilation.

Anaesthetic developments

As surgical techniques advanced (particularly in thoracic surgery), traditional anaesthetic techniques using spontaneous or negative pressure ventilation were inadequate. Very few doctors were trained, or even interested, in anaesthesia, and the task was often allocated to an untrained junior surgeon or nurse. The operative mortality was high. The pressure for advanced anaesthesia techniques led to:

- Translaryngeal insufflation of anaesthetic gases and manual ventilation by face mask (the preferred technique)
- Endotracheal intubation. After experience during World War I, Sir Ivan Magill and Stanley Rowbotham (London) established endotracheal intubation, initially with two catheters, and subsequently with a cuffed

endotracheal tube. Their developments in airway techniques helped to gain respect for anaesthesia and to establish it as a stand-alone medical specialty.

Positive pressure ventilation

- 1906—Heinrich Dräger (Lübeck, Germany) designed the first positive pressure ventilator, the Pulmotor, for resuscitation in mines.
- Positive pressure ventilation was not widely accepted into anaesthetic practice until the1940s, with some resistance from surgeons in the USA even into the late 1950s.
- 1947—John Blease (Liverpool, UK) designed and built one of first anaesthetic positive pressure ventilators to become widely used, the Blease Pulmoflator. He had an unusual career path. Blease was an untrained car mechanic who produced anaesthetic apparatus for Dr Henry Roberts, a GP who provided dental anaesthesia. After Dr Roberts' sudden death Blease took over his duties and was appointed to an anaesthetic post in Birkenhead General Hospital!
- 1948—During the Los Angeles polio epidemic a physician, A. Bower, demonstrated respiratory acidosis in patients ventilated in Drinker's 'iron lung'. With the engineer Ray Bennett, he developed an intratracheal attachment to supplement negative pressure ventilation with positive pressure ventilation, which increased tidal volume and dramatically improved survival.

Modern history

1950s

1952 Copenhagen poliomyelitis epidemic

The response to this epidemic is often hailed as 'the birth of intensive care medicine'.

A turning point in respiratory support occurred in 1950 when Carl-Gunnar Engstrom (Stockholm) used blood gas analysis to show that the high mortality among polio patients with respiratory and bulbar paralysis was due to hypoventilation, with aspiration and inadequate clearance of secretions. He designed a volume-controlled positive pressure ventilator to ensure adequate tidal volumes were achieved even with sputum retention and bronchial plugging.

The poliomyelitis epidemic which followed in Copenhagen in 1952–53 was marked by both very large numbers of patients and also by the exceptionally large proportion of patients who presented with a combination of respiratory and bulbar involvement. Early in the epidemic tank ventilators and uncuffed tracheostomy tubes were used, with a mortality of 87%. Bjørn Ibsen, an anaesthetist, was asked to advise on the management of a 12-year-old girl who appeared to be dying of respiratory failure. In conjunction with Poul Astrup, head of clinical biochemistry, they demonstrated severe hypercapnia, despite normal oxygenation, undertook a tracheostomy using a cuffed tube, performed bronchial toilet, and subsequently achieved adequate ventilation with manual positive pressure ventilation. On returning her to a cuirass ventilator all the clinical signs of hypercapnia and high arterial CO_2 returned. When they resumed manual ventilation she improved again and subsequently made an excellent recovery.

Following this demonstration all polio victims with ventilatory failure were supported with positive pressure ventilation, but as there were no such ventilators available the work had to be done by hand. Professor Lassen (head of communicable diseases) organized shifts of thousands of helpers, including hundreds of medical students, dental students, and student nurses. Up to 75 patients received manual ventilation simultaneously. The mortality for respiratory failure patients fell from 87 to 30%.

In addition, Ibsen recognized that some patients were dying before they could reach hospital because of the very rapid progression of respiratory failure, and developed mobile teams who were rushed to patients' homes, where they successfully implemented manual ventilation and stabilization before transfer.

Other factors probably also contributed to the fall in mortality. The clinical teams consisted of skilled nurses, anaesthetists, physicians, ear, nose, and throat (ENT) surgeons, clinical biochemists, physiotherapists, and others. Routine humidification, suctioning, chest physiotherapy, and blood gas analysis became established. Ibsen subsequently developed an ICU in the Kommune Hospital in Copenhagen, probably the first of its type in the world, where he demonstrated the benefits of a multidisciplinary team approach to critically ill patients concentrated in a specified area.

As a result of the improved outcomes with positive pressure ventilation Engstrom's ventilator was produced commercially and was ready in time for a further polio outbreak in Stockholm in 1953, where a similar fall in mortality to 27% of ventilated cases was demonstrated.

During the 1950s a number of mechanical positive pressure ventilators were produced in response to the polio epidemics. They had no alarms, were powered by gas or electricity, and were designed for either volume control (Europe) or pressure control (USA), but not both.

- 1952—Mask CPAP was first used to treat pulmonary contusion.
- 1959—Frumin immersed the expiratory limb of a ventilator under a few centimetres of water and showed improved gas exchange, thus demonstrating the first use of PEEP.
- 1959—The 'sigh' was described, i.e. a few breaths of approximately twice normal tidal volume per minute, which had already been found to relieve the sensation of dyspnoea in polio patients and is currently being advocated again by some in the management of acute respiratory failure.
- By 1960 polio vaccination had almost eradicated the disease in the developed world and ventilators were increasingly used for other emergencies, such as crushed chest, spinal injuries, and drug overdose.
- There was no continuous sedation, so respiratory depression was created by overventilation giving a respiratory alkalosis.

1960s

- 1967—Adult (later 'acute') respiratory distress syndrome (ARDS) was described by D. Ashbaugh, although it had been previously noted in World War II as 'wet lung' and in the Vietnam war as 'Da Nang lung' or 'shock lung'.

- 1967–70—The first electronically controlled ventilators, by both Bennett and Siemens, were produced. The Servo 900A was equipped with a PEEP valve and the ability to monitor airway pressure and gas flow.

Patients were sedated with intermittent doses of long-acting opiates, sedatives and muscle relaxants. Damage to the tracheal mucosa and long-term stenosis was common from the use of red rubber endotracheal or tracheostomy tubes and high-pressure cuffs.

1970s
Attention turned to weaning the patient from ventilation. Intermittent mandatory ventilation (IMV) was developed in 1971 but spontaneous breaths through the ventilator were unsupported, required considerable effort to open the inspiratory valve, and could be interrupted by a mandatory breath.

1980s
- Synchronous intermittent mandatory ventilation (SIMV) was developed in Norway and first introduced on the Servo 900B. It had advantages in improving patient synchrony and comfort, and possibly in preventing respiratory muscle wasting.
- Sedation techniques progressed to continuous infusions of short-acting anaesthetic agents and opiates with less need for muscle relaxation.
- Although developed many years earlier, pulse oximetry and capnography became more available for routine monitoring as the technology became less bulky and more affordable.

1990s
- During the 1990s the rapid development of electronics and computerization enabled the almost countless options in ventilator controls, monitoring, and display available today.
- Pressure support modes became almost routine to aid weaning and offset the additional WOB through a ventilator.
- Percutaneous tracheostomy was described in the late 1980s and became established practice over the following decade. The value and optimal timing of tracheostomy are still controversial.
- High-frequency ventilation was developed in the 1970s and accepted into neonatal practice by the 1990s, but has been slow to establish a firm position in adult ventilation.
- NIV became an established practice in patients with exacerbations of COPD.
- Prone ventilation was initially shown to improve oxygenation in ARDS and was rapidly accepted in many ICUs. It has yet to demonstrate a benefit in terms of mortality.

2000s
The majority of equipment developments have been software enhancements which allow improved patient–ventilator interaction or automated weaning. More recently NAVA (📖 Neurally adjusted ventilatory assist, p 178) has allowed patient–ventilator interaction without the encumbrance of pneumatic triggers.

In addition, the importance of clinical measures to reduce the incidence of complications related to ventilation (such as ventilator-induced lung injury and ventilator-associated pneumonia) as well as protocol-driven weaning, avoidance of over-sedation, and many other 'bundles' of care have generally over-shadowed further technical advances in ventilator design.

Further reading

Trubuhovich RV (2003) In the beginning. The 1952–3 Danish epidemic of poliomyelitis and Bjørn Ibsen. *Crit Care Resusc* **5**, 227–230.
A detailed account of the response to the epidemic and its relationship to the development of the specialty of intensive care medicine.
Mørch E (1990) *History of Mechanical Ventilation in Clinical Applications of Ventilatory Support*, eds Kirby R and Banner M. Churchill Livingston Inc., New York.
A fascinating and extremely comprehensive (over 700 references) history from the personal perspective of a Danish freedom-fighter and pioneer of positive pressure ventilation who took his innovations from Nazi-occupied Copenhagen to the USA and became Professor of Anesthesiology in Chicago.

3.2 **Triggering and cycling**

Triggering

Ventilators measure pressure, volume, flow, and time. Inspiration is started (triggered) when one of these variables reaches a preset value. Breaths may be triggered by the patient or the ventilator.

The site of measurement of these variables may affect the triggering characteristics. Changes may be measured on the inspiratory limb of the circuit (where any resistance in the ventilator circuit from humidifiers etc. adds to the work of triggering), the Y piece, or the expiratory limb.

Pressure triggering

With pressure triggering, patient effort results in isometric contraction of the inspiratory muscles, decreasing the pressure in the circuit. When this pressure drop reaches a predetermined value, a breath is triggered and the inspiratory valve opens.

Flow triggering

Basic flow triggering is similar to pressure triggering. Flow at end expiration is zero and all valves are closed. Patient effort results in inspiratory flow, detected by the ventilator.

In more modern ventilators, there is a continuous flow around the circuit during expiration; all valves are open. The ventilator measures a change in this base flow to trigger inspiration. The continuous flow serves two purposes: it keeps valves open, and it meets the patient's initial demand for inspiratory flow. This should decrease the imposed WOB, and flow triggering is now the default trigger on most ventilators. However, on new-generation ventilators both flow and pressure triggers are probably equally effective.

Flow waveform triggering

This is a modification of flow triggering in which the expiratory flow waveform is monitored by the ventilator. Triggering occurs when the patient's inspiratory effort modifies the expiratory flow waveform, and flow waveform triggering has been shown to decrease triggering delay and ineffective efforts compared to pressure or flow triggering. Auto-triggering is increased.

Time triggering

In controlled modes of ventilation the ventilator will initiate a breath after a set period of time. Most modes attempt to avoid these breaths during patient effort.

Other triggers

Neurally adjusted ventilatory assist (NAVA) uses diaphragmatic electrical activity to trigger inspiration (and cycle to expiration) (see 📖 Neurally adjusted ventilatory assist, p 178). An oesophageal catheter monitors diaphragmatic EMG. It is reported to reduce trigger delay and asynchrony, but catheter placement can sometimes be unreliable. The mode uses pneumatic triggers as a backup.

Alternative methods of triggering the ventilator include chest wall motion or chest wall impedence in children.

Cycling

Expiration starts when a preset value of flow, time, and volume (or pressure) is reached.

Time cycling

Mandatory modes using pressure control are usually time cycled. The time can be set manually (e.g. T_{insp} is set in BIPAP) or by manipulating respiratory rate and I:E ratio.

Volume cycling

In volume-controlled ventilation, the ventilator cycles to expiration when a target volume has been reached. Ventilators that appear to be volume cycled may actually use a combination of flow rate and inspiratory time to work out inspiratory volume rather than measure volume directly. Strictly, they are time cycled.

Flow cycling

Spontaneous supported breaths (pressure support ventilation, PSV) are typically flow cycled. When inpiratory flow falls to a set percentage of peak inspiratory flow (usually 25–33%), the ventilator cycles to expiration. This ETS is adjustable in some ventilators and can be titrated according to the underlying disease (see 📖 Pressure support ventilation, p 144). Adjusting the ETS upwards will result in earlier cycling and longer expiration, and is useful in obstructive disease. Adjusting the ETS downwards will prolong inspiration and is useful in conditions of low compliance.

Pressure cycling

Pressure cycling is now only used as a safety backup for other forms of cycling, i.e. it will terminate the breath if pressure rises to the preset level.

Limit

Variables (e.g. pressure) may be limited by the ventilator. The terms 'limiting' and 'cycling' are sometimes used interchangeably. Strictly speaking, limited variables are those which are raised to a preset value before inspiration ends and used to sustain inspiration. They are not cycling variables.

Confusion arises when pressure 'limits' are set as a safety backup: the breath is terminated at a preset pressure level and this is properly referred to as pressure cycling.

Problems with triggering and cycling

Asynchrony is common and difficulties with triggering or cycling are frequent contributors to it (see 📖 Asynchrony, p 267, and Pressure support ventilation, p 144). It can result in:

- Inspiratory trigger delay
- Ineffective triggering
- Double (or triple) triggering
- Auto-triggering
- Inspiratory time extension
- Expiratory trigger cycling
- 'Hang-up' phenomenon.

3.3 Pressure vs volume delivery

Volume-controlled ventilation

Ventilators are classified as pressure, flow, or volume controllers. Practically, flow and volume controllers behave almost identically. Direct control of flow means indirect control of volume and vice versa, and both can deliver volume-controlled ventilation (VCV). Most VCV uses flow control with constant inspiratory flow (a square wave flow–time profile). Fig. 3.3 illustrates the typical flow, pressure, and volume changes seen during VCV and PCV.

Settings

In VCV, the clinician can alter the:
- Tidal volume (V_t)
- Machine rate

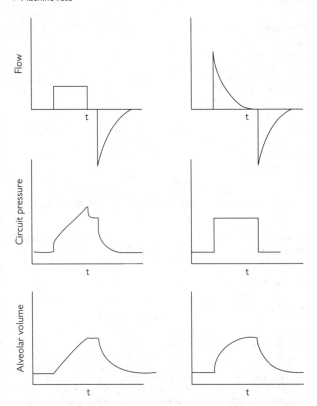

Fig. 3.3 Typical flow, pressure, and volume changes in VCV (L) and PCV (R).

- Inspiratory time/I:E ratio
- Flow–time profile.

Tidal volume

Excessive V_t results in volutrauma (see 📖 Complications of ventilation, p 244). Acceptable V_t can be estimated using patient height and sex. Without this correction, women are at greater risk of having an acceptable V_t overestimated.

Machine rate

The required minute ventilation for desired CO_2 elimination is estimated. Normal minute ventilation of 100mL/kg/min may be a useful starting value, but $PaCO_2$ is affected by CO_2 production and physiological dead space.

With limited V_t ventilation strategies, the most appropriate way of increasing minute ventilation is often by increasing respiratory rate. An increased rate may increase peak airway pressure (the same tidal volume is delivered in a shorter time), and the shorter expiratory time may lead to the development of intrinsic PEEP ($PEEP_i$) because of incomplete emptying.

Inspiratory time/I:E ratio

Many ventilators allow direct setting of the I:E ratio. In others it is set by manipulating the inspiratory time (T_i) and expiratory time (T_e), or by altering the inspiratory flow rate. Incomplete expiration may occur as Te reduces, resulting in $PEEP_i$ (see 📖 Positive end expiratory pressure, p 119, and 📖 Pressure support ventilation, p 144).

Flow–time profile

Various profiles have been described, for example decelerating or sinusoidal. Definitive advantages of specific flow–time profiles (lower peak pressures or more homogeneous gas distribution) are not clearly established.

Pressure changes in VCV

In VCV, delivered V_t is assured, but the resulting airway pressure is variable. During constant flow VCV with a brief inspiratory hold in an 'ideal' relaxed patient, pressure at the tracheal tube (P) is described by the equation

$$P = P_{res} + P_{el}$$

where $P_{res} \approx$ resistive pressure (flow × resistance of the tube and thorax) and $P_{el} \approx$ elastic pressure (elastance of the thorax × volume).

The relative contributions of resistive and elastic pressures change during inspiration (Fig. 3.4):
- Initial pressure rise is related to $P_{res} + PEEP_i$ (A – B).
- Ramp is related to rising P_{el} (B – C).
- Peak pressure is determined by both P_{res} and P_{el}.
- Plateau pressure (P_{plat}) is a function of P_{el} at equilibrium V_t.

During the inspiratory hold there is a rapid fall from peak pressure (C – D) then slow decay to static P_{el} (D – E). The initial drop reflects airway resistance (R_{aw}); the slow decay reflects the dissipation of stored energy in viscoelastic tissues and, in diseased lungs, intrapulmonary gas redistribution between lung units with a heterogeneous time constant (Pendelluft).

The relationship between lung volume and pressure generated during inspiration is complex because airway resistance is variable and viscoelastic

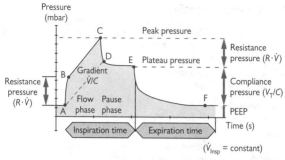

Fig. 3.4 Pressure changes during VCV. See text for explanation.

tissue components store energy imperfectly and in a time-dependent fashion. Normally energy lost per breath (the area of the hysteretic P–V loop) is ~60% due to airway resistance and ~40% due to tissue resistance.

Narrowed airways increase resistance to airflow. Energy is lost by convective inertia and gas compression, and at boundary layers where turbulence is made more likely by faster flows. Increasing end expiratory lung volume (EELV), e.g. with PEEP, may increase airway caliber and reduce resistance. By contrast, tissue resistance is increased by EELV, atelectasis, consolidation, oedema, and fibrosis, but remarkably, as inspiratory flow is increased up to ~1L/s, tissue resistance falls.

Increasing airway resistance may be obvious when flow is increased because peak pressure rises, but in patients whose tissue resistance predominates, increasing inspiratory flow may act to decrease total resistance, dynamic compliance, and energy lost.

Changes in resistance and compliance that might appear to be treatment-related are therefore only meaningful if conducted at the same flow and from the same EELV. Despite constant flow from the ventilator, pressure is highly dependent on starting conditions, which can change unpredictably between breaths. Several cycles may need to be observed.

In addition, after days of ventilation at supranormal end expiratory or inspiratory volumes, changes in viscoelastic tissue elements may mean that acute reduction of PEEP and V_t may induce greater atelectasis and airway closure than expected. Gradual restoration of normal EELV and V_t may be required.

Using pressure changes to inform ventilator settings

Quasi-static P–V loops (low flow VCV breaths) have been used to set ventilators in ARDS and airway pressure–time profiles (stress indices) have also been proposed to detect intrabreath recruitment and hyperinflation. Given the complexity of thoraco-abdominal mechanics, the flow, volume, and time dependency of resistance, and the ability of very different model pathologies to produce similar traces, these tools must be used very carefully.

Pressure control ventilation

In pressure control ventilation (PCV) breaths are delivered using a constant inspiratory pressure. The resulting tidal volume depends on the patient's respiratory mechanics and the inspiratory time.

Settings

In PCV the clinician can alter the:
- Target pressure (P_{set})
- Machine rate
- Inspiratory time/I:E ratio
- Inspiratory rise time (time to P_{set}), 'the ramp'.

Target pressure

In PCV, pressure is constant during inspiration ('square wave' pressure-time profile). This constant pressure regulation is achieved by:
- Rapid (ms) circuit pressure feedback
- Monitoring the rate of pressure change (avoiding overshoot).

The clinician must be clear whether the set inspiratory pressure is an absolute pressure or is relative to PEEP. Driving pressure = P_{set} – PEEP or $PEEP_i$ if greater.

Increasing P_{set} will usually increase V_t but it should prompt an examination of the I:E ratio (see below).

Immediate pressure reduction and emergency opening of the exhalation valve should occur if a critical circuit pressure limit is exceeded.

Machine rate

- With P_{set} and I:E fixed, stepwise increases in machine rate may initially increase minute volume.
- As the respiratory rate increases further, there is insufficient time for full inspiratory and expiratory equilibration.
- The maximum achievable minute ventilation depends on the patient's respiratory mechanics (see below).
- Further increases in respiratory rate will then decrease minute ventilation.
- Even when overall measured minute ventilation rises with increased rate, alveolar ventilation may fall because of a higher proportion of dead space with $PEEP_i$.
- Increases in respiratory rate should be assessed by monitoring V_t, minute ventilation and $PaCO_2$.
- Low impedance and rapid respiratory rate test the limits of ventilators. Machine performance may not be adequate to achieve the desired effects.

Inspiratory time

T_i should be sufficiently long to allow equilibration between alveolar and circuit pressure, and for intrapulmonary flow to stop. Shorter T_i may result in discontinuation of inspiratory flow before equilibrium occurs, and maximal V_t at that pressure will not be achieved.
- 95% equilibration takes ~ three inspiratory time constants (normally <1.5s but may be >5s in obstructive disease).

- The easiest method of identifying lack of equilibration is the persistence of gas flow at the end of inspiration.

Extending T_i beyond equilibration increases mean airway pressure but not V_t unless elastance changes or alveolar recruitment develops.

I:E ratio
- Maximal V_t will only be delivered in inspiration if there is also sufficient time to complete expiration (indicated by expiratory flow–time curve falling to zero before onset of next breath).
- When T_e is too short, $PEEP_i$ develops, reducing driving pressure.

Resulting flows and tidal volume
Flows
The resulting flow–time curves have a uni-exponential decay pattern in patients with high impedance, and a linear deceleration pattern in patients with low impedance.

Tidal volume
V_t in PCV depends on:
- Driving pressure
- T_i
- T_e and I:E ratio
- Thoracic resistance and compliance.

Effects of thoracic mechanics
Resistance
Increasing *expiratory* resistance reduces expiratory flow, prolongs the expiratory time constant, predisposes the patient to $PEEP_i$, and is easily unrecognized. Expiratory resistance is normally ~1.4 × inspiratory resistance but it is increased in COPD and markedly elevated in asthma. Where expiratory resistance is increased, long I:E ratios will allow:
- More complete expiration
- Lower EELV and $PEEP_i$
- Larger driving pressure and V_t.

Increasing *inspiratory* resistance reduces flow, prolongs the inspiratory time constant, and therefore increases the time required for equilibration between P_{set} and alveolar pressure.
- In adult patients with increased airway resistance, respiratory rates >12/min are not likely to increase alveolar minute ventilation.
- Falling expiratory resistance with successful treatment will reduce $PEEP_i$ and increase driving pressure.
- The increase in V_t and fall in $PaCO_2$ and $PaCO_2$-end tidal CO_2 gradient can be used to monitor the response to treatment.
- V_t should be closely monitored, and appropriate alarms set for high and low tidal volumes.

Compliance
- Falling compliance will reduce V_t.
- Reduced compliance will also decrease thoracic time constants, allowing faster equilibration with shorter T_i.

- In patients with reduced compliance, increasing machine rate is more likely to successfully increase minute ventilation (shorter expiratory time constant and less predisposition to $PEEP_i$ with shorter T_e).
- Rising compliance with successful treatment may produce higher V_t but increases thoracic time constants and risks development of $PEEP_i$.

Possible advantages of PCV over VCV

The theory that PCV *per se* is 'better' than VCV for injured lungs is unproven.

- The effects of ventilator settings on the patient are more important than the mode. Unfortunately, ventilator-derived measures of thoracic mechanics, P–V curves, and arterial blood gases do not reliably predict CT-apparent regional lung unit hyperinflation or atelectrauma.
- Trials comparing equivalent PCV and VCV settings in ARDS do not show consistent clinical effects or reduced mortality.
- Modern VCV with a decelerating flow profile, pressure limit, and inspiratory hold can mimic PCV.

Despite these caveats, there are a number of potential advantages to PCV when compared to VCV.

PaO$_2$ and compliance

Compared with VCV delivering similar V_t, T_i, and PEEP in patients with ALI/ARDS, PCV may modestly improve:

- PaO_2/FiO_2
- Compliance
- WOB.

PCV delivers most of the V_t early in inspiration, raising mean airway pressure. This recruits alveoli with slow time constants, providing more homogeneous gas distribution and better $\dot{V}/\dot{Q}$.

Caveat

- High or even normal PaO_2 is rarely a primary goal. Permissive hypoxaemia is acceptable in many conditions and may be preferable to VILI.
- Recruitment affects intrathoracic pressure, venous return, pulmonary vascular resistance, and cardiac output. Alterations in O_2 delivery affect SvO_2, therefore changes in PaO_2 associated with ventilator settings may be related to SvO_2 and not $\dot{V}/\dot{Q}$.

PaCO$_2$

The use of PCV in ALI/ARDS may reduce dead space fraction when compared with VCV. An associated fall in $PaCO_2$ of 0.25–0.5kPa has been reported.

Caveat

Lung units opened with airway pressures higher than pulmonary vascular pressures (West zone 1) may increase dead space and worsen $\dot{V}/\dot{Q}$.

Ventilator-induced lung injury

- To avoid VILI, ventilator settings should keep alveoli within normal elastic limits. With the development of $PEEP_i$, PCV still limits end inspiratory lung volume but this will rise with VCV.

- PCV-reduced peak pressure may reduce the pressure and volume in fast time constant lung units especially near central airways.
- In obstructive diseases a slower flow profile will reduce laminar shear stress.
- PCV with PEEP as part of a lower V_t strategy may produce less pulmonary inflammation than a historically 'normal practice' VCV.

Caveats

- Recruitment and oxygenation do not necessarily equal lung protection.
- Stretching alveoli beyond an acceptable elastic limit, and recurrent collapse and inflation, are injurious regardless of ventilatory mode.
- Models of lung injury suggest faster initial inspiratory flow typical of PCV, and resulting laminar shear stress is inflammatory and can adversely affect mechanics.
- In obstructive disease, EELV is related to barotrauma. With normal or increased compliance in these diseases, VCV with restricted V_t may more reliably control EELV and limit gas trapping.

Leaks and tubing

- Small V_t and uncuffed tubes with variable leak complicate paediatric V_t measurement.
- Unknown portions of the prescribed V_t in VCV distend and compress the breathing system.
- In PCV, breathing system and patient get the same prescribed pressure.
- Breathing system distension will reduce the peak flow, but with sufficient T_i the effect on V_t will be minimized.

WOB and patient comfort

- Patient inspiratory flow rates and V_t are variable. Negative intrathoracic pressure generation (patient work) and 'gasping' occur if the fixed flow and V_t of VCV are exceeded ('scooping' the pressure–time curve). PCV may avoid 'low flow suffocation' by meeting flow and volume demands.
- Fast flows, short T_i, and low V_t can cause spontaneous tachypnoea, hypocapnia, and PEEP$_i$ through reflexes affecting respiratory cycling. At the bedside, attempting to synchronize the ventilator to the patient's I:E and flow demands may be simpler with PCV.

Caveat

- Reducing WOB does not always reduce dyspnoea or respiratory drive. Multiple pathological drives (acidosis, lung inflammation/irritation, CNS dysfunction, and thoracopulmonary distortion are not removed by 'unloading' the diaphragm (e.g. inspiratory WOB in asthma might be reduced by volume or pressure assistance) but this may exacerbate hyperinflation, adversely effect ABGs and increase dyspnoea.
- Neither mode can provide consistently effective neuromechanical coupling.

Possible advantages of VCV over PCV

Reliable V_t control

In obstructive disease, inspiratory resistance and $PEEP_i$ reduce V_t in PCV. If resistance increases or improves, or if patient effort alters, V_t changes, with potentially important clinical consequences. Appropriate alarms are essential.

Simplicity

The ARDS Network chose VCV for their landmark trial of low V_t partly for simplicity.

Sleep quality

Synchronized VCV may provide better sleep quality than PSV. The relative effect of PCV is unknown.

3.4 Positive end expiratory pressure

Definitions

Positive end expiratory pressure

Airway pressure maintained above atmospheric pressure throughout the respiratory cycle by pressurizing the ventilator circuit.

Continuous positive airway pressure

Positive airway pressure applied during spontaneous ventilation where there is no IPPV.

Expiratory positive airway pressure

Synonymous with PEEP. EPAP is usually the term used during turbine-driven BiPAP.

Basics

Hypoxia caused by hypoventilation is easily corrected by mechanical ventilation or compensated for by increased FiO_2. PEEP is primarily a technique used to improve arterial hypoxia resulting from intrapulmonary shunt and venous admixture by recruiting additional alveoli for ventilation. PEEP increases FRC relative to closing capacity (CC). This reduces venous admixture as well as moving tidal ventilation to the most compliant portion of the pressure–volume relationship, reducing WOB and so total body oxygen consumption.

Physiological effects

Gas exchange

In responsive diseases, PEEP recruits alveoli and increases FRC. As FRC rises above closing volume (the volume at which end expiratory alveolar collapse occurs), $\dot{V}/\dot{Q}$ increases and shunt reduces. As lung volume rises, there may be a reduction in pulmonary vascular resistance and airway resistance. The response to PEEP may be variable in different conditions:

- Some diseases will respond better to PEEP than others. If the lung is not recruitable (e.g. pulmonary fibrosis or consolidation due to infection rather than oedema or atelectasis), then the potentially harmful cardiovascular effects of PEEP may predominate (heart lung interactions are discussed fully in 📖 Heart–lung interactions, p 275).
- PEEP may cause over-distension of areas of normal or high compliance, leading to increased dead space by compression of alveolar capillaries or by decreased cardiac output and reduced lung perfusion.
- PEEP may increase the shunt fraction in lobar or unilateral disease by diverting blood flow to less compliant non-ventilated areas of lung.
- The greater the heterogeneity of the lung disease the less predictable the effect of PEEP.

Ventilator-induced lung injury

- By moving FRC above the closing volume, there should be a reduction in repetitive tidal opening and closing of alveoli (atelectrauma), and resultant biotrauma.
- If lung units are over-distended, there may be an increase in volutrauma or barotrauma.

Work of breathing

Fig. 3.5 illustrates a typical inspiratory pressure volume (P–V) curve. Reduced compliance is seen in zones A (derecruitment) and C (over-distention). Maximal compliance is seen in zone B.

- Ventilation in zone A is thought to result in cyclical opening and closing of alveoli, causing lung damage (repetitive alveolar collapse expansion (RACE) injury or atelectrauma).
- Although lung recruitment may also take place during ventilation in zone B, the majority of alveoli are stable.
- In zone C there is over-distension of an increasing number of alveoli.

Ventilation on a steep part of the curve (B) is achieved at a lower WOB than ventilation at less compliant lung volumes (A and C). PEEP can be used to increase FRC above the lower inflection point at B. Providing lung volumes are kept below C this will have the effect of reducing WOB. In a spontaneously breathing patient with high WOB, this may result in:

- Reduced WOB and oxygen consumption
- Increased mixed venous saturation and therefore reduced consequences from venous admixture or shunt.

Unfortunately this is too simplistic an explanation. A whole series of compliance curves can be plotted from recruitable lungs depending on the initial PEEP. A compliance curve plotted from zero PEEP (ZEEP) will have a lower lung volume at $15cmH_2O$ than if the lungs were stably ventilated with $15cmH_2O$. This increased volume A–B (Fig. 3.6) represents recruited lung.

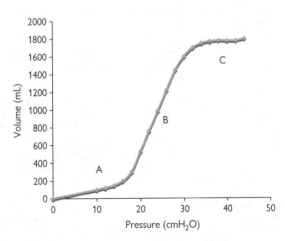

Fig. 3.5 Typical static inspiratory pressure volume curve.

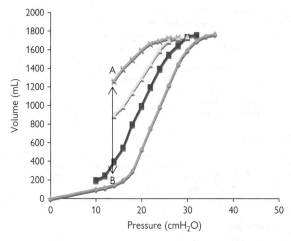

Fig. 3.6 Inspiratory pressure volume curves in recruited lungs (A) and derecruited lungs (B).

Threshold load
In the presence of PEEP$_i$ (see below), extrinsic PEEP (PEEP$_e$) reduces threshold load, the work required to initiate a breath or trigger the ventilator (see Fig. 3.7).

Cardiovascular system (see also 📖 Heart–lung interactions, p 275)
Preload
PEEP reduces cardiac output predominantly because of decreased preload. The precise mechanism for reduced preload is not certain. It may be due to effects on peripheral venous circulation rather than a decreased pressure gradient for venous return. The decrease in venous return has less effect in volume overloaded patients and can be counteracted by volume loading a normovolaemic patient.

RV performance
PEEP increases lung volumes and may cause direct compression of alveolar vessels. This increases pulmonary vascular resistance (RV afterload) and may increase tricuspid regurgitation and move the interventricular septum towards the LV cavity. Theoretically this will reduce LV compliance and contribute to the reduction in LV cardiac output. Some workers have suggested that the reduction in LV compliance is most attributable to direct compression of the pericardium by the lungs.

LV performance
PEEP increases the intrathoracic pressure (ITP) and therefore decreases
LV afterload by decreasing transmural pressure (the difference between
intracavity pressure and ITP). In normal patients this is a small effect relative to the fall in venous return, but in patients with LV failure and volume
overload, who are relatively protected from the fall in venous return,
this reduction in transmural pressure enhances ventricular ejection and
cardiac output. PEEP also reduces alveolar oedema (but not extravascular
lung water), by promoting movement of oedema fluid from the alveolar
space into the compliant interstitial space. It may be seen on CXR as an
increase in perivascular cuffing.

Oxygen delivery
The effect on oxygen delivery is unpredictable because of the opposing
effects of increased oxygenation and decreased cardiac output. The extent
to which PEEP is transmitted from the lungs to the heart and other great
vessels is greatly affected by lung compliance and the homogeneity of lung
disease. In conditions of poor compliance in homogenous lung disease as
little as 30% of PEEP may be transmitted.

Intracranial pressure
PEEP can increase right atrial and central venous pressure. This will
increase ICP and reduce cerebral perfusion pressure. This effect is most
marked in supine patients and is to a great extent mitigated by elevation of
the patient's head. Use of moderate levels of PEEP in head-injured patients
is generally safe and is likely to be beneficial if hypoxia is reduced.

Renal and splanchnic perfusion
PEEP is associated with a reduction in renal blood flow, urine output,
sodium excretion, creatinine clearance, hepatic blood flow, and gastric
mucosal pH. Experimentally it is difficult to know whether this is solely
a consequence of reduced cardiac output or if additional mechanisms
are involved. These effects are reduced by increasing cardiac output
with inotropes. PEEP-induced hormonal effects such as the activation of
sympathetic nerves, increased catecholamines, increased ADH, and up-
regulation of the renin-angiotensin system may be involved in mediating
or compensating for the observed effects.

Intrinsic PEEP
During passive expiration, airflow is described by an exponential decay
curve. The time constant of this process is the product of respiratory
system compliance and expiratory airway resistance with three to five
time constants required to complete expiration. In conditions of increased
expiratory airway resistance, low elastic recoil (increased compliance), or
reduced expiratory time, lung volume does not return to FRC by end
expiration. The volume of trapped gas exerts an intra-alveolar pressure (the amount depends on respiratory compliance) called auto PEEP
or $PEEP_i$. This results in dynamic hyperinflation, where inspiration starts
before the lungs have reached their resting volume.

$PEEP_i$ may also occur if expiratory muscle effort is high and expiration
is no longer passive. Expiratory flow limitation arises because ITP exceeds

intrabronchial pressure and creates a 'choke point', so that the difference between alveolar pressure and mouth or ventilator pressure is no longer the driving force. This is common in COPD, but has been reported in asthma, ARDS, and obesity.

Measurement of PEEP$_i$

Examination of the flow curve allows qualitative detection of PEEP$_i$. If end expiratory flow persists, PEEP$_i$ is present (see Fig. 3.8).

- Quantitative measurement is relatively straightforward during controlled ventilation in a passive patient.
  - Static PEEP$_i$ is measured with an end expiratory occlusion manoeuvre.
  - Dynamic PEEP$_i$ is the difference between PEEP$_e$ and the airway pressure at which inspiratory flow starts. Dynamic PEEP is lower than static PEEP$_i$ in airway obstruction, and similar if PEEP$_i$ is due to shortened expiratory time or large tidal volume.
- In spontaneously breathing patients an oesophageal balloon (and a gastric balloon for those with expiratory muscle recruitment) is required to accurately measure PEEP$_i$.

Effects of PEEP$_i$

PEEP$_i$ increases WOB by increasing the threshold load, i.e. the amount of work required to commence inspiratory flow or trigger the ventilator (see Fig. 3.7). This can account for 40% of the total WOB in ventilated patients with COPD. By the same mechanism it leads to wasted inspiratory efforts because of missed triggering. Reducing pressure support or increasing PEEP$_e$ may help (see 📖 Pressure support ventilation, p 144).

The effects of PEEP$_i$ on cardiovascular performance, gas exchange, and VILI are similar to those of PEEP$_e$.

PEEP$_i$ and PEEP$_e$

- In patients who are triggering the ventilator or spontaneously breathing, application of PEEP$_e$ will reduce the threshold load and WOB, and may reduce missed triggering (Fig. 3.7).
- In ventilated patients with COPD, PEEP$_e$ does not affect lung volumes until it approaches PEEP$_i$.
- In ventilated patients with asthma, because resistance to expiratory flow is not due to dynamic airway collapse, PEEP$_e$ has a greater effect on lung volumes. In ventilated asthmatic patients, if PEEP$_e$ is to be used at all, low levels should be used cautiously.
- If the application of PEEP$_e$ in a ventilated patient leads to over-distension, compliance will be reduced. If the tidal volume falls in pressure-controlled modes or airway pressure rises in volume-controlled modes, PEEP$_e$ is having a detrimental effect on lung mechanics. In the absence of these consequences, PEEP$_e$ can be safely applied.

Setting PEEP

In the considerable literature on PEEP, many superlatives have been used: optimal, ideal, best etc. This promotes the idea that there is a single 'best' value of PEEP for a patient. It also makes discussion of setting PEEP difficult as some readers will associate a specific term with a specific strategy

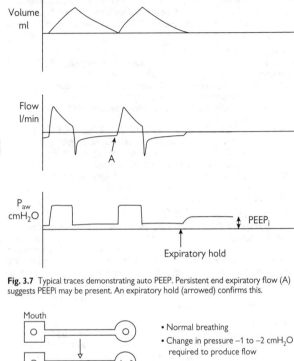

Fig. 3.7 Typical traces demonstrating auto PEEP. Persistent end expiratory flow (A) suggests PEEPi may be present. An expiratory hold (arrowed) confirms this.

Fig. 3.8 How $PEEP_i$ increases threshold load and how $PEEP_e$ reduces threshold load and reduces ineffective triggering.

of PEEP setting. Different principles are used for setting PEEP in different conditions.

ARDS/ALI

The rationale for using PEEP in ARDS has three strands:
- Improvement of oxygenation by decreasing intrapulmonary shunt.
- Increasing compliance and decreasing WOB (especially in spontaneously ventilated patients) by recruiting lung volume.
- Decreasing VILI cause by RACE (atelectrauma).

To date there is no clear consensus about the best level of PEEP or how to set PEEP. Many of the more recent studies have compared different ventilator strategies (including different levels of PEEP). It is widely accepted that low V_t and plateau pressure $<30cmH_2O$ confer a survival benefit. The ARDS Network (ALVEOLI)[1] trial randomized patients to the same lung protective ventilation, varying only in the combinations of PEEP and FiO_2. It was stopped early because there was no difference between groups. Post-hoc subgroup analysis suggests some difference occurred after a protocol change that made the PEEP difference between the groups bigger and this has left some thinking that this may have been a false negative trial.

Numerous approaches to setting PEEP have been advocated: maximal static compliance, best oxygenation, lowest intrapulmonary shunt fraction, maximal oxygen delivery, and maximal recruitment. Intellectually satisfying methods for setting PEEP, such as at, or just above, the lower inflection point on a static compliance curve, have been compared to a more conventional approach by Ranieri of targeting normal gas exchange.[2] The better outcome group not only had higher PEEP but also lower V_t.

There is no evidence to support a partisan 'high' or 'low' PEEP strategy in clinical practice. In particular, differing underlying pathophysiology in individual patients makes response to PEEP difficult to predict. In practice PEEP can be titrated to SpO_2, $PaO_2:FiO_2$ ratio, compliance, or oxygen delivery (taking into account adverse haemodynamic effects), or set using the static compliance curve (see below).

Static compliance curve

This approach requires a static compliance curve for each patient, with PEEP being set just above the lower inflection point. However, this is not universally available and unless the compliance curve is plotted from ZEEP there may be no lower inflection point.

When considering compliance in response to PEEP, the inspiratory compliance curve is less relevant than the expiratory curve. Indeed we should be aiming to ventilate a patient on the expiratory compliance curve after full recruitment.

Decremental PEEP trial
A decremental PEEP trial has the advantage of not requiring special equipment to plot a static compliance curve and yet it still pays intellectual homage to this cornerstone of respiratory physiology. It has not been shown to be better than any other method.
- Recruitment manoeuvre ($40cmH_2O$ maintained for 40s), which may be repeating to maximize PaO_2.
- Set PEEP to $20cmH_2O$ and decrease FiO_2 until SpO_2 92–94%.
- Reduce PEEP in decrements of $2cmH_2O$ every 2min until SpO_2 <90%.
- Repeat the recruitment manoeuvre.
- Set PEEP at the level before SpO_2 fell to 90%.

Much work is being done by ventilator manufacturers to develop breath-by-breath or rapid adjustments to PEEP. If beneficial this might create problems for clinicians using ventilators from a different manufacturer.

Cardiogenic pulmonary oedema
CPAP has been extensively studied in cardiogenic pulmonary oedema (CPO). The overwhelming majority of the published evidence is concordant. CPAP produces a more rapid resolution of CPO than conventional treatment and reduces the number of patients who require invasive ventilation. Meta-analysis suggests mortality is reduced (relative risk 0.64, 95% CI 0.44–0.92).[3] This effect is especially prominent when CPO was caused by myocardial infarction or ischaemia. Compared to BiPAP most studies have shown equivalence in outcome and one has shown CPAP to be superior. Thus CPAP is widely accepted to be the first-line mode of ventilatory assistance in CPO.

CPAP should be high enough to abolish negative swings in ITP (see 📖 Heart–lung interaction, p 275, and Continuous positive airway pressure, p 95).

COPD and asthma
COPD and asthma represent different pathophysiological processes but share some similarities when considering the effects of PEEP. Both diseases may be associated with dynamic hyperinflation during ventilation. When dynamic hyperinflation is caused solely by expiratory resistance and not flow limitation (common in asthma) the addition of external PEEP is transmitted to the distal airway and is additive to $PEEP_i$, increasing EELV and muscle load and further decreasing the mechanical advantage of the diaphragm. However, if there is flow limitation caused by dynamic airway compression (common in COPD), external PEEP (up to about 85% of $PEEP_i$) will not add to $PEEP_i$ or EELV and may actually decrease it.

During spontaneous ventilation, adding external PEEP may reduce inspiratory load, ease triggering, and improve patient–ventilator synchrony. Thus, in spontaneous modes of ventilation, especially in patients with COPD, external PEEP may be helpful.

Prophylaxis and postoperative PEEP

Atelectasis, pulmonary shunt, and consequent arterial hypoxia have been recognized after surgery for many years. It is only recently that good RCTs have shown outcome benefits such as lower rates of pneumonia or intubation for prophylactic PEEP. This has been demonstrated following oesophageal surgery and major abdominal surgery, but required continued CPAP for approximately 24h post operatively. This has important logistical and resource implications.

There is no good evidence for CPAP preventing the development of ARDS in patients thought to be at risk. There might be a benefit in immunocompromised patients with pulmonary infiltrates, although this is far from clear.

Contraindications

There are few contraindications to PEEP but understanding the underlying physiology identifies circumstances where disadvantageous side-effects outweigh the benefits. These include bronchopleural fistula, elevated intracranial pressure, dynamic hyperinflation without flow limitation, and hypovolaemia. Perhaps the only absolute contraindication is a tension pneumothorax.

It is noteworthy that it is prudent to discontinue all positive pressure to the airway when inserting an intercostal drain.

1 Brower RG, Lanken PN, MacIntyre N, *et al.* (2004). Higher versus lower positive end-expiratory pressures in patients with the acute respiratory distress syndrome. *N Engl J Med* **351**, 327–36.

2 Ranieri VM, Suter PM, Tortorella C, *et al.* (1999). Effect of mechanical ventilation on inflammatory mediators in patients with ARDS. *JAMA* **282**(1), 54–61.

3 Weng C, Zhao T, Liu Q, *et al.* (2010). Meta-analysis: Non-invasive ventilation in acute cardiogenic pulmonary edema. *Ann Int Med* **152**(9), 590–600.

Invasive ventilation modes

4.1 Synchronized intermittent mandatory ventilation

Introduction

Intermittent mandatory ventilation (IMV) is a mode in which mandatory breaths are ventilator or patient triggered, and delivered at a set volume or pressure, with a minimum frequency. Between the mandatory ventilator breaths, spontaneous patient breaths are facilitated but not assisted by the ventilator.

IMV was developed as an alternative to CMV and assist control ventilation (ACV). By allowing spontaneous breathing, it was thought that the $\dot{V}/\dot{Q}$ ratio at the lung base would be improved, that mean airway pressure and pulmonary vascular resistance (PVR) would decrease, cardiovascular stability would be enhanced, and respiratory muscle function maintained.

However, the patient's spontaneous breaths frequently coincided with ventilator-triggered breaths, leading to patient–ventilator asynchrony. To overcome this limitation, synchronized intermittent mandatory ventilation (SIMV) was introduced. SIMV allows the ventilator to synchronize with patient-triggered breaths, leading to significantly improved patient–ventilator interaction.

Basics

In IMV, mandatory breaths are volume or pressure controlled, ventilator triggered, and can be volume or time cycled. There is no attempt to synchronize with the patient's spontaneous effort. Depending on where the spontaneous breath occurs in the ventilator cycle, this can lead to:
- An augmentation of the patient breath (early inspiratory phase)
- Breath stacking (late inspiratory phase)
- An interruption of expiration (expiratory phase).

Synchronization

In SIMV, the mandatory breaths have similar characteristics to those in IMV. To improve patient–ventilator interaction, SIMV incorporates a 'synchronization' window in mid–late expiration during which spontaneous effort is augmented and turned into a mandatory breath. In effect, the next mandatory breath is delivered early to coincide with the patient's spontaneous respiratory effort.

The rules regarding the duration of this synchronization window vary between ventilator manufacturers and the clinician should be familiar with their particular ventilator. The longer the duration of the synchronization window, the more SIMV resembles ACV (see 📖 Assist control ventilation, p 140).

Spontaneous breaths outside this 'synchronization' window may be unsupported or pressure supported (SIMV + pressure support (PS)).

There are therefore three types of breath possible in (S)IMV + PS (see Fig. 4.1):
- Mandatory breaths: time triggered, volume or time cycled
- Supported breaths: patient triggered, flow cycled
- Synchronized breaths: patient triggered, volume or time cycled.

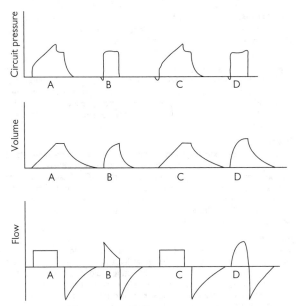

Fig. 4.1 The pressure–volume and flow traces for a patient ventilated with volume-controlled, volume-cycled SIMV + PS. Breath A is a mandatory volume-controlled, volume-cycled breath. Breath B is a spontaneous, patient-triggered breath, sensed outside the synchronization window. It is pressure supported and flow cycled. Breath C is a spontaneous effort sensed within the synchronization window. It is volume controlled and volume cycled. Breath D is a spontaneous effort, sensed outside the synchronization window with greater patient inspiratory effort. It is pressure supported and flow cycled, but the flow pattern resembles a spontaneous breath in a non-ventilated patient.

Physiological effects

Respiratory muscle strength and tone
Spontaneous patient-triggered breaths outside the synchronization window require use of respiratory muscles, theoretically maintaining their tone and function. Clinically, this is useful as the underlying indication for ventilation resolves and the proportion of respiratory work the patent undertakes is increased. A balance needs to be struck between preserving respiratory muscle strength and muscle fatigue caused by excessive WOB.

Reduced airway pressures
Spontaneous breaths and/or improved patient ventilator synchrony result in lower mean and peak airway pressures compared to ACV or CMV. This may be useful in some conditions (see below).

Indications

SIMV has been used to support patients with all causes of respiratory failure. More specific indications are listed below.

Post operative

In patients who have undergone surgery under general anesthesia with paralysis, SIMV provides reliable minimum mandatory ventilation as they regain their full spontaneous respiratory function. Periodic assessment of the patient's improving spontaneous breath characteristics assists the clinician with the reduction in mandatory breaths and the timing of extubation.

Airway injury

Patients with respiratory system anatomical injuries who need ventilator support and whose injuries may be worsened by high airway pressures may be treated more safely by SIMV rather than ACV. Examples of such injuries include tracheal tears and broncho-pleural fistulas. Other modes of ventilation (e.g. PSV) may provide even lower mean airway pressures than SIMV, and high-frequency oscillatory ventilation (HFOV) has been used successfully in this context.

Weaning

Soon after its development, SIMV became a popular mode for liberating patients from the ventilator. Although at least two studies[1,2] have shown that PSV or spontaneous breathing trials using T-pieces are both superior to (S)IMV, SIMV is still useful for facilitating transition from full mandatory ventilation to a spontaneous mode. It is also helpful in specific patients who do not tolerate weaning from mechanical ventilation by T-piece or PSV with PEEP, and in patients who require overnight ventilation.

Troubleshooting

Problems arising from SIMV can be divided into those arising during mandatory/synchronized breaths and those arising during spontaneous breaths.

Problems relating to mandatory breaths are covered in the chapter on ACV (see 📖 Assist control ventilation, p 140) and this section will only cover problems relating to spontaneous breaths.

Level of pressure support

Spontaneous breaths can be unsupported or pressure supported. The level of pressure support chosen is often titrated clinically.
- Unsupported or under-supported breathing will lead to increased WOB as circuit and tube resistance must be overcome.
- Over-support will lead to increased respiratory muscle atrophy and predispose the patient to dynamic hyperinflation.

See also 📖 Pressure support ventilation, p 144.

Asynchrony

SIMV performs much better than IMV or CMV. There are still potential problems, particularly when a spontaneous effort coincides with peak or plateau airway pressure of a controlled ventilator breath. In this circumstance, airway pressures rises and early termination of the breath is likely.

BIPAP has addressed this problem by allowing spontaneous breathing at any point during the respiratory cycle (if breaths coincide, the expiratory valve opens and airway pressures are controlled).

Reduced respiratory failure detection

A significant degree of respiratory muscle fatigue and failure can go undetected because the mandatory component of SIMV may provide just enough ventilation to prevent breaching traditional alarm limits (for low minute ventilation or respiratory rate). This can be avoided by setting appropriate alarm limits.

Trigger problems

See 📖 Patient ventilator asynchrony, p 267, Triggering/cycling, p 109, and Pressure support ventilation, p 144.

Initial set up

Full ventilatory support

SIMV is often the initial mode of ventilation used in ICU for respiratory failure and for patients who are recovering from surgery and anaesthesia. Each patient and disease is different and the ventilator settings should be adjusted to the individual. A useful starting set up for volume-controlled SIMV is:

- FiO_2 1.0. Wean to ≤0.6 as soon as possible.
- Frequency of 14–16/min.
- Tidal volume 6–8mL/kg of ideal body weight.
- Plateau pressure ≤30cmH$_2$O.
- I:E ratio 1:1.5.
- PEEP 5–10cmH$_2$O.

Setting up pressure-controlled SIMV is similar, although tidal volume is achieved by titrating inspiratory pressure.

Partial ventilator support

When SIMV is used in previously well patients recovering from general anesthesia, the goal is to provide just enough ventilatory support to prevent significant respiratory acidosis but not so much that their respiratory centres will be blunted by hypocapnia.

When patients are ready to commence spontaneous breathing:
- Set the mandatory breaths to give 50% of their predicted requirements, e.g. 50mL/kg/min, using a tidal volume of 8–10mL/kg.
- Set a flow trigger at 2–5L/min.
- Adjust the pressure support to achieve the desired tidal volume.
  This will normally be slightly less than the inspiratory pressure set for mandatory breaths.

Minimizing airway pressures

The goal is to provide enough ventilatory support to produce acceptable gas exchange, while reducing overall peak and mean airway pressures by providing a proportion of that support as spontaneous breaths. The higher the proportion of spontaneous breaths, and the lower the set airway pressures, the better.

The degree of mandatory support will depend on the nature and degree of the injury and the stage of recovery.

Ventilator weaning

When used for weaning, SIMV is usually augmented with pressure support.

The goal is to initially reduce the mandatory component of SIMV to 60–70% of the minute volume the patient required while on full ventilatory support. Mandatory breaths are further reduced depending on the patient's tolerance and the clinician's periodic assessment of the trend in the patient's spontaneous breath characteristics.

1 Esteban A, Frutos F, Tobin MJ, *et al.* (1995) A comparison of four methods of weaning patients from mechanical ventilation. *N Eng J Med* **6**, 345–50.
2 Brochard L, Rauss A, Benito S, *et al.* (1994) Comparison of three methods of withdrawal from ventilatory support during weaning from mechanical ventilation. *Am J Resp Crit Care Med* **150**, 896–903.

4.2 Pressure control ventilation

Pressure controlled ventilation (PCV) delivers a constant inspiratory pressure; the resulting volume and flow are variable. This is in contrast to volume controlled ventilation (VCV) where constant flow (or volume) results in variable pressure.

VCV allows the clinician to set the desired minute ventilation and to control $PaCO_2$. However, when compliance is low or resistance is high, elevated airway pressures may be required to deliver this tidal volume. Different lung unit time constants also mean that VCV may lead to regions of alveolar overdistension.

In PCV, alveolar pressure cannot be higher than the set ventilator pressure, but since tidal volumes and minute ventilation are not precisely controlled, $PaCO_2$ may rise.

The differences between PCV and VCV are dealt with in 📖 Pressure vs volume delivery, p 111.

Basics

The terms used for PCV include:
- Pressure limited
- Pressure targeted.

These terms are used interchangeably.
- When referring to PCV, convention dictates that at least some breaths are mandatory (i.e. ventilator rather than patient cycled).
- The clinician sets the inspiratory airway pressure, PEEP, respiratory rate, and inspiratory time.
- Tidal volume, flow, and alveolar ventilation depend on the respiratory system compliance and resistance.

Inspiratory flow
- Delivered airway pressure rises quickly, leading to a rapid increase in inspiratory flow. The pressure ramp or 'rise time' can be set on some ventilators. As the alveolar pressure rises, the pressure gradient between the ventilator and the alveolus falls, and the flow decreases in an exponential fashion. If the inspiratory time is long enough, ventilator and alveolar pressures equilibrate and inspiratory flow will cease (Fig. 4.2).

Tidal volume
Tidal volume will depend on:
- The pressure gradient between the ventilator (P_{insp}) and the alveolus (including intrinsic and extrinsic PEEP)
- Inspiratory time—if the inspiratory time is too short, alveolar and ventilator pressures do not equilibrate
- Inspiratory resistance—as resistance rises, the inspiratory time required for equilibration between circuit and alveolar pressures will increase
- Respiratory system compliance—as compliance falls, the tidal volume resulting from a set pressure will reduce.

Intrinsic PEEP
Since the tidal volume depends partly on the pressure difference between the delivered pressure and the alveolar pressure, increased PEEPi will reduce tidal volume.

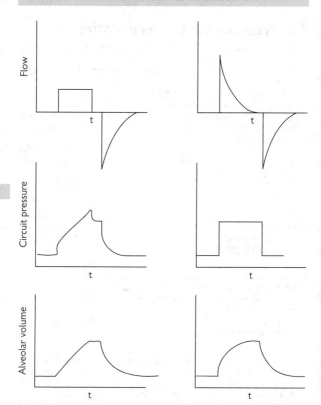

Fig. 4.2 Typical flow, pressure, and volume traces seen in VCV (L) and PCV (R).

PEEPi rises with respiratory frequency, increasing I:E ratio, and in patients with expiratory airflow limitation. It is recognized most easily by the persistence of end expiratory flow.

Alveolar ventilation and dead space

Alveolar ventilation may be paradoxically reduced by increasing the respiratory rate.

- Increasing respiratory frequency may cause a reduction in tidal volume:
  - Shorter inspiratory times may preclude equilibration of ventilator and alveolar pressure (look for persistent end inspiratory flow).
  - The development of PEEPi reduces the inspiratory pressure gradient.
- The relative proportion of dead space per breath increases with reduced tidal volume.

As a rule of thumb, if tidal volumes fall by more than 25% with an increase in frequency, there will be no gain in alveolar ventilation.

Advantages

PCV has several theoretical advantages over VCV.

- Alveolar pressure is limited and cannot be higher than the set inspiratory pressure.
- For a given peak airway pressure, the mean airway pressure is higher (see Fig. 4.3).
- For a given tidal volume, peak (and possibly plateau) airway pressure will be reduced.
- There may be improved distribution of ventilation because there is less end inspiratory gradient of pressure among regional units with heterogeneous time constants. CO_2 elimination is improved.
- Oxygenation may be improved (but will also depend on the plateau pressure and PEEP, see 📖 Effect of mechanical ventilation on oxygenation, p 282).

Disadvantages

- Tidal volume and minute ventilation vary with lung compliance or resistance.
- $PaCO_2$ is not strictly controlled.
- Requires monitoring of tidal volumes with appropriate alarms.
- If there is vigorous patient inspiratory effort, the intrapleural pressure may fall and transpulmonary pressure (and, potentially, VILI) may increase.

Setting the ventilator

P_{insp} or P_{set}

The clinician should be clear in setting P_{insp} whether it is relative to PEEP (i.e. ΔP) or an absolute pressure. The nomenclature varies between manufacturers.

Start at 12–$16cmH_2O$ above PEEP. Monitor the volume achieved and vary pressure to optimize tidal volume with a peak/plateau $<30cmH_2O$.

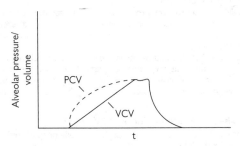

Fig. 4.3 For the same plateau pressure PCV increases alveolar pressure and volume compared with (square flow wave) VCV.

T_{insp} and respiratory rate

To realize the potential gas exchange advantages, T_{insp} should be long enough for alveolar pressure to equilibrate with ventilator pressure. End inspiratory flow should be zero.

The expiratory time is a function of T_{insp} and respiratory rate (e.g. respiratory rate 12 and T_{insp} 2s results in a breath cycle of 5s and I:E ratio 1:1.5).

Increasing respiratory rate without altering T_{insp} will change the I:E ratio. In the example above, increasing the respiratory rate to 20/min will result in a breath cycle time of 3s and I:E ratio of 2:1.

Most ventilators will display the I:E ratio as T_{insp} is altered.

Inverse ratio ventilation

Inverse ratio ventilation (IRV) is defined as an inspiratory time greater than expiratory time (I:E > 1:1). It results in improved oxygenation and reduced peak airway pressures compared with traditional VCV. IRV results in the following.

Higher mean airway and alveolar pressures

IRV allows mean airway pressure to be increased without increasing peak airway pressures.

Mean airway pressure (P_{aw}) can be approximated by the equation:

$$P_{aw} = (P_{insp} - PEEP)(T_{insp}/\text{breath cycle time}) + PEEP$$

Increasing the I:E ratio therefore increases mean airway pressure without changing PEEP or P_{insp}. Increased mean airway pressure may improve oxygenation and/or cause haemodynamic compromise (see 📖 Effect of mechanical ventilation on oxygenation, p 282). There seems to be no particular advantage when compared to other modes of ventilation that raise mean airway pressure.

Higher total PEEP (extrinsic PEEP plus intrinsic PEEP)

Because of the limited expiratory time, PEEPi often develops when IRV is used. Although some authors argue that PEEPi is advantageous compared with PEEPe, studies suggest little difference or a slight advantage for PEEPe in terms of gas exchange improvement.

Improved gas distribution

This is discussed above. The prolongation of the inspiratory time will lead to more complete equilibration between alveolar units of different time constants. There are theoretical advantages, but little evidence for significant clinical differences.

Use of IRV has declined in recent years. As the mechanisms of gas exchange improvement have become clearer, other solutions to increase total PEEP and mean airway pressure have emerged. These alternatives are usually clearer in their objectives and may have less haemodynamic consequences.

Spontaneous breathing during PCV

PCV may be delivered as a purely mandatory mode or synchronized with patient effort (P-SIMV).

P-SIMV and PCV are identical in a passive patient. In a patient making respiratory effort, the synchronization algorithm for P-SIMV functions in the same way as volume-controlled SIMV (see 📖 Synchronized intermittent mandatory ventilation, p 130). There is a synchronization window in expiration prior to the following breath.

If the ventilator is triggered during this period, the mandatory breath due to be delivered is synchronized with patient effort. This mandatory breath is pressure controlled and time cycled.

If patient effort is detected outwith the synchronization window, this breath is often pressure supported (P-SIMV + PS). This resulting breath is flow cycled.

Conclusion

- Although no change in important outcomes has ever been demonstrated, PCV is a popular mode of ventilation. As clinicians have moved form precise control of minute volume (MV) and $PaCO_2$ towards lung protection as an important goal of mechanical ventilation, the potential gas exchange advantages have convinced many that pressure control should be the default method of ventilation.

4.3 Assist control ventilation

Assist control ventilation (ACV) is a mandatory mode of ventilation where breaths can be ventilator or patient triggered, delivered with a set volume and at a minimum frequency. It is a technological evolution from CMV, where breaths are solely ventilator triggered.

The patient-triggered breaths are sometimes called assisted breaths and this mode has also been called CMV with assist or assisted mechanical ventilation.

Basics

Inspiratory triggering

Breaths can be time or patient triggered.

• Patient-triggered breaths are initiated by flow or pressure triggers.
• Time triggering depends on the set frequency and is automatically inhibited if there is an ongoing patient-triggered breathing cycle.

Inspiratory phase

Although ACV may be used in flow-volume or pressure-targeted modes, most ventilators delivering ACV are flow controllers. The flow pattern is usually constant (square wave), although modern microprocessors allow some variation to this pattern (e.g. a decelerating flow waveform).

The inspiratory phase characteristics are determined by the frequency, volume, and inspiratory flow set by the clinician and their relationship to the respiratory system compliance and resistance. Peak and plateau airway pressures and the breathing cycle time depend on the interaction of these factors.

Inspiratory pause

Many ventilators allow for the setting of an inspiratory pause. The inspiratory pause may produce additional alveolar recruitment. It also allows determination of plateau airway pressure.

Cycling

All breaths are volume or time cycled (i.e. mandatory breaths) regardless of the trigger.

Expiratory phase

Expiration is passive and exponential. The speed of expiration is determined by the expiratory time constant. Expiratory time should be sufficiently long to allow complete emptying (> three expiratory time constants, minimal end expiratory flow).

Indications

ACV is indicated whenever a patient needs invasive positive pressure ventilation and is one of the most common initial modes of invasive ventilation in the USA because of its relative conceptual simplicity. This is particularly useful in locations where mechanical ventilation is often commenced by non-physician healthcare personnel.

It unloads the respiratory muscles, improves gas exchange, and allows complete respiratory muscle rest without having to paralyse or significantly sedate the patient.

It may be used whenever full mechanical ventilation is needed for any reason and is particularly useful as initial full ventilator support for most forms of respiratory failure. Once the underlying cause of respiratory failure begins to resolve, patients are switched to a weaning mode of ventilation such as PSV or intermittent T-piece.

It differs from (S)IMV because with ACV every breath, whether triggered by the patient or by the machine, is a full, mandatory breath. With (S) IMV, the patient may breathe spontaneously (supported or unsupported) between mandatory breaths.

Physiologic effects
- $\uparrow \dot{V}/\dot{Q}$ ratio by alveolar recruitment.
- $\downarrow PaCO_2$ by increasing minute ventilation.
- $\downarrow$WOB.
- $\downarrow$RV preload, $\downarrow$LV afterload.

In addition, ACV has been reported to cause less sleep fragmentation and central apnoea than PSV, especially in heart failure patients.

Adverse effects
- May compromise cardiac output and oxygen delivery, especially if there is significant patient ventilator asynchrony.
- Significant dynamic hyperinflation may develop with rapid respiratory rates and/or large tidal volumes. This can be severe and the potentially unrecognized increases in $PEEP_i$ may lead to considerable cardiovascular instability.
- As with all controlled modes of positive pressure ventilation, it may cause ventilator induced diaphragmatic dysfunction.

Troubleshooting
The majority of problems with ACV arise from patient–ventilator asynchrony (see 📖 Patient ventilator asynchrony, p 267, and Pressure support ventilation, p 144).

Auto triggering
The ventilator delivers a breath without patient effort. Causes include:
- Trigger too sensitive
- Presence of a ventilator circuit leak
- Movement of fluid or debris in the ventilator circuit, leading to significant changes in circuit flow and pressure
- Cardiac oscillations.

Solutions
- Make flow or pressure trigger less sensitive. Balance any increase in WOB with the reduced number of autotriggers.
- Clear ventilator circuit of fluid, condensate, and any debris.

Ineffective triggering
The ventilator does not detect the patient's efforts. May be caused by:
- Dynamic hyperinflation and high $PEEP_i$
- Weak respiratory muscle strength.

Solutions
- Make inspiratory trigger more sensitive. Use a flow trigger.
- If dynamic hyperinflation or high $PEEP_i$ is the problem, adjust the frequency and tidal volume downwards until the expiratory flow wave form is approaching baseline on every breath and the peak airway pressure is not increasing with successive breaths.
- In the presence of expiratory flow limitation (e.g. COPD), consider increasing extrinsic PEEP ($PEEP_e$). This will reduce the effort required to trigger the ventilator and WOB. Ensure compliance does not decrease (i.e. that end *inspiratory* airway pressure does not rise with the increase in end *expiratory* pressure, signifying an increase in $PEEP_e$ above $PEEP_i$) (see ⏍ Positive end expiratory pressure, p 119).

Double triggering
- Auto-triggering (as above).
- Inspiratory flow too low.
- Tidal volume too low.

Solution
- Adjust inspiratory flow and then tidal volume upwards. Each inspiratory flow wave should have a smooth ascent. Patient comfort should improve (decreased respiratory rate, heart rate, blood pressure, agitation, and sedation requirements).

Premature inspiratory flow cessation
- Inspiratory flow too low.
- Tidal volume too low.
- Peak airway pressure above set maximum limit.
- Patient generating reverse airway flow, e.g. from cough, hiccough.
- Airway occlusion.
- Ventilator circuit leak.

Solutions
- Adjust inspiratory flow and then tidal volume upwards.
- Check alarm settings.
- Identify leak.

Absence of inspiratory pause
- Large airway leak, e.g. bronchopleural fistula, ET-tube cuff deflated.
- Ventilator circuit leak.

Solution
- Locate and correct the leak.

Incomplete expiration
Recognized as persistent end expiratory flow at the start of the next inspiration.
- Tidal volume too large.
- Frequency too high.
- New bronchospasm.
- Patient agitated.

Incomplete expiration leads to $PEEP_i$—see below.

Solutions
- Give bronchodilators for bronchospasm.
- Adjust tidal volume then inspiratory flow downwards until expiratory phase flow consistently reaching baseline.
- Lengthen expiratory time (increase inspiratory flow rate, reduce respiratory rate or tidal volume).

Dynamic hyperinflation and PEEP$_i$

Although PEEP$_i$ usually implies dynamic hyperinflation, the two terms are not identical. Dynamic hyperinflation is the start of inspiration before the respiratory system has reached its resting volume. PEEP$_i$ can be present in the context of normal lung volumes if expiratory muscle recruitment is high (for example in COPD).

Dynamic hyperinflation is a particular hazard with ACV because the ventilator will attempt to deliver the set tidal volume with each triggered breath. The limiting factor at this point is the upper maximum airway pressure alarm limit, and indeed the diagnosis is often made because of a continually sounding maximum airway pressure alarm.

It can lead to ineffective triggering, excessively elevated airway pressure, increased WOB, and cardiovascular compromise.

Solutions
- Lengthen expiratory time (increase inspiratory flow rate, reduce respiratory rate or tidal volume).
- Consider disconnecting the patient from the ventilator for no more than 10s, reconnecting with reduced tidal volume, and then adjusting inspiratory flow downwards until successive expiratory flow wave forms reach baseline.
- If dynamic hyperinflation is severe enough to cause haemodynamic compromise, disconnect the patient from the ventilator for 5–10s and let the lungs deflate to baseline. Reconnect at a much reduced frequency and/or tidal volume.
- If the combination of excessive patient triggers and pulmonary pathology is leading to dynamic hyperinflation, consider a brief period of increased sedation or paralysis, or another mode of ventilation.

Initial set up
- FiO$_2$ 1.0. Wean to ≤0.6 as soon as tolerated.
- Frequency of 14–16/min.
- Tidal volume 8–10mL/kg of ideal body weight if ALI/ARDS is not an anticipated diagnosis, tidal volume 6mL/kg if ALI/ARDS anticipated.
- Peak inspiratory flow rate at 50–60L/min initially and then titrated to achieve a peak airway pressure of ≤30cmH$_2$O. Since plateau airway pressure is by definition always less than peak airway pressure, this early titration ensures one is within the safe airway pressure zone.
- Flow trigger sensitivity 2L/min.
- Adjust either the peak inspiratory flow or tidal volume to achieve the desired I:E ratio.
- If the patient is conscious and triggering the ventilator, adjust the tidal volume and/or inspiratory flow to match the patient's demand.
- Consider the inspiratory flow pattern (square wave versus decelerating) if the ventilator allows such adjustments. Many clinicians prefer decelerating flow.

4.4 Pressure support ventilation

Pressure support ventilation (PSV) is a widely used, well-tolerated, synchronized mode of ventilator support. There are no mandatory breaths. It is one of the most commonly used weaning modes.

PSV may reduce sedation requirements, decrease respiratory muscle disuse atrophy, and compensate for the additional WOB imposed by the underlying disease process, the ETT, and the breathing circuit.

Precise control of tidal volume, MV, mean P_{aw}, and I:E ratios is not possible. Under-recognized disadvantages include unidentified ventilator patient dysynchrony, excessive support, and poor sleep.

PSV is patient triggered, pressure targeted, and flow cycled.

Basics

Inspiratory triggering
Inspiration is triggered by the patient, or by changes in pressure or flow (see 📖 Triggering and cycling, p 109).

Inspiratory pressure delivery
- When inspiration has been triggered, the ventilator raises airway pressure to the set PS level.
- The speed of initial pressurization (the pressure 'ramp') may be adjusted on some ventilators.
- Flow pattern can vary between a decelerating flow pattern in mainly passive patients and a sine wave flow pattern in patients making effort throughout inspiration.

Cycling (expiratory triggering)
- PSV is flow cycled.
- Inspiration ends when inspiratory flow falls below a certain percentage of the peak flow (usually 25%).
- The expiratory trigger sensor (ETS) may be adjusted on some ventilators.

Indications

With non-invasive ventilation
- Exacerbation of COPD with respiratory acidosis.
- No proven efficacy in other forms of acute respiratory failure (ARF), although it is commonly used.
- Long-term ventilation.

With invasive ventilation
- Exacerbation of COPD with respiratory acidosis.
- Any form of ARF where partial ventilatory support is required.

Not suitable when precise control of tidal volume, MV, mean P_{aw}, or I:E ratios required.

Physiological effects

CO_2, breathing pattern, and WOB

The introduction of PSV usually causes an increase in tidal volume and a decrease in respiratory rate while overall MV increases. Further increases in PS often increase tidal volume and reduce respiratory rate without an overall increase in MV.

- Dead space ventilation is reduced.
- There is a reduction in hypercapnia and respiratory acidosis.
- As PS increases, WOB reduces in proportion up to a point where no further reduction occurs, but problems with over-support begin.

The mechanisms for these changes are discussed in depth in 📖 Effect of mechanical ventilation on control of breathing, p 257.

O_2

- Oxygenation often improves. Generally overall $\dot{V}/\dot{Q}$ increases and there is some alveolar recruitment, reducing shunt and improving $\dot{V}/\dot{Q}$ mismatch. This is affected by the underlying disease process and cardiovascular status.
- PEEP and FiO_2, as well as changes in WOB, oxygen consumption, and SvO_2 are also important.

The effect of mechanical ventilation on oxygenation is discussed in detail in 📖 Effect of mechanical ventilation on oxygenation, p 282.

Problems with synchronization

Ventilator inspiration and expiration should start and finish as closely as possible to neural inspiration and expiration. It is easy to assume that, since PSV is patient triggered and flow cycled, synchronization is straightforward. While modern ventilators perform much better than older ventilators, problems still exist.

Trigger delay

Trigger delay is recognized when the patient seems to be attempting to inspire but there is no inspiratory flow for a period at the start of inspiration. Some trigger delay is inevitable. See 📖 Patient ventilator asynchrony, Fig. 5.12, p 267.

- Check that the rate of pressurization is not too slow.
- Try the solutions for ineffective triggering (below).

Ineffective triggering

Ineffective triggering occurs when there is no PS provided for a patient's inspiratory effort.

- It is often unrelated to the sensitivity of the trigger (i.e. turning down the pressure or flow required to initiate a breath makes no difference).
- Recognition is most accurately done with an oesophageal pressure monitor, but these are rarely used outside clinical trials.
- On the pressure and flow waveform (see 📖 Patient ventilator asynchrony, Fig. 5.13, p 267) small perturbations may occur (a small reduction in pressure and increase in flow in the expiratory portion of the waveform), not followed by a positive pressure breath.

- Comparing the patient's breathing pattern with the ventilator breathing pattern is a sensitive method of detection.
- A respiratory rate of <20 should make the clinician check carefully for wasted efforts.

Causes
- $PEEP_i$ is the most common cause of ineffective efforts. A much greater inspiratory effort must be generated by the patient to overcome the $PEEP_i$ and trigger a breath (see 📖 Positive end expiratory pressure, p 119, and Fig. 3.8).
- Over-supported breaths. Ineffective breaths are more common immediately following breaths with large tidal volumes where expiration takes longer, particularly with long expiratory time constants. Also, ventilator inspiratory time (vTi) may extend into neural expiratory time (nTe), thereby lowering the time before the next neural (and ventilator) inspiration.

Treatment
The possible solutions to wasted efforts/ineffective triggering and trigger delay are:
- Alter trigger sensitivity
- Change to flow triggering—with flow triggers there is a statistically (although perhaps not clinically) significant reduction in WOB (📖 Triggering and cycling, p 109).
- Increase $PEEP_E$ to help overcome the effects of $PEEP_i$.
- Decrease PS to reduce the chance of over-support.
- Adjust ETS if set at a low level (see below).
- Reduce instrumental dead space (HME, catheter mounts).

Auto-triggering
Auto-triggering is the triggering of inspiratory support by something other than the patient's respiratory effort. For example:
- Leaks in the circuit or round a mask (interpreted as patient respiratory effort by the ventilator)
- Motion of liquid that has collected in the ventilator tubing
- Cardiac oscillations (especially in high output states).

Recognition and treatment
- The clue is a high respiratory rate without apparent patient effort or any decrease in the pressure tracing preceding delivery of positive pressure (see 📖 Patient ventilator asynchrony, Fig. 5.15, p 267).
- The diagnostic test is to remove the potential cause or decrease the sensitivity of the trigger (make it more difficult to trigger a breath).
- These manoeuvres are also the treatment. This will result in slightly increased effort to initiate inspiration, but improved synchrony.

Double cycles
Double cycles are two episodes of ventilator support during only one patient effort. They may be intermittent. See 📖 Patient ventilator asynchrony, Fig. 5.14, p 267.

Causes
- Premature cycling to expiration because the expiratory trigger is too high. The first ventilator expiration occurs during neural inspiration,

patient inspiratory effort continues and triggers a second breath in rapid succession. Reduce the ETS.
- Too rapid early pressurization (very fast pressure ramp) may lead to a reduction in vTi compared with nTi. Slow the ramp speed.
- Auto-triggering can also present as double breaths.

Cycling
- Ideally the end of vTi should perfectly coincide with the patient's nTi. This is rarely the case.
- Even with a system that could recognize the neural output from the respiratory centre, there would be some delay as the machine recognized and produced a response to the neural changes.
- The closest available system (neurally adjusted ventilatory assist) uses the diaphragmatic EMG signal and is discussed on 📖 Neurally adjusted ventilatory assist, p 178.
- The expiratory trigger is usually set at 25–30%. It may be fixed or adjustable (see below).

Problems with pressure delivery
Pressure ramp

Increased patient effort should result in increased delivered flow and volume. The initial inspiratory flow rate will alter the rate of pressurization (pressure ramp). This is adjustable on many ventilators.

When the patient demand is high, WOB may be increased if the rate of pressurization is too low, i.e. the patient is 'sucking' against the ventilator. However, too fast a rate may cause initial pressure overshoot, an early termination of inspiration, and double breaths or an increased respiratory rate (increasing inspiratory flow increases respiratory rate through an immediate neural mechanism). This is poorly tolerated by patients.

Over-support

At high levels of support there is a tendency to encourage hyperventilation, resulting in a respiratory alkalosis. This alkalosis leads to apnoeas, desaturations, and micro arousals, resulting in more sleep disturbance than is seen in other ventilatory modes and is the reason many weaning units fully ventilate patients overnight. This problem is exacerbated by increasing the PS level to compensate for the natural increase in CO_2 that occurs in sleep. Over-support also results in ineffective triggering (see above).

Practicalities
Initial setup
- Use a flow trigger routinely. Start at 5L/min.
- Adjust trigger sensitivity to a lower level if trigger delay or missed efforts are a problem. Intermittent use of a pressure trigger allows measurement of $P_{0.1}$ (See 📖 Monitoring on a ventilator, p 231).
- P ramp should be set to avoid pressure overshoot, allow patient comfort, and prevent increased WOB: 50ms is a reasonable starting figure.

The PS level should be adjusted using the following indices: none are known to be superior so assessing a mix is the best compromise:
- Respiratory rate <35.

- Tidal volume 6–8mL/kg unless respiratory rate low, patient comfortable.
- $P_{0.1}$ <5cmH$_2$O.
- No use of accessory muscles or signs of respiratory distress.
- No wasted efforts or PEEP$_i$.

Expiratory trigger sensitivity

Set to 25–30%.

Adjust upwards

- In obstructive diseases ETS should be set higher (~50%).
  - A low ETS will increase inspiratory time (vTi), which will encroach into neural expiratory time (nTe).
  - This will shorten vTe and produce expiratory muscle activation during vTi.
  - End inspiratory airway pressure will increase, and dynamic hyperinflation and PEEP$_i$ may develop.
  - Ineffective triggering may result.
- If neural expiration starts significantly before ventilator expiration (sudden increase in airway pressure curve just pre expiration).
- In NIV, ETS should be set high (~50%) with additional backup time cycling.
- In NIV leaks are common (even desirable).
  - The criteria for cycling to expiration may not be reached because flow continues at a high level through the leak.

Adjust downwards

- In diseases with low compliance the ETS should be set low (5%).
  - This should increase tidal volume and reduce respiratory rate by extending inspiratory time.
- If there are double breaths.
  - In bronchospasm it may not be possible to lengthen expiration enough to avoid breath stacking and the development of PEEP$_i$.
  - A controlled form of ventilation may be necessary.

The effect of ETS adjustment in practice is often disappointing. This mainly results from a sine wave flow pattern as opposed to a decelerating flow pattern, or because active expiration is started by the patient before cycling. In these circumstances, the down slope of the expiratory flow curve is so steep that the time between, for example, 50% and 5% is minimal and changes do not have a clinically significant impact.

Pressure support, respiratory rate, and triggering

When adjusting PS, the clinician should be clear that the adjustments are having the desired effect.

- An increase in PS will often reduce respiratory rate. This may be due to a neural mechanism secondary to extension of vTi into nTe (📖 Effect of mechanical ventilation on control of breathing, p 257).
- However, a reduction in measured respiratory rate may also be due to the development of ineffective efforts.

- Conversely, an increase in respiratory rate with reducing pressure support may *not* be due to respiratory distress, but previously unrecognized wasted efforts now triggering the ventilator.

No matter how diligent a clinician is in setting these parameters, the limiting factors may be the electronic logic, the patient's physiology and pathology, and the underlying assumptions made in the inspiratory and expiratory triggers. It is not always possible to achieve satisfactory synchronization, gas exchange, or reduction in WOB.

Use of PSV as a weaning mode

Reduction of ventilatory support

PSV is one of the most common weaning modes. Levels of support are titrated to breathing pattern, signs of respiratory distress, and arterial blood gases. In general, support is reduced as the patient's respiratory function improves. Some ventilators will automatically reduce support according to pre-programmed algorithms (Adaptive Support Ventilation, SmartCare).

Use of PSV to aid the decision to extubate
- Once PS has been reduced to 5–8cmH$_2$O, extubation may be considered.
- This level of support is designed to overcome the resistance of the ETT and the breathing circuit.
- Theoretically, if the correct level of support is chosen, the WOB pre extubation should be the same as that post extubation.
- Therefore, if a patient tolerates breathing with these low levels of support, and is otherwise ready for extubation (📖 Extubation, p 350), extubation may proceed safely.
- Judging the likely post-extubation WOB is difficult. It will vary with the underlying disease as well as the upper airway anatomy.

The decision to extubate is sometimes difficult. It is dealt with in detail in 📖 Extubation, p 350. Automatic tube compensation is sometimes used with PSV (see 📖 Software enhancements, p 165)

Troubleshooting

Hypercapnia

This is a common blood gas abnormality when using PSV. An integrated approach to management can be found in 📖 Hypercapnia while on a ventilator, p 296, but there are a few points specific to PSV that are worth special mention here:
- Increased pressure support (within safe limits) will in general reduce CO$_2$, as explained above.
- Compared with controlled ventilation, during PSV the patient's efforts and the ventilatory support are more likely to be additive. In controlled ventilation the chest wall is often passive, reducing the compliance of the respiratory system. Therefore it is usually possible to deliver a higher tidal volume and minute ventilation for a given airway pressure.
- It may not be possible to equal the minute ventilation achieved by PSV using a controlled ventilator mode (e.g. converting to SIMV or BIPAP). If the MV is already high, carefully think about the tidal volume

and respiratory rate you need to set in order to increase the MV significantly.
- An over-sedated patient will always have a tendency to be hypercarbic despite the level of PS because of reduced respiratory drive.
- High ITPs may paradoxically increase the $PaCO_2$ by increasing physiological dead space.
- A slight overnight increase in CO_2 does not usually require any alteration in PS.

Hypoxaemia

An integrated approach to the management of hypoxaemia in ventilated patients can be found in 📖 Effect of mechanical ventilation on oxygenation, p 282. Points specific to PSV:
- In PS, flow cycling tends to shorten the inspiratory time and increase the expiratory time, and therefore reduce MP_{aw} compared with controlled ventilation.
- In diseases that respond to increases in MP_{aw}, increasing PEEP or prolonging inspiration (by lowering ETS or by changing ventilatory mode) may help.
- The converse is also true. When changing a patient from a time-cycled controlled ventilation mode to PSV a deterioration in gas exchange is often seen despite identical support and control pressure levels.
  - This results from a reduction in MP_{aw}, causing an increase in shunt and a reduction in overall $\dot{V}/\dot{Q}$ ratio with associated gas exchange deterioration.
  - This is often interpreted as a failure of spontaneous ventilation with a resultant return to a controlled mode of ventilation.
  - The simplest way to counteract this fall in MP_{aw} is to increase PEEP.

4.5 Airway pressure release ventilation and biphasic positive airway pressure

Airway pressure release ventilation (APRV) combines high CPAP levels with brief pressure releases and unsupported spontaneous breathing. APRV has been shown to improve oxygenation at lower peak airway pressures and have similar (surrogate) outcomes to conventional ventilator strategies in ARDS and ALI.

Reported advantages include reduced shunt and dead space, reduced sedation requirements, and improved cardiovascular function and end organ perfusion.

Biphasic positive airways pressure (BIPAP) utilizes similar principles and is properly considered in conjunction with APRV.

APRV

APRV is a time-cycled pressure-controlled mode that allows unsupported spontaneous respiration throughout the respiratory cycle. Rather than a conventional ventilatory mode in which tidal volumes are intermittently delivered, it is useful to think of APRV as high-level CPAP with short pressure drops or 'releases' to facilitate ventilation and CO_2 clearance. Advantages include:

- Improved $\dot{V}/\dot{Q}$ matching
- Lower peak airway pressure for a given mean airway pressure
- CO_2 clearance maintained with lower MV
- Cardiovascular stability
- Reduced vasopressor requirements
- Preserved renal and splanchnic blood flow
- Reduced sedation and paralysis requirements.

Basics

Hypoxaemia in ALI or ARDS is largely due to $\dot{V}/\dot{Q}$ mismatch and intrapulmonary shunting in areas of consolidation and alveolar collapse. This occurs predominantly in the postero-basal portions of the lung as a result of hydrostatic forces, raised intra-abdominal pressure, and diaphragmatic elevation. Recruiting this area of collapsed lung may be achieved by a combination of:

- CPAP with moderate to high levels of airway pressure
- Spontaneous breathing—contraction of the posterior part of the diaphragm assists in recruiting the postero-basal lung (Fig. 4.4).

Recruitment of alveoli continues throughout inspiration. As alveoli open, compliance improves. Conventional ventilation may allow cyclic expiratory derecruitment of alveoli. There is therefore no improvement in compliance, and the next inflation requires similarly high pressures. APRV may be considered to be an almost continuous, mild recruitment manoeuvre.

In addition, alveolar recruitment reduces PVR and improves right ventricular function.

Spontaneous breathing

Diaphragmatic contraction in unsupported spontaneous breathing preferentially recruits the postero-basal areas of the lung (Fig. 4.4). As pressure

(A)

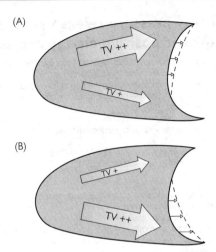

(B)

Fig. 4.4 Distribution of ventilation in a controlled mechanical breath (A) and a spontaneous breath (B).

support is added, this effect becomes less pronounced, the inspiratory flow waveform becomes decelerating, and the gas distribution of the resulting breath becomes more ventral (Fig. 4.4). At high levels of pressure support, the gas distribution eventually mirrors that of mandatory ventilator breaths and the recruitment advantage is lost.

Diaphragmatic contraction also reduces intrapleural and ITP. This increases venous return, augments cardiac output, and improves splanchnic and renal perfusion.

Unsupported spontaneous breaths are more likely to produce a sinusoidal flow pattern similar to normal unintubated breathing, where flow and pressure are linked to patient effort. Because the patient can breathe at any point in the respiratory cycle, this is a well-tolerated mode, reflected in the reduced sedation requirements. Some ventilators attempt to synchronize the changes from the high-pressure level (P_{high}) to the low-pressure level (P_{low}) and vice versa with patient's inspiratory and expiratory efforts.

The cardiovascular, splanchnic, renal, and sedative sparing effects are only seen when spontaneous respiration is unsupported.

Using tube-resistance compensation does not pose the same problems as adding PSV, and may help to reduce the additional WOB imposed by the breathing circuit.

Pressure releases

The WOB required to maintain sufficient minute ventilation with unsupported breaths will be too great for many patients. To assist with CO_2 clearance, the high CPAP levels in APRV are 'released' momentarily, to a lower level (P_{low}). To prevent de-recruitment, this release time is kept as short as possible and by definition in APRV is less than 1.5s. The I:E ratio is irrelevant because APRV is best thought of as CPAP (with short releases).

Effects on $\dot{V}/\dot{Q}$ mismatch, shunt, and deadspace

The combination of sustained airway pressure and unsupported spontaneous breathing recruits previously atelectatic alveoli, reducing shunt fraction and improving oxygenation.

APRV improves CO_2 clearance for a given minute ventilation. Several mechanisms have been postulated:

- Cardiac pulsation may improve CO_2 diffusion into large airways during T_{high}, reducing the CO_2-free expired gas.
- Unventilated alveoli are recruited, and ventilation to previously well perfused alveoli is improved.
- As lung volume increases, pulmonary vascular resistance decreases and blood flow to previously hypoperfused alveoli increases, reducing physiological dead space.
- Unsupported spontaneous breathing increases cardiac output, which will also improve $\dot{V}/\dot{Q}$ matching and reduce physiological dead space.

It may take up to 16h to achieve these effects on gas exchange. There is little additional gain after 24h.

Indications

APRV has been designed to 'open the lung and keep it open' in patients with ALI/ARDS. The short release periods use intrinsic rather than extrinsic PEEP to maintain FRC.

APRV should be considered in patients in whom oxygenation is difficult and patient ventilator interaction is problematic (the ability to breathe through all phases of the respiratory cycle makes this a surprisingly well-tolerated mode). Before muscle relaxation, prone position, or nitric oxide, consider APRV.

It should be used with caution in:

- Head injury (CO_2 control)
- Bronchopleural fistulae
- Severe obstructive lung disease.

Practicalities

P_{high} = *high pressure level*

- Initial setting 25–30cmH$_2$O.
- Consider up to 35cmH$_2$O if reduced chest wall/abdominal compliance.
- Set at 30cmH$_2$O if P_{plat} greater than this on conventional ventilation.

P_{low} = low pressure level
- 0cmH$_2$O. Allows maximum ΔP and therefore maximum flow during expiration.
- Lung collapse is avoided by manipulating T_{low} rather than P_{low}.

T_{high} = time spent at high pressure
- Initial setting 4–6s.
- Progressively increase to 10–15s.
- Target is oxygenation.

T_{low} = time spent at low pressure
- Initial setting 0.6s.
- Restrictive lung disease: 0.2–0.8s.
- Obstructive lung disease: 0.8–1.5s.

The most common method described for setting T_{low} uses the expiratory flow waveform (Fig. 4.5). T_{low} should end when expiratory flow falls to 50–75% of PEFR. In poorly compliant lungs, emptying occurs more quickly and T_{low} should end earlier in the expiratory cycle (~75% of PEFR). The opposite occurs in obstructive diseases, where T_{low} should end at ~50% of PEFR. The expiratory flow curve should be displayed at all times to allow adjustment of T_{low} as lung compliance changes. As the lungs recover, compliance improves and T_{low} can be increased in 0.1s increments.

Others have described setting T_{low} using optimal PEEP. A P–V curve is used to determine optimal PEEP. This pressure maintains sufficient volume (FRC) to prevent derecruitment. The tidal volume generated by

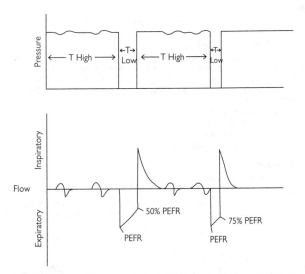

Fig. 4.5 Pressure and flow traces during APRV. The expiratory flow waveform can be used to set T_{low} (explanation in text).

moving from optimal PEEP to T_{high} is noted. T_{low} is then set to deliver an equivalent expiratory volume.

Titrating settings in APRV

Hypoxia
- Increase FiO_2.
- Increase P_{high}.
- Increase T_{high} (watch CO_2).
- Consider reducing T_{low} (effects on PEEPi, but watch CO_2).

Hypercapnia
- Increase alveolar ventilation ('increase' APRV)—increase P_{high}, or increase P_{high} and T_{high} together.
- Increase minute ventilation—decrease T_{high} and increase P_{high}
- Check T_{low} (Can you lengthen it?).

Hypocapnia
- Increase T_{high}.
- Decrease P_{high} (play-off against oxygenation).

Weaning APRV

There is no requirement to change to any other mode of ventilation; weaning may be achieved by the 'drop and stretch' method.
- FiO_2 should be 0.4 before attempting any reduction in airway pressure.
- P_{low} remains at 0 for as long as the patient remains on APRV.
- Only adjust T_{low} in response to changes in lung compliance.
- Reduce P_{high} in 2cmH_2O increments, guided by oxygenation. Eventual target 8–10cmH_2O.
- In tandem, increase T_{high} in 2s increments. Monitor $PaCO_2$. This effectively reduces the release rate and CO_2 clearance is achieved by spontaneous ventilation.
- At CPAP 8–10cmH_2O with few, if any, releases, an assessment of suitability for tracheal extubation may be appropriate (see Extubation, p 350).

Should the patient's condition deteriorate at any stage during this process, increase P_{high} (for deterioration of oxygenation) or reduce T_{high} (for unacceptable rise in CO_2). This avoids switching from one mode to another with potentially deleterious effects.

BIPAP

APRV and BIPAP were described by groups working independently in the USA and Europe in the latter half of the 1980s. The modes were similar when initially described (i.e. support at two pressure levels with spontaneous breathing throughout the respiratory cycle). Over time APRV has remained the generic term for high-level CPAP with intermittent pressure releases and unsupported spontaneous breathing, while BIPAP has evolved the way it handles spontaneous breathing. In addition, the I:E ratios in BIPAP are often similar to those used in conventional ventilation.

Nomenclature

Commercial trademarking means that BIPAP is also termed:
- Bi-Vent (Servo *i*)
- BIPAP (Drager Evita XL)
- BiLevel (Puritan Bennett)
- BiPhasic (Viasys Avea)
- DuoPAP (Hamilton).

It is not to be confused with bilevel positive airway pressure (BiPAP), a non-invasive ventilation system offered by Respironics (Carlsbad, CA).

Basics

I:E ratio

The major difference between BIPAP and APRV is in the duration of time spent at the lower pressure level (T_{low}). This has effects on the I:E ratio, the mean airway pressure for a given peak airway pressure, and the potential for derecruitment.

In practice, this means BIPAP functions more like PCV (see 📖 Pressure-controlled ventilation, p 135) and PEEP needs to be set conventionally to prevent end expiratory collapse.

Spontaneous breathing

Because T_{low} is much longer than in APRV, spontaneous ventilation can occur at P_{low}. Depending on the presence or absence of spontaneous breathing, BIPAP may be subdivided into (Fig. 4.6):
- CMV style—no spontaneous breathing
- IMV style—spontaneous breathing at lower pressure level
- True BIPAP—spontaneous breathing at both pressure levels
- APRV style—spontaneous breathing at the upper pressure level (due to the very short duration of time spent at the low pressure level).

The role of unsupported spontaneous breathing has not achieved the same importance in BIPAP as it has in APRV. Some BIPAP modes have attempted to synchronize cycling between pressure levels and others have added pressure support to spontaneous efforts at P_{low}.

In practice, BIPAP is sometimes used simply as a better synchronized form of P-SIMV, with *supported* spontaneous breaths, rather than true BIPAP.

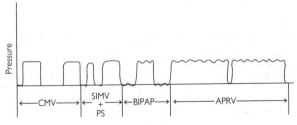

Fig. 4.6 Breathing patterns possible during BIPAP. See text for explanation.

Practicalities

Setting the ventilator for BIPAP

The parameters used in BIPAP are the same as those used in APRV, but it is easier to think of them in terms of setting conventional pressure control ventilation:

- P_{high} = P_{insp}. Initial setting 20–25cm H_2O. Titrate to deliver TV 6–8ml/kg. Avoid $P_{high} \geq$ 30cm H_2O.
- P_{low} = PEEP. Initial setting 5–10cm H_2O (see 📖 Positive and expiratory pressure, p 119).
- T_{high}:T_{low} = I:E ratio. Initial setting 1:15. Adjust accordingly to inspiratory and expiratory flows (see 📖 Pressure control ventilation, p 135).
- T_{high} + T_{low} = breath cycle time (60/respiratory rate). Initial setting ~45 i.e. respiratory rate 15 bpm.
- P_{Supp} = P_{Supp}. Titrate according to TV delivered, patient inspiratory effort and WOB.

Weaning BIPAP

It is not necessary to change to any other mode to facilitate weaning. Provided gas exchange remains satisfactory, P_{high} can be reduced in 2cmH_2O increments until it reaches the same value as P_{low}, at which point the patient is effectively breathing spontaneously on CPAP. The P_{low} value is then weaned incrementally until it is possible to switch to a dedicated T-piece CPAP system or a decision is made for tracheal extubation.

Further reading

Habashi N. (2005) Ventilator strategies for posttraumatic acute respiratory distress syndrome: airway pressure release ventilation and the role of spontaneous breathing in critically ill patients. *Crit Care Med* **33**(3) (suppl.), S228–S240.

Putensen C, Hering R, and Wrigge H. (2002) Controlled versus assisted mechanical ventilation. *Curr Opin Crit Care* **8**, 51–57.

4.6 High-frequency oscillatory ventilation

High-frequency oscillatory ventilation (HFOV) is a mode of ventilation that uses high respiratory rates (3–10Hz) and extremely low tidal volumes (1–4mL/kg). Pressurization is achieved by using an oscillating piston that periodically compresses a constant inspiratory gas to generate pressure waveforms.

HFOV differs from conventional ventilation techniques in that the tidal volumes delivered are less than dead-space volume and both the inspiration and expiration phases are active. This results in reduced peak airway pressure for a given mean airway pressure, and a reduced tendency for derecruitment.

Other methods of high-frequency ventilation, such as high-frequency jet ventilation and high-frequency positive pressure ventilation, have been described, but these are rarely used in ICU and are not discussed here.

Basics

Physiology of gas transport in HFOV

As the tidal volume delivered by HFOV is less than dead-space volume, gas transport within the airways cannot be explained by a simple 'in and out' model. Inspiratory and expiratory gas streams must coexist in the airways and at least six modes of gas transport may occur:

- *Bulk convection*: Inspired gas directly reaches alveolar regions more proximal to conducting airways. CO_2 is cleared when V_t is 50–75% of the anatomical dead space.
- *Convective dispersion due to asymmetric (inspiratory and expiratory) velocity profiles*: The more central particles are propelled down the length of the airway during inspiration, while the peripheral expiratory gas is streamed away from the alveoli along the airway's wall.
- *Pendelluft*: Asynchronous filling of adjacent lung units with different time constants. Gas flows from fast- to slow-filling regions at end inspiration. The reverse occurs at end expiration.
- *Augmented diffusion (Taylor-type dispersion)*: Interplay between convective forces and molecular diffusion generating high-energy eddies and vortices, which enhances gas mixing.
- *Cardiogenic mixing*: Cardiac contractions promote peripheral gas mixing up to five-fold along the concentration gradient. May account for up to half of the oxygen uptake in apnoeic respiration.
- *Molecular diffusion*: Brownian motion in the alveoli with a large cross-sectional area and gas velocities that approximate zero.

HFOV parameters

- Bias flow: This is the rate of fresh gas entering the HFOV circuit. It facilitates CO_2 clearance and establishes a continuous distending pressure or mean airway pressure (mP_{aw}).
- Continuing distending pressure or mean airway pressure (mP_{aw}): This determines lung volume, recruitment, and therefore oxygenation.
- Frequency: The rate of pressure oscillations in Hertz (1Hz = 60 breaths per minute).

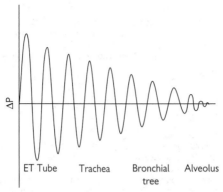

Fig. 4.7 Attenuation of ΔP from oscillator to alveolus.

- Oscillatory pressure amplitude (ΔP): Describes the 'peak to trough' pressure excursions around the mP_{aw} (usual range 60–90cmH$_2$O). These pressure changes are measured at the ventilator and do not reflect pressure changes within the lungs (see Fig. 4.7). The pressure waveform is attenuated by the compressibility of the gas, the frequency of the respiratory cycle, the resistance to flow within the tubing and proximal airway, and the mechanical properties of the airways.
- Inspiratory time: Percentage of the respiratory cycle allocated to inspiration—routinely set at 33% (I:E ratio 1:2).

Indications

The use of HFOV has been described and shown to be safe and effective in numerous conditions, although it has not yet been shown to be statistically superior to conventional ventilation. Its use has been described in:

- ARDS on CMV when:
  - FiO$_2$ > 0.7 and/or SpO$_2$ < 88% with PEEP > 15cmH$_2$O, or
  - Plateau pressures > 30cmH$_2$O, or
  - mP_{aw} > 24cmH$_2$O.
- Pulmonary contusion.
- Bronchopleural fistulas and massive air leaks.
- Bronchial injury.
- Neuro-critical care: HFOV seems to be safe and effective in severe ARDS and raised ICP secondary to acute brain injury because it:
  - Avoids large swings in peak inspiratory pressure.
  - Increases PaO$_2$ and therefore tissue brain oxygenation.
  - Controls PaCO$_2$ (and ICP).
  - Often requires the use of paralysis and heavy sedation, which helps the management of ICP.

- Burns
  - Facilitates early excision and closure of the burn wounds by reversing hypoxaemia and can serve as an intra-operative mode of ventilation in burn patients with severe ARDS.
  - Less effective in burns patients with smoke inhalation injury.

Practicalities

Initial settings
- FiO_2 1.0.
- Frequency 4–6Hz.
- I:E 33%.
- Bias flow 30–60L/min.
- mP_{aw} 3cmH$_2$O above the mP_{aw} on CMV prior to HFOV.
- ΔP 80–90cmH$_2$O. Reduce in severe proximal air leaks.
  - In the 3100B oscillator, ΔP is controlled by the power-setting measured in arbitrary units ranging from 1 to 10. The relationship between power and ΔP is not fixed but depends on the mechanical characteristics of the respiratory system.
  - In the Vision Alpha oscillator ΔP is controlled by setting the cycle volume.
- HFOV controls oxygenation and ventilation (CO_2 removal) separately.

Management of oxygenation
- Oxygenation is controlled via FiO_2 and mP_{aw}.
- Increasing mP_{aw} will increase aerated lung volume (recruitment).
- Establishing 'optimal mP_{aw}' relies on the combination of clinical and haemodynamic parameters, radiological data, and gas exchange.
- ⚠ Worsening of gas exchange, particularly an increase in $PaCO_2$, with hypotension or reduction in CO may indicate over-distention or low potential for lung recruitment.

Management of ventilation (CO_2 removal)
As in conventional ventilation, CO_2 clearance is increased with greater tidal volumes. Increases in V_t are seen with with:
- Increased internal diameter ETT
- Increased ΔP
- Reducing frequency (Hz).

Ventilation efficiency (Q) is more dependent on V_t and is expressed as: $Q = f \times V_t^2$. Ventilation using larger ΔP and higher frequency seem more protective to lungs than that with smaller ΔP and lower frequency. The goal of HFOV is to achieve adequate CO_2 elimination with the highest frequency tolerated.
- Higher frequencies result in the peak airway pressure being applied for such a short time that over-distension will not occur in compliant areas (which have long time constants).
- High frequencies can increase alveolar recruitment as higher gas velocities generate pressures that can exceed the thresholds for alveolar opening.

If the patient is still hypercapnic with a ΔP of 90cmH$_2$O, reduce the frequency by 1Hz to a minimum of 3–5Hz and consider potential causes:
- Derecruitment
- Increased intra-abdominal pressure

- ETT obstruction
- Pneumothorax.

If there is refractory hypercapnia (pH <7.20), the use of a deliberate cuff leak of 5–7cmH$_2$O may be considered to achieve CO$_2$ clearance.

⚠ Monitor mP$_{aw}$ to protect the patient from a sudden increase in mP$_{aw}$ as a result of a decreased cuff leak (e.g. tracheal oedema, secretions, body positioning). Also be aware of micro-aspiration and tube dislodgement.

Weaning
Consider returning to CMV when mP$_{aw}$ <22cmH$_2$O and FiO$_2$ is 0.4 for 24h.

Airway leak
Use the highest frequency, the lowest ΔP, the lowest mP$_{aw}$, and the shortest inspiratory time (IT%) possible.

Patient monitoring
- Chest wiggle and chest auscultation: depends on ΔP, lung compliance, or airway resistance. Sudden loss of wiggle may indicate:
  - ETT obstruction
  - Mucous plugging
  - Accidental extubation
  - Bronchial intubation
  - Pneumothorax.
- Haemodynamic monitoring.
- ABGs.
- CXR.
- Monitoring changes in mP$_{aw}$ and ΔP.

Currently no bedside monitoring is available to determine best mP$_{aw}$. Newer techniques such as electrical impedance tomography and respiratory inductance plethysmography may represent useful bedside tools for assessing lung volume.

Recruitment manoeuvres
Recruitment manoeuvres (RM) aim to open or recruit all available alveolar units. In HFOV, RM are recommended:
- On the initiation of HFOV.
- Following circuit disconnection or endotracheal suction.
- Following bronchoscopy.
- In response to patient desaturations.

They should be avoided if there is:
- Significant hemodynamic instability.
- Intractable respiratory acidosis.
- An unstable air leak with multiple recurrences.

Sustained inflation
Increase mP$_{aw}$ to 40–45cmH$_2$O for 40–60s with the oscillator piston turned off to avoid transmission of the ΔP at high mP$_{aw}$. Decrease mP$_{aw}$ by 2cmH$_2$O every 15min until optimal mP$_{aw}$ is found using the PaO$_2$:FiO$_2$ ratio.

Slow RM

Increase mP_{aw} by $3cmH_2O$ every 10min until mP_{aw} is 45–50cmH$_2$O or there is haemodynamic instability. Reduce mP_{aw} by $2cmH_2O$ every 5min until optimal mP_{aw} is found using the PaO_2:FiO_2 ratio.

Reported advantages

HFOV delivers lung protective ventilation, minimizing VILI by providing:
- High mP_{aw} that maintains lung recruitment and prevents shear stress injury from repetitive opening and closing of atelectatic lung units (atelectrauma).
- Small tidal volumes (volutrauma).
- Reduction in peak pressure swings (barotrauma).
- More uniform, compliance-independent distribution of ventilation.
- Reduced lung inflammation (biotrauma).

Complications and limitations

- Pneumothorax.
- Haemodynamic compromise (haemodynamic monitoring and fluid challenges may be required on commencing HFOV and when performing RM).
- Migration of ETT (due to high mP_{aw} and oscillations).
- Prolonged sedation and neuromuscular blockade.
- Infection control.
- Aerosol delivery.
- Transport.
- Monitoring.
- Staff training.

Troubleshooting

Humidification and suction

Humidification of the bias flow is required to prevent:
- Inspissated airway secretions.
- Thermal injury of the airway mucosa.
- Damage to the piston diaphragm.

Tracheal suctioning reduces carinal airway pressure and promotes alveolar derecruitment. It is best avoided during the first 12h on HFOV. After that time it should be performed with a closed in-line suction system and only when clinically indicated, that is:
- Visible secretions.
- Decrease in chest wiggle.
- Desaturation and unexplained increase in PaCO$_2$.

Endotracheal tubes

ETT obstruction should be suspected in the presence of:
- A sudden increase in PaCO$_2$
- Increase in ΔP (>5–10cmH$_2$O) coupled with a decrease in chest wiggle, breath sounds, desaturation, and hypercapnia.

To ensure ETT patency, the in-line tracheal suctioning catheter can be passed (without turning on suction) along with instillation of a small volume of sterile saline (2–3mL). If a suction catheter cannot be passed and manual ventilation produces no air movement, emergent reintubation is required.

The ETT position should be recorded to allow early detection of tube migration.

Sedation and neuromuscular blockade agents

HFOV cannot synchronize or augment a patient's inspiratory effort. Spontaneous respiratory efforts during HFOV may produce large inspiratory flow rates and pressure swings that cause a drop in the mP_{aw} and derecruitment, so deeper sedation, analgesia, and neuromuscular blockade agents (NMBAs) may be necessary.

- Assess sedation regularly with Richmond agitation–sedation scale or equivalent.
- Try to maintain shallow spontaneous breaths if they do not interfere with the delivery of HFOV.
- Future gas flow controller (demand-flow system) may allow gas flow compensation and allow continuous spontaneous ventilation during HFOV.
- In patients receiving NMBA:
  - Use the smallest dose for the shortest time or intermittent boluses.
  - A train-of-four peripheral nerve stimulators should be used, aiming for one or two thumb twitches.
  - Consider using a bispectral index (BIS) monitor.
  - Frequent clinical evaluation of muscular tone (e.g. tendon reflexes, muscular activity, respiratory efforts) should be performed.

HFOV and aerosol delivery

Aerosol generators that use vibration to produce low-velocity, small-droplet drug delivery may improve drug delivery without affecting HFOV parameters.

Patient transport

No HFOV transport ventilators are currently available and HFOV should only be used during transport if absolutely necessary. The ETT should be clamped during any disconnection to maintain alveolar recruitment.

Infection control

HFOV was previously a high-risk intervention for infection control because of the difficulty filtering exhaled respiratory secretions. Staff treating patients at risk of infection without an expiratory filter required protective equipment (goggles, N95 mask, gown, and gloves) and scavenger systems over the mP_{aw} control diaphragm. A suitable filter is now available from SensorMedics and for the Vision Alpha machine.

Further reading

Bennett SS, Graffagnino C, Borel CO, and James ML (2007) Use of high frequency oscillatory ventilation (HFOV) in neurocritical care patients. *Neurocrit Care* **7**(3), 221–226.

Fessler HE, Derdak S, Ferguson ND, Hager DN, Kacmarek RM, Thompson BT, and Brower RG (2007) A protocol for high-frequency oscillatory ventilation in adults: results from a roundtable discussion. *Crit Care Med* **35**(7), 1649–1654.

Hager DN, Fessler HE, Kaczka DW, Shanholtz CB, Fuld MK, Simon BA, and Brower RG (2007) Tidal volume delivery during high-frequency oscillatory ventilation in adults with acute respiratory distress syndrome. *Crit Care Med* **35**(6), 1522–1529.

Higgins J, Estetter B, Holland D, Smith B, and Derdak S (2005) High-frequency oscillatory ventilation in adults: respiratory therapy issues. *Crit Care Med* **33**(3) (suppl.), S196–S203.

Rose L (2008) High-frequency oscillatory ventilation in adults: clinical considerations and management priorities. *AACN Adv Crit Care* **19**(4), 412–420.

4.7 Software enhancements

Dual-control ventilatory modes

Principles

Normal ventilator modes control pressure, flow, or volume. Dual-control or hybrid modes of ventilation can control both pressure and volume at different points in the breathing cycle (they cannot control both at the same time). They aim to provide the assured minute ventilation of volume control with the potential advantages of a decelerating inspiratory flow pattern. There are two methods of delivering dual control:
- Dual control within a breath.
- Dual control from breath to breath.

Dual control within a breath

This principle is used by Volume-Assured Pressure Support on Bird® ventilators and Pressure Augmentation on Bear® ventilators (both Viasys).

The initial breath is patient or time triggered and pressure controlled. If the software calculates that the minimum tidal volume (or greater) will be delivered, the breath is flow cycled, that is, the equivalent of a pressure support breath.

If it is calculated that the desired tidal volume will not be reached, a flow controller is activated which maintains a constant inspiratory flow until the desired tidal volume is attained. Airway pressure may rise above set ventilator pressure during this portion of the breath. The breath has therefore become a flow-controlled, volume-cycled breath. There is automatic time cycling as a safety default to prevent prolonged inspiration.

Dual control from breath to breath

These modes measure tidal volume and adjust the pressure delivered in subsequent breaths to reach a predefined target.

Pressure limited, flow cycled

This is closed-loop pressure support, using tidal volume to adjust inspiratory pressure. Examples include:
- Volume Support (Siemens).
- Flow-Cycled Pressure Regulated Volume Control (Viasys).

This type of support is patient triggered. The ventilator starts with a $5cmH_2O$ test breath and compliance is calculated. In subsequent breaths, pressure is increased gradually until the desired tidal volume is achieved or the set pressure limit is breached. Changes in pressure support of $1–3cmH_2O$ per breath are then made in response to measured compliance in order to keep tidal volume constant. Just as with normal pressure-support breaths, flow cycling terminates the breath.

Pressure limited, time cycled

This is closed-loop pressure control ventilation, using tidal volume to adjust inspiratory pressure. Examples include:
- Pressure Regulated Volume Control (Siemens and Viasys).
- Autoflow (Drager).
- Adaptive Pressure Ventilation (Hamilton Medical).
- Volume Control+ (Puritan Bennett).

There are minor differences between the modes, but all operate on similar principles. They can be patient or time triggered. The ventilators deliver a test breath of 5–10cmH$_2$O, determine compliance, and then gradually increase the pressure until the desired tidal volume is delivered or the set pressure limit is breached. Pressure is then adjusted (by 1–3cmH$_2$O per breath) on the basis of measured compliance in order to keep the tidal volume constant. Breaths are time cycled.

Automode

Automode from Siemens combines the two methods of between breath dual control. If the patient is breathing spontaneously, breaths will be flow cycled, and if the patient is apnoeic, breaths will be time cycled.

Problems

- If there is major patient ventilator asynchrony during the test breaths calculated compliance will be erroneous. Subsequent breaths are delivered at the new, falsely calculated, pressure.
- Significant leaks may be misinterpreted (by some ventilators) as increased lung compliance, leading to reduced delivered pressures.
- In patients with high compliance or a very high respiratory drive, the tidal volume target may be met without additional pressure support from the ventilator. If WOB is very high, alternative modes may be more suitable.

Flow patterns produced by the ventilator

VCV usually delivers positive pressure using constant flow. Some ventilators allow the clinician to adjust this flow profile. These breaths are not dual-control breaths since airway pressure is secondary to the flow delivery and respiratory mechanics, and is not controlled by the ventilator.

Decelerating flow (descending ramp)

Although designed to mimic a pressure-controlled breath, decelerating flow breaths cannot adjust for conditions of changing resistance. For example, in airway obstruction the slope of deceleration should be much gentler. Ventilators are unable to make these adjustments and on average airway pressures will still be slightly higher with these modes than with a true pressure-controlled breath.

Sinusoidal

This type of flow pattern more closely replicates the flow pattern of normal breathing.

Accelerating (ascending ramp)

This flow pattern tends to produce higher peak pressures and lower mean pressures, and its use is therefore limited.

Automatic tube compensation

The pressure drop along an ETT, and therefore the additional WOB attributable to the tube, varies with the diameter of the tube and the inspiratory flow rate (see Fig. 4.8).

As resistance is non-linear, setting a fixed pressure support to overcome this additional WOB will lead to over-support at low flow rates and under-support at increased flow rates.

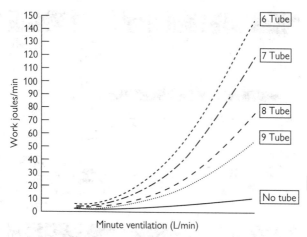

Fig. 4.8 Measured WOB as a function of ETT diameter and minute ventilation.

Automatic tube compensation (ATC) uses instantaneous flow, as well as the diameter and length of the ETT, to calculate the pressure drop along the tube and the resultant additional WOB. It then adjusts the circuit pressure to overcome this additional work.

The pressures set by the clinician are therefore the calculated pressures at the tracheal end of the tube (P_{trach}). The compensation may be applied during inspiration alone (increased circuit pressure) or also during expiration (decreased circuit pressure). This effectively removes the ETT as a source of resistance and it has been described as an 'electronic extubation'.

Fig. 4.9 is a screenshot of a patient breathing at CPAP 5cmH$_2$O. The grey line on the pressure trace (P_{trach}) is the tracheal airway pressure calculated by the ventilator. It can be seen to dip below atmospheric pressure during inspiration. Fig. 4.10 shows the same patient with ATC applied. The tracheal pressure is kept much more constant.

Prediction of successful extubation in trials, however, has not been improved. This may be because ATC does not take account of:

• The breathing circuit resistance
• Changes with underlying lung disease
• Instrumental dead space (for example, HMEs can add significant dead space, requiring additional PS to compensate).

The underlying assumption made during the use of ATC is that the WOB post extubation will be similar to the WOB the patient would have if the tube was not *in situ*. This is not true in some patients, where upper airway anatomy is altered by the illness and the recent presence of an ETT, so that the WOB post extubation is, for that patient, unnaturally high. In this case, use of ATC will *underestimate* the post-extubation WOB.

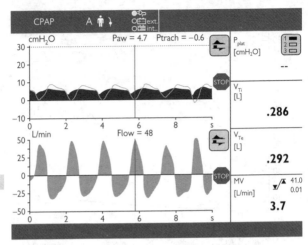

Fig. 4.9 Tracheal (grey) and circuit (black) pressure trace of patient breathing spontaneously at CPAP 5cmH$_2$O.

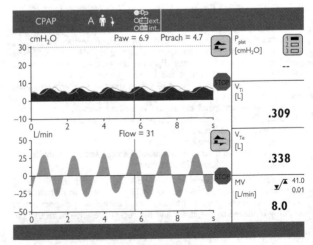

Fig. 4.10 Same patient as Fig. 4.9 with ATC applied.

Other software enhancements

Adaptive Support Ventilation

Adaptive Support Ventilation from Hamilton Medical is a sophisticated form of dual control and closed-loop feedback. It is considered in 📖 Adaptive support ventilation, p 170.

Proportional Assist Ventilation

See 📖 Proportional assist ventilation, p 174.

4.8 Adaptive support ventilation

Introduction

Adaptive support ventilation (ASV) is a patented mode of ventilation available on Hamilton Medical machines. It delivers a mandatory minute volume while attempting to minimize WOB.

It is a closed-loop system that automatically escalates or reduces both pressure support and mandatory breaths, depending on patient effort. It is capable of delivering any level of support from CPAP to full PCV.

Basics/principles

ASV targets a minute volume set by the clinician. This can be delivered by pressure-supported spontaneous ventilation, volume-targeted PCV, or a combination of both depending on patient effort. The mode preference is for spontaneous respiration, but if the respiratory rate is below the desired rate, mandatory breaths are gradually introduced.

- The ideal respiratory rate and V_t are calculated based on the 'minimum WOB' (see box).
- Three test breaths measure compliance and airways resistance using a least-squares fit technique (the mathematical procedure commonly used in statistics for multiple linear regression).
- Compliance and resistance are monitored on a breath-by-breath basis. The WOB is recalculated every three to five breaths, and adjustments made for any change in respiratory mechanics.
- In full controlled mode, breaths are pressure-controlled and time-cycled.
- Support breaths are pressure-supported and flow-cycled.
- During both spontaneous and controlled breaths, inspiratory pressure is adjusted to achieve the desired tidal volume.

Targets and limits

ASV targets the minute volume set by the clinician.

- Normal minute ventilation is estimated at 100mL/kg IBW or 7L for a 70kg patient. This corresponds to 100%MinVol. %MinVol can be increased or decreased by the clinician (e.g. adjusting %MinVol to 150 will deliver 150mL/kg minute ventilation).
- Dead space is calculated as 2.2mL/kg IBW.

The mode attempts to avoid some of the problems encountered with delivering a mandatory minute volume and has integrated a number of safe guards. They are represented by the rectangular box on the screen-shot (Fig. 4.12)

- Minimum tidal volume (min V_t) = 4.4 × IBW, reducing excessive dead-space ventilation.
- Maximum ventilator respiratory rate is the lowest of:
  - Target minute volume/min V_t
  - 20/expiratory time constant
  - 60 breaths/minute
- Maximum V_t is $(P_{max} - PEEP) \times C$ or 22mL/kg.
- Maximum delivered pressure is 10cmH$_2$O below the set pressure limit.
- Expiratory time >2 × expiratory time constant minimizing breath stacking and PEEP$_i$.

Minimum WOB concept

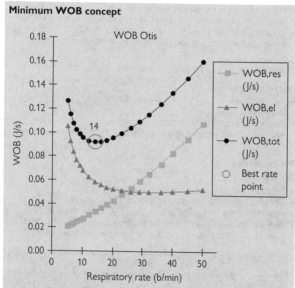

Fig. 4.11 Relationship between respiratory rate and WOB.

In the 1950s Otis hypothesized that respiratory rate was dictated by the need to achieve the minimum inspiratory WOB.

For any minute ventilation, there are an infinite number of combinations of V_t and respiratory rate. There is a J-shaped relationship between respiratory rate and WOB (see Fig. 4.11). As the respiratory rate rises for the same MV, resistive WOB increases (faster air flow) and elastic WOB falls (less respiratory system expansion).

This relationship is expressed mathematically as

$$RR = (1 + 4\pi^2 RC(V_A/V_D) - 1)/(2\pi^2 RC)$$

where RR is respiratory rate, R is airways resistance, C is compliance, the product RC gives the expiratory time constant, V_A is alveolar minute ventilation, and V_D is dead-space ventilation.

This equation is used as the basis for the ASV algorithm.

Indications

ASV is a relatively new mode and few indications have been clearly established.

- Postoperative patients. Capable of supporting transition from full mechanical ventilation to pressure supported spontaneous breathing without intervention by clinical staff.

- Has been used in respiratory failure from a variety of causes. There is little evidence available to support its preferential use in this setting.
- Weaning. Appears to allow timely extubation after cardiac surgery with fewer interventions and ventilator adjustment compared with SIMV.

Contraindications
- ASV cannot be used for NIV.

Not recommended
- Significant airleaks, e.g. bronchopleural fistula.
- During bronchoscopy.
- May not be appropriate for restrictive tidal volume ventilation in ARDS. In clinical practice, it has been shown to deliver tidal volumes closer to 8mL/kg.

Practicalities

Initial set up
- Set PEEP and FiO_2 as for regular ventilation.
- Upper pressure limit must be at least $25cmH_2O$ above PEEP. The maximum pressure applied will be $10cm\ H_2O$ *below* this limit.
- IBW should be calculated from height. Increase IBW by 10% if HME filter incorporated into circuit (allows for increased dead space).

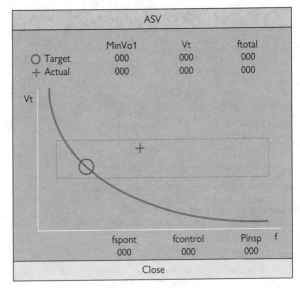

Fig. 4.12 Screenshot for ASV. The curve represents the combination of V_t and respiratory rate which will deliver the desired minute volume. The dotted rectangle is formed by the maximum and minimum allowed respiratory rate and tidal volume. See text for calculation of these values.

- Choose the minute ventilation in the normal fashion, and then calculate the %MinVol required to deliver it. 100%MinVol = 100mL/kg/min.
- Initial %MinVol should be higher in patients known to have increased dead space or if there is increased CO_2 production (e.g. pyrexia).
- Use %MinVol to alter tidal volume not IBW.
- Enter trigger method (pressure or flow), sensitivity, P-ramp, and ETS (see 📖 Pressure support ventilation, p 144).

Using ASV

- ASV will preferentially allow spontaneous breathing so that patients will wean from controlled ventilation automatically.
- For a particular MV, ASV will adjust the respiratory rate and inspiratory pressure provided according to changes in compliance and resistance. For example, if resistance increases and %MinVol is unchanged then the respiratory rate will fall and the tidal volume will increase (both to reduce WOB and to avoid $PEEP_i$).
- If initial chosen %MinVol is reasonable, weaning to low levels of respiratory support may occur automatically. If minute volume is high, reduction of %MinVol allows weaning of respiratory support. Assess respiratory pattern and patient effort, blood gases, and inspiratory pressure before adjustment.
- When P_{insp} <8 and frequency of spontaneous breaths acceptable, extubation may be considered. If %MinVol is significantly greater than 100, then it should be considered whether extubation with high minute ventilation is desirable.
- Even if the respiratory pattern is optimized there is no guarantee of acceptable gas exchange. Arterial blood gas monitoring is still essential.
- Although ASV is able to automatically adjust the level of ventilatory support, it should not replace clinician input and assessment.

Problem solving

- Least-squares fit measurement of respiratory mechanics is only applicable in relaxed or nearly relaxed patients. If $P_{0.1}$ is high, increasing the pressure support temporarily by 10cmH$_2$O may allow more accurate measurement.
- Respiratory mechanics measurements are also invalid in patients with small airways collapse (e.g. COPD)—compliance and $PEEP_i$ are both underestimated.
- The ability of the ventilator to adjust respiratory rate, tidal volume, and I:E ratio according to underlying pathology is more pronounced in fully ventilated rather than spontaneously breathing patients.
- Patients with a high respiratory drive may breathe well above the set %MinVol. If reversible causes of high respiratory drive have been excluded, PSV should be considered as an alternative mode of ventilation.
- When %MinVol is set at a high level to compensate for increased dead space (e.g. fibrotic ARDS), the ideal respiratory pattern calculated by ASV often means that support remains high and respiratory rate relatively low. Weaning is slow. PSV should be considered as an alternative mode of ventilation.

4.9 Proportional assist ventilation

Proportional assist ventilation (PAV, sometimes called proportional pressure support) is a mode of spontaneous ventilatory support in which the degree of assist varies according to patient effort. Rather than targeting a set pressure level, tidal volume, or respiratory rate, it targets a set level of respiratory muscle offloading. There are no mandatory breaths.

Basics

Principles

PAV is a mode of support in which the ventilator pressure (P_{aw}) is proportional to instantaneous inspiratory flow (V') and volume (V), which in turn are determined by the patient's inspiratory muscle pressure (P_{mus}).[1,2] With this mode the clinician sets the respective flow and volume gain signals, the *flow assist* (FA) and *volume assist* (VA). As a result, P_{aw} is a function of V' and V according to the equation:

$$P_{aw} = VA \times V + FA \times V'$$

VA has units of elastance (cmH_2O/L) and FA units of resistance ($cmH_2O/L/s$) and may be expressed as a percentage of the elastance (E_{rs}) and the resistance (R_{rs}) of the patient's respiratory system. If VA/E_{rs} and FA/R_{rs} represent similar fractions (K) the equation above can be rewritten

$$P_{aw} = K (E_{rs} \times V + R_{rs} \times V') (2)$$

When VA and FA are set to lower values than the E_{rs} and R_{rs} of the respiratory system, respectively, the patient always contributes to total inflation pressure. Under these conditions, Paw increases with increasing $Pmus_l$ and decreases with decreasing P_{mus}. It follows that the inspiratory muscles cope, after triggering, with an afterload (E_{rs} and R_{rs}) that is reduced by an amount equal to VA and FA: 50% assist should reduce inspiratory muscle output by 50% (in reality the measured reduction is usually slightly lower than the set assist level). Therefore, with this mode the ventilator simply amplifies patient inspiratory effort without imposing any target for flow, volume, or P_{aw}, and the patient is able to retain considerable control of the desired breathing pattern.

Proportionality

In PAV the clinician sets the assist level, K. For example, in setting K to 80% the ventilator provides 80% of the elastic and resistive work, while the patient contributes the remaining 20%. The proportionality between the ventilator (P_{aw}) and patient inspiratory muscle (P_{mus}) is 4:1 (80/20).

The relative contributions of resistive and elastive components to the overall WOB varies during inspiration (resistive work predominates, with greater flows in early inspiration, elastive work rises with increased stretch at end inspiration). If the proportionality is different for VA and FA the correlation between P_{mus} and P_{aw} is lost. In order to maintain this relationship, *there must be similar levels of support for VA and FA*.

This proportionality between P_{mus} and P_{aw} also ensures:

• Expiratory synchrony—as P_{mus} falls, P_{aw} falls and zero flow (the end of ventilator inspiration) occurs as near to the end of neural inspiration as it does even without ventilator support.

- Matching of patient effort with delivered tidal volume—the harder the patient tries to breathe (increased P_{mus}), the higher the P_{aw}.

In some ventilators, the resistance and compliance are calculated manually during volume-controlled, constant-flow mandatory ventilation, and the VA and the FA are set individually. In others, software has been developed (PAV+) that calculates semi-continuously the respiratory system mechanics and automatically adjusts the FA and VA so that they always represent constant fractions of the measured values of R_{rs} and E_{rs}.[2,3] In these ventilators, there is a single control for proportionality (%support).

Indications

PAV+ has been successfully used as the main mode of respiratory support in critically ill patients.[4] It has been demonstrated to increase the probability of patients remaining on a spontaneous breathing mode and it reduces the incidence of patient–ventilator asynchronies (Fig. 4.13). Compared to PSV, it has been shown that PAV/PAV+:

- Decreases triggering delay
- Decreases the likelihood of ineffective efforts
- Decreases expiratory asynchrony
- Increases sleep efficiency
- Promotes breathing stability
- Increases the efficiency of the respiratory system compensation for any added mechanical load.

Limitations

Low respiratory effort

PAV/PAV+ is dependent on inspiratory effort to drive the ventilator. It should be applied with caution in patients with low respiratory drive.

Leaks

With PAV/PAV+ the command signal for pressure delivery is instantaneous flow and volume. Circuit leaks will cause the ventilator to overestimate the patient's inspiratory effort, with the risk of over-support. The proportionality between P_{mus} and P_{aw} is lost.

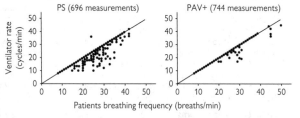

Fig. 4.13 Relationship between patient's breathing frequency and ventilator rate during PS and PAV+. Each closed circle represents a measurement at a particular time. The disagreement between the patient's breathing frequency and ventilator rate is mainly due to the presence of ineffective efforts. From reference 4 with permission.

Dynamic hyperinflation
In the presence of dynamic hyperinflation, patient inspiratory effort is required to overcome $PEEP_i$. This effort is not apparent to the ventilator and the level of inspiratory support will be inappropriately reduced.

Setting the ventilator
PEEP and O_2 are set as for a conventional ventilation mode. The ETT size should be entered, and alarms and limits set carefully (see below—Runaway).

Assist level
Usually the percentage assist should start at 60%.

Some ventilators calculate E_{rs} and R_{rs} on a breath-by-breath basis and adjust the VA and FA to maintain constant levels of support. WOB is calculated and displayed graphically to assist in titrating percentage support levels.

In ventilators where E_{rs} and R_{rs} are calculated manually, it is essential that VA and FA:
• Are set to lower values than E_{rs} and R_{rs}, respectively, and
• Represent similar fractions of E_{rs} and R_{rs}.

Only under these conditions does the patient always contribute to total pressure, while P_{aw} has a constant and predictable relation to P_{mus}.[2]

As E_{rs} and R_{rs} change with the clinical condition, there must be frequent remeasurements to ensure the conditions above are met.

Weaning
If the patient is comfortable and respiratory rate and blood gases satisfactory, the percentage assist may be reduced in 10–20% increments.

Troubleshooting
Runaway
Excessive pressure or volume delivery will lead to runaway. This occurs when the pressure provided by the ventilator is greater than the sum of elastic and resistive pressures (i.e. K> 100%). As a result the ventilator continues to deliver volume despite the fact that the patient has terminated their inspiratory effort. Theoretically, over-distension and barotrauma may occur, but sensible setting of alarms and limits on the ventilator prevent this problem. The biggest issue is constant ventilator alarming. This is a common phenomenon with PAV and occurs when VA and/or FA are set to values higher than E_{rs} and R_{rs} (due to overestimation of the actual values). Decreasing VA and/or FA may solve this problem.

With PAV+, however, runaway occurs rarely and only when the percentage assist (K) approaches 90–95%.[4] This is because with PAV+ the ventilator adjusts the VA and FA in the face of changing respiratory system mechanics, so that they represent a constant fraction of E_{rs} and R_{rs}.[3]

Abnormal breathing patterns
It is important for the physician to realize that breathing pattern varies greatly among patients on PAV/PAV+.[2,4] If the clinician is unhappy with the tidal volume (V_T) or breathing frequency and attempts to increase or decrease the assist (K), the patient might undertake an opposite action to

maintain the desired breathing pattern. The spontaneous breathing frequency varies considerably in intubated patients, with respiratory rates of up to 45/min seen in undistressed patients. If the respiratory rate is high, set the percentage assist to 85%; if the respiratory rate does not change, it is unlikely to be related to respiratory distress and under-support.

This is not the case with other assisted modes, where V_T and ventilator rate are considerably modified by the ventilator settings. It follows that with PAV/PAV+ settings the level of assist based solely on the patient's breathing pattern may be misleading.

1 Younes M (1992) Proportional assist ventilation, a new approach to ventilatory support theory. *Am Rev Respir Dis* **145**, 114–20.

2 Younes M (2006) Proportional assist ventilation, in Tobin MJ (ed.), *Principles and practice of mechanical ventilation*, 2nd edn. McGraw-Hill, pp.335–64.

3 Kondili E, Prinianakis G, Alexopoulou C, Vakouti E, Klimathianaki M, and Georgopoulos D (2006) Respiratory load compensation during mechanical ventilation – Proportional assist ventilation with load-adjustable gain factors vs. pressure support. *Intensive Care Med* **32**, 692–9.

4 Xirouchaki N, Kondili E, Vaporidi K, Xirouchakis G, Klimathianaki M, Gavriilidis G, Alexandopoulou E, Plataki M, Alexopoulou C, and Georgopoulos D (2008) Proportional assist ventilation with load-adjustable gain factors in critically ill patients: comparison with pressure support. *Intensive Care Med* **34**, 2026–34.

4.10 Neurally adjusted ventilatory assist

Absence of spontaneous breathing during mechanical ventilation quickly results in disuse atrophy of the respiratory muscles.[1] Modern ventilatory strategies favour the promotion of spontaneous respiratory effort and the reduction in unnecessary use of paralytic and sedative agents.[2] They have been shown to reduce the duration of ventilation, but the combination of spontaneous breathing and reduced sedation requires focused attention on patient ventilator synchrony (see 📖 Patient ventilator asynchrony, p 267).

Patient ventilator interaction is influenced by the co-ordination of ventilator triggering and off-cycling with the patient's breathing efforts. In addition, patient–ventilator interaction involves adjusting the magnitude of assist in relation to the degree of patient effort. Asynchrony can result in trigger failure or, at the other extreme, 'fighting the ventilator' and has been associated with prolonged duration of mechanical ventilation.

Traditionally, the patient communicates with the ventilator through pneumatic triggers. As Fig. 4.14 demonstrates, this trigger system will be subject to delays, even in a fully intact respiratory system. In critical illness, with neuromuscular dysfunction, reduced compliance, and increased resistance, these delays will be compounded, with consequent effects on patient–ventilator synchrony.

Neurally adjusted ventilatory assist (NAVA) is controlled by the diaphragm electrical activity.[3] Not only does this facilitate more accurate ventilator triggering and cycling, but the quantitative nature of the electrical activity allows the magnitude of support to alter according to patient effort.

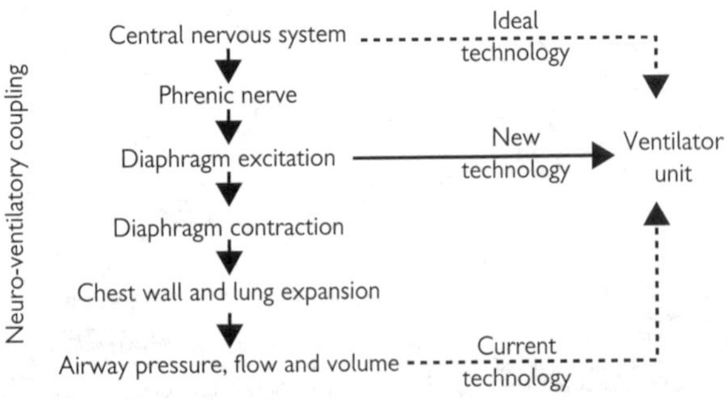

Fig. 4.14 Description of the new technology (NAVA) in perspective with current technology. The steps necessary to transform central respiratory drive into an inspiration are shown (that is, the neuro–ventilatory coupling with indications for the levels at which technology able to control a mechanical ventilator could be implemented). NAVA uses the electrical activation of the diaphragm to control the timing and assist delivery. (From reference 3).

Basics

NAVA is a synchronized mode of ventilator support. It unloads inspiratory muscles while upholding spontaneous breathing in patients with acute respiratory failure. As the respiratory muscles and the ventilator receive the same signal, synchronization is improved compared with other spontaneous modes of ventilatory support. The patient–ventilator synchrony is equally efficient during both invasive and non-invasive application of NAVA.

Diaphragm electrical activity

- The electrical activity of the diaphragm (EAdi, measured in μV) is measured trans-oesophageally with microelectrodes situated near the tip of the NAVA catheter.
- The electrodes are positioned at the level of the oesophageal hiatus, using esophageal ECG to assist placement.
- The NAVA catheter also functions as a standard feeding tube.
- The EAdi comprises the temporo-spatial summation of the neural output to the diaphragm transmitted via the phrenic nerves, and hence is a representation of the neural drive to the diaphragm.
- The EAdi can be used to monitor spontaneous respiratory activity (also in conventional modes).

Triggering

- Breaths are triggered by the EAdi.
- Breaths can also be triggered by a conventional pneumatic signal (should the EAdi signal be late or inadequate).
- The trigger settings in NAVA are adjustable.

Cycling

- The assist is cycled off when the EAdi decreases to a percentage of the peak EAdi (40–70% of the peak EAdi, depending on the amplitude of the signal).
- The cycling-off criterion during NAVA are non-adjustable.

Pressure delivery

- Pressure delivery is controlled by the EAdi signal.
- Setting the NAVA level (cmH$_2$O/μV) determines the scale of support.
- The pressure delivered (cmH$_2$O above PEEP) is proportional to the EAdi (μV).
- The proportionality can be adjusted by changing the NAVA level (e.g. increasing the NAVA level: for a given EAdi, the pressure delivered increases).
- This allows ventilatory demand and neural afferents to regulate the assist, but within limits set by the caregiver.

Indications

Ventilatory assist

NAVA is indicated in all patients with acute respiratory failure in whom spontaneous respiratory activity is present or desired. NAVA can be used on all patients who qualify for partial ventilator assist and who generate an EAdi signal. NAVA may:

- Improve patient–ventilator interaction.
- Prevent disuse atrophy.

- Increase patient comfort.
- Reduce sedative requirements.
- Improve sleep.

When using NAVA, it is not possible to force a preferred tidal volume, respiratory rate, or minute ventilation on the patient.

NAVA cannot be used in the absence of EAdi, e.g. due to neuromuscular pathology or trauma.

Monitoring

The EAdi monitoring function can be used even if the patient is ventilated in a mode other than NAVA. Using this, it is possible to perform bedside evaluation of patient–ventilator interaction and determine if spontaneous breathing is present. It also allows the clinician to:

- Verify the presence of respiratory drive—EAdi amplitude changes in response to pressure support titration and sedation level alterations will help to ensure maintenance of respiratory drive.
- Verify the response to unloading—if reduction in EAdi is absent despite significant increase in assist, look for causes of respiratory drive that are not associated with respiratory muscle loads and assisted ventilation, e.g. metabolic acidosis, trauma to respiratory centers, delirium.
- Quantify the response to unloading—when expressed in relation to the EAdi obtained without assist, the EAdi obtained during assist represents the relative neural down-regulation of respiratory drive to the diaphragm.
- Quantify the ventilatory efficiency—the ratio of tidal volume to EAdi indicates efficiency to generate volume.

Problems

Pathological central respiratory drive

NAVA is integrated with the respiratory centres and therefore depends on their adequate response. Particular care should be taken if using NAVA in the presence of:

- Respiratory centre trauma
- Loss of lung-vagal afferents (e.g. heart–lung transplant).
- Delirium.
- Other neurological disturbances related to sedation and critical illness.
- Pathological respiratory drive due to other causes (e.g. acidosis).

The monitored EAdi signal will reveal atypical breathing efforts and can be used to guide and evaluate changes of ventilator settings and/or pharmaceutical interventions.

Circuit dead space

Rebreathing caused by insufficient tidal volume relative to anatomical/ physiological and respiratory circuit dead space may result in:

- Excessive minute ventilation.
- Elevated tidal volume and/or respiratory rate.
- Increased $PaCO_2$.

Limitation of the external (respiratory circuit) dead space is hence very important to ensure adequate respiratory feedback and avoid unnecessary load and stress on the respiratory system.

Air trapping
- During PSV, intrinsic PEEP or over-supported breaths can prevent the ventilator sensing patient effort, causing trigger failure (see 📖 Pressure support ventilation, p 144).
- One of the most attractive features of NAVA is a reduction in this problem, but there are some limitations to its application. In situations of severe dynamic hyperinflation and severely increased respiratory drive, the neural expiratory time can become too short to allow full expiration. Improved synchrony between patient and ventilator may paradoxically exacerbate this incomplete emptying and aggravate dynamic hyperinflation.
- In these circumstances, increasing NAVA levels may not reduce respiratory drive. There may also be discomfort and abrupt termination of expiratory flow.

Practicalities

Inserting catheter and verifying position
Inserting tube/NAVA catheter:
- Verify predicted and actual insertion distance of NAVA catheter.
- Confirm electrode array position (oesophageal ECG tracing should show P and QRS waves on upper leads, but only QRS on lower).
- Perform end-expiratory occlusion and ensure that positive EAdi and negative airway pressure deflections occur simultaneously.

Setting NAVA level
As NAVA is controlled by EAdi, which in turn is affected by the patient's respiratory feedback, it is important to understand the physiological response to increasing NAVA levels. The NAVA level can be set in three ways.

Using EAdi response
As NAVA levels are titrated upwards, the patient initially welcomes the unloading of their failing respiratory muscles. Eventually a level of assist is reached where the WOB associated with the required minute ventilation is sustainable, without significant reduction in respiratory effort or EAdi.

Further increases in the NAVA level will reduce patient effort and EAdi via a respiratory feedback loop. This dynamic reduction of EAdi results in a plateauing of the delivered support. At this point, there is little or no benefit in increasing NAVA levels as transpulmonary pressure and tidal volumes tend to stabilize.

Aiming for a target pressure
- Suppose we aim for $10cmH_2O$ above PEEP. If EAdi is $20\mu V$, then a NAVA level of $0.5cmH_2O/\mu V$ would reach the target pressure. If the target pressure is reached and the EAdi is still $20\mu V$, one can assume that the patient 'welcomed' the assist. Since, to unload the patient, a reduction in EAdi is required, a second increase of, for example, $10cmH_2O$ could then be attempted, by increasing the NAVA level to $1.0cmH_2O/\mu V$. If this second increase results in a pressure well below $20cmH_2O$, this indicates that the patient is 'satisfied' with the unloading and has reduced his or her respiratory drive (i.e. EAdi) in response to the unloading. Similar to other modes of assisted ventilation,

the targeted steps of pressure increase should be performed at the discretion of the caregiver and be appropriate for the type of patient (infant/adult) and pathologies involved.

Using overlay tool
- If a patient is ventilated in a mode other than NAVA, the 'overlay' tool may be used. This tool allows the EAdi waveform to be multiplied by the proposed NAVA level, and the estimated NAVA pressure waveform can be superimposed on the current airway pressure waveform. The NAVA level can then be adjusted to match the peak airway pressure. This also allows optimization of patient–ventilator synchrony in the conventional mode.

Upper pressure limits
As delivered pressure is a function of patient effort, upper pressure limits need to be manually set to avoid the risk of barotrauma.

Backup settings
NAVA is dependent on successful detection of EADi. Should this signal be lost, the backup ventilator settings allow the patient to be ventilated using traditional pneumatic triggers and inspiratory pressure support.

PEEP
Setting the level of PEEP during NAVA currently does not differ from that of other modes of partial ventilatory assist. However, if the EAdi signal persists into the exhalation phase, as commonly observed in infants[4] (so-called 'tonic activity' or EAdi min), this may suggest that adjustment of PEEP is required.

Troubleshooting
Absence of EAdi
- Verify catheter position.
- Reduce trigger sensitivity and assist level.
- Reduce sedation.

Triggering of breath in synchrony with ECG
- Verify electrode position.
- If the signal appearing between QRS complexes is unstable, try advancing the electrode by one inter-electrode distance.

Non-responsiveness to unloading
If testing the physiological response to increasing NAVA levels, ensure the upper pressure limit is set at an adequate level. NAVA does not deliver pressure higher than 5cmH$_2$O below the upper pressure limit.

---

1 Levine S, Nguyen T, Taylor N, et al. (2008) Rapid disuse atrophy of diaphragm fibers in mechanically ventilated humans. *N Engl J Med* **358**, 1327–35.

2 Girard TD, Kress JP, Fuchs BD, et al. (2008) Efficacy and safety of a paired sedation and ventilator weaning protocol for mechanically ventilated patients in intensive care (Awakening and Breathing Controlled trial): a randomised controlled trial. *Lancet* **371**, 126–34.

3 Sinderby C, Navalesi P, Beck J, et al. (1999). Neural control of mechanical ventilation in respiratory failure. *Nat Med* **5**, 1433–6.

4 Emeriaud G, Beck J, Tucci M, Lacroix J, and Sinderby C. (2006) Diaphragm electrical activity during expiration in mechanically ventilated infants. *Pediatr Res* **59**, 705–10.

4.11 Extracorporeal membrane oxygenation

Extracorporeal membrane oxygenation (ECMO) uses modified cardiopulmonary bypass (CPB) technology to provide prolonged respiratory, cardiac, or cardiorespiratory support to patients in ITU who are dying despite optimal conventional treatment. It can be used in patients from 34 weeks gestation up to the elderly for any form of potentially reversible respiratory or cardiac failure. This chapter will concentrate on the use of ECMO to treat adults with respiratory failure.

Patient selection

There are three main questions to be answered during the selection process:
- Does the patient's pre-morbid condition preclude recovery, i.e. what is their physical level of function, which will predict their physiological reserve to survive the current illness?
- Is the current acute disease process potentially reversible or is this the terminal stages of a chronic irreversible illness?
- Are there any absolute contraindications, e.g.
  - High pressure/FiO_2 ventilation for longer than 7 days (peak inspiratory pressure (PIP) > $30cmH_2O$ or FiO_2 > 80%) leads to severe VILI, which makes recovery extremely unlikely
  - Contraindication to limited anticoagulation, e.g. intracranial bleeding
  - Moribund condition, i.e. rigor mortis, prolonged cardiac arrest, brain death (all examples taken from actual ECMO patient referrals).

It is important to emphasize that one-third of adult ECMO patients have multiorgan failure and this is not a contraindication.

The ECMO centre

ECMO is not a treatment that should be offered on an *ad hoc* basis, so patients should be referred to centres with a formal ECMO programme. To find your local centre check the Extracorporeal Life Support Organization (ELSO) website (www.elso.med.umich.edu). ECMO centres are usually tertiary referral hospitals with cardiothoracic units.
- The ECMO co-ordinator manages the programme. The co-ordinator is usually a senior nurse who handles referrals and allocates appropriate personnel.
- The medical team consists of consultants in either cardiothoracic surgery or critical care with specific training in the use of ECMO, and junior staff (ECMO Fellows) from the same specialities.
- ECMO specialists are senior intensive care nurses with additional training who manage the ECMO circuit. They are the most important members of the team.

Each patient has an ECMO specialist and a nurse present 24h a day. All ECMO patients are reported to the ELSO registry. Each programme is supported by perfusion technicians, blood transfusion, cardiology, radiology, physiotherapy, and other specialities. Each ECMO centre has its own retrieval team experienced in the air and ground transport of patients referred for ECMO. This can include establishing ECMO at the referring hospital and then transporting the patient back to base on ECMO (mobile ECMO).

The ECMO circuit

The circuit is designed to eliminate areas of stasis and is much simpler than a CPB circuit, having no reservoir. The ECMO circuit can therefore be run with much less heparin than CPB, typically 10–30u/kg/h, to give a whole blood activated clotting time (ACT) of 140–200s (vs 500–1000s on CPB). The circuit consists of vascular access cannulae, tubing, a pump, an oxygenator with integral heat exchanger, and monitoring devices (see Fig. 4.15). Heparin is adjusted hourly according to the ACT measured at the bedside.

Cannulae

For respiratory support veno-venous access is preferred, usually through a double lumen cannula (27-31F) placed percutaneously via the right internal jugular vein under X-ray control.

Pump

This can be a roller pump (which must have a compliance chamber, servo-regulation, and super-durable raceway tubing) or a centrifugal pump (which must have inlet pressure monitoring), depending on institutional preference.

Bridge

This is a short length of tubing joining the drainage tube (blood from the patient) to the return tubing (blood to the patient). It is kept clamped during ECMO, but can be used to bypass the ECMO circuit, allowing the patient to be clamped off from the circuit. This is necessary when air is being removed from the circuit or components are being changed. Recently, many teams have removed the bridge from the circuit and have it as a component that can be added as required: this eliminates a potential area of clot formation.

Oxygenator

The oxygenator must be specifically designed for long-term support. Polymethylpentene (PMP) hollow-fibre design has low resistance and priming volume with good biocompatibility, and eliminates the plasma leak seen with polypropylene microporus oxygenators. PMP supersedes the previous solid silicone oxygenators. Sweep gas flows through the oxygenator in a counter-current direction to the blood, controlled by a flowmeter. Increasing the sweep gas flow is analogous to increasing the minute volume during mechanical ventilation, causing more CO_2 to be removed but having no effect on oxygenation. Adjusting the FiO_2 of the sweep gas can alter the amount of oxygenation, but many centres use 100% O_2 to simplify management and also to reduce the risk of nitrogen embolus in the event of a membrane rupture. Oxygenation is improved by increasing the ECMO blood flow rate.

Monitoring

Monitoring should consist of a minimum of:
- Inlet pressure monitoring and ultrasonic flow meter for a centrifugal pump
- Servo-regulation alarm for a roller pump
- Pre- and post-membrane pressure monitoring
- Gas supply disconnection alarms for all circuits

Optional extras such as in-line blood gas analysis (i.e. CDI500) can also be added.

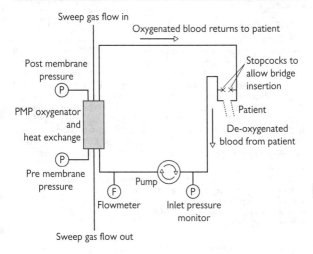

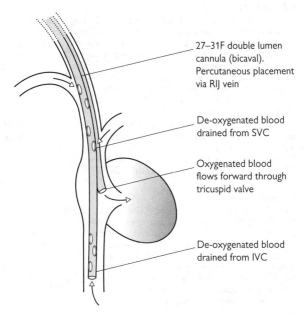

Fig. 4.15 Adult venovenous ECMO circuit for respiratory failure.
PMP = poly-methyl pentene.

ECMO patient management

ECMO circuit

Respiratory patients are managed on veno-venous ECMO. Extracorporeal flow is increased until the venous line pressure is around –50 to –70mmHg (centrifugal pump) or until 4–5L/min flow is obtained. The ventilation is then weaned (see below). Once lung rest is achieved, the ECMO flow is adjusted to give a PaO$_2$ of 6–8kPa. Sweep gas is started at the same rate as the blood flow and then adjusted to maintain a PaCO$_2$ of 5–7kPa. Blood and products are transfused to maintain Hb 12–14g/dL, international normalized ratio (INR) <1.5, fibrinogen >2g/dL and platelet count of >75,000/mL. Invasive procedures are avoided because of the risk of bleeding. If they are absolutely necessary they are undertaken by the most skilled operators available.

Lung rest

Once the patient is established on ECMO, ventilation is reduced to prevent further lung injury. Typical 'rest settings' are:

- PEEP 10–15cmH$_2$O
- Peak airway pressure 20–25cmH$_2$O
- Respiratory rate 10
- FiO$_2$ 0.3.

High-frequency oscillation can also be used to achieve lung rest with the same FiO$_2$ and a mean airway pressure of around 15cmH$_2$O.

General ITU care

This is continued as usual. Full nutrition is provided, a negative fluid balance is initiated and maintained, and antibiotics are given as appropriate. Activated protein C should not be used on ECMO due to the risk of haemorrhage. If renal support is needed a continuous veno-venous haemofiltration (CVVH) machine can be connected to the ECMO circuit. Tracheostomy is usually performed for patients who need more than a week of ECMO.

Other interventions (such as steroids for sepsis or for late stage ARDS) are used as per institutional protocols.

Weaning from ECMO

As the patient recovers the ECMO flow is reduced. When 1L/min is sufficient to maintain blood gas parameters on rest settings, the patient is ventilated with lung protective settings (PIP <30cmH$_2$O, FiO$_2$ <0.6) and the sweep flow is disconnected from the oxygenator while blood flow is maintained. If the patient achieves PaO$_2$ 8-10kPa and PaCO$_2$ 5–7kPa during this 'trial-off' then they can be decannulated.

Complications

Apart from the usual complications of ITU, ECMO has additional risks due to cannulation, anticoagulation, and circuit management. ELSO registry data shows that approximately half of ECMO runs have problems with clots or air in the circuit and a similar incidence of bleeding complications. ECMO teams are well versed in preventing these problems and dealing with them when they occur. A survey of paediatric cardiac ECMO done in non-ECMO centres showed a survival of roughly half that seen in ECMO centres. Complications are also significantly reduced when ECMO is performed by trained teams in dedicated centres.

Results

Approximately 50–70% of adult respiratory patients supported with ECMO can be expected to survive to hospital discharge.

CESAR trial

In the CESAR trial, a strategy of transferring patients to a single centre for advanced respiratory support, including ECMO where necessary, increased survival without disability at 6 months post randomization (47% vs 63%, p = 0.03, number needed to treat (NNT) 6). CESAR was a pragmatic study comparing the actual care given in UK ITUs to that delivered in a single ECMO centre. Although it would have been more elegant to design a study where both groups have carefully regulated treatment, this is practically nearly impossible.

The authors believe that improvement was demonstrated because the patients had such severe lung disease they could not receive lung protective ventilation without the benefit of ECMO. Hopefully the debate that has been generated by CESAR and the 2009 H1N1 epidemic (where ECMO was used extensively and successfully world wide) will lead to improved care for the small minority of patients who develop severe respiratory failure that is refractory to conventional ventilation. ECMO is currently the only adjunct to protective mechanical ventilation shown to improve outcome in severe respiratory failure in adults.

$AVCO_2R$

Artero-venous carbon dioxide removal (AVCO2R) is a simple technique where extracorporeal flows of around 1L/min are generated by the patient's own circulation via a 13F cannula in the femoral artery. Blood is routed through a low-resistance PMP membrane and then returned to the contralateral femoral vein. The circuit requires very little training or supervision to install and operate, and is a very effective method of CO_2 elimination. It has minimal effect on oxygenation and is therefore only suitable for patients with hypercapnoeic respiratory failure. There is a 10% incidence of leg ischaemia associated with the arterial cannulation. Worldwide experience with this technique is much smaller than with ECMO, and cases are not reported to the ELSO registry. Investigations are ongoing, but there is no current evidence of efficacy. Even if effective CO_2 removal is possible, associated hypoxia often continues to deteriorate and requires intervention. It is essential that clinicians recognize the limitations of this device for them to use it successfully; AVCO2R is not a substitute for ECMO.

Conclusion

We know that lung rest and avoidance of tissue oedema result in improved survival for adults with respiratory failure. Unfortunately, a small minority of patients with aggressive disease can quickly end up in a viscous spiral of increasing ventilator pressures, fluid loading, hypoxia, and acidosis, which eliminates any prospect of lung recovery and leads to multiorgan failure and death. ECMO is a tool that allows this spiral to be broken, allows ventilation to be reduced in order to facilitate lung recovery, and allows homeostasis to be restored. ECMO is a complex treatment with enormous potential for harm if not conducted by properly configured and trained teams.

Further reading

Peek GJ, Mugford M, Tiruvoipati R, et al. (2009) Randomized controlled trial and economic evaluation of Conventional Ventilatory Support vs Extracorporeal Membrane Oxygenation for Severe Adult Respiratory Failure (CESAR) [ISRCTN47279827]. *Lancet* **374**, 1351–1363.

Van Meurs K, Lally KP, Peek GJ, and Zwischenberger JB (eds) (2005) *Extracorporeal life support in cardio-pulmonary critical care*, 3rd edn. Extracorporeal Life Support Organization, Ann Arbor, MI.

4.12 Adjuncts to ventilation

Management of the critically ill is complicated, with many confounding factors and treatments influencing the final outcome. It is of the utmost importance to remember two important tenets:

"Primum non nocere" (*Hippocrates*) and
"The art of medicine consists of amusing the patient while nature cures the disease." (*Voltaire*)

The following pages will put in perspective some of the novel additional therapies tested over the last 20 years and whether they have stood the test of time.

In our current world of evidence-based practice it may be depressing to find that none of these therapies has produced a significant reduction in mortality. There may be many reasons for this: the studies are often small, the variation in study design makes direct comparison difficult, and changes in ventilation strategy over the last 20 years may have overtaken the impact of these novel therapies.

However, most of the therapies improve gas exchange, and this may allow some extra time for other proven interventions to work.

Many of the trials into these interventions have used surrogate outcome measures such as length of stay or time on a ventilator. We have to consider whether significant changes in these surrogate end points can be used as a justification for integrating the use of novel therapies into everyday practice.

Prone positioning

First proposed in 1974, prone positioning during ventilation was thought to lead to better expansion of dorsal regions of the lung. Bryan went on to produce two randomized controlled studies (1976 and 1977) showing benefit in oxygenation.

Concepts

Prone position produces transpulmonary pressure gradients sufficient to exceed the opening pressure in dorsal and juxtadiaphragmatic regions where atelactasis and shunt are most severe. Alveolar recruitment with improved oxygenation follows.

- It reduces the compliance of the anterior chest wall, decreasing the over-ventilation of apical areas seen in supine patients, and redistributes ventilation to dorsal regions.
- Perfusion of the lung has a predominantly anatomical distribution, i.e. optimal in the bases. Gravity does not influence blood flow as much as was once thought, and so as ventilation is redirected dorsally, blood flow to this region remains high.
- Improvements in $\dot{V}/\dot{Q}$ matching follow with improved ventilation to the optimally perfused areas.
- When supine PEEP can over-distend apical lung units and divert blood flow to dependent collapsed areas. When prone this effect is reduced.
- Lung compression from the mediastinum is eliminated.
- There is a reduction in incidence of VILI, decreased parenchymal stress and strain, and reduced cytokine release.
- There is a reduction in VAP from better postural drainage of secretions.

Techniques

Prone positioning has become a relatively common procedure. Care should be taken when positioning to avoid pressure areas, particularly to the face and eyes, but also to ensure the thorax and hips are elevated high enough off the bed on supports such that the neck is slightly flexed and the abdomen is free. If there is significant pressure against the abdominal wall, intra-abdominal pressure will be elevated and recruitment will not occur at the bases.

Absolute contraindications are pregnancy and spinal injuries. Relative contraindications include morbid obesity, profound haemodynamic instability, and recent abdominal surgery.

The logistics of proning a patient need to be considered and the process well drilled and practiced.

- Is sedation adequate?
- Muscle relaxation?
- Four or five personnel need to be available for the turn.
- Can patient tolerate circuit disconnection from ETT?

What the evidence shows

- Gattinoni:[1] 304 patients with ARDS/ALI were randomized to conventional ventilation with or without prone ventilation, 6h a day for 10 days. The ICU mortality difference was not significant (48% vs 51%).
- Gattinoni:[2] *Post hoc* analysis of 225 patients proned for 6h a day for 10 days. Mortality outcomes analysed according to PaO_2 response and $PaCO_2$ response. An improvement in oxygenation of >20mmHg not associated with improvement in mortality. Mortality was significantly lower in patients whose $PaCO_2$ fell by >1mmHg compared with those in whom $PaCO_2$ did not fall (35% vs 52%). The fall in $PaCO_2$ was thought to represent evidence of lung recruitment.
- The largest trial[3] of prone ventilation in respiratory failure used 791 patients (413 with ALI/ARDS). Intervention group proned for 8h per day vs control. PaO_2/FiO_2 improved. No mortality benefit (32% vs 32%) and complications increased (pressure sores, extubation, tube obstruction) with proning.
- How quickly should prone positioning commence?[4] 136 patients randomized within 48h to conventional or prone ventilation for 20h per day. Mortality difference (43% vs 58%) not significant. Significant improvements in compliance PaO_2/FiO_2, ventilator days, and ICU length of stay.
- The most recent trial[5] studied 342 patients randomized to conventional or 20h per day prone ventilation. Subgroup stratification into moderate and severe hypoxaemia. There was no difference in the 28-day mortality independent of severity of illness classification.

Summary

No study to date has demonstrated a significant reduction in mortality, but all of them show significant improvements in the PaO_2/FiO_2 ratio which increase with proning duration. The study that gets closest to a significant mortality benefit started proning early and sustained it for 20h a day.

It may be a useful rescue therapy for severe hypoxaemia.

1 Gattinoni L, Tognoni G, Pesenti A, et al. (2001) Effect of prone positioning on survival of patients with acute respiratory failure. *New Engl J Med* **345**(8), 568–73.
2 Gattinoni L, Vagginelli F, Carlesso E, et al. (2003) Decrease in PaCO₂ with prone position is predictive of improved outcome in acute respiratory distress syndrome. *Crit Care Med* **31**(12), 2727–33.
3 Guerin C, Gaillard S, Lemasson S, et al. (2004) Effects of systematic proning in hypoxaemic respiratory failure a randomized controlled study. *JAMA* **292**(19), 2379–87.
4 Mancebo J, Fernandez R, Blanchet L, et al. (2006) A multicenter trial of prolonged prone ventilation in severe acute respiratory distress syndrome. *Am J Respir Crit Care Med* **173**, 1233–9.
5 Taccone P, Pesenti A, Latini R, et al. (2009) Prone postioning in patients with moderate and severe ARDS. *JAMA* **302**(18), 1977–84.

Alveolar recruitment and high PEEP

It is now widely accepted that reducing over-distension of heterogeneous lung units by limiting end-inspiratory volume has a beneficial effect on outcome. Prevention of alveolar collapse and cyclical reopening reduces the production of lung cytokines and may also be beneficial.[1] The extent of end-expiratory collapse, the primary determinant of oxygenation, is a function of both the inspiratory pressure (recruitment) and the level of PEEP (anti-derecruitment). It is implicit that the RM cannot be separated from use of PEEP.

Concepts

Alveolar closing pressures in ARDS vary according to the distribution of lung unit damage. Recruitment is a dynamic process in inspiration to aerate previously collapsed lung units, accomplished by raising the transpulmonary pressue above that used in tidal ventilation.

Returning to the same level of PEEP after a' successful' RM may result in the loss of lung units that have a closing pressure higher than the baseline level of PEEP. Each RM requires a strategy to optimize PEEP, and RMs may need to be repeated to sustain alveolar recruitment. (see 📖 Positive end expiratory pressure, p 119 for further details on the determination of optimal PEEP).

RMs should be considered following techniques which reduce PEEP, for example patient disconnection or physiotherapy and suctioning.

Techniques

Various techniques for performing an RM have been described. In essence they all involve a breath hold in inspiration, usually delivered using a pressure-controlled or CPAP mode. The RM may be limited by haemodynamic compromise or hypoxia. The methods described include:

- Three consecutive 'sigh' breaths every minute for 1h
- PEEP increased to 15cmH$_2$O and two inspiratory pauses of 7s every minute for 15min
- Progressive elevation of PEEP in tandem with peak airway pressure
- Progressive elevation of PEEP with peak airway pressure limited
- Sustained inflation of 40cmH$_2$O applied to patient's airway for up to 1min
- 'Ramping' procedure involving a slow increase in airway pressure up to 40cmH$_2$O.

The act of proning a patient has been described as an RM because of its effects on basal collapse. Performing an RM in the prone position when the anterior chest wall is splinted may reduce the risk of over-distension of apical regions and optimize basal recruitment.[2]

Techniques involving sustained inflation have been reported to result in more transient improvements in oxygenation, and are associated with more haemodynamic compromise and the potential for barotrauma.

What the evidence shows

- Amato[3] demonstrated improved outcome in ARDS with a protective ventilation strategy. The study also included an RM, optimization of PEEP from a static compliance curve, and increasing mean airway pressure using inverse ratio settings. The specific contribution of the RM to the overall outcome is unclear. A more recent study[4] confirms these findings.

- The assessment of low tidal volume and elevated end expiratory pressure to obviate lung injury (ALVEOLI) study[5] assessed 549 patients, randomized to high PEEP (12–24cmH$_2$O) or low levels of PEEP (5–24cmH$_2$O). All patients were ventilated at 6mL/kg. High PEEP improved PaO$_2$/FiO$_2$ but there was no improvement in important outcomes such as mortality (28% v 25%) or length of time on mechanical ventilation.

- ALVEOLI[5] also studied RMs in the first 80 randomized to the high PEEP group. Patients were recruited with CPAP 40cmH$_2$O for 30s. Transient hypotension and hypoxaemia were noted, with no benefit on mortality.

- Badet[6] showed that sigh breaths superimposed on lung-protective mechanical ventilation with optimal PEEP improved oxygenation and static compliance in patients compared with either optimal PEEP alone or optimal PEEP plus one sustained inflation (40cmH$_2$O for 30s).

- Recently published work suggests that if lung can be recruited and recruitment sustained, PVR decreases and improvements in right ventricular function follow.

- All of the studies on protective ventilation with high PEEP and limited plateau pressures encourage a raised mean airway pressure. It may be that recruitment is happening already in these studies over a longer time scale than a single breath, particularly if inverse ratio strategies with pressure control modes are employed to further raise and sustain the mean airway pressure.[2]

Summary

RMs are of interest as an additional tool to manage ARDS. There is no evidence of benefit on important outcomes when used in isolation.

As their purpose is to open the lung, each RM should be followed by an appraisal of the PEEP level. Intermittent sigh breaths appear to be more useful in keeping the lung open after an RM than high PEEP alone.

RMs have less benefit in primary ARDS with more heterogeneous lung units than with the diffuse injury of secondary ARDS.

1 Ranieri VM, Suter PM, Tortorella C, et al. (1999) Effect of mechanical ventilation on inflammatory mediators in patients with ARDS. *JAMA* **282**, 54–61.

2 Galiatsou E, Kostanti E, Svarna E, et al. (2006) Prone position augments recruitment and prevents alveolar overinflation in ALI. *Am J Respir Crit Care Med* **174**(2), 187–197.

3 Amato MB, Barbas CS, Medeiros DM, et al. (1998) Effect of a protective ventilation strategy on mortality in ARDS. *New Engl J Med* **338**, 347–354.

4 Villar J, Kacmarek RM, Pérez-Méndez L, and Aguirre-Jaime A (2006) A high PEEP low tidal volume strategy improves outcome in persistent ARDS. *Crit Care Med* **34**(5), 1311–1318.

5 Brower RG, Lanken PN, MacIntyre N, et al. (2004) Higher versus lower positive end expiratory pressure in patients with ARDS. *New Engl J Med* **351**, 327–336.

6 Badet M, Bayle F, Richard J, and Guerin C (2009) Comparison of optimal positive end-expiratory pressure and recruitment maneuvers during lung-protective mechanical ventilation in patients with acute lung injury/acute respiratory distress syndrome. *Respir Care* **54**(7), 839–840.

Fluid management in acute respiratory failure

The day-to-day management of fluid balance in the critically ill presents a conundrum for the intensivist between optimal perfusion of tissues and the prevention of excess lung water. This debate has been longstanding and continues to be controversial. What about the subgroup of patients with ARDS/ALI?

Concepts
- For each value of the filtration coefficient (capillary leakiness), the balance of pericapillary hydrostatic pressure and colloid osmotic pressure (COP) governs the extravasation of fluids from capillaries.
- The effects of a rise in hydrostatic pressure are mitigated by:
  - Increased lymph drainage in lung compared with normal tissue
  - Simultaneous rise in COP because of the increased loss of fluid to the tissues.
- The shape of the Starling curve describes an initial rapid rise in CO (y-axis) for a small increase in pulmonary artery occlusion pressure (PAOP) (x-axis). In this part of the curve the choice of fluid (crystalloid v colloid) is unlikely to influence formation of pulmonary oedema as the hydrostatic pressure (surrogate PAOP) is low and changes in COP will have negligible impact. The final part of the curve at higher PAOP sees little or no improvement in CO. COP and type of fluid may now be important in countering the higher hydrostatic pressure.
- In ARDS/ALI, the filtration coefficient or capillary leakiness is increased with greater fluid flows into the interstitium.
- In mechanically ventilated patients the increase in pleural pressure may impede fluid reabsorption. Pleural fluid will often accumulate as a result of increased pulmonary filtration, particularly if lymph flow is then exceeded.

Measurement of lung water
- Extravascular lung water (EVLW) measured by a single transpulmonary thermodilution technique is the accepted standard for measurement and monitoring.
- EVLW + pulmonary blood volume correlates well with lung tissue weights estimated from CT scans.
- Increased EVLW is associated with a worse ICU outcome. However, the relationship may be association rather than causation, and there is no evidence that specifically targeting EVLW improves outcome.

What the evidence shows
- Evidence from two large ARDS studies[1,2] shows overall fluid balance while on IPPV accumulated by 1000mL/day.
- FACTT[3] compared two fluid management strategies in ALI in 1000 patients who were randomized to be 'dry' (CVP <4 or PAOP <8) or 'wet' (CVP 10–14 or PAOP 14–18). If the MAP was <60mmHg and the CVP and PAOP were below the upper limits patients were treated with fluid; if CVP or PAOP were above these limits then vasopressors

were used. If MAP was >60mmHg then furosemide would be used when necessary to maintain targets for CVP and PAOP in each of the groups. At the end of 7 days in the dry vs wet groups fluid balance was 0 vs 7000mL, and furosemide used was 1000 vs 45mg. There was no significant difference in primary outcome 60-day mortality (25% vs 28%), but there was a significant reduction in ventilator days with no increase in non-pulmonary-organ failures.

- FACTT[4] also compared PA vs CVP catheters in the management of patients with ALI. Fluid balance was equivalent in the two groups. There were no significant differences in any end point. There was a higher incidence of minor complications associated with the use of PA v CVP catheters, but no excess mortality.
- Another study[5] took 40 patients with ALI (mainly from trauma) and total protein <5g/dL, randomized to a 5-day protocol of 25g albumin every 8h or saline. Both groups received a continuous furosemide infusion, which was discontinued if systolic pressure <90 for >30min, Na >154mmol/L and K <2.6mmol/L. The treatment group had 5.3kg weight loss, were less tachycardic, with a higher mean arterial pressure (MAP) and cardiac output (CO). PaO_2/FiO_2 ratio improved by 40% in first 24h. The improvement was not significant at 7 days.
- Use of traditional PAOP to target optimal fluid resuscitation tends to overestimate the fluid required compared with use of EVLW.

Summary

- Initial fluid loading is essential in hypotensive or shocked patients.
- Judicious fluid resuscitation can be guided by markers of fluid reponsiveness, e.g. an increase in stroke volume or cardiac output until a point of improved or acceptable tissue oxygenation is reached.
- Continuous cardiac output monitoring allows titration of fluid administration to cardiac output response. Measurement of EVLW adds additional information.
- Once initial resuscitation has taken place, a conservative fluid strategy improves lung function and shortens the duration of ventilation. Target values for CVP should be <4 (it does not appear necessary to measure PAOP). Furosemide can be used safely to achieve this together with vasopressors if MAP is low and fluid targets are being sustained.
- Albumin may provide an alternative to vasopressors.[6]
- Hypoproteinemia is an independent prognostic risk factor in ALI/ARDS and contributes to worsening pathophysiology. Fluid balance and oncotic pressure alterations induced by diuretic and colloid therapy improve respiratory physiology (including PaO_2/FiO_2) and are likely to alter net flux of fluid across the injured capillary-alveolar membrane. This strategy will achieve a greater net negative fluid balance and better haemodynamic stability.
- There is unreliable data about the role of other colloids. Some evidence suggests that starches may affect lung water less adversely than gelatins or saline in healthy lungs.[7] However, certain starches at high dose have been shown to cause renal failure in critically ill patients, and currently their use should be restricted.

1 ARDS Network (2000) Ventilation with lower tidal volumes as compared with traditional tidal volumes for ALI/ARDS. *New Engl J Med* **342**(18), 1301–8.

2 Brower RG, Lanken PN, MacIntyre N, *et al.* (2004) Higher versus lower positive end expiratory pressure in patients with ARDS. *New Engl J Med* **351**, 327–36.

3 FACTT NIH ARDS Network (2006) Comparison of two fluid management strategies in acute lung injury. *New Engl J Med* **354**(24), 2564–75.

4 FACTT NIH ARDS Network (2006) PA catheter versus CV catheter to guide treatment for acute lung injury. *New Engl J Med* **354**(21), 2213–24.

5 Martin G, Moss M, Wheeler A, Mealer M, Morris J, and Bernard G (2005) A randomized, controlled trial of furosemide with or without albumin in hypoproteinemic patients with acute lung injury. *Crit Care Med* **33**, 1681–7.

6 Dubois M, Orellana-Jimenez C, Melot C, *et al.* (2006) Albumin administration improves organ function in critically ill hypoalbuminemic patients: a prospective, randomized, controlled, pilot study. *Crit Care Med* **34**(10), 2536–40.

7 Verheij J, van Lingen A, Raijmakers P, *et al.* (2006) Effect of fluid loading with saline or colloids on pulmonary permeability, oedema and lung injury score after cardiac and major vascular surgery. *Br J Anaesth* **96**(1), 21–30.

Nitric oxide

The pathophysiology of ARDS involves mismatching of ventilation/perfusion and pulmonary hypertension. Nitric oxide (NO) may ameliorate these pathophysiological changes. Unfortunately there was a rapid uptake of its use prior to peer review of outcome. Sixty-three per cent of European ITUs were using NO in 1997, and despite evidence of some potential harm 32% of Canadian ICUs continued to use it in 2004.

Concepts

- NO is known to be a local vasodilator released by the endothelium of pulmonary vasculature and probably accounts for the low resting pulmonary vascular tone.
- Hypoxic pulmonary vasoconstriction helps optimize $\dot{V}/\dot{Q}$ matching. It depends on a balance of NO, endothelins, and prostaglandins.
- If inhaled, NO causes selective vasodilatation of pulmonary vasculature at sites of ventilation. This should improve $\dot{V}/\dot{Q}$ matching and hence oxygenation.
- Pulmonary hypertension will also be reduced. NO synthase inhibitors (decrease inducible NO) worsen pulmonary hypertension.
- NO has a very short half-life and systemic effects are minimized. This is probably dose dependent.
- NO is a renal vasodilator and may improve renal blood flow.
- NO reduces leucocyte adhesion.
- NO is known to inhibit mitochondrial and enzymatic function. It can damage DNA, cell membrane permeability and platelet function.

Techniques

NO can be added to the inspired gases at various stages:

- Premixing—usually proximal to the ventilator delivered in the high pressure gas supply.
- Internal mixing—blends NO, O_2, and air within the ventilator.
- Injection techniques—into the ventilator circuit or ETT.

NO is very reactive, and at higher concentrations is readily converted into NO_2 when exposed to oxygen. In order to minimize the available time for this reaction, injection devices are common.

Levels are monitored using an NO analyser, which allows control of the blender. There is no traditional dose-response curve. Doses between 4 and 8ppm appear to improve PaO_2/FiO_2 maximally.

What the evidence shows

- Industry-sponsored studies of 177, 180, and 385 patients, randomized to receive NO or controls. No benefit in mortality (may trend towards worse outcome). Increased end organ damage.
- There are numerous studies from 1995 to 2004. These have been summarized in two meta-analyses:
  - Sokol (2003)—Five randomized studies, no benefit in mortality or ventilator-free days.[1]
  - Adhikari (2007)—12 randomized studies, 5 of which were blinded, no improvement in mortality or ventilator-free days.[2]

- There appears to be a worsening of liver and renal function. There is an increased incidence of renal failure in several of the larger studies.
- Above 80ppm of NO, methaemoglobinaemia becomes significant.

Summary

- NO is associated with a limited improvement in PaO_2/FiO_2 ratio predominantly in first 24h. No firm evidence of harm, but worries persist about consistent trends to increased mortality and incidence of renal failure.
- Improvement in PaO_2/FiO_2 is a poor surrogate marker for mortality. Most patients with ARDS die from multiple organ failure.
- Tachyphylaxis is common.
- Some of these studies were performed in an era when the benefits of protective ventilation were not widely practiced or controlled for.
- The use of NO cannot be recommended in the routine management of ARDS/ALI. Some units continue to use NO as a rescue therapy for profound hypoxaemia.
- NO may have a place for the management of pulmonary hypertension.

1 Sokol J, Jacobs S, and Bohn D (2003) Inhaled nitric oxide for acute hypoxaemic respiratory failure in children and adults: a meta-analysis. *Anesth Analg* **97**, 989–98.
2 Adhikari N, Burns K, Friedrich J, Granton J, Cook D, and Meade M (2007) Effect of nitric oxide on oxygenation and mortality in acute lung injury: systematic review and meta-analysis. *Brit Med J* **334**, 779–86.

β2-agonists

There is limited evidence of the role of any pharmacological strategy to enhance the benefits from improved ventilation strategies over the last 10 years. Following BALTI 1,[1] a phase II study using intravenous β2-agonists for 7 days in patients with ARDS, interest has now turned to a potential role for β2-agonists.

Concepts

Inflammatory modulation

After an inflammatory insult to the lung, neutrophils rapidly aggregate in pulmonary capillaries and then migrate into the alveolar spaces. Pre-treatment with β2-agonists has been shown to modify this process by:

- Increasing neutrophil apoptosis, which may increase clearance of reactive neutrophils from alveolar cells
- Reducing oxygen free radical formation
- Attenuating inflammatory cytokine cascades.

Fluid clearance

Very early in ARDS microvascular thrombosis occurs, with subsequent damage to the alveolar epithelial membrane. This leads to increased fluid crossing into the alveoli and non-cardiogenic pulmonary oedema.

β2-agonists increase the rate of alveolar fluid clearance through effects on sodium and chloride channels and Na/K ATPase pumps.

Techniques

- Nebulised—Evidence suggests that the drug distributes down to the alveoli effectively, but there is little information on doses or efficacy.
- Intravenous therapy—Studies so far have tried an infusion rate around 15ug/kg/h, but again no firm evidence exists around the actual doses that may be effective.
- Potential side effects include tachyarrhythmias, myocardial ischaemia, loss of hypoxic pulmonary vasoconstriction, and metabolic effects such as hypokalaemia and hyperglycaemia.

What the evidence shows

- ALTA[2] (ARDSnet) use of nebulized β2-agonists vs control was stopped due to futility in 279 patients with ALI, no significant difference in ventilator-free days, or 60-day mortality.
- BALTI-2, a UK multicentre placebo-controlled double-blinded study using intravenous salbutamol, for 7 days or until extubated in patients with ARDS, has just been stopped after interim analysis demonstrated excess mortality in the treatment group.

Summary

- Current evidence does not support the routine use of β2 agonists in ARDS.

1 Perkins G, McAuley D, Thickett D, and Gao F (2006) Beta agonist lung injury trial (BALTI): A randomized placebo controlled trial. *Am J Respir Crit Care Med* **173**, 281–7.
2 Matthay M, Brower R, Thompson B, et al. (2009) Randomised placebo-controlled trial of aerosolized albuterol for the treatment of acute lung injury. *Am J Respir Crit Care Med* **179**, A2166.

Rotational therapy

To manually turn critical patients every 2h is part of core practice in critical care. This will reduce the incidence of pressure sores and DVT/PE but may also modify basal atelectasis. Head-up positioning (30–45°) is equally recognized as important to reduce the incidence of VAP. These two strategies are not completely compatible. On average patients undergo 9.6 turns in a 24h period. In the original studies compared with no movement, significant reductions in VAP and length of stay in ICU were achieved.

Concepts
- Increase in FRC in ventilated patients due to an increased critical opening pressure to the uppermost lung. Improved $\dot{V}/\dot{Q}$ matching.
- Enhanced drainage of secretions.
- Baboons[1] ventilated for 11 days' continuous rotation to 45° on each side had better PaO_2/FiO_2 ratios and showed less lung injury (CXR/lavage and post Mortem).

Techniques
- 'Continuous lateral rotation' is the generic term to describe using a bed that rotates through its longtitudinal axis in either a continuous or intermittent motion.
- 'Kinetic therapy' describes an arc of 80° (>40° either side).
- Most commercial beds work in the arc of 50–120° (25–60° either side).
- Other therapies that can be delivered by these beds include percussion, vibration, and pulsation.
- Potential disadvantages include disconnection of ETT or CVC and intolerance by patients (often require increased levels of sedation).
- Contraindicated in spinal injury and with agitated or awake non-ventilated patients.

What the evidence shows
First studies reported in 1967.
- There are 15 non-randomized studies. These tend to be descriptive, with relatively small numbers of patients and comment on reductions in complications.
- Twenty prospective randomized studies exist in the literature. In all of these studies the degree of rotation, the number of rotations per hour, and duration of rotation were variable. No real comment can be made except that there is possibly greater benefit with greater arc of rotation.
- The best review, by Sahn,[2] looks at two retrospective analyses, the best four randomized studies, and a meta-analysis.[3] All the studies reviewed compared RotoRest (KCI) vs standard manual turning every 2h. There were significant reductions in the incidence of VAP in the first 2 weeks, ventilator days, and ICU length of stay. No significant difference in the primary end points of length of hospital stay and mortality.
- Staudinger and colleagues[4] compared prone ventilation with rotational therapy in 26 ARDS patients. They found no difference in physiology or outcome.

- In a review of VAP,[5] no recommendation could be made for prone positioning or rotational therapy compared with a 45° head-up position.
- Reported reduced risk of DVT/PE.

Summary

- Rotational therapy has the theoretical benefits of prone positioning, with increased FRC, and optimized V̇/Q̇ matching.
- Improved drainage of secretions, reduction in VAP rate relative to manual turning.
- There is a trend to do better if >40° for more than 18h a day. Overall difficult to make specific recommendations about strategy, angle, frequency, pause time, or use of adjuncts such as vibration, percussion, and pulsation.
- Limited evidence of overall benefit. Probably need to target specific patients where other more proven strategies are not possible.

1 Anzueto A, Peters J, Seidner S, et al. (1997) Effects of continuous rotation and prolonged mechanical ventilation on healthy adult baboons. Crit Care Med **25**, 1560–4.
2 Sahn S (1991) Continuous lateral rotational therapy and nosocomial pneumonia. Chest **99**, 1263–7.
3 Choi S and Nelson L (1992) Kinetic therapy in critically ill patients: Combined results based on meta-analysis. J Crit Care **7**, 57–62.
4 Staudinger T, Kofler J, Müllner M, et al. (2001) Comparison of prone positioning and continuous rotation of patients with ARDS: Results of a pilot study. Crit Care Med **29**, 51–6.
5 Dodek P, Keenan S, Cook D, et al. (2004) Evidence based clinical practice guideline for the prevention of VAP. Ann Intern Med **20**, 225–32.

Surfactant

Surfactant (phospholipid 90%/surfactant proteins 10%) is produced by type II alveolar cells. It is fundamental in reducing alveolar surface tension and preventing alveolar collapse. It may also help in local immune function.

Concepts

- Surfactant production is impaired in ARDS and pneumonia.
- In theory, replacing surfactant should reduce surface tension and alveolar collapse.
- Surfactant in use is either synthetic (no surfactant proteins) or recombinant with added surfactant proteins B and C.

Techniques

- Nebulization of surfactant has been tried and is a component of many studies. No real benefit has been demonstrated and it is likely that the delivered dose of drug by this route is inadequate.
- Direct instillation of liquid surfactant (+postural changes to aid distribution if tolerated) seems more effective and allows larger doses of drug to be delivered. A variant of this is targeted instillation with a bronchoscope.

What the evidence shows

Over 250 studies of varying sophistication exist in the literature.

- Use of exogenous surfactant in the respiratory distress syndrome of premature infants is of proven benefit and part of standard practice.
- In ARDS, many case series or pilot studies report safety and improved PaO_2/FiO_2. Heterogenicity exists between the origin of the surfactant in use, dose, mode of delivery, duration of therapy, and study end points. This makes useful comparison particularly difficult.
- A multicentre randomized double-blind study[1] in 725 patients using nebulized synthetic surfactant for 5 days failed to demonstrate a significant difference.
- A small, prospective randomized controlled trial (32 patients) of bovine surfactant down ETT,[2] showed a significant reduction in mortality (18% vs 44%).
- Meta-analysis[3] reduced the available literature down to six trials (1270 patients) of suitable standardization and quality. There was no significant difference in any measured end point.

Summary

- Not all the isoforms of synthetic surfactants have the same mechanical properties in the lung as human surfactant.
- In neonates there is a deficiency of surfactant. In ARDS there is an abnormality of surfactant.
- There is no evidence of benefit for use of surfactant in adults. Enthusiasts for surfactant find this surprising, point to the lack of standardization in study designs, and call for further studies to be performed.

1 Anzueto A, Baughman R, Guntupalli K, *et al.* (1996) Aerosolised surfactant in adults with sepsis induced ARDS. *New Engl J Med* **334**, 1417–21.
2 Gregory T, Steinberg K, Spragg R, *et al.* (1997) Bovine surfactant therapy for patients with ARDS. *Am J Respir Crit Care Med* **155**, 1039–1315.
3 Davidson W, Dorscheid, D, Spragg R, *et al.* (2006) Exogenous surfactant for treatment of ARDS. *Crit Care* **10**(2), R41.

Helium

Helium is an inert gas whose density is one-seventh that of air, with a slightly higher viscosity. Breathing helium reduces resistance to flow. Theoretically this could be of benefit in upper airways obstruction, COPD, and asthma.

Concepts

- Gas flow in airways is complex. Turbulent flow occurs in the larynx and trachea. The transition to laminar flow occurs in the main stem and lobar bronchi at low flow, and at fifth-generation bronchi at high flow rates (2L/s).
- Reynolds number (Re =2 × flow × density/π × radius × viscosity) predicts laminar flow (Re < 2000) or turbulent flow (Re > 4000). Reducing density and increasing viscosity reduces the Reynolds number and favours laminar flow.
- With laminar flow: flow ∝ driving pressure; density has no effect on pressure–flow relationships.
- With turbulent flow: flow ∝ √driving pressure; lower density significantly lowers the driving pressure needed at a given flow.
- Breathing Heliox (see below) allows more rapid transit of gas, shorter inspiratory and expiratory times and specifically a reduction in gas trapping. In certain circumstances, it may considerably reduce WOB.
- Effects are lost if helium concentration falls much below 65%. This means that FiO2 is limited to <35%.

Techniques

- Helium is commercially available as pure Helium (used in respiratory function labs), but more practically as Heliox, a mix of 21% oxygen and 79% helium
- Heliox can be blended with oxygen and breathed spontaneously. If an oxygen analyzer is in use then the ideal blend helium and oxygen can be obtained.
- There are 4 commercially available ventilators that can deliver helium to ventilated patients. Helium has a very high specific heat capacity and cools heated wire flow sensors. Flow is calculated using a pressure drop across a narrowed orifice.

What the evidence shows

- The traditional indication for Heliox is upper airway obstruction. Concentrations <60% may be effective.
- More recently it has been used for bronchoscopic procedures where instrumentation narrows the airway, particularly in patients with respiratory failure.
- In asthma, Heliox may be useful if the patient is deteriorating with respiratory acidosis and slow response to normal therapy. Heliox reduces WOB and may delay the need for ventilation. There are reports of reduction in gas trapping and doubling tidal volume in ventilated patients. $PaCO_2$ and H^+ may fall. These manoeuvres aim to provide extra time for normal pharmacological manipulation to work.

Systematic review of 554 adults with acute asthma failed to show any improvement in lung function or other outcomes.

- In COPD faster inspiratory and expiratory flows reduce dynamic hyperinflation, move the lung volumes to a more mechanically advantageous volume for the start of inspiration, and potentially reduce $PaCO_2$. The largest randomized trial (n = 204) of Heliox added to NIV for COPD exacerbations did not demonstrate any difference in measured outcomes.[1]
- Using Heliox as the driving gas for nebulisers improves the delivery of drug to the alveoli.

Summary

- The benefits of the use of helium in upper airway obstruction are uncontested.
- Benefits in other conditions have not yet been demonstrated.

1 Maggiore S, Richard J, Abroug F, et al. (2010) A multicenter, randomized trial of noninvasive ventilation with helium-oxygen mixture in exacerbations of chronic obstructive lung disease. Crit Care Med 38(1), 145–51.

Tracheal gas insufflation

Over the last 20 years the concept of permissive hypercapnia has become part of the management of ARDS/ALI. This phenomenon followed a better understanding of the actual physiological effects of an elevated $PaCO_2$. It allows us to practice protective ventilation with lower plateau pressures and higher PEEP but smaller targeted tidal volumes. The patient's ability to tolerate permissive hypercapnia is compromised in particular by concomitant metabolic acidosis. In this situation strategies have been employed to try and lower $PaCO_2$, e.g. NovaLung and tracheal gas insufflation.

Concepts

- The delivery of fresh gas close to the carina washes CO_2 out of the large airways, effectively reducing dead-space ventilation.
- The higher the flow of insufflated gas the more turbulent the flow close to the carina, the more gas mixing takes place, and the better the $PaCO_2$ clearance.

Technique

- Fresh gas is delivered down a catheter positioned close to the carina.
- The gas must be humidified.
- Conventional ventilation is delivered via the ETT.
- Tracheal Gas Insufflation is not easily synchronized and so takes place throughout the respiratory cycle. It therefore increases tidal volume and airway pressures in inspiration and may cause volutrauma.
- If the jet of gas is too high in expiration, auto PEEP occurs and may cause barotrauma.
- There is a risk of trauma to the airway directly from the catheter.

What the evidence shows

There are no large randomized controlled studies, only small series (<10 patients reporting physiological changes).

- Studies reliably show an ability to lower $PaCO_2$ and decrease V_d/V_t ratios.[1]
- Modification of the technique to synchronize with expiration (expiratory washout) will avoid the rise in tidal volume and airway pressures, but may still generate auto PEEP.[2] No such device exists commercially at present.

Summary

- The widespread acceptance of permissive hypercapnia has obviated the need to aggressively reduce $PaCO_2$.

1 Ravenscraft S, Burke W, Nahum A, et al. (1993) Tracheal Gas Insufflation augments CO_2 clearance during mechanical ventilation. Am J Respir Crit Care Med **148**(2), 345–51.
2 Kalfon P, Rao G, Gallart L, et al. (1997) Permissive hypercapnia with and without expiratory washout. Anesthesiology **87**(1), 6–17.

Partial liquid ventilation

Perfluorocarbons have a high affinity for binding oxygen and carbon dioxide. They are also physiologically inert and do not undergo degradation in the body. Animal studies demonstrate that mice can survive and breathe submerged in a tank of oxygenated perfluorocarbons.

Concepts

Perfluorocarbons have been studied in patients with ARDS/ALI.[1,2] If inhaled they remove the air/fluid interface at the alveolar epithelial membrane.

- They gravitate to the dependent areas (of optimal perfusion) as they are heavier than water. $\dot{V}/\dot{Q}$ matching will benefit.
- They reduce surface tension in alveoli, improve FRC, and hence recruit alveoli.

Technique

- The lung is degassed and filled with liquid perfluorocarbon. 'Tidal volumes' of perfluorocarbon are then added and removed. Carbon dioxide is extracted from, and oxygen added to, the perfluorocarbon before 'reventilation'.
- It is also possible to partly fill the lung (low-dose perfluorocarbon) and then ventilate the patient conventionally. Problems exist with viscid sputum clearance, constant evaporation of the perfluorocarbon, and inability to use chest radiographs as perfluorocarbons are radio-opaque.

What the evidence shows

- Numerous animal studies and some phase 1 and 2 studies on humans have shown improvements in lung compliance and $\dot{V}/\dot{Q}$ ratio without increase in mortality.
- Two randomized studies in over 400 patients with ALI have shown no benefit in mortality or duration of mechanical ventilation.

Summary

Although considerable novelty exists around this technique, the use of perfluorocarbons cannot be recommended at present.

1 Kacmarek RM, Wiedemann HP, Lavin PT, et al. (2006) Partial liquid ventilation in adult patients with acute respiratory distress syndrome. *Ann J Respir Crit Care Med* **173**(8), 882–9.
2 Hirschl RB, Croce M, Gore D, et al. (2002) Prospective, randomized, controlled pilot study of partial liquid ventilation in adult respiratory distress syndrome. *Am J Respir Crit Care Med* **165**(6), 781–7.

The ventilated patient

5.1 Tracheal tubes

The presence of a cuffed ETT secures the airway for ventilation and allows the generation of much higher ITPs during invasive ventilation than are possible during NIV. ETTs also facilitate airway toilet and provide some protection against gas and fluid leakage.

Ventilator-associated pneumonia

Recently, the role of tracheal tubes in the pathogenesis of VAP has been highlighted. Indeed, some assert that this common complication could be better termed intubation-associated pneumonia. Two aspects of tracheal intubation lead to VAP:
- Aspiration of contaminated oro-pharyngeal secretions
- The development of a biofilm on the surfaces of the tube.

The following modifications to tracheal tubes help prevent lower airway contamination and colonization, reducing the risk of VAP.[1]

Subglottic drainage

Some tracheal tubes have been adapted to incorporate a subglottic drainage port, situated above the cuff. Suctioning this channel removes contaminated oro-pharyngeal secretions and reduces aspiration.
- Six RCTs have demonstrated that subglottic drainage prevents VAP.
- Meta-analysis has confirmed that the incidence of VAP is halved in patients with a subglottic drainage port.[2]

Despite the weight of evidence, few ICUs use subglottic drainage. There are a number of reasons postulated for this reluctance:
- There are logistical problems in ensuring that patients requiring ventilation for more than 1 day receive a subglottic drainage tube.
- Replacement of conventional tubes would expose the patient to the risk of re-intubation, including aspiration and pneumonitis.
- There are anecdotal reports of mucosal damage and suction channel blockages.

Tracheal tube cuffs

- Conventional tracheal tube cuffs have a high volume and low internal pressure, designed to prevent tracheal wall damage. The cuff wall is >50µm thick. Small folds in the cuff permit micro-aspiration of contaminated oro-pharyngeal secretions, colonizing the lower airways.
- Recently, high-volume low-pressure cuffs with thin (7µm) walls have been introduced. This structure avoids the formation of folds in the cuff wall.
- Another solution has been a silicone low-volume, low-pressure cuff.
- Leakage past these cuffs is minimized, and there is some evidence that the combination of these cuffs with subglottic drainage reduces VAP.

Routine cuff pressure measurement

- Cuff pressures <20cmH$_2$O are associated with the development of VAP. Pressures >30cmH$_2$O may cause ischaemic injury to the tracheal mucosa.
- Routine cuff pressure measurement should ensure that pressures are kept within the range 20–30cmH$_2$O.
- Automatic cuff pressure controllers are available.

Impregnated tracheal tubes

The formation of biofilm on tracheal tubes is implicated in the pathogenesis of VAP. In 70% of cases of VAP, genotypically identical organisms have been recovered from tracheal tubes and the lungs. Bacteria in biofilm reside in a protective extracellular matrix and behave more like a sessile multicellular organism. They are resistant to antibiotics and are continually dispersed into the lower airways by ventilation and suctioning.

Recently silver-coated tracheal tubes have been developed. Silver ions have broad-spectrum antibacterial actions and inhibit biofilm formation. Silver-impregnated tubes reduce bacterial colonization of the airways and have been shown to reduce the rate of VAP in patients ventilated for >24h.[3]

It seems prudent to consider the use of subglottic drainage, aspiration-resistant cuffs, or silver-coated tubes in patients at high risk of developing VAP. These technologies would be attractive in ICUs with a high incidence of VAP, despite the introduction of other preventative measures.

Mechanical complications

Position of tracheal tube

The critically ill patient requiring tracheal intubation presents challenges that require expertise and the immediate availability of the adjuncts for difficult intubation.

- Immediately after intubation, correct placement of the tracheal tube is confirmed both clinically and by capnography.
- Chest radiography may reveal right main bronchial intubation. The tip of the tracheal tube should lie in the middle third of the tracheal with the head and neck in the neutral position. This avoids cord damage and extubation on neck extension, and bronchial intubation on flexion.

Inadvertent extubation is common, perhaps more so with lighter levels of sedation and positional changes. No method of securing the tube is absolutely safe and care must be taken during changes of the patient's position.

Occlusion

Tracheal tubes will partly occlude with respiratory secretions.

- Using larger tubes delays this process, but they are more uncomfortable and cause more mucosal damage.
- Recognition of partial tube occlusion is difficult, especially with the use of pressure support and automatic tube compensation.
- Difficulty in ventilation, or weaning, and a rise in respiratory resistance, indicated by high peak pressures, should lead one to suspect obstruction.
- If a flow trigger is used, a large negative pressure may be required to generate sufficient flow to initiate inspiration.

Post-extubation stridor

Post-extubation stridor is more common in patients after a traumatic intubation, in those with laryngeal oedema, and those ventilated for more than 3 days.

- A leak past the deflated tracheal tube cuff of less than 25% of the tidal volume helps predict stridor.

- Prophylactic steroids may be given at least 4h before extubation to reduce the risk of stridor and re-intubation.
- Voice hoarseness, a bovine cough, and difficulty swallowing are common after extubation. These symptoms usually settle over 1–2 days. If symptoms persist, an ENT consultation is helpful.
- Serious complications, such as laryngeal injury, arytenoid dislocation, subglottic stenosis, and laryngeal nerve injury are uncommon.

1 Lorente L, Blot S, and Rello J (2007) Evidence on measures for the prevention of ventilator associated pneumonia. *Eur Respir J* **30**, 1193–207.
2 Lorente L, Lecuona M, Jimenez A, Mora ML, and Sierra A (2007) Influence of an endotracheal tube with polyurethane cuff and subglottic secretion drainage on pneumonia. *Am J Respir Crit Care Med* **176**, 1079–83.
3 Kollef MH, Afessa B, Anzueto, A, et al. (2008) Silver-coated endotracheal tubes and incidence of ventilator-associated pneumonia. The NASCENT Randomized Trial. *J Am Med Assoc* **300**(7), 805–13.

5.2 Tracheostomy

A tracheostomy is an artificial opening in the trachea, formed surgically or using a percutaneous technique, through which a tracheostomy tube is placed.

Tracheostomy may be temporary or permanent, and placed electively or as an emergency. This chapter will concentrate on planned, temporary tracheostomy in the critically ill.

Indications for temporary tracheostomy in the critically ill

- To allow prolonged invasive ventilation.
- To protect and maintain the airway in patients with neurological disease, e.g. head trauma, bulbar palsy.
- To maintain an airway, e.g. upper airway obstruction.
- To facilitate reduction in sedation and weaning from the ventilator.
- For ongoing bronchial toilet (e.g. inadequate cough, profuse secretions) when there is no longer a need for ventilatory support.

Reported advantages of tracheostomy over endotracheal intubation

- Reduced need for sedation with improved patient comfort.
- Assisted weaning due to reduced dead space. However, the decrease in dead space has been measured at <20mL.
- Reduced tube resistance and WOB.
- Improved mouth care.
- Decreased incidence of sinusitis (particularly compared to naso-tracheal intubation).
- Enables speech (with use of a speaking valve).
- Reduced risk of inadvertent decannulation.
- Ability to move patient to a lower dependency area.

Timing of tracheostomy

The optimal timing for tracheostomy in the critically ill is not known and the evidence to date is conflicting. Current practice in most ICUs is to site a tracheostomy for those patients who are likely to require prolonged translaryngeal intubation, but this is based on personal preference and received wisdom rather than evidence of superiority. There are advocates of early tracheostomy, delayed tracheostomy, and occasional proponents of prolonged translaryngeal intubation.

A recent UK multicentred trial (Tracman) randomized over 900 patients to either early (<4 days) or late (>10 days) tracheostomy. It demonstrated that tracheostomy timing had no effect on 30-day mortality, antibiotic usage, ICU or hospital length of stay, although sedation requirements were reduced in survivors.

Further interpretation of the results suggested that in every 100 patients predicted to be ventilated for 1 week or longer, performing an early tracheostomy would result in 48 unnecessary tracheostomies and three procedural complications. ICU survivors, however, would require 2.4 days less sedation (D. Young, personal communication).

Percutaneous dilational tracheostomy vs surgical tracheostomy

Meta-analyses have concluded that, in comparison to surgical tracheostomy, percutaneous dilational tracheostomy (PDT) results in less frequent wound infections, with equivalent rates of bleeding and procedural complications. Consequently, PDT is now recommended as the procedure of choice for critically ill adult patients.

In some patients surgical tracheostomy may be preferred:

- Coagulopathy—direct haemostasis reduces post-procedural bleeding.
- Obesity—tracheostomy in general is more hazardous in the very obese, and is associated with more life-threatening complications. Comparison between PDT and surgical tracheostomy in the morbidly obese reveals similar rates of adverse events. Carefully consider the suitability of the available percutaneous kit in the very obese, as depth of insertion may exceed the capacity of the dilator.
- High ventilatory requirements/high PEEP—the loss of PEEP associated with the technique of PDT has led some to consider PEEP >10cmH$_2$O a contraindication to tracheostomy. In surgical tracheostomy, when a bronchoscope is not used and the ETT is not withdrawn until the trachea is exposed, the loss of PEEP may be less than using a PDT technique.
- Anatomical variance/proximity to previous surgery—patients with a deep lying trachea or reduced crico-sternal distance are often inappropriate for PDT, as are patients who have a large goitre or previous surgery to the neck.

Performing a tracheostomy

The most common technique for performing PDT was described by Ciaglia (pronounced 'Shy-ia') in 1985, involving serial dilatation over a wire. This has now developed into a single 'rhino horn' dilator system. Other techniques include Griggs' single forceps dilatation, the PercuTwist single dilator with a screw thread, and the Fantoni translaryngeal tracheostomy technique. Description of a standard technique for performing percutaneous tracheostomy may be found in the UK Intensive Care Society's *Standards for the care of adult patients with a temporary tracheostomy*.

Practical advice

- Bronchoscopy should be available and used routinely.
- Two trained medical practitioners are required—one to manage the airway and anaesthesia, and one to perform the procedure. Both should wear eye protection against aerosolized blood and respiratory secretions.
- Choose the tracheostomy tube that is most suitable for the individual patient (see below).
- Visualize the anterior neck with ultrasound prior to the procedure to identify blood vessels in the line of the proposed stoma.
- Extend the neck with a rolled towel or similar under the shoulders and remove the pillow.
- Elevate the head of the bed to minimize bleeding.
- Allow adequate time for local anaesthetic (and vasoconstrictor) to work.
- Ensure surgical anaesthesia and neuromuscular blockade.

- Set inspired oxygen concentration to 100% and aspirate the NGT.
- In slim patients with minimal respiratory support, the ETT may be replaced with a laryngeal mask airway or a ProSeal laryngeal airway.
- Swabs soaked in 1% lidocaine with adrenaline placed in the wound minimize ooze between dissection and cannulation of trachea.
- Attach a syringe containing saline to the introducer needle to easily detect aspiration of air once the trachea is entered.
- If bronchoscopically guided and uncomplicated, CXR may not be required post procedure.
- Documentation of the process should include the staff involved, the technique employed, the size and type of tube inserted, and difficulties or immediate complications.

Complications in tracheostomy care

Complications may be minimized by monitoring cuff pressure, humidification of inspired gases, regular suctioning, cleaning/changing of inner tubes, and good wound care of the stoma. The most common complications are shown in Table 5.1.

Table 5.1 Common complications in tracheostomy care

Immediate	Early	Late
Bleeding	Bleeding	Bleeding
Misplacement of tube	Misplacement of tube	Infection
Pneumothorax	Pneumothorax	Tracheal ulceration
Surgical emphysema	Surgical emphysema	Tracheal stenosis
	Blockage	Blockage
		Stoma granulation
		Fistula formation • Oesophageal • Innominate artery • Cutaneous (persistent stoma)

Choice of tracheostomy tube

Care should be taken in choosing the correct tube for each patient. The assessment should include the depth and angle of the trachea relative to skin, the length of the trachea (may be related to patient height), and the proposed site of insertion. Inappropriate insertion can lead to tube displacement, local erosion, cutaneous infection, vascular and oesophageal fistulation, and tracheal stenosis (Table 5.2).

Tracheostomy tubes are constructed from a variety of materials and vary considerably in rigidity, durability, and kink resistance. Tubes are usually chosen according to their inner diameter, with less consideration to external diameter, angulation, and length. Often, these choices are only considered following assessment of a poorly fitting tube.

Most adult patients who require a temporary tracheostomy during their critical illness will initially need a semi-soft, cuffed, non-fenestrated tube, ideally with an inner cannula.

Table 5.2 Potential problems arising from insertion of an inappropriate tracheostomy tube

Intratracheal tube length too short	Misplacement, pressure on anterior or posterior tracheal wall, leading to erosion or later stenosis formation
Intratracheal tube length too long	Bronchial placement, pressure on anterior or posterior tracheal wall
Intrastomal tube length too short	Misplacement, pressure on anterior neck structures
Intrastomal tube length too long	Risk of tube kinking or becoming misplaced
Incorrect angulation	Airway obstruction, tracheal erosion
Tube too small	High cuff pressures needed, leading to tracheal erosion/stenosis, increased WOB
Tube too large	Difficulty in insertion, no leak when cuff down precludes use of speaking valve and hinders swallowing

Inner diameter
Trachestomy tubes are usually chosen according to their inner diameter. The inner diameter will be reduced by an inner cannula (see below). Smaller tubes are associated with greater resistance to airflow and increased WOB.

The sizing of tubes varies markedly between manufacturers, leading to confusion. Table 5.3 shows the inner diameters of three different tracheostomy tubes, all size 7.

Table 5.3 Inner diameters of tracheostomy tubes

Tracheostomy tube	Inner diameter (mm)
Portex® Blue Line®	5.0
Portex® Blue Line Ultra®	5.5
Kapitex® Tracoetwist®	7.0

External diameter
External diameter is (obviously) larger than inner diameter. It determines the size of the defect to be made in the anterior tracheal wall and may affect the degree of long-term tracheal stenosis. The choice of tube therefore is a compromise between sufficient internal diameter and excessive

external diameter. A thorough understanding of manufacturers' sizing schemata is important.

Inner cannula

Tracheostomy tubes with inner cannulae are inherently safer than single cannula tubes, as they allow immediate relief of airway obstruction should the tube become blocked with encrusted secretions, blood clot etc. In addition, a non-fenestrated inner cannula may allow assisted ventilation in a patient with a fenestrated tracheostomy *in situ*, without the need for a full tracheostomy tube change.

The presence of an inner cannula causes an inevitable reduction in the functional internal diameter. This results in an increase in airway resistance and WOB.

Patients should not be discharged from a critical care setting with a tracheostomy tube that has no inner cannula.

Angulation

Insertion of a tracheostomy whose angulation is not properly matched to the individual patient's anatomy can lead to the tip of the tube abutting either the posterior or anterior tracheal wall. This may lead to airway obstruction and tracheal erosion. Most tubes have a fixed angulation, but flexible/armoured tubes are also available.

Length/adjustable flange

The distance between skin incision and trachea varies considerably between patients. Consequently, the length of tracheostomy tube that is intrastomal rather than intratracheal will vary. Failure to appreciate this is a common cause of poor fit. In the obese, for example, the intratracheal portion of the tube is often too short, leading to problems with tube obstruction against the posterior tracheal wall, tube displacement, and tracheal erosion. Similarly, in patients with very thin necks, the tracheal segment of the tube may be too long. The use of a flexible tracheostomy tube, or one with an adjustable flange, may be useful in these situations, but it must be remembered that these tubes have no inner cannula.

Cuff

Cuffs allow effective mechanical ventilation and protect the lower respiratory tract against aspiration. The cuff should effectively seal the trachea at pressures of 20–25cmH$_2$O. Regular monitoring of this pressure is important in reducing late tracheal erosion and stenosis. Excessive cuff pressures may result if the tube is poorly positioned within the trachea or if the tracheostomy tube itself is too small.

Fenestration

Fenestrated tubes have a single large window or multiple small perforations in the posterior wall of the tracheostomy tube, above the cuff but within the trachea. They should not be used without an inner cannula when positive pressure ventilation is necessary, as they carry a significant risk of surgical emphysema. They are primarily used in weaning and to aid phonation. In reality, the fenestrations are often poorly positioned within the trachea and down sizing or deflating the cuff of a standard tracheostomy is more effective.

Subglottic suction ports
Subglottic suction ports allow aspiration of secretions from the trachea above the cuff and may contribute to a reduction in VAP. However, they necessitate a larger stoma, and may lead to tracheal stenosis and unsightly scars.

Changing a tracheostomy tube

- Changing a tracheostomy tube is potentially hazardous and should only be attempted by staff who are competent in the procedure.
- Time to closure of tracheostomy stoma is directly related to duration of cannulation, occurring almost immediately if a newly placed tracheostomy is removed, and taking up to a couple of days if cannulation has lasted over 2 weeks.
- Changes within the first 72h should be avoided unless absolutely essential, and should only be performed in an environment in which translaryngeal intubation could immediately be secured if necessary. The first tracheostomy change should take place between 7 and 10 days after a percutaneous tracheostomy as the risk of stoma closure lessens after this time. The use of a bougie or airway exchange catheter should be considered for the first tube change.
- Tracheostomy tubes without inner cannulae should be changed every 7–14 days.
- Subsequent tube changes are likely to be easier, but should still be performed by appropriately trained staff, in a safe environment, with a back-up plan if the tube cannot be inserted or is misplaced.
- Tracheostomy tubes with inner cannulae require the inner cannula to be changed daily, or more frequently if secretions are thick and there is risk of tube obstruction, but there is usually no need to change the outer tube routinely.
- Indications for changing an outer cannula would be to downsize or to change for a fenestrated tube.

Tracheostomy emergencies

Blockage
A blocked tracheostomy usually presents with respiratory difficulty or an inability to pass a suction catheter. Most patients on the ICU with a temporary tracheostomy in place will have normal upper airway anatomy. A systematic approach to management is important:
- If the cuff is up, and the patient can breathe spontaneously, deflate the cuff to allow breathing past the tracheostomy via the nose and mouth.
- If the tracheostomy has an inner tube, remove it. Depending on the type of tracheostomy, it may be necessary to replace the inner tube to allow connection of the tube to a breathing circuit.
- If the tracheostomy tube is completely blocked, it is safer to remove the tube and ventilate via the face (assuming normal upper airway anatomy), remembering to occlude the stoma site with gauze swabs or similar.
- If the tracheostomy tube appears partially patent attempt to pass a suction catheter. If this is possible, it may be feasible to change the tube over a bougie.

- If it is impossible to pass a suction catheter, attach a Waters' circuit to the tracheostomy tube to make an assessment of airflow through the tube.
- Attempts to oxygenate the patient via a bag/valve/mask at the face may not be successful with a tracheostomy tube *in situ*.
- If the tube is fully blocked, attempts to change the tracheostomy should only be made by experienced personnel.
- Oral intubation may be necessary. In this case, use an uncut tube and inflate the cuff distal to the stoma site.

Displacement

A partially displaced tube is as dangerous as, if not more so, a fully displaced one. Displacement may result from moving the patient or from ventilator tubing pulling on the tracheostomy. Restless or agitated patients may displace their own tubes.

- A displaced tracheostomy usually presents with respiratory difficulty or the inability to pass a suction catheter.
- If a trachestomy tube becomes partially displaced, it is safer for the inexperienced practitioner to fully remove the tube and maintain the airway by other methods rather than attempt to replace it.
- CXR does not give useful information about the position of a tracheostomy tube in this situation.
- A spontaneously breathing patient may be able to breathe through their nose or mouth if the tracheostomy tube is partially displaced. The patient may also breathe through the stoma site. Listening over the nose, mouth, and stoma site will clarify where to apply supplemental oxygen. If assisted ventilation is needed, occlude the stoma and assist breathing via the face.
- Experienced staff may attempt to re-insert a tracheostomy via the stoma, especially if the tracheostomy was formed more than 7 days previously. This is likely to be easier if the tracheostomy tube is inserted with the introducer in place.
- If insertion of a pre-formed tracheostomy tube is difficult, an ETT may be passed through the stoma, taking care not to insert it too far.
- Oral intubation may be necessary, as above.

Bleeding

Bleeding is the most common complication of tracheostomy and can occur early (within 48h) or late (days later). It may be minor or major, requiring transfusion.

- Minor bleeding may be controlled with pressure, infiltration with dilute adrenaline (1:100 000), or application of Kaltostat® around the stoma site.
- Major bleeding may require surgical exploration.
- Bleeding may be accompanied by occlusion of the tracheostomy tube by blood clot. If direct suction fails to clear this, the airway should be secured by trans-laryngeal intubation, inflating the cuff distal to the stoma, pending surgical exploration.
- A bleeding tracheostomy should be managed by senior personnel (surgeon and anaesthetist), as the combination of major vessel bleeding and a compromised airway is a hazardous one.

Swallowing

Tracheostomy affects swallowing in several ways:

- The tracheostomy tube reduces hyoid movement and laryngeal elevation as it effectively tethers the trachea to the anterior neck skin.
- The presence of the tube increases extrinsic oesophageal pressure, causing regurgitation and aspiration.
- The lack of airflow over the glottis and the pooling of pharyngeal secretions reduce the sensitivity of airway protective reflexes, resulting in an increased risk of aspiration.

Despite this, many patients can swallow with a tracheostomy. Fluoroscopic studies have suggested that cuff inflation reduces the effectiveness of swallowing and increases the risk of aspiration compared with swallowing with the cuff deflated. Clinical assessment by speech and language therapists is often conservative, and a pragmatic, graduated approach to allowing the introduction of oral intake may be more appropriate. Our unit uses water, followed by blackcurrant cordial, observing tracheal secretions for evidence of aspiration. The psychological benefits to the patient of re-starting oral intake should not be underestimated.

Speaking valves

A speaking valve is a one-way valve that is attached to the tracheostomy tube and allows airflow in during inspiration, then closes on expiration to re-direct air past the vocal cords and out through the nose and mouth. For this reason, speaking valves can only be used with uncuffed or fenestrated tubes, or with cuffed tubes *after* the cuff has been deflated.

Several designs exist, including Passy-Muir (closed position) and Rusch (open position) valves. Passy-Muir valves are always in a closed position until the patient inhales, thus allowing generation of a positive airway pressure and a more physiological 'closed respiratory system'. The valve opens easily with less than normal inspiratory pressures and closes automatically at the end of the inspiratory cycle without air leak and without patient expiratory effort.

Patients with tracheostomies are often frustrated at their inability to communicate. Use of a speaking valve once the patient is beginning to wean, even for short periods of time, can markedly reduce this frustration.

Weaning and decannulation

Tracheostomy tubes should be removed as soon as they are no longer required. Weaning usually involves a gradual increase in periods spent off the ventilator, followed by periods of self-ventilation with the cuff down. An inflated cuff provides protection from oral secretions. Cuff deflation is often associated with increased coughing and altered sensation associated with tracheal airflow.

Following deflation of the cuff, briefly occluding the tracheostomy tube with a gloved finger will allow an assessment of flow around the tube through the upper airway.

Weaning may progress to the use of a speaking valve, and then to use of a decannulation cap, which occludes the tracheostomy tube completely and forces the patient to breathe around the trachestomy tube. This stage of weaning actually requires more effort than after decannulation, as airflow resistance is high.

Successful weaning from the ventilator may then be followed by decannulation. In deciding to remove a tracheostomy the following should be considered:

• The patient is able to cough effectively and protect their airway.
• The patient has adequate ventilatory reserve.
• The pathological process necessitating the insertion of the tracheostomy has resolved.
• Pulmonary secretions are not excessive.
• Nutritional status and respiratory muscle strength are adequate.
• The airway is patent above the level of the stoma.

Decannulation should take place in a safe environment, in a controlled fashion, with the facilities to rapidly re-institute ventilatory support if necessary.

The presence of a tracheostomy tube may cause persistent respiratory secretions. In some instances, the tracheostomy tube may be downsized or replaced with a mini-tracheostomy.

Mini-tracheostomy

A mini-tracheostomy (mini-trach) is a 4-mm, percutaneous cricothyroidotomy device that is used for the treatment (or prevention) of sputum retention. Its use has been shown to reduce sputum retention and the need for re-intubation (but only in thoracic surgical patients). These tubes are also occasionally used as a 'step-down' tool in patients who have had a tracheostomy for weaning from mechanical ventilation, who have an ongoing, but temporary, need to access the airway to assist secretion clearance. They can be placed, non-traumatically, through an already-formed stoma at the time of decannulation.

In non-intubated patients, insertion of a mini-trach to facilitate tracheal suction is hazardous, as these patients are often hypoxic and in respiratory extremis. Sedation in these patients is dangerous, and the technique is often complicated by bleeding or misplacement. It may be wiser in these cases to opt for intubation and ventilation, and early percutaneous dilational tracheostomy.

Further reading

De Leyn P, Bedert L, Delcroix M et al. (2007) Tracheotomy: clinical review and guidelines. *Eur J Cardiothorac Surg* **32**, 412–421.

Intensive Care Society (2008) *Standards for the care of adult patients with a temporary tracheostomy.* Available at: http://www.ics.ac.uk/intensive_care_professional/standards_and_guidelines/care_of_the_adult_patient_with_a_temporary_tracheostomy_2008.

5.3 Humidification and suction

Humidification

During normal breathing, the upper airway plays an important role in modifying inspired gases. This includes:
- Warming to 32–35°C
- Humidification to 100% relative humidity
- Filtering of particles >2–5μm—this reduces the exposure of the lower airways to contamination. Particles trapped on the epithelium are transported upwards on the muco-ciliary escalator. Respiratory mucus is rich in antimicrobials, such as interferon and immunoglobulin.

Tracheal intubation allows inspired gas to bypass the upper airway, avoiding the natural processes of humidification, warming, and filtering.

Mechanical ventilation with dry medical gases damages the tracheal epithelium and dries respiratory secretions. This interferes with normal mucociliary function and may cause airway obstruction, 'mucous plugging', alveolar collapse, and ventilation–perfusion mismatch. Sedation, intubation, and ventilation with dry gases all impair innate immunity, increasing the risk of respiratory infection.

The optimal humidity of inspired gases to avoid such complications is not known. The International Standards Organization recommends an absolute humidity of >30mgH₂O/L (this corresponds to a relative humidity of 68% at 37°C at sea level) (see box).

> ### Assessment of humidification
>
> The humidity of inspired gases is rarely measured. Useful clinical rules of thumb are:
> - A tracheal connecting tube that is dry, misty, or has a few water drops on it indicates inadequate humidification and the method of humidification should be changed.
> - Many water drops, or dripping, implies adequate humidification.

Two types of device are used to humidify and warm inspired gases during mechanical ventilation (Table 5.4):
- Heated humidifiers
- Heat and moisture exchangers.

Heated humidifiers

Heated humidifiers (HHs) work by heating sterile water in a chamber attached to the inspiratory tubing. Theoretically, these devices achieve 100% relative humidity and a variable outlet temperature up to 40°C.

Cooling of inspiratory gas in the ventilator tubing causes precipitation of water (rainout). Bacterial colonization of the ventilator tubing is promoted and inadvertent tipping of contaminated water down the patient's airway may be a cause of VAP.

Rainout may be overcome by the use of heated wire elements in the inspiratory tubing. Two temperatures are set, typically 37°C at the humidification chamber and 40°C at the patient connector. This will help prevent rainout and theoretically provides inspiratory gas at 37°C and an absolute humidity of 44mgH$_2$O/L.

Independent bench and clinical tests demonstrate differences between the manufacturers' specifications and show that performance varies between manufacturers. Further impartial, longer-term studies are needed to assess these devices.

Heat and moisture exchangers

HMEs passively conserve airway heat and moisture. They are made with hydroscopic and hydrophobic materials that allow water vapour to condense on their surface during expiration. During inspiration, evaporation humidifies the inspired gas and heat is conserved in the water vapour.

Independent bench tests of 48 HMEs demonstrated considerable variability in their humidification properties.[1] Only 12 devices maintained an absolute humidity >30mgH$_2$O/L. There were many discrepancies between measured performance and the manufacturers' data. There are less clinical data on the performance of HMEs over several days. Most modern HMEs also filter out microbes and prevent contamination of the ventilator tubing.

Frequency of changing HMEs

HMEs ought to be changed if they become damaged or soiled. Changing HMEs more frequently than every 48h does not affect the performance of tested devices or the incidence of VAP.

Dead space and the use of HMEs

HMEs add to apparatus dead space. The effect on carbon dioxide elimination can become significant, especially when low tidal volumes are used as part of a lung-protective strategy. HHs improve carbon dioxide elimination in these circumstances.

Humidification and airway occlusion

Inadequate humidification can cause fatal occlusion of the airway with dried respiratory secretions. However, inappropriate use of humidification devices can also precipitate airway occlusion.

- The simultaneous use of an HH and an HME will lead to condensation on the HME and circuit occlusion.
- Using a bacterial filter at the expiratory limb of the ventilator circuit with an HH may cause condensation within the filter and expiratory obstruction. There is no evidence that bacterial filters positioned at the ventilator expiratory port prevent VAP as the ventilator is rarely the source of VAP. However, their use is recommended in patients with infectious pneumonia, e.g. TB or influenza.

Humidification device and the risk of pneumonia

The ability of HMEs to avoid condensation and contamination of the ventilatory circuit has led to speculation that their use may prevent VAP. Several trials have compared the occurrence of VAP in patients randomized to having HMEs or HHs. A meta-analysis of 13 RCTs, with 2580 patients, showed no difference in the rate of VAP between HH and HME groups.[2]

In conclusion there is no firm evidence that the choice of humidification device affects the risk of pneumonia in ventilated patients.

Table 5.4 Summary

	HH	HME
Pro	Effective	Inexpensive
	No dead space	Convenient
Con	Expensive	Less effective
	Labour intensive	Increased circuit dead space
	Performance may vary	Increased circuit resistance
	Condensation in the circuit	Performance varies widely between manufacturers

Suctioning

Tracheal suctioning is needed to remove respiratory secretions that accumulate because of the impaired muco-ciliary escalator and cough reflex. It should be used only when indicated. Suctioning is performed frequently, often without considering the potential disadvantages. These include loss of airway pressure with lung collapse, contamination of the airway or environment, pain/distress, and airway trauma.

- Pre-emptive sedation and analgesia alleviate pain and distress.
- Pre-oxygenation helps prevent hypoxaemia.
- Alveolar collapse may be reduced by using short bursts of intermittent suction rather than continuous aspiration. Intermittent suctioning also avoids mucosal trauma.
- The suction pressure should be the minimum necessary to aspirate secretions, and some authors have recommended a 'maximum' negative pressure of $-30cmH_2O$.
- Larger suction catheters are more effective but may cause trauma.
- Recruitment manoeuvres may be required afterwards.

Closed vs open systems

Closed suction catheters have advantages:
- Convenient
- Less contamination of environment and healthcare workers
- Theoretically there should be a smaller drop in PEEP, with less derecruitment.

Meta-analysis of studies comparing closed and open systems found little evidence of clinically significant differences in oxygenation and no reduction in VAP.

Instillation of normal saline

It is controversial whether or not normal saline should be instilled down the tracheal tube before suctioning. Instillation may wash biofilm further down the airways. On the other hand, improved clearance of secretions may reduce lower airway contamination. One recent RCT comparing

VAP in ventilated cancer patients showed benefit in patients receiving saline instillation. Before recommending this practice, further studies in a more general sample, with blinding of the person initiating microbiological testing, would be welcome.

Further reading

Lorente L, Blot S, and Rello J (2007) Evidence on measures for the prevention of ventilator-associated pneumonia. *Eur Respir J* **30**, 1193–1207.

1 Lellouche F, Taille S, Lefrancois F, *et al.* (2009) Humidification performance of 48 passive airway humidifiers. Comparison with manufacturer data. *Chest* **135**, 276–86.
2 Siempos II, Vardakas KZ, Kopterides P, and Falagas ME (2007) Impact of passive humidification on clinical outcomes of mechanically ventilated patients: A meta-analysis of randomized controlled trials. *Crit Care Med* **35**, 2843–51.
3 Caruso P, Denari S, Ruiz SAL, Demarzo SE, and Deheinzelin D (2009) Saline instillation before tracheal suctioning decreases the incidence of ventilator-associated pneumonia. *Crit Care Med* **37**, 32–8.

5.4 **Physiotherapy in intensive care units**

Physiotherapy plays an important role as part of the MDT approach to the management of the critically unwell patient. The most recognized role of the physiotherapist in the ICU is to help optimize respiratory function—this has been shown to increase ventilator-free days.[1] Physiotherapy is not a generic treatment for all causes of deteriorating respiratory function (Table 5.5). It has specific indications, and the inappropriate use of physiotherapy outside these indications may worsen respiratory function.

Table 5.5

Physiotherapy indicated	Conditions not helped by physiotherapy
Pulmonary collapse	Bronchospasm without infection
Sputum retention	Pulmonary oedema
Tracheostomy management	Uncontrolled pain
Slow respiratory wean	Pleural effusion/empyema
Rehabilitation	Pneumothorax

Physiotherapy is integral in:[2]
- Reducing the unwanted effects of immobility through maintenance of strength, function, and co-ordination
- The rehabilitation of patients to full potential.

Physiotherapy techniques

Positioning

Positioning is used to manipulate $\dot{V}/\dot{Q}$, increase FRC, and facilitate gravitational drainage of secretions.
- Care should be taken in patients with cardiovascular instability or raised ICP.
- Consider a spinal or tilting bed in patients with uncleared/unstable spine or pelvic injuries.

Mobilization

This is the treatment of choice for volume loss and sputum retention. The effects of mobilization on respiratory function include:
- Increased lung volumes and FRC
- Large increase in FRC in moving from supine to standing
- Mobilization of secretions to larger airways, enhancing expectoration
- Prevention of deconditioning, muscle weakness, and the detrimental effects of bed rest.

Airway clearance techniques

These are used to increase tidal volumes and facilitate collateral ventilation, aiding sputum clearance. They can be used with manual techniques and postural drainage positions.

- Active cycle of breathing technique (ACBT). This involves cycles of thoracic expansion exercises to increase tidal volume used in conjunction with diaphragmatic breathing control. It can be adapted to suit both ventilated and self-ventilating patients, for example the use of forced expiratory technique rather than cough in patients with bronchospasm and sputum retention.

Manual techniques

These consist of percussion, vibrations, and shakes of the chest to mobilize secretions proximally and therefore aid sputum clearance.

Caution should be taken when using these techniques in patients with chest trauma, osteoporosis, and bronchospasm.

Assisted cough

This is a manual technique designed to augment a cough in patients with neuromuscular weakness or spinal cord injury. The technique involves compressing the abdomen (and diaphragm) to augment the patient's effort. The technique should be used with caution in patients with unstable spinal injuries, rib fractures, paralytic ileus/abdominal distension, and osteoporosis.

Incentive spirometry

Incentive spirometry uses a device that incorporates visual feedback on performance when carrying out thoracic expansion exercises. There is a limited evidence base when compared to airway clearance techniques. It is indicated mostly in a paediatric population or in patients struggling with thoracic expansion exercises.

Positive pressure adjuncts

Intermittent positive pressure breathing

Intermittent positive pressure breathing (or Bird®) is used to augment the patient's respiratory effort by using positive pressure. It is usually patient triggered (pressure drop in circuit), but can be time triggered or manually triggered. The expiratory trigger is pressure or time. It can be used with a mouthpiece or facemask interface. It will help to:

- Increase lung volume
- Reduce work of breathing
- Mobilize secretions.

It is a passive technique with a transient effect on tidal volume, therefore it is not as effective as mobilization, which is active and increases FRC. It is indicated in patients with poor lung volume and retained secretions who are unable to mobilize.

Cough assist device

This is used to increase tidal volume and augment cough by using positive and then negative pressures. It can be used via a catheter mount, mouthpiece, or facemask (e.g. CPAP mask). There is evidence of benefit in patients with neuromuscular disease, but it should also be considered in patients with low lung volumes and sputum retention, for example critical care illness polyneuropathy.

Manual hyperinflation

Manual hyperinflation (MHI) uses a waters circuit (Mapleson C) to increase tidal volume to promote collateral ventilation and sputum mobilization in intubated patients or those with a tracheostomy. It is usually incorporated in manual techniques and positioning to optimally facilitate sputum clearance. It is not recommended as a first-line treatment for sputum retention because of the risks associated with loss of PEEP and cardiovascular instability. PEEP can be maintained by adding an expiratory valve to the waters circuit.

Relative contraindications for positive pressure adjuncts

- CVS instability.
- Recent upper airway or oesophageal surgery.
- Undrained pneumothorax.
- Haemoptysis.
- Emphysematous bullae.
- Broncho-pleural fistula.
- Surgical emphysema.
- Lung abscess.
- Facial trauma.

Other techniques

Humidification

- Adequate humidification is essential in the prevention and management of sputum retention. Its use in ventilated patients is discussed in 📖 Humidification and suctioning, p 222.
- In self-ventilating patients humidification can be administered using either hot or cold water systems.

Nebulization

- Saline nebulizers can be used to further facilitate sputum clearance.
- They may precipitate bronchospasm in patients with hyper-reactive airways.

Mucolytics

- Mucolytics can also be considered. There is limited evidence outside COPD and CF.
- Nebulized *N*-acetylcysteine has anecdotal benefit in the critical care population, but it is not in widespread use because of perceived risk of bronchospasm.

Suction

- In self-ventilating patients, nasopharyngeal or oropharyngeal (Guedel) airway may help insertion of a suction catheter if all other airway clearance techniques failed.
- Consider mini-tracheostomy if repeated suctioning required and other airway adjuncts not tolerated.
- Use caution with deranged clotting and CVS instability.

Techniques for management of breathlessness in chronic pathology

- Optimize the position of the patient to increase the quality of the respiratory pattern. Consider forward leaning and high side lying, and ensure arms are supported if sitting.
- Encourage diaphragmatic respiratory pattern and also relaxation of shoulder girdle.
- If the patient is using a venturi device, increase the flow rate to match the patient's inspiratory flow rate.
- Consider using a very high flow oxygen delivery device to match the inspiratory flow requirements (e.g. the Whisper® Flow without a PEEP valve can provide up to 140L/min).

Rehabilitation

Rehabilitation should be considered from the point of admission to help prevent the musculoskeletal complications of critical illness, such as muscle and soft tissue shortening.[2] A full social history should be obtained from the family or patient to establish what the rehabilitation goals are for the long term. The rehabilitation of the patient should begin as soon as the patient's cardiovascular and respiratory system allows. Rehabilitation will include:

- Strengthening work, with weights if appropriate
- Sitting over the edge of the bed:
  - Improves respiratory function
  - Strengthens core muscles
  - Challenges balance
- Sitting out of bed (active transfer if possible, passive if not)
- Mobilizing around bedspace, then ward.

All of these manoeuvres can be safely carried out on ventilated patients. When patients are weaning, decisions need to be made on an individual basis, with the MDT, about the benefits of exercise versus the potential effects on weaning.

Weaning and tracheostomy management

An MDT approach is integral to the management of patients with tracheostomy. Physiotherapists are especially equipped to assist/advise in the weaning of patients requiring prolonged ventilation because of their specialist knowledge of fatigue and exercise physiology. Physiotherapists also have the advantage of providing continuity of care to patients because they still work in an on-call structure rather than a shift pattern.

Speaking valves

Communication for patients in the critical care setting is a challenge. Poor communication may cause psychological and emotional frustrations that might affect progress. Speaking valves can be used with tracheostomies in patients on or off the ventilator (depending on the design of the valve). Speaking valves rely on the cuff being deflated to allow airflow over the vocal cords.

The use of the speaking valve will need to be carefully managed and constantly re-evaluated to complement ventilatory weaning and decannulation.

The assessment and application of a speaking valve should only be carried out by a skilled and competent practitioner. Patients should:

- Be co-operative and able to follow commands
- Be medically stable and tolerate weaning if ventilated
- Not have copious secretions
- Be able to tolerate cuff deflation
- Have adequate air flow around the tracheostomy.

The on-call physiotherapist

On-call physiotherapy is indicated in patients at risk of deterioration in the following situations:

- Volume loss such as lobar collapse secondary to sputum retention.
- Sputum that is not clearing with basic techniques such as suction.
- Respiratory function deterioration related to either of the above.

The provision of an on-call physiotherapy service and the call-out criteria will vary nationally and local guidelines will therefore need to be sought. Points to consider prior to calling out the on-call physiotherapist are:

- Is the patient adequately analgesed?
- Is the patient on optimal humidification?
- Is the patient cardiovascularly stable enough for treatment?
- Is the patient compliant?
- Is the patient for active management?

1 Schweickert WD, Pohlman MC, Pohlman AS, et al. (2009). Early physical and occupational therapy in mechanically ventilated, critically ill patients: a randomised controlled trial. *Lancet* **373**, 1874–82.
2 NICE (2009). *Rehabilitation after Critical Care.* www.nice.org.uk.

5.5 Monitoring on a ventilator

The ICU ventilator provides a wide range of both continuous and intermittent measurements that allow a comprehensive assessment of the respiratory system of the ventilated patient. These measurements assist the clinician in the following ways:

- They ensure that the optimal ventilatory settings are used, enhancing efficacy and safety.
- They allow assessment of the mechanical properties of the respiratory system, which can assist in determining the underlying cause of respiratory failure.
- They assess the response to therapeutic interventions.
- They predict readiness for weaning from ventilatory support.

Transducers

Ventilators incorporate accurate transducers to measure pressure and flow. Integration of the flow measurement with time allows calculation of volume. A range of transducers are used to measure flow, including:

- Pneumotachograph
- Mechanical flow transducer
- Hot wire anemometer.

Accuracy

Transducers are prone to drift (e.g. hot wire anemometers). In addition, when measurements are made within the ventilator, inaccuracies can result from humidification (increases the volume of gas by increasing temperature and saturating it with water vapour) and expansion of the breathing circuit with pressure (creates an effective volume loss). To maintain accuracy:

- Flow and pressure transducers are calibrated at the ventilator start-up initial check
- Respiratory circuit compliance is measured as part of this initial check, allowing for compensation of the respiratory circuit expansion during patient use
- Some ventilators supplement proximal flow and volume measurement with a pneumotachograph at the breathing circuit 'Y' piece to allow compensation for humidification and circuit expansion
- Recalibration of transducers prone to drift should be undertaken regularly to ensure the accuracy of displayed measurements.

Basic measurements

The following measurements are typically displayed and updated on a breath-by-breath basis:

- Volumes
  - Inspired tidal volume
  - Expired tidal volume
  - Minute volume (total, set, spontaneous)
- Pressures
  - Peak
  - Plateau

- Mean
- PEEP
- FiO_2.

Depending on the ventilator, additional measurements may be displayed, including compliance, resistance, and $PEEP_i$ (see below).

Volumes

Tidal volume should be based on ideal body weight (predicted from the patient's height and sex) and the underlying lung pathology. It is usually 8–10mL/kg in unintubated individuals, but should be 6–8mL/kg in ventilated patients. The measured expired tidal volume may be slightly higher than the inspired volume as expired gas has been warmed and humidified compared to dry inspired gas. If expired tidal volume is significantly lower than inspired volume, this suggests a leak within the respiratory circuit (e.g. cuff leak) or a leak within the lungs (e.g. broncho-pleural fistulae).

Minute volume in health is approximately 100mL/kg. If a high minute volume is required to maintain normocapnia one of the following is likely:
- High CO_2 production (e.g. high metabolic rate associated with fever, sepsis)
- Increased dead space
  - Alveolar dead space ($\dot{V}/\dot{Q}$ mismatch)
  - Equipment dead space
  - Low tidal volume strategy (V_d/V_t increases).

Pressures

Peak pressure is influenced by inspired volume, flow rate, flow pattern, and airway resistance (including ETT diameter).

Plateau pressure is measured at the end of inspiration following an end inspiratory pause. Plateau pressure reflects the end inspiratory lung volume and is therefore the most appropriate predictor of lung over-distension. Plateau pressure depends on delivered tidal volume and respiratory system compliance, and should be <30cmH$_2$O in the majority of patients. If chest wall or abdominal compliance are significantly reduced (e.g. morbid obesity or raised intra-abdominal pressure), higher plateau pressures may be acceptable as they will not be associated with lung over-distension. In these conditions, intrapleural pressure increases and transpulmonary (distending) pressure may remain within acceptable limits.

Mean pressure (mP_{aw}) depends on plateau pressure, I:E ratio, and PEEP. Increasing the mean airway pressure is associated with improved oxygenation but greater haemodynamic effects due to reduction in venous return. The mean airway pressure can be used as an indicator of how aggressively the lungs are being ventilated and is included in the oxygenation index:

$$\text{oxygenation index} = FiO_2 \times mP_{aw}/PaO_2$$

Ventilation curves

The continuous graphical display of pressure, flow, and volume is a standard feature of most ICU ventilators that can provide important information to the clinician at the bedside. The display provides the clinician with an immediate visual confirmation of the mode of support and the ventilatory settings.

Graphical information is provided about the respiratory frequency, spontaneous respiratory efforts, tidal volume, airway pressures, inspiratory time, and I:E ratio. This enables experienced clinicians to assess the appropriateness of ventilator settings and allows early identification of certain problems. Specific issues that may be recognized are detailed below.

Pressure–time curves

Volume control

- In conventional VCV inspiratory flow is delivered at a constant rate and therefore volume increases linearly throughout the inspiratory phase.
- Airway pressure increases to a peak at the end of the active inspiratory phase.
- If an inspiratory pause is set, the airway pressure will fall to the plateau pressure (see Fig. 3.4, p. 113).

Peak airway pressure and peak to plateau pressure difference

- Peak pressure depends on the set inspiratory flow rate and respiratory system resistance (airway and lung).
- High airway resistance results in a high peak airway pressure with a large peak to plateau pressure gradient.
- Reducing the inspiratory flow rate or increasing the diameter of the ETT will reduce the peak airway pressure.
- The peak to plateau pressure gradient can be used to assess response to bronchodilators in acute asthma, with the gradient reducing as airway resistance falls in response to treatment.

Plateau pressure

- Reflects the tidal volume and respiratory system compliance.
- Correlates with the end inspiratory lung volume and is used to monitor lung distension.
- Values >30cmH$_2$O are associated with an increased risk of VILI.
- Low compliance is associated with an increase in peak and plateau pressures.

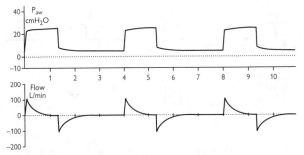

Fig. 5.1 Pressure control flow–time waveform (adequate inspiratory time).

Pressure control
- Constant inspiratory pressure is applied. In a passive patient the inspiratory flow curve has a characteristic decelerating profile (Fig. 5.1).
- The corresponding volume–time curve is an exponential build-up curve, representing the fall in pressure gradient between ventilator and alveolus as inspiration progresses (see 📖 Pressure vs volume delivery, Fig. 3.3, p 111).
- Dual-control modes are discussed in 📖 Software enhancements, p 165. The pressure and flow patterns depend on the precise type of dual control.

During PCV it is not possible to assess the mechanical properties of the respiratory system from inspection of the pressure–time curve as inspiratory pressure is constant during inspiration.

Pressure support
- A pressure-supported breath may have a similar appearance to a pressure-controlled breath with a constant inspiratory pressure and a decelerating flow profile (Fig. 5.2).
- Increased patient contribution to inspiration, particularly at low levels of pressure support, will produce a sine wave pattern more in keeping with the flow profile of an unsupported breath.
- A scooped appearance of the inspiratory pressure rise may occur with high respiratory drive. It may also suggest a 'rise time' that is too long or inadequate pressure support.
- A slight reduction in airway pressure immediately before the onset of inspiration may be observed, reflecting patient triggering of each breath. Exaggerated dips may be seen with high respiratory drive, inadequate pressure support, a partially obstructed ETT, or incorrect trigger sensitivity (see below).
- Cycling from inspiration to expiration occurs when the inspiratory flow rate falls below a set percentage of the peak inspiratory flow rate (typically 25%). Some ventilators allow this cycling threshold (ETS) to be adjusted (see 📖 Pressure support ventilation, p 144).

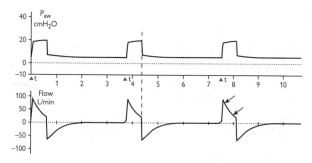

Fig. 5.2 Airway pressure trace pressure support. Pressure support ends when inspiratory flow falls to 25% of peak inspiratory flow (arrows).

Use of pressure–time curve to assess patient–ventilator synchrony
The pressure–time curve can provide information about spontaneous patient respiratory efforts and their synchrony with the ventilator.

Trigger sensitivity
Spontaneous efforts should result in a small and transient drop in the end expiratory pressure. A large fall in pressure may occur if the trigger sensitivity is set too low and is addressed by increasing the sensitivity of the trigger.

Inspiratory flow rate (volume modes)
A large and sustained drop in pressure during inspiration may occur if the flow rate is set too low to match the patient's efforts during volume-controlled modes with a constant inspiratory flow. Increasing the flow rate to match the patient's effort will improve comfort.

Rise time (pressure modes)
The inspiratory rise time in pressure modes is adjusted to match the patient's inspiratory effort. If the patient makes large efforts the rise time can be shortened to prevent a significant fall in inspiratory pressure after triggering.

Inspiratory to expiratory cycling in pressure support
A transient increase in airway pressure at the end of the inspiratory phase may occur if the patient has to actively exhale in order to force the ventilator to cycle to expiration (Fig. 5.3).

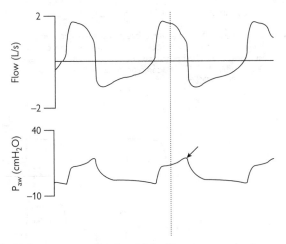

Fig. 5.3 Pressure support with active exhalation. The pressure trace is not square wave but increases towards end inspiration (arrow).

This is common in patients with severe COPD where inspiratory flow starts at a low level, decreases slowly, and does not reach the normal ETS of 25% unless the patient actively exhales. This results in patient discomfort, intolerance of pressure support, and possible failed attempts to wean. Some ventilators allow the ETS to be adjusted. Titrating the ETS upwards in obstructive diseases may improve patient comfort.

Flow–time curve
Careful inspection of the inspiratory and expiratory flow curves allows optimal setting of inspiratory and expiratory times.

Inspiration
The shape of the inspiratory flow curve may be used to guide the setting of pressure-controlled modes (and dual modes).
- If an adequate inspiratory time is set, the inspiratory flow rate should fall to zero (Fig. 5.1).
- If inspiratory time is too short or airway resistance is high, flow may not fall to zero before the onset of the expiratory phase (the flow curve will look more like Fig. 5.2 (persistent end inspiratory flow) than Fig. 5.1). In these circumstances, increasing the inspiratory time to allow flow to reach zero may improve gas exchange by allowing adequate time for all lung units to fill.
- However, care needs to be taken as any resulting reduction in expiratory time may cause gas trapping (Fig. 5.4).

Expiration
- A high expiratory flow rate with rapid return of flow to zero is associated with reduced compliance and high recoil pressure within the lungs.
- A low expiratory flow rate with decreased slope resulting in a prolonged expiratory phase occurs when airway resistance is increased. Causes include include bronchospasm, obstructive airways disease, blockage within the ETT, and saturation of a heat and moisture exchange filter (HMEF).

Intrinsic PEEP

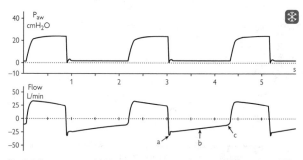

Fig. 5.4 Pressure control: high airway resistance with signs of PEEP-initial rapid fall in flow (a); second slow redirection in flow (b); persistant and expiratory flow (c). Similar expiratory pattern seen in Fig. 5.9B.

- If there is inadequate time for expiration, flow does not reach baseline before the onset of the inspiratory phase, resulting in dynamic hyperinflation (gas-trapping) (Fig. 5.4).
- This may occur due to increased airway resistance or if expiratory time is very short (e.g. inverse ratio ventilation see 📖 Pressure control ventilation, p 135).
- The additional volume causes increased alveolar pressure at the end of expiration (PEEP$_i$), which may have effects on the cardiovascular system and on gas exchange (see below).

Ventilation loops

Dynamic loops

The clinical utility of dynamic loops plotting pressure, flow, and volume is limited as they cannot distinguish the resistive and elastic properties of the respiratory system.

Flow–volume loop

The flow volume loop displayed on a ventilator is not the same as that performed in the respiratory function laboratory. The latter is performed under conditions of maximal spontaneous effort while the former is performed during normal tidal breathing. Most information is obtained by inspection of the expiratory phase. In severe airway obstruction there is a characteristic appearance of two-compartment emptying (a fast compartment followed by a slow compartment, Fig. 5.8). A similar appearance is seen in the flow–time curve (Fig. 5.4).

Pressure–volume loop

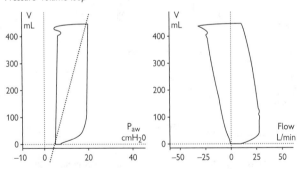

Fig. 5.5 Pressure– and flow–volume loops PCV. Slope of dotted line in pressure volume curve represents dynamic compliance.

The dynamic pressure–volume loop should not be confused with the static pressure–volume loop (see below). It is difficult to differentiate the effects of the changes in the resistive and elastic properties of the lung in a dynamic loop. Pressure-targeted ventilation results in a square pressure–volume loop. Changes in compliance will alter the height of the loop, but the shape of the inspiratory limb is unchanged. Assuming that flow is zero at end inspiration and expiration, the slope of a line drawn through the loop will reflect the dynamic compliance (Fig. 5.5).

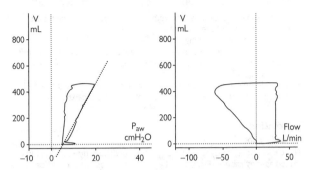

Fig. 5.6 Pressure–volume loop VCV. The slope of the inspiratory PV curve (dotted line) is linear, reflecting constant dynamic compliance during inspiration.

More information may be obtained from the pressure–volume curve during constant flow ventilation (classical volume control). Assuming inspiratory resistance is constant, the gradient of the inspiratory limb of the pressure–volume curve will reflect changes in dynamic compliance (Fig. 5.6). If airway resistance or inspiratory flow rate increase, the curve is offset to the right-hand side, as demonstrated in Fig. 5.8. The shape of the inspiratory limb is unchanged.

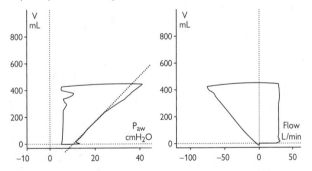

Fig. 5.7 Pressure– and flow–volume loops: low compliance. Note that the slope of the PV curve (dotted line) is reduced compared to Fig. 5.6 and not constant, reflecting a further reduction in compliance at the end of inspiration, suggesting lung over-distension.

If lung over-distension occurs during tidal ventilation, the slope of the inspiratory limb will reduce towards the end of the inspiratory phase (Fig. 5.7). This is the equivalent of the upper inflection point on a static pressure–volume loop. It is not possible to interpret the lower inflection point. A change in airway resistance (with a constant flow rate) will shift

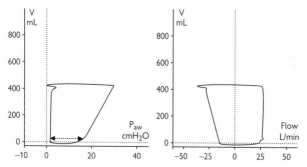

Fig. 5.8 Pressure– and flow–volume loops: high resistance. Compared to Fig. 5.6 note the right shift of the inspiratory PV curve, reflecting increased airway resistance. Increasing inspiratory flow rate will produce a similar shift in PV curve.

the inspiratory curve to the left (reduced resistance) or right (increased resistance) (Fig. 5.8).

Static loops

Pressure–volume loop

The classic static pressure–volume loop is obtained using the 'super syringe' method where the lung is progressively inflated in a stepwise manner with small increments of volume (50mL) and the associated change in airway pressure measured during conditions of no gas flow. Under these conditions, the effects of resistance are removed and the pressure–volume curve reflects the elastic properties of the lung. This allows the zone of maximum compliance to be identified, with lower and upper inflection points representing lung volumes where compliance is significantly reduced due to de-recruitment and over-inflation respectively (Fig. 5.9).

Many ventilators now offer the facility to perform a 'quasi-static' pressure–volume curve using the slow inflation technique. The lung is slowly inflated using a low flow rate over 15–20s. The low flow rate limits the pressure changes required to overcome the resistive forces such that the pressure–volume curve generated is a reasonable reflection of the true static pressure–volume curve. Both inspiratory and expiratory curves may be constructed. The procedure generally requires that the patient is deeply sedated and paralysed to ensure no spontaneous respiratory effort during the manoeuvre. Upper and lower inflection points may then be identified, although their clinical utility remains debated. It has been proposed that PEEP should be set at a value greater than the pressure of the lower inflection point, whilst the pressure of the upper inflection point should not be exceeded during tidal breathing to avoid lung over-distension. In a significant number of patients these inflection points are not clearly identified.

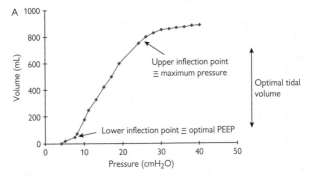

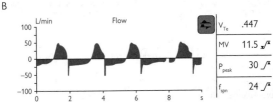

Fig. 5.9 A, Static pressure volume curve. B, Flow–time curve in patient with severe airflow limitation (COPD). Note characteristic expiratory flow pattern.

Respiratory system mechanics

Compliance and resistance

Static compliance (CRS) and resistance (R_{aw}) are easily measured during VCV with constant flow inspiration using the following equations:

$$\text{static CRS (mL/cmH}_2\text{O)} = \text{tidal volume/P}_{plat} - \text{PEEP}_{tot}$$

and

$$R_{aw} \text{ (cmH}_2\text{O/L/min)} = (P_{peak} - P_{plat})/\text{inspiratory flow}$$

where P_{plat} = plateau pressure measured after an end inspiratory pause and $PEEP_{tot}$ = total PEEP ($PEEP_e + PEEP_i$) measured after an end expiratory pause.

Accurate measurements require that the patient is sedated and making no spontaneous respiratory efforts.

Many ventilators now display breath-by-breath dynamic measurements of compliance and resistance. These are derived from the continuous analysis of the pressure–, flow–, and volume–time curves. One form of analysis used is multiple linear regression to derive values of compliance, resistance, and total PEEP to fit the equation of motion for the lung:

$$P_t = (F_t \times R_{aw}) + (V_t/CRS) + PEEP_{tot}$$

where P_t, F_t, and V_t are pressure, flow, and volume at time t.

All measurements of compliance and resistance assume that patients are not making significant respiratory efforts (see box). Any values measured during periods when patients make effective respiratory efforts will not be accurate and should be interpreted with caution.

Typical compliance values

Normal compliance*	100mL/cmH$_2$O
Ventilated and sedated patient	50mL/cmH$_2$O
Severe ARDS	20mL/cmH$_2$O

Typical resistance values

Normal resistance*	0–5cmH$_2$O/L/s
Cardiogenic pulmonary oedema	10–20cmH$_2$O/L/s
ARDS	10–20cmH$_2$O/L/s
COPD	15–30cmH$_2$O/L/s
Severe asthma	20–40cmH$_2$O/L/s

*Normal values in healthy spontaneously breathing subject.

Compliance measurements may be useful in setting the correct tidal volume and PEEP level. Lung recruitment following the application of PEEP will result in an increase in compliance, while an excessive tidal volume that results in lung over-distension will cause a reduction in compliance.

Serial measurements of resistance are useful for assessing the response to bronchodilators.

Intrinsic PEEP

PEEP$_i$ should be monitored whenever its presence is suggested by examination of the expiratory flow waveform (Fig. 5.4). PEEP$_i$ is likely to be significant in:

- Patients with severe airflow limitation (e.g. asthma and COPD)
- High set respiratory frequency resulting in short expiratory time
- Inverse ratio ventilation with short expiratory time.

A static measurement of PEEP$_i$ is obtained by recording the increase in airway pressure after an end expiratory pause with both inspiratory and expiratory valves closed.

This produces conditions of no flow and the pressure within the lungs equilibrates with that in the ventilator. The patient must be relaxed and not make any respiratory effort during the measurement, which usually requires deep sedation and often a muscle relaxant.

$PEEP_i$ of up to $20cmH_2O$ is not uncommon in severe airflow limitation. Measurement of $PEEP_i$ is essential to ensure that the most appropriate ventilator settings are used in patients with severe COPD or asthma. A reasonable aim is to maintain $PEEP_i$ <10 cmH_2O.

Static $PEEP_i$ cannot be measured during spontaneous breathing and a dynamic measurement may be derived from the pressure changes before the onset of inspiratory flow. This requires the insertion of an oesophageal balloon to estimated pleural pressure and is not commonly undertaken.

Other measurements

Maximal inspiratory pressure

This is the maximum negative inspiratory pressure that can be generated by a patient during occlusion of the airway and is used to assess respiratory muscle strength. A value less negative than $-20cmH_2O$ has been used to predict failure to wean. Predictors of successful weaning are listed in the box. However, the measurement does not have adequate specificity or sensitivity for routine use in clinical practice. The measurement is very effort dependent and false negatives are common.

Inspiratory occlusion pressure

Inspiratory occlusion pressure ($P_{0.1}$) is the maximum pressure developed during a spontaneous respiratory effort during a 100ms occlusion at the beginning of inspiration. There is correlation between $P_{0.1}$ and WOB. A high value (>$6cmH_2O$) reflects a high WOB and predicts failure to wean. However, low values may also be associated with failure to wean due to either inadequate respiratory drive or severe respiratory muscle weakness.

Predictors of successful weaning	
Respiratory frequency	<35/min
Tidal volume	>5mL/kg
Rapid shallow breathing index (F/V_t)	<80
Occlusion pressure ($P_{0.1}$)	<$6cmH_2O$
Vital capacity	>10mL/kg
Maximal inspiratory pressure	<$-20cmH_2O$

Dead space

Volumetric capnography describes the continuous measurement of exhaled CO_2 tension, combined with simultaneous measurement of exhaled volume. Accurate measurements use a transducer that is placed at the 'Y' piece that combines in-line capnography with a pneumotachograph. Anatomical dead space (from Fowler's method) and physiological dead space (if $PaCO_2$ is also recorded) can then be measured. In addition, total CO_2 production can also be calculated as a measurement of metabolic activity.

- Physiological dead space may be considerably increased in patients with respiratory failure and is indicated by a high minute ventilation to maintain normocapnia.
- Dead space is usually expressed as a fraction of the tidal volume (V_d/V_t) with a value <0.3 considered normal.

- V_d/V_t elevation in ARDS (mean value 0.58) has been reported to be an independent predictor of mortality.
- The physiological dead space may be useful in optimizing PEEP, with lung recruitment being associated with a reduction in V_d/V_t.
- Lung over-distension will increase physiological dead space.

A sudden and marked increased in physiological dead space in a ventilated patient may indicate a pulmonary embolus. However, other causes of increased alveolar dead space should be considered, including low cardiac output and gas trapping ($PEEP_i$).

Further reading

Macnaughton PD (2006) New ventilators for the ICU: usefulness of lung performance reporting. *Br J Anaesth* **97**, 57–63.

Grinnan DC and Truwit JD (2005) Clinical review: Respiratory mechanics in spontaneous and assisted ventilation. *Crit Care* **9**, 472–484.

5.6 Complications of ventilation

Ventilator-induced lung injury

VILI is defined as lung damage caused by mechanical ventilation. In clinical practice it is difficult to distinguish the effects of mechanical ventilation from those of the underlying disorder, and ventilator associated lung injury (VALI) may be a more appropriate term.

Historically, numerous other terms have been used to describe what we now call VILI and an appreciation of these terms provides the rationale for current ventilation strategies.

Barotrauma

In the early days of positive pressure mechanical ventilation large (10–15mL/kg) tidal volumes were recommended to prevent alveolar collapse. It was soon recognized that the use of large tidal volumes was associated with high airway pressures, which could cause the rupture of lung parenchyma. As this was initially thought to be primarily a pressure effect, the term 'barotrauma' was used to describe the associated lung injury.

Volutrauma

In 1988 Dreyfuss et al. demonstrated that alveolar over-distension was the primary mechanism for the development of VILI,[1] and that this can occur at low airway pressures (volutrauma).

Histological studies have confirmed that over-inflation of normal lung units during mechanical ventilation produces stress fractures at the alveolar–capillary interface that can allow alveolar gas to escape into the pulmonary parenchyma and beyond.

Atelectrauma

PEEP markedly reduces lung oedema and preserves lung ultrastructure in experimental models of ARDS. Cyclical de-recruitment/re-recruitment of alveolar units results in shear stress in the parenchyma between adjacent units (atelectrauma). PEEP is thought to reduce atelectrauma and the subsequent lung injury.

Biotrauma

Molecular biological studies have demonstrated that stress fractures at the alveolar–capillary interface cause an inflammatory lung injury that is indistinguishable from ARDS. This inflammatory reaction may also spill cytokines into the systemic circulation and produce a systemic inflammatory response syndrome. The production and release of inflammatory mediators in response to the mechanical stress of ventilation is termed 'biotrauma'.

These findings led to the adoption of a lung protective ventilation (LPV) strategy, which aimed to avoid over-distension (high end inspiratory pressures/volumes) and repetitive collapse of unstable lung units (low end expiratory pressures/volumes). This strategy was shown to decrease mortality and reduce the duration of mechanical ventilation, but the rates of pneumothorax and air leaks were unchanged. The current working hypothesis is that LPV improves survival by decreasing biotrauma.

Prevention

Many strategies have been tried to prevent VILI in patients with ARDS (Table 5.6).

Table 5.6 Strategies used to prevent VILI in patients with ARDS

Ventilatory strategies

- LPV
- Recruitment manoeuvres
- High PEEP
- Prone ventilation

Strategies to 'rest the lungs'

- Permissive or deliberate hypercapnia
- Extracorporeal lung support (ECMO, $ECCO_2R$)

Pharmacotherapy

- Steroids
- Exogenous surfactant use
- Partial liquid ventilation (with perfluorocarbons)
- Nitric oxide
- Adrenergic β2-agonists
- Miscellaneous agents, e.g. non-steroidal anti-inflammatory agents, N-acetylcysteine, pentoxifylline

General measures

- Fluid management (usually aimed at reducing extravascular lung water using diuretics)

Despite initial enthusiasm for various interventions, to date only LPV has been shown to improve survival in patients with ALI/ARDS.

The ARDSNet trial published in 2000[2] compared LPV with a standard ventilation strategy in over 800 patients. Hospital mortality was reduced from 40% to 31%.

There is emerging evidence to suggest that LPV is probably beneficial for patients at risk of ARDS, such as patients undergoing thoracic or major abdominal surgery.

Wherever possible the principles of LPV should be used, even if it results in hypercapnia (see 📖 Hypercapnia while on a ventilation, p 296) or a reduction in oxygenation. Under certain circumstances this may not be possible. For example, in closed head injuries, tight control of $PaCO_2$ is desirable, and a balance must be struck.

In other conditions higher airway pressures may be necessary. The transpulmonary pressure (the pressure difference between the alveoli and the pleural space) determines alveolar distension. Alveolar pressure equals proximal airway pressure when there is no gas flow, such as at the end of inspiration (end inspiratory pause pressure or plateau pressure) or during an inspiratory hold. In patients with bronchospasm *peak* airway pressures are a result of high airways resistance and do not translate into transpulmonary pressures. Similarly, in diseases with reduced chest wall compliance (e.g. raised intra-abdominal pressure) the airway pressure measured at the mouth is higher than the transpulmonary pressure. While overall transpulmonary pressure in these circumstances may be acceptable, regional differences in lung mechanics mean that it is less certain that all distal lung units are protected to the same degree.

Pneumothoraces and air leaks

VILI can result in alveolar rupture. This usually occurs deep within the lung and the air dissects along fascial planes to produce pulmonary interstitial emphysema. The air may track into the mediastinum to produce pneumo-mediastinum and pneumopericardium. In turn, mediastinal gas can move into the neck to produce subcutaneous emphysema or pass below the diaphragm to produce pneumoperitoneum.

If the visceral pleura ruptures, air will collect in the pleural space and produce a pneumothorax. Tension pneumothoraces occur when pleural air, under pressure, displaces mediastinal structures (heart and great vessels), resulting in cardiovascular collapse.

Diagnosis
Clinical features
Clinical features may be non-specific, subtle, or absent, and gas exchange may not change markedly. A high index of suspicion is required.
- Subcutaneous emphysema implies an air leak and is highly suggestive of a pneumothorax.
- Worsening hypoxaemia, increasing airway pressures, tachycardia, hypotension, and rising CVP strongly suggest the development of a tension pneumothorax.

Radiographic features
See 📖 Pleural disease, p 481

Treatment
Tension pneumothoraces should be decompressed as an emergency. Classical management involves needle decompression in the second inter-costal space, mid clavicular line, followed by formal drainage.

Almost all pneumothoraces in mechanically ventilated patients require drainage. There is often a rush of air on insertion of an intercostal chest drain. This is usually a consequence of positive pressure ventilation rather than evidence of a tension pneumothorax.
- If there is no direct communication between the airways and the pleural space, the bubbling usually stops within a few hours when the lung is fully re-expanded.
- If the bubbling continues for 24h or more, a broncho-pleural fistula (BPF) is said to be present.

Broncho-pleural and alveolo-pleural fistulae

An air leak persisting for more than 24h is often termed a bronchopleural fistula (BPF). A true BPF is a communication between the central airways and the pleural space. Most persistent air leaks in mechanically ventilated patients are due to parenchymal necrosis and an air leak distal to a seg-mental bronchus. These are more accurately described as alveolo-pleural fistulae (APF).

In the patient receiving mechanical ventilation air leaks can be classified as:
- A forced expiratory leak, which occurs only on coughing
- An inspiratory air leak, which occurs during the inspiratory cycle of positive pressure ventilation
- A continuous air leak, which is present throughout the ventilatory cycle. This is the largest type of air leak but even so most are not of sufficient magnitude (i.e. >100–150mL per breath) to result in differences between inspired and expired tidal volumes as detected by the ventilator.

APF complicating acute respiratory failure usually resolves as the patient's underlying lung injury improves. There is no evidence that any of the measures outlined below affect mortality or any other outcome. Experience with APF complicating acute respiratory failure also indicates that measures directed at reducing the leak generally prove unsuccessful until the patient's underlying lung injury improves. Once the underlying lung injury improves and there is diminished requirement for positive-pressure ventilation and PEEP, the APF nearly always resolves without specific therapy.

Ventilation strategies for APF
The aim is to maintain adequate alveolar ventilation and oxygenation while minimizing fistula flow. The particular mode of ventilation is of less importance. Peak airway pressure and transpulmonary pressure (alveolar minus intra-pleural pressure) should be minimized by using:
- The lowest effective tidal volume
- The minimum PEEP
- The least number of positive-pressure breaths
- Discontinuation of negative suction on chest drains as early as possible.

With severe lung disease, where relatively high pressures are required in order to keep the patient alive, a large air leak may have to be tolerated.

Problems
- Gas exchange may deteriorate. Permissive hypercapnia, an increase in FiO_2, and perhaps permissive hypoxia may have to be accepted.
- Auto-triggering. Air leaks may be interpreted by the ventilator as the initiation of a breath. This may result in hyperventilation, respiratory alkalosis, the inappropriate escalation of sedatives, and the use of neuromuscular blocking agents.

High-frequency ventilation
High-frequency ventilation (HFV) is superior to conventional ventilation in patients with proximal BPF and otherwise normal lung parenchyma. Its efficacy in patients with APF and abnormal lung parenchyma is controversial. During conventional mechanical ventilation, gas flows preferentially through a fistula because it has low airway impedance. HFV redirects flow away from a fistula because airway impedance is increased with increased respiratory rate. However, this increase in airway impedance becomes less important in patients with reduced compliance in the rest of the lung. In addition, reduced peak airway pressure in HFV is less of a concern in a peripheral APF because pressure changes are blunted by intervening resistances (see 📖 High-frequency oscillatory ventilation, p 158).

Independent lung ventilation

A double-lumen ETT may be necessary to isolate a large BPF. The affected side can be maintained inflated on PEEP, ventilated with pressure limitation or with HFV.

The majority of double lumen tubes are designed to sit in the left main bronchus. This is because of the proximity of the lobar ostia to the carina on the right main bronchus. Right-sided tubes are available and may need to be used in disease of the proximal left main bronchus.

Disadvantages include the additional skills required at placement, tube displacement, bronchial ischemia, stenosis, and rupture from the high pressure generated by the endobronchial cuff.

Chest drain

Large air leaks may require large chest tubes. The use of suction is debatable. It has been common practice to place thoracostomy tubes on suction on the assumption that this promotes early resolution of air leaks by eliminating residual space and encouraging pleural apposition.

• Current opinion is that water seal is superior to suction in small air leaks, but large leaks require suction.
• When suction is used, early conversion to water seal is advised because prolonged use of suction may retard resolution of the air leak.

Intermittent inspiratory chest tube occlusion

This synchronizes chest tube occlusion on inspiration, potentially reducing the leak and facilitating distribution of tidal volume to the rest of the lung. The underwater seal is connected to the inspiratory limb of the ventilatory circuit through a pressure-amplifying valve. The positive pressure generated on inspiration closes the outlet of the underwater seal and thereby the chest tube. Pulmonary gas exchange may be improved.

Chest tube pressurization

Chest tube pressurization applies positive pressure equivalent to PEEP to the intrapleural space by connecting the underwater seal to the expiratory limb of the ventilatory circuit. This limits air leak on expiration and maintains intrapulmonary PEEP, which is necessary to prevent hypoxemia in some patients.

Other measures

Surgical repair may be the only option for a large proximal BPF, for example post pneumonectomy.

Surgical closure of an APF is fraught with problems. Lung resection (or 'blebectomy') may be technically possible when there is a single leak site, but is not an option as the size and number of leaks increases, as occurs frequently in ARDS.

Also, many of these patients are too ill to risk surgical repair, and non-surgical methods need to be considered.

Pleurodesis

In chemical pleurodesis, a sclerosant is instilled through the chest tube when the lung is fully re-expanded. However, the chest tube needs to be clamped after instillation of the sclerosant (contraindicated in the presence of an air leak). One way around this is to elevate the connecting tube between the chest tube and the underwater seal up to 60cm above the level of the chest. Raising the tubing (but not the bottle containing the underwater seal) prevents the sclerosant immediately trickling out of the chest drain but still allows air to escape. Because of the relatively high failure rates (in the region of 10%) with pleurodesis compared with surgical pleural stripping procedures, pleurodesis is usually only considered for those patients who are either unwilling or too unwell to undergo surgery.

Pleurectomy

This involves stripping the parietal pleura to encourage the lung to stick to the chest wall in an attempt to obliterate the pleural space and achieve symphysis. The pleurectomy may be total or partial (where the mediastinal and diaphragmatic pleural surfaces are just abraded rather than stripped) and it can be performed thoracoscopically or via open thoracotomy. Video-assisted thoracoscopic pleurectomy has been shown to be a successful intervention with a relatively low risk of complication (recurrence, bleeding, chronic chest wall pain) in patients with recurrent primary spontaneous pneumothoraces (a pneumothorax arising in an otherwise healthy person without any lung disease). However, open thoracotomy is still recommended in patients with secondary pneumothoraces (secondary to underlying lung disease), which would include most critically ill patients with a pneumothorax. Pleurectomy is usually performed under general anaesthesia with one-lung ventilation and unfortunately many critically ill patients are too sick to tolerate this.

Endoscopic repair

If the leak can be identified it may be amenable to endoscopic or endobronchial closure. A number of methods have been described, including:
• Balloons (Fogarty or Swan-Ganz catheter)
• Plugs (Gelfoam, fibrin, autologous clot, or tissue glue)
• Nd:YAG laser
• Endobronchial valves primarily designed for endoscopic lung volume reduction in emphysema
• Amplatzer device (originally used for closure of atrial septal defects).

None of these methods have been subjected to rigorous, systematic clinical evaluation and the decision to use any one of them is usually based on local experience and expertise.

Ventilator-associated pneumonia

VAP is the most common nosocomial infection encountered in the ICU. It is associated with both increased mortality and ICU length of stay, although it is not clear if VAP functions as an independent risk factor for these outcomes.

The diagnostic approach and diagnostic criteria are not standardized and at least six different diagnostic methods have been described:
• Quantitative and qualitative cultures of tracheal aspirates
• Bronchial brushings with and without bronchoscopy
• Bronchoalveolar lavage with and without a bronchoscopy.

Such diagnostic uncertainty leads to lack of consensus on basic information such as incidence (quoted incidence ranges from 9% to 28%), treatment, and outcome.

VAP is defined as an inflammation of the lung parenchyma occurring 48h or more after intubation of the trachea because of organisms not present or incubating at the time mechanical ventilation was commenced.

Early-onset VAP occurs within the first 4 days of intubation and is usually due to antibiotic sensitive bacteria.

Late-onset VAP develops 5 or more days after intubation and is commonly caused by opportunistic and multidrug-resistant pathogens.

Pathophysiology

VAP is thought to develop as a result of aspiration of pathogenic organisms from the oropharynx.

The normal flora of the mouth and oropharynx are harmless saprophytes (e.g. α haemolytic streptococci). In illness, this flora is replaced by pathogenic organisms, most notably enteric aerobic Gram-negative bacilli and *Staphylococcus aureus*. This change in microbial flora is directly related to the severity of illness of the patient, rather than environmental factors (healthy individuals who work in hospitals do not become colonized) or antibiotic use (it occurs in patients who have not received antibiotics). Bacteria may gain access to the lower respiratory tract either at or following intubation. In intubated patients contaminated secretions pool above ETT cuffs and leak into the trachea along wrinkles in the cuff. The inner surface of the tracheal tube also acts as a nidus for biofilm formation, which protects the colonizing pathogens. Ventilator cycling and the frequent passage of suction catheters through these tubes introduce the pathogens into the lower airway.

Risk factors

Studies employing multivariate analysis have identified many variables as independent risk factors for the development of VAP (Table 5.7).

Table 5.7 Independent risk factors for the development of VAP

Host factors

- Advanced age
- Co-morbidities (alcoholism, renal impairment, pre-existing pulmonary disease, diabetes mellitus, cigarette smoking, malnutrition)
- Severity of illness
- Hypoalbuminaemia

Intervention related factors

- Stress ulcer prophylaxis (with proton pump inhibitors or H_2 antagonists) is thought to promote gastric colonization with pathogens
- Enteral feeding (probably increases the risk of regurgitation); post pyloric feeding is thought to decrease the risk
- Presence of a tracheal tube
- Failed extubation

Pathogens

The predominant organisms responsible for infection are *Staphylococcus aureus*, *Pseudomonas aeruginosa*, and Enterobacteriaceae (e.g. *E. coli*, Proteus, Enterobacter, Klebsiella, Serratia). The range of organisms found varies according to patient population, duration of hospital stay, and prior antimicrobial therapy (see also 📖 Microbiology, p 49).

Diagnosis

The diagnosis of pneumonia in ventilated patients using clinical and radiological criteria alone is difficult.

- Clinical signs of infection such as fever, leucocytosis, and purulent secretions have a low specificity for confirmation of VAP.
- The presence of infiltrates on CXR is not specific to VAP.
- CXR may be normal in the face of VAP.

The Clinical Pulmonary Infection Score

The Clinical Pulmonary Infection Score (CPIS) was developed to increase the diagnostic accuracy for VAP (Table 5.8). It relies on four components:

- Clinical signs of infection (fever, leucocytosis, purulent secretions)
- Impaired gas exchange
- Radiological signs of new or worsening infiltrates on CXR
- Microbiological evidence of infection.

Table 5.8 Clinical Pulmonary Infection Score

	CPIS points		
	0	1	2
Temperature	36.5–38.4	38.5–38.9	≤36 or ≥39
Leucocyte (cells/µL)	4000–11000	<4000 or >11000	Band forms ≥50%
PaO$_2$/FiO$_2$ (mmHg)	>240 or ARDS		≤240 and no evidence of ARDS
CXR	No infiltrates	Diffuse/patchy infiltrate	Localized infiltrate
Tracheal secretions	None	Non-purulent secretions	Purulent secretions
Culture	Minimal or no growth	Moderate growth of pathogenic organisms	Moderate or greater growth of pathogenic bacteria consistent with that seen on original Gram stain

Points are allocated according to the presence or absence of the components and a score >6 is suggestive of a diagnosis of VAP.

In clinical trials, a CPIS score >6 has been demonstrated to be 89% sensitive but only 47% specific when compared to bronchoscopic specimen culture. It is poorly predictive of VAP in certain patient groups, such as trauma patients and those with burns.

Antibiotic prescribing based on the CPIS score would result in unnecessary treatment, so in clinical practice a CPIS score >6 should prompt further sampling and microbiological analysis of pulmonary secretions (see below).

Investigation

Tracheal aspirates

Tracheal aspirates have a high sensitivity (>90%) but a very low specificity (<60%) for the diagnosis of pneumonia. The poor positive predictive value of tracheal cultures is due to contamination of tracheal aspirates with secretions from the ETT.

Microscopic analysis of tracheal aspirates is unreliable in predicting culture results and should not be used to guide antibiotic therapy. Even the presence of white blood cells on microscopy is of limited value. The presence of macrophages indicates that the specimen is from the lower respiratory tract. As neutrophils comprise up to 20% of the cells recovered from a routine mouthwash, they must be present in abundance on microscopy in order to be used as evidence of infection.

Quantitative cultures can be used to determine the number of colony-forming units (CFU) present in a specimen. They are less sensitive but more specific. The threshold for positivity is 10^5CFU/mL. Isolates that do not meet the threshold are considered to be contaminants.

Bronchoalveolar lavage

BAL cultures have a high sensitivity and specificity, resulting in a high positive predictive value.

Between 60 and 120mL of sterile saline is instilled in 20mL aliquots. Usually less than 25% of the instilled volume is recovered. The first aliquot is discarded on the assumption that it may be contaminated by organisms carried down from the ETT; the remaining specimens are pooled and quantitatively cultured. A threshold of 10^4CFU/mL is usually applied to BAL cultures.

Protected specimen brush

The PSB is designed to minimize microbiological contamination from the ETT, only collecting uncontaminated specimens from the distal airways.

A gelatine plug seals the sampling brush in the inner lumen of a catheter, preventing upper airway contamination. When in the distal airway, the brush is advanced, displacing the gelatine seal. After sampling, the brush is retracted before withdrawing the apparatus.

Catheters are usually placed by brochoscopic control, although blind sampling devices are now available (protected catheter specimen).

PSB has a low sensitivity but a very high specificity. A threshold of 10^3CFU/mL is usually used for PSB cultures.

Which diagnostic method is best?

- Most studies show that the mortality in VAP is not influenced by the diagnostic method therefore it is hard to argue that any one method is better than another.
- Treatment based solely on cultures of tracheal aspirates may result in excessive use of antibiotics due to the high false-positive rate.

Treatment

There is often pressure to start antibiotics in suspected VAP because delay in receiving effective antibiotics has been shown to be associated with a worse outcome for a number of infections.

- If at all possible antibiotics should be withheld until specimens have been collected from the respiratory tract.

- Antibiotic choice should be based on local recommended empiric guidelines rather than on microscopy findings.
- Antibiotics should be discontinued after 2–3 days if the cultures are negative.

Antibiotic guidelines

A variety of factors should influence the choice of initial antibiotic therapy, including knowledge of the likely organisms and their sensitivities, local microbial epidemiology, and the results of surveillance cultures from the patient. Multidrug-resistant pathogens are more likely in patients who have had a prolonged hospitalization, those receiving mechanical ventilation for >7 days and those who have received prior antibiotic therapy.

Guidelines for the empirical treatment of VAP have been produced by the British Society for Antimicrobial Chemotherapy (Table 5.9). Seven days of appropriate antibiotic therapy is generally considered adequate for most patients with VAP.

Table 5.9 Guidelines for the empirical treatment of VAP

Early onset VAP	
First line	Cefuroxime or co-amoxiclav
If recent antibiotic therapy consider	Third generation cephalosporin or fluoroquinolone or piperacillin/tazobactam
Late onset VAP	
Choose from	Ceftazidime or ciprofloxacin or meropenem or piperacillin/tazobactam
Consider therapy for MRSA	Glycopeptide or linezolid

Prevention of VAP

Prevention of any nosocomial infection in the ICU requires a multidisciplinary approach. However, a number of specific interventions have been shown to reduce the incidence of VAP. These interventions broadly fall into three groups.

Minimising the duration of intubation

- Sedation breaks are effective in reducing the duration of mechanical ventilation.
- Weaning protocols—although viewed with suspicion by a number of clinicians, these protocols have been demonstrated to reduce time on a ventilator.
- NIV is associated with decreased VAP rates and is increasingly being used successfully as an alternative to invasive ventilation in patients with acute respiratory failure.

Reducing colonization of the oropharynx

- Nursing the patient head up—unless specifically contraindicated all mechanically ventilated patients should be nursed in a semi-recumbent position (30° to 45° head up) to decrease regurgitation of gastric contents into the oropharynx.

- Selective decontamination of the digestive tract (SDD) and selective oral decontamination (SOD) aim to reduce the pathogenic microbiological load while maintaining normal gut flora. In SOD topical pastes (typically amphotericin B, tobramycin, and polymyxin) are applied to the orophaynx until ICU discharge. In SDD the pastes are also administered nasogastrically and combined with systemic antibiotics for 4 days (typically cefotaxime). Although there is some conflicting evidence, several studies have shown that SDD and SOD reduce mortality.
- Oral decontamination with topical oral antiseptics—oropharyngeal decontamination with antiseptics such as chlorhexidine 1–2% or povidone iodine 10%, have also been shown to significantly reduce the incidence of VAP.

Reducing aspiration

The introduction of recent advances in ETT design have been associated with reduced incidence of VAP (see 📖 Tracheal tubes, p 210).

- Subglottic suction channels allow the aspiration of subglottic secretions, reducing the incidence of VAP.
- Wrinkle-free cuffs—the LoTrach system uses a special ETT with a wrinkle-free cuff that is maintained at a constant pressure of 30cmH$_2$O. This reduces the channelling of subglottic secretions.

There are practical and safety issues with changing previously sited standard ETTs after admission to ICU, e.g. in hypoxaemic patients and in patients with elevated intracranial pressure following traumatic brain injury.

It has been suggested that heated water humidifiers (HWHs) may be associated with a higher incidence of VAP because of the build up of condensation within the ventilator tubing, subsequent bacterial colonization, and the potential for aspiration of this contaminated water. The evidence supporting this hypothesis is weak.

Ventilator-associated tracheobronchitis

The term 'ventilator-associated tracheobronchitis' (VAT) has been used to describe the clinical situation of a patient who fulfils all of the criteria for VAP without CXR evidence of new or worsening infiltrates. Although its existence as an entity in its own right is debatable, post-mortem studies *do* sometimes find high bacterial counts in lung samples without histological pneumonia.

This creates a dilemma: should patients with fever, purulent secretions, and a bacterial isolate in tracheal secretions be treated with a course of antibiotics? When the diagnostic criteria for a condition are imprecise or subjective, such as the presence of purulent secretions or the presence of new or worsening infiltrates on CXR, decisions to treat are a matter of clinical judgment.

Cardiovascular effects

This is fully discussed in 📖 Heart–lung interactions, p 275.

Renal and other organ systems

The immediate effects of positive pressure ventilation on other organ systems relate to a reduced cardiac output and increased venous pressures.

The resulting venous congestion increases end-capillary pressure and alters fluid dynamics within organs.

Renal
Reduced cardiac output will cause:
- Decreased glomerular filtration rate
- Diversion of intrarenal blood flow.

Pulmonary lymphatics
Mechanical ventilation increases pulmonary interstitial fluid, some of which will make its way into the lymphatics.
- The positive pressure on the interstitium may compress some peripheral lymphatics, aiding flow, but it may also occlude these thin-walled vessels, impeding flow.
- Elevated CVP associated with positive pressure ventilation will impede drainage from the thoracic duct.
- PEEP helps to remove fluid from the alveoli but the reduction in thoracic duct drainage results in fluid retention in the interstitium.
- Impaired lymphatic drainage may also predispose to infection.

Fluid homeostasis
Positive pressure ventilation is associated with salt and water retention. Several mechanisms may be involved, including a fall in cardiac ouput, sympathetic activation, the renin–angiotensin–aldosterone system, increased antidiuretic hormone, and reduced atrial natriuretic peptide.

Ventilator-induced diaphragmatic dysfunction
Ventilator-induced diaphragmatic dysfunction (VIDD) causes a reduction in the force-generating capacity of the diaphragm. It has been demonstrated in animal models following mechanical ventilation both histologically and physiologically (*in vivo* and *in vitro*). In humans phrenic nerve elicited transdiaphragmatic twitch pressures were reduced by half following mechanical ventilation, and diaphragm myofibril atrophy has been shown after 18h of mechanical ventilation in brain-dead organ donors.[3]

To date disproportionate diaphragmatic atrophy when compared to other muscle groups has not been demonstrated, and similar histological changes have been shown in unloaded muscles.
- The prime mechanism is suspected to be disuse atrophy.
- Nutritional state, oxidative stress, steroid use, and muscle relaxants have all been implicated.
- It has been postulated as a major cause of delayed weaning and weaning failure.
- The effects may be attenuated by spontaneous rather than controlled modes of ventilation.

The clinical significance of VIDD is not clear, but it would seem logical to minimize conditions causing muscle atrophy (e.g. inadequate nutritional intake, muscle relaxant use) and to minimize disuse atrophy by the use of spontaneous ventilatory modes rather than controlled modes wherever possible.

Sinus infections

The use of nasotracheal tubes in the past was associated with sinus infection rates of 5–8%. Although these tubes are no longer routinely used in adults, nasogastric tubes or some monitors may still occlude the paranasal sinus ostia and predispose patients to infection (paranasal sinus opacification and air-fluid levels are common findings on CT scans of critically ill patients).

Sinus infection may be an important consideration when all other causes of fever have been eliminated. However, it is not routinely looked for, rarely treated, and there are few reports of apparent adverse consequences, all of which suggests that the incidence of clinically significant sinus infection is minimal.

Diagnosis
- The typical symptoms of sinusitis (facial pain, nasal obstruction, loss of smell, purulent nasal discharge) are usually obscured in the critically ill patient. Physical examination is also of limited benefit.
- Positive radiographic findings include an air-fluid level, opacification, and mucosal thickening. CT is recommended, although portable sinus films are also helpful.
- Aspiration of the maxillary antrum is considered the gold standard technique for the diagnosis of purulent maxillary sinusitis.
- Common infecting organisms include Gram-negative bacilli (particularly *P. aeruginosa*) and Staphylococci. Up to half have multiple organisms.

Treatment
- Antibiotics.
- Methods to improve drainage:
  - Removal of nasal tubes
  - Semi-recumbent nursing
  - Decongestants.

Complications
The complications of acute sinusitis are rare but often rapidly fatal.
- Orbital infection.
- Intracranial involvement:
  - Meningitis
  - Epidural abscess
  - Subdural empyema
  - Cavernous sinus thrombosis
  - Cerebral abscess.

1 Dreyfuss D, Soler P, Basset G, and Saumon G (1988) High inflation pressure pulmonary edema. Respective effects of high airway pressure, high tidal volume, and positive end-expiratory pressure. *Am Rev Respir Dis* **137**(5), 1159–64.
2 Acute Respiratory Distress Syndrome Network (2000) Ventilation with lower tidal volumes as compared with traditional tidal volumes for acute lung injury and the acute respiratory distress syndrome. *N Engl J Med* **342**(18), 1301–8.
3 Levine S, Nguyen T, and Taylor N et al. (2008) Rapid disuse atrophy of diaphragm fibers in mechanically ventilated humans. *N Engl J Med* 2008, **358**(13), 1327–35.

5.7 Effects of mechanical ventilation on control of breathing

The respiratory control system consists of a control centre located in the medulla, a motor arm that executes respiratory effort, and various feedback mechanisms that convey information to the control centre (Fig. 5.10). During assisted mechanical ventilation the respiratory control centre interacts with the ventilator and this interaction determines the ventilatory output, which in turn influences feedback to the patient's control centre.

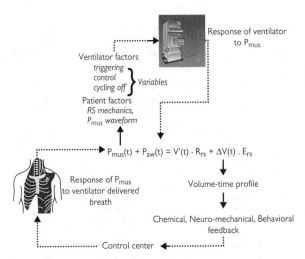

Fig. 5.10 Schematic representation of variables that determine the volume–time profile during mechanical ventilation. $P_{mus}(t)$ is instantaneous respiratory muscle pressure. $P_{aw}(t)$ is airway (ventilator) pressure. $V'(t)$ is instantaneous flow. $\Delta V(t)$ is instantaneous volume relative to the passive functional residual capacity of respiratory system. R_{rs} is resistance and E_{rs} is elastance of the respiratory system (RS). Neuromechanical, chemical, and behavioural feedback systems are the main determinants of P_{mus}. The functional operation of the ventilator mode (triggering, control, and cycling-off variables) and patient-related factors (respiratory system mechanics and P_{mus} waveform) determine the response of the ventilator to P_{mus}.

Effects of mechanical ventilation on feedback systems

Behavioural feedback

The effects of mechanical ventilation on behavioural feedback in awake, ventilated patients are unpredictable and depend on:
- Individual patient and environmental factors
- The degree to which the ventilator unloads the patient's respiratory effort
- Patient–ventilator synchrony.

Behavioural feedback, along with other cortical input (collectively termed 'the wakefulness drive to breathe'), is a potent stimulus that maintains breathing activity even in the absence of chemical or any other stimuli, preventing the occurrence of apnoea.

Chemical feedback

Chemical feedback is the response of respiratory muscle pressure (P_{mus}) mainly to $PaCO_2$ and, to a lesser degree, to PaO_2 and pH. Mechanical ventilation influences chemical feedback by altering these variables, not only by its effect on ventilation, but also on the gas-exchange properties of the lung and cardiac function.

$PaCO_2$ stimulus

- Respiratory drive. The intensity of respiratory effort increases progressively as a function of $PaCO_2$. This is evident even in the hypocapnic range, but the response slope increases progressively with increasing $PaCO_2$. This response is independent of the wakefulness state of the patient.
- Respiratory rate in awake subjects. Manipulation of $PaCO_2$ over a wide range has no appreciable effect on respiratory rate. Despite hypocapnia, subjects continue to trigger the ventilator with a rate similar to that of eupnea and slight hypercapnia.
- Respiratory rate in asleep subjects. During non-REM sleep (or sedation) an increase in ventilation sufficient to decrease $PaCO_2$ by only a few mmHg below eupneic $PaCO_2$ causes abrupt apnoea. Respiratory rhythm is not restored until $PaCO_2$ has increased significantly above eupneic levels. The $PaCO_2$ value when apnoea occurs is termed *apnoeic threshold* and the difference between eupneic $PaCO_2$ and $PaCO_2$ at apnoeic threshold ($\Delta PaCO_2$) is termed *CO_2 reserve*. This reserve determines the propensity of an individual to apnoea and thus breathing instability, and it is influenced by many factors.
- Apnoeic threshold and CO_2 reserve are extremely important in asleep patients ventilated with pressure support or assist VCV. Increasing the support level gradually decreases eupneic $PaCO_2$ to levels approaching the apneic threshold, so that further random minor increases in ventilation will induce apnoea. This is particularly common in patients with congestive heart failure and brain damage, who exhibit inherently increased propensity to unstable breathing.

When asleep or sedated, PSV or ACV may induce intermittent apnoeas because CO_2 falls below the apnoeic threshold.

PaO_2 and pH stimulus

In a steady state during wakefulness, the effects of PaO_2 and pH on breathing pattern are qualitatively similar to those observed with CO_2: changes in PaO_2 and pH mainly alter the intensity of patient effort whereas respiratory rate is considerably less affected. Although the effects of mechanical ventilation on the response of respiratory motor output to stimuli other than CO_2 have not been adequately studied, there is no reason to expect a different response pattern.

It is important to note that during mild hypocapnia the hypoxic ventilatory response is attenuated. At moderate hypocapnia (end-tidal PCO_2 ~4.1kPa) the response is negligible. The latter observations may be clinically relevant because ventilated patients do not always keep $PaCO_2$ at eucapnic levels.

> During hypocapnia any hypoxic response will be blunted and the control centre will be dangerously 'unresponsive'.

Chemical stimuli and unstable breathing

During non-REM sleep (or sedation), when the respiratory control system is predominantly governed by chemical stimuli feedback, it becomes susceptible to unstable (periodic) breathing. By altering this feedback system, mechanical ventilation may promote breathing instability.

Neuromechanical feedback

Intrinsic properties of respiratory muscles

For a given neural output, P_{mus} decreases with increasing lung volume and flow, as dictated by the force–length and force–velocity relationships of inspiratory muscles, respectively. Therefore, for a given level of muscle activation, P_{mus} should be smaller during mechanical ventilation than during spontaneous breathing if the pressure provided by the ventilator results in greater flow and volume. This type of feedback is of minimal clinical significance.

Reflex feedback

The P_{mus} characteristics of each breath are influenced by various reflexes, which are related to lung volume or flow and mediated by receptors located in the respiratory tract, lung, and chest wall.

The best studied is the Hering–Breuer or inflation reflex, where excessive lung inflation leads to decreased frequency due to increased neural expiratory time. Mechanical ventilation, as well as any changes in ventilator settings, may stimulate these receptors by changing flow and volume, and elicit acute reflex P_{mus} responses.

For example, a decrease in V_t (in ACV) or pressure support (in PSV) leads to a decrease of neural expiratory time, whereas an increase in inspiratory flow leads to a decrease of neural inspiratory time. Both result in increased respiratory frequency. Additionally, expiratory asynchrony (i.e. the extension of mechanical inflation into neural expiration) causes the expiratory time to increase proportionally to the asynchrony time.

The final response to any planned ventilation strategy may be unpredictable depending on the magnitude and type of lung volume change, the level of consciousness, and the relative strength of the reflexes involved. Two examples:
- If pressure support is decreased during weaning, the resulting lower V_T will cause a reflex decrease of neural expiratory time and increase in respiratory frequency. Increased respiratory rate is therefore not necessarily patient intolerance to weaning.

- Consider ventilatory strategies to decrease dynamic hyperinflation in a patient with COPD. If pressure support (in PSV) or V_T at a constant inspiratory flow (in ACV) is decreased, it will decrease expiratory asynchrony and will by reflex cause the neural expiratory time to also decrease. Alternatively, if inspiratory flow is increased at constant V_T (in ACV), it will by reflex cause the neural inspiratory time to also decrease. Both strategies will result in *reflex increased neural respiratory frequency*, limiting their effectiveness in reducing dynamic hyperinflation.

Neuromechanical inhibition
Mechanical ventilation at relatively high tidal volume and ventilator frequency above spontaneous respiratory rate results in a non-chemically mediated decrease in respiratory motor output, which is manifested both in respiratory frequency and amplitude of respiratory motor output. This decrease is termed 'neuromechanical inhibition' and is of questionable clinical relevance.

Entrainment of respiratory rhythm to ventilator rate
Entrainment of respiratory rhythm to the ventilator rate implies a fixed, repetitive, temporal relationship between the onset of respiratory muscle contraction and the onset of a mechanical breath. Human subjects exhibit one-to-one entrainment over a considerable range above and below the spontaneous breathing frequency. Cortical influences (learning or adaptation response) and the Hering–Breuer reflex are postulated as the predominant mechanisms of entrainment. Studies of the entrainment response in critically ill patients are lacking.

> **Increased respiratory rate** may occur as a *reflex* if:
>
> PS is reduced in PSV (reduces nTe)
> V_T is reduced in ACV (reduces nTe)
> Inspiratory flow is increased in ACV (reduces nTi).
>
> For example, if $PEEP_i$ has developed in COPD, a reduction in PS in PSV, or V_T in ACV, may lead to reflex increase in respiratory rate, counteracting any reduction in $PEEP_i$.

Patient factors that may influence control of breathing by altering the patient–ventilator interaction

Mechanics of the respiratory system
The mechanical properties of the respiratory system may influence the pressure delivered by the ventilator independently of patient effort, and thus may modify the effects of mechanical ventilation on the various feedback loops. For example, excessive triggering delay and ineffective triggering are common in patients with obstructive lung disease and dynamic hyperinflation.

Characteristics of the P_{mus} waveform
The characteristics of the P_{mus} waveform influence the ventilator-delivered volume in a complex manner, depending on several patient

and ventilator factors. As a simplified summary, a low rate of initial P_{mus} increase will predispose the patient to triggering delays or ineffective triggering, whereas a vigorous inspiratory effort that extends beyond mechanical inflation time may trigger the ventilator more than once during the same inspiratory effort.

It follows that changes in these patient-related factors may influence the ventilator rate and total ventilatory output despite no change in the patient's intrinsic breathing frequency. In turn, alterations in ventilatory output may significantly modify the patient's respiratory effort secondary to changes in feedback loops.

1 Georgopoulos D (2008) Effects of mechanical ventilation on control of breathing, Tobin MJ (ed.) *Principles and Practice of Mechanical Ventilation*. McGraw-Hill, New York, pp 715–28.

5.8 Patient ventilator asynchrony

The word 'synchrony' derives from the Greek σύν (with) and χρόνος (time), and, in the context of mechanical ventilation, it refers to the agreement between the patient's own (neural) and the ventilator (mechanical) inspiratory and expiratory times. It also includes the matching of patient effort with delivered tidal volume.[1]

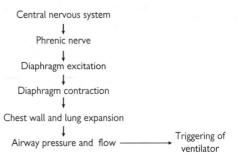

Fig. 5.11 Actions during spontaneous breathing.

During spontaneous breathing, there is a physiological time lag between the stimulus to breathe generated by the CNS and the contraction of the inspiratory muscles that results in the generation of airflow and therefore of tidal volume (Fig. 5.11). All ventilators that use pneumatic triggers are affected by this time lag and are susceptible to patient ventilator asynchrony.

Theoretically the ventilator should cycle in synchrony with the activity of the patient's respiratory rhythm. There are three major sites of possible asynchrony:

- Triggering of the ventilator
- The phase of inspiration after triggering
- The passage from inspiration to expiration (cycling or expiratory triggering).

Detection of asynchronies

The more obvious forms of patient–ventilator mismatching, such as wasted efforts, auto-cycled breaths, and double triggering, may be assessed at the bedside using ventilator waveforms and monitors (see below). Automatic detection of major patient/ventilator interaction problems using closed visual monitoring of the ventilator screen has been recently proposed.

Asynchrony may also be subtle and detected only with more advanced monitoring techniques. Precise recording of the neural respiratory timing can be achieved by using oesophageal catheters, which measure pressure changes (the transdiaphragmatic pressure (Pdi)) or monitor diaphragm electrical activity (diaphragmatic EMG). Pdi is probably used more frequently in clinical practice, since it requires less sophisticated technology, although it is more prone to errors.

Triggering of the ventilator
Inspiratory trigger delay (Fig. 5.12)
The diaphragm contraction is represented by the positive deflection in Pdi. The time (T_1) elapsed between the onset of Pdi and the reaching of the zero flow is due to the presence of $PEEP_i$, while the following delay of 360ms (T_2) is due to the slow response of the machine to provide an inspiratory flow (i.e. opening of the valve, increased dead space).

This T_2 delay may also be picked out on the ventilator screen by the flow trace, as an unusually prolonged flat signal before the pressurization of the ventilator begins.

Ineffective triggering (Fig. 5.13)
This is as an inspiratory effort that does not trigger the ventilator. This phenomenon may be simply picked out using the Pdi trace. It can also be easily recognized as a notch on the pressure and flow traces.

Double (or triple) triggering (Fig. 5.14)
This is two or more breath cycles separated by a very short expiratory time, the first cycle being a patient-triggered one. Double and triple triggering can be easily depicted on the flow and airway pressure recordings.

Auto-triggering (Fig. 5.15)
This is a breath delivered by the ventilator without a prior airway pressure decrease, indicating that the ventilator delivered a breath that is not triggered by the patient. It is more difficult to recognize auto-triggering when the ventilator mode includes time-cycled mandatory breaths.

The phase of inspiration after triggering
Inspiratory time extension (Fig. 5.16)
The end of the patient's effort, as assessed by the peak Pdi, is much shorter than the ventilatory inspiratory time. The machine provides flow even when the patient has relaxed his diaphragm. This difference between the neural and mechanical inspiratory times is called T_i extension and it is almost impossible to detect from screen traces.

The passage from inspiration to expiration
Expiratory trigger cycling (Fig. 5.17)
In this case the ventilator ceases its inspiratory support before the patient has finished the inspiratory phase.

'Hang-up' phenomenon (Fig. 5.18)
This may happen during NIV in the presence of large air leaks, when the inspiratory flow remains higher than the threshold value set for the expiratory trigger because the ventilator tries to compensate for leaks. In this case the flow signal reaches a sort of plateau after an initial brisk decay.

Causes of ventilator asynchrony
$PEEP_i$ and excessive tidal volume
When PSV is used to provide respiratory support in intubated patients with COPD, some of the patient's inspiratory efforts may fail to trigger the ventilator.[2] These ineffective efforts are very common phenomena, especially when dynamic hyperinflation is present, and may be dependent on an excessive inspiratory pressure delivered by the ventilator. It has

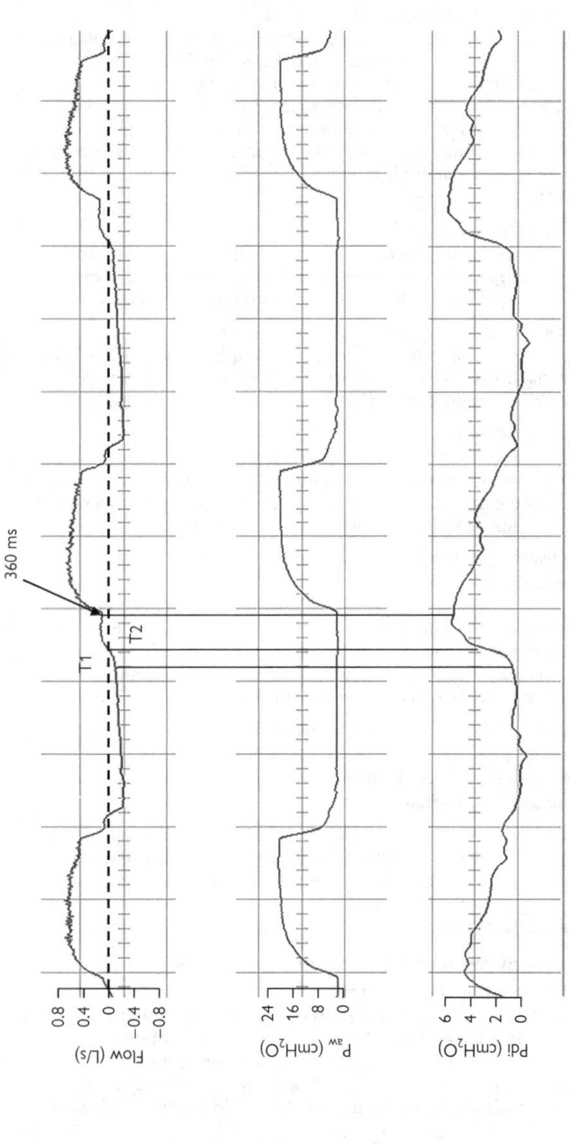

Fig. 5.12 Inspiratory trigger delay.

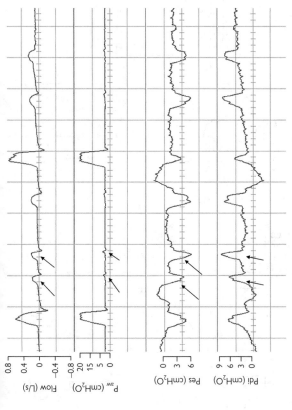

Fig. 5.13 Ineffective triggering.

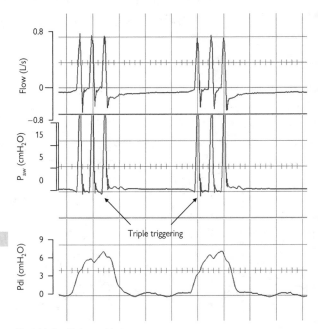

Fig. 5.14 Double (or triple) triggering.

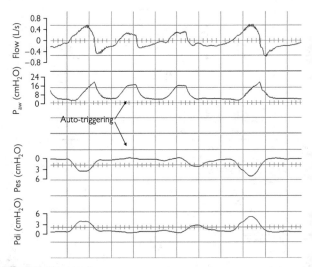

Fig. 5.15 Auto-triggering.

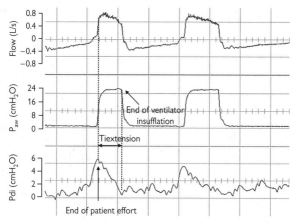

Fig. 5.16 Inspiratory time extension.

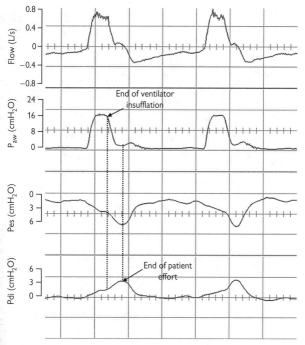

Fig. 5.17 Expiratory trigger cycling.

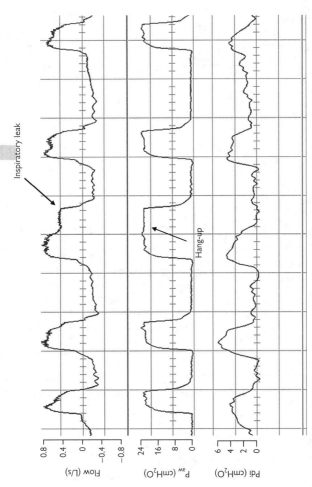

Fig. 5.18 'Hang-up' phenomenon.

been demonstrated that almost half of the patients using PSV and NIV had ineffective efforts. Interestingly, the use of a more sophisticated technique, with the insertion of gastric and esophageal balloons to record the respiratory mechanics, reduced asynchrony to 30%, but did not eliminate it. Applying extrinsic PEEP should theoretically reduce the effects of PEEP$_i$, but is often ineffective in practice (see 📖 Pressure support ventilation, p 144, and Positive end expiratory pressure, p 119).

These problems are common also to other modes of assisted ventilation.

Air leaks

In the setting of NIV air leaks are common and may even be desirable. If air leaks are excessive, however, end-inspiratory flow may be greater than the flow required to cycle the ventilator to exhalation and the patient becomes stuck in inspiration. This often results in an active expiratory effort by the patient to force the ventilator into expiration with the use of accessory muscles and increased WOB. Under these circumstances, the patient is seen to 'fight' the ventilator. Cycling to exhalation may only occur after the fixed maximum ventilator inspiratory time has passed.

This may be a cause of NIV failure and/or intolerance, especially using older ventilators.

Ventilator trigger delays

Matching the 'neural start' of inspiration and the 'ventilator start' is difficult, particularly for NIV. Ventilatory modes, apart from NAVA (see below), share similar inspiratory triggering systems, regulated by flow, pressure, volume, or complex algorithms including all of these.

Several bench studies have looked the 'inspiratory trigger variables' using NIV or ICU ventilators. Trigger delays range between 50 and 300ms, although delays of up to 500ms have been recorded. Varying the settings of the ventilator and the mechanical characteristics of the system has an inconsistent but generally small effect on triggering times, suggesting that there is a largely unavoidable element to the triggering delays intrinsic to the design of the ventilators.

Although these studies did not examine in detail the problem of patient ventilator interaction, most of the ventilators commercially available have an 'acceptable' intrinsic delay (<120ms) in the inspiratory trigger. Flow triggering is usually preferred because of a slight reduction in WOB.

Pressure rise time

The effect of the initial flow rate has been mainly studied in intubated patients. Variation has no effect on tidal volume, respiratory frequency, or arterial blood gases, but a high pressure rise time is associated with a reduction in the inspiratory effort.

During NIV, however, different initial flow rates affect patient–ventilator interaction. The ratio of neural inspiratory time to mechanical inspiratory time is significantly shorter with the highest flow rate. This suggests that although inspiratory effort is reduced, the mechanical breath delivered by the ventilator exceeds what is required by the patient.

Expiratory trigger

The manipulation of the expiratory trigger during PSV may also deeply influence patient–ventilator interaction. During PSV, the ventilator cycles into expiration when inspiratory flow decreases to a given percentage of peak inspiratory flow. In obstructive disease, the slower rise and decrease of inspiratory flow will lead to delayed cycling, an increase in $PEEP_i$, and non-triggering efforts. Setting the expiratory trigger at a higher than usual percentage of peak inspiratory flow attenuates the adverse effects of delayed cycling, improves patient–ventilator synchrony, and reduces inspiratory muscle effort.

Endotracheal and tracheostomy tubes

Kinked or partially blocked tubes increase the frequency of ineffective efforts and increase WOB.

Interfaces for NIV

- The internal volume of the masks has no apparent short-term dead-space effect on gas exchange, minute ventilation, or patient effort. Interfaces are therefore interchangeable in clinical practice, although adjustment of the ventilator settings may be required.
- Although helmets are better tolerated as an interface for CPAP, the increased apparatus dead space and compliance associated with the helmet leads to problems with trigger delay and CO_2 clearance if used for NIV. Higher PS and PEEP may partially compensate for this problem.

Ventilator tubing

Excessive dead space in the tubing between the 'Y' piece and the patient should be avoided.

Condensate in dependent parts of the ventilator tubing can lead to auto-triggering.

Humidification

Very little is known about the impact of the humidification system on patient–ventilator synchrony, especially during NIV, where this problem seems to be more important.

- Inadequate humidification may cause patient distress, but available data are too scarce to allow specific recommendations.
- Mouth leaks during CPAP lead to high unidirectional nasal airflow. Subsequent increases in nasal resistance may be prevented by humidification.
- HMEs increase the apparatus dead space compared with HHs. HMEs may produce less of a reduction in inspiratory effort during NIV for hypercapnic respiratory failure.
- HMEs may make triggering more difficult.
- HHs may cause water 'drop out' in the circuit and lead to auto-triggering.

Improved synchrony with newer ventilator modes?

Modes of ventilation have attempted to match the patient's inspiration and expiration to the ventilator inspiration and expiration, and to ensure that the patient receives more assistance when demand is high and less assistance when demand is low.

Proportional assist ventilation

PAV (see 📖 Proportional assist ventilation, p 174) is a ventilatory mode where the inspiratory support more closely mirrors the patient's effort, i.e. when effort is high, pressure support increases and when the patient's neural output ends, so does inspiration.

Several studies have shown both in the acute and chronic settings that PAV delivered non-invasively may improve gas exchange, reduce dyspnoea, and decrease the inspiratory efforts in the same fashion as PSV. In intubated patients PAV has been shown to reduce WOB and be better tolerated than PSV.

The triggering system for PAV is identical to PSV and other modes of ventilation, and is subject to the limitations described above. Therefore, in conditions of elevated $PEEP_i$, this mode is also subject to ineffective triggering and trigger delay.

Neurally adjusted ventilatory assist

In NAVA (see 📖 Neurally adjusted ventilatory assist, p 178), the patient's neural output is quantified with the electrical activity of the crural diaphragm (the EAdi).[3] In this manner, cycling on and off are determined directly by the EMG. The final pressure support delivered is governed by the size of the EAdi. The operator sets 'cmH_2O of pressure support per μV of EAdi'. The bigger the diaphragmatic contraction, the more support is given. With this ventilatory technique the synchrony between the neural and mechanical inspiratory times should be guaranteed at any phase of respiration, irrespective of $PEEP_i$ and respiratory mechanics.

Theoretically air leaks should not be a problem during NIV, and synchrony improved. The insertion of an esophageal catheter is considered a semi-invasive procedure, and this may limit uptake of this mode during NIV. NAVA is a very promising mode of ventilation, but data are currently lacking about its clinical use.

Clinical importance of ventilator asynchrony

The most important example of asynchrony is the mismatch between the patient's (neural) inspiration and the ventilator's inspiratory time. This generates 'wasted' or ineffective efforts. If severe, this can lead to:

- Fighting against the ventilator
- Increased use of sedatives
- Prolonged duration of mechanical ventilation and increased frequency of tracheotomy.[4]

The most immediate and common consequence of these ineffective efforts is the extra load on the respiratory muscles. These muscles already have to cope with increased elastic, resistive, and threshold workload. This increased load can be overcome with ease in patients with well-preserved muscular force, but in difficult-to-wean patients this force–load imbalance can significantly hamper the process of weaning from mechanical ventilation.

Asynchrony has mostly been studied during daytime. Poor patient–ventilator interaction during sleep can lead to sleep fragmentation, frequent arousals, and inadequate correction of nocturnal hypoventilation.[5]

The asynchrony literature focuses on patients with COPD, and especially in those with low elastance and/or high levels of auto-PEEP.

There are also studies in patients with restrictive thoracic disorders, but ARDS and pneumonia are under-represented. This may be partly due to the different mechanical properties of the respiratory system, and partly because the higher frequency of asynchrony in COPD patients makes it easier to study. It does not mean that asynchrony does not present a problem in patients with other diseases.

Problem solving
The ventilatory mode
In approximately 70% of patients the most common assisted modes of ventilation do not cause major asynchronies. In the more complex patients, if the manipulation of the settings (see below) does not improve this phenomenon, one may consider more sophisticated modes like PAV and NAVA. These modes have advantages but are more difficult to set and titrate.

In the presence of airleaks during NIV, time cycling may improve synchrony. Pressure support may be primarily time cycled or time cycling may be set as a backup if flow cycling fails. Time-cycled pressure support is essentially assisted synchronized PCV.

The characteristics of the ventilator
Most available ventilators synchronize satisfactorily in most cases. There are several studies comparing the *in vitro* characteristics of the various ventilators, and the knowledge of these results may eventually drive the decision of the clinician to use a specific ventilator. For NIV, the use of dedicated NIV ventilators, or ICU ventilators with an NIV module, is strongly recommended.

Ventilator settings
Alteration of the ventilator settings is the best available method to improve patient–ventilator interaction.
- The inspiratory trigger. A flow trigger is likely to be more sensitive than a pressure trigger. Very sensitive triggers can, however, produce autotriggering.
- The set or generated tidal volume. High tidal volumes (i.e. >8mL/kg) or high inspiratory support may lead to significant asynchrony, especially if there is airflow limitation. In COPD patients the reduced elastance of the respiratory system may lead to a large expired tidal volume ($\approx$10mL/kg) if the level of inspiratory support is elevated (i.e. >18–20cmH$_2$O). Ventilator inspiration continues into patient (neural) expiration when the inspiratory muscles have stopped contraction. This leaves inadequate time for expiration and leads to 'breath stacking' and dynamic hyperinflation. The following inspiration starts at a high lung volume, when the pressure at the airway opening is still significantly positive. Therefore, the inspiratory effort does not create a pressure gradient capable of being sensed by the ventilator.
- The initial flow rate during PSV. In the intubated patient with high respiratory demand, an elevated pressurization rate may reduce WOB. During NIV, very fast inspiratory flow (i.e. square wave) may increase air leaks, with the associated problems. During NIV, the pressurization rate should be set considering both the compliance of the patient and the size of the air leak.

- The cycling from inspiration to expiration during PSV. Expiratory triggering usually takes place at around 25% of peak inspiratory flow. In some ventilators this may be varied. In the presence of severe expiratory flow limitation, a more sensitive trigger (expiration staring at a higher percentage of peak flow) may reduce the number of ineffective efforts.

The apparatus used

HHs reduce the dead space compared with HMEs, and they may be preferentially used in those patients with CO_2 retention.

If using a helmet, increasing the 'usual' baseline inspiratory and expiratory pressures by 50%, and increasing the pressurization rate, reduces the number of asynchronies. Even with these adjustments, oro-facial masks perform better.

Sedation

Agitation and diaphoresis may result in ventilator asynchrony or NIV treatment failure.

However, pharmacological sedation should be used cautiously, since confusion and agitation may also be caused by hypoxia and hypercapnia.

Opioids such as morphine and fentanyl are powerful analgesics, but even at therapeutic doses will cause respiratory depression. Other adverse effects include hypotension, bradycardia, ileus, delirium, and agitation. Newer opiods (e.g. sufentanil) have a favourable pharmacokinetic profile and are suitable for 'awake' sedation during partial ventilatory support. In intubated patients an infusion of 0.2–0.3mcg/kg/h did not change respiratory drive or ventilatory pattern.

It is reasonable to administer small doses of opioids (fentanyl, morphine) where blunting of respiratory drive is desirable. Remifentanil-based sedation may be used successfully even with NIV.

If benzodiazepines are required, lorazepam (0.5–1mg) has fewer drug interactions than diazepam or midazolam because of its metabolism via glucuronidation. It is indicated for younger patients, for chronic benzodiazepine users, and for patients with preserved lean mass and muscular force, where a mild muscle relaxant effect elicited by benzodiazepines can be desirable.

Conclusions

Patient–ventilator asynchrony is underestimated in clinical practice. Particularly in patients with airflow limitation it may cause increased duration of mechanical ventilation and increased frequency of tracheostomy. Air leaks mean that asynchrony is also common during NIV and may interfere with the treatment success.

The clinician should consider how best to correct this harmful interaction between the 'two brains' (i.e. the patient and the clinician who is responsible for the ventilator settings).

Recommended reading

Thille AW, Cabello B, Galia F, Lyazidi A, and Brochard L (2008) Reduction of patient–ventilator asynchrony by reducing tidal volume during pressure-support ventilation. *Intensive Care Med* **34**, 1477–1486.

1 Tobin MJ, Jubran A, and Laghi F (2001) Patient–ventilator interaction. *Am J Respir Crit Care Med* **163**, 1059–63.
2 Nava S, Bruschi C, Rubini F, Palo A, Iotti G, and Braschi A (1995) Respiratory response and inspiratory effort during pressure support ventilation in COPD patients. *Intensive Care Med* **11**, 871–9.
3 Sinderby C, Navalesi P, Beck J, et al. (1999) Neural control of mechanical ventilation in respiratory failure. *Nat Med* **5**, 1433–6.
4 Thille AW, Rodriguez P, Cabello B, Lellouche F, and Brochard L (2006) Patient–ventilator asynchrony during assisted mechanical ventilation. *Intensive Care Med* **32**, 1515–22.
5 Fanfulla F, Delmastro M, Berardinelli A, Lupo ND, and Nava S (2005) Effects of different ventilator settings on sleep and inspiratory effort in patients with neuromuscular disease. *Am J Respir Crit Care Med* **172**, 619–24.

5.9 Heart-lung interactions

The cardiovascular and respiratory systems are not separate but tightly integrated. Acute respiratory failure and forced ventilatory efforts can profoundly alter cardiovascular function, just as heart failure can alter ventilation and gas exchange. Many of these effects are predictable and can also be used to diagnose cardiovascular status. For example:

- Both lung under-inflation and hyperinflation increase pulmonary vascular resistance, heart–lung interactions, and WOB.
- Spontaneous inspiratory efforts during acute bronchospasm and acute lung injury induce markedly negative swings in ITP.[1] These negative swings increase venous return and impede LV ejection, causing intrathoracic blood volume to increase.
- Positive pressure ventilation increases ITP during inspiration, decreasing both venous return and LV afterload. This differs from normal spontaneous ventilation, where inspiration is accompanied by a reduction in ITP.

Heart–lung interactions involve four basic concepts:

- Inspiration increases lung volume.
- Spontaneous inspiration decreases ITP.
- Positive pressure ventilation increases ITP.
- Ventilation is exercise; it consumes O_2 and produces CO_2.

Haemodynamic effects of changes in lung volume

Lung inflation:

- Alters the flow characteristics of venous return
- Affects pulmonary vascular resistance
- Compresses the heart in the cardiac fossa—at high lung volumes this can limit cardiac volumes in a similar fashion to cardiac tamponade
- Alters autonomic tone.

Each of these processes may predominate in determining the final cardiovascular state.

Venous return

The major determinants of the hemodynamic response to increases in lung volume are mechanical in nature. Lung inflation, independent of changes in ITP, primarily affects cardiac function and cardiac output by altering:

- Right ventricular (RV) preload and afterload
- LV preload.

Inspiration alters right atrial pressure and induces diaphragmatic descent, both of which alter venous return.

Venous return is a function of:

- The ratio of the pressure difference between the right atrium and the systemic venous reservoirs
- The resistance to venous return.

There are four main changes induced by inspiration:

- RA pressure is lowered by spontaneous breaths and raised by positive pressure breaths.

- A large proportion of the venous blood volume is in the abdomen. Increased intra-abdominal pressure (diaphragmatic descent) increases abdominal venous pressure and augments venous blood flow.[2]
- Diaphragmatic descent also compresses the liver. This increases hepatic outflow resistance, decreasing splanchnic venous reservoir flow.
- Inspiration shifts venous flow from high-resistance splanchnic circuits, which drain through the liver, to low-resistance systemic venous circuits, making the venous return greater for the same driving pressure.

Thus, increasing lung volume may increase, decrease, or not alter venous return depending on which of these factors are predominant.

Usually:
- Spontaneous inspiration increases venous return
- Positive pressure inspiration decreases venous return in normo- and hypovolemic states and in patients with hepatic cirrhosis
- Positive pressure inspiration increases venous return only in volume overloaded states.

Pulmonary vascular resistance
RV output is sensitive to changes in pulmonary outflow resistance. Decreased pulmonary artery pressure reduces RV afterload and improves RV ejection.

Low lung volumes
Alveolar collapse often occurs in ALI/ARDS and is associated with increased pulmonary vascular tone induced by hypoxic pulmonary vasoconstriction. Alveolar recruitment restores end-expiratory lung volume back to FRC and may reverse this process. However, during the recruitment manoeuvres, RV dysfunction often occurs.

High lung volumes
Increasing lung volume above FRC also increases RV outflow resistance. This is due to progressive increases in transpulmonary pressure (airway pressure relative to ITP). Since the heart and great vessels (extra-alveolar vessels) exist in the thorax and sense ITP as their surrounding pressure, increases in transpulmonary pressure will induce pulmonary vascular collapse as transpulmonary pressure approaches pulmonary artery pressure. Hyperinflation therefore increases pulmonary vascular resistance and pulmonary artery pressure.

Hyperinflation may be reversed by:
- Prolonging expiration
- Reducing levels of PEEP
- Reducing tidal volumes
- Bronchodilation.

The use of smaller tidal volumes and less PEEP has reduced the incidence of acute cor pulmonale seen in critically ill patients.[3]

In addition to the changes in PVR induced by changes in lung volume, mechanical ventilation may also reduce PVR by correcting hypoxia, reducing respiratory acidosis, and attenuating sympathetic tone (sedation and reduced WOB).

Effects on LV function

LV end-diastolic volume (preload) can be altered by ventilation:
- Decreasing RV volume must eventually decrease LV volume because the two circulations are in series.
- Changes in RV end-diastolic volume inversely alter LV diastolic compliance because of ventricular interdependence.[4]
- Increasing lung volume restricts absolute cardiac volume by tamponade-like direct compression.

Autonomic tone

Small tidal volumes (<10mL/kg) increase heart rate by vagal withdrawal (respiratory sinus arrhythmia). Larger tidal volumes (>15mL/kg) decrease heart rate, arterial tone, and cardiac contractility by increased vagal tone and sympathetic withdrawal. These effects are probably only relevant in the diagnosis of dysautonomia and in the care of neonatal subjects where autonomic tone is high.

Haemodynamic effects of changes in intrathoracic pressure

The heart within the thorax is a pressure chamber within a pressure chamber. Changes in ITP affect the pressure gradients for both systemic venous return to the RV and systemic outflow from the LV, independent of the heart itself.[1]
- Increases in ITP reduce these pressure gradients, decreasing venous return and aiding LV ejection. Intrathoracic blood volume is decreased.
- Decreases in ITP augment venous return and impede LV ejection. Intrathoracic blood volume is increased.

Since the pressure gradient for venous return is small relative to LV ejection, similar changes in right atrial and transmural LV pressures will have a disproportionately greater effect on venous return than on LV ejection.

Venous return

Variations in right atrial pressure represent the major factor determining the fluctuation in pressure gradient for systemic venous return during ventilation.[2] Changes in mean systemic pressure (the pressure in the upstream venous reservoirs) due to intra-abdominal pressure fluctuations mitigate the detrimental effect of positive pressure ventilation on venous return.

Increases in ITP with positive pressure ventilation or hyperinflation during spontaneous ventilation decrease venous return. Decreases in ITP during spontaneous inspiration increase venous return.

LV ejection

$$\text{LV afterload} \propto \text{transmural systolic LV pressure} \times \text{LV volume}$$

Thus, increasing ITP will decrease transmural LV pressure (if arterial pressure is constant) and will unload the LV. Increases in ITP actually may increase cardiac output in congestive heart failure states. Decreases in ITP have the opposite effect.[1]

Spontaneous ventilatory efforts against a resistive (bronchospasm) or elastic (acute lung injury) load decrease LV stroke volume. This manifests as pulsus paradoxus caused by both ventricular interdependence[4] and increased LV afterload.[1]

Increases in ITP have the opposite effect, decreasing LV afterload. The effect on LV ejection is limited because of the obligatory decrease in venous return.

Negative swings in end inspiratory intrathoracic pressure

From a mechanical perspective, there is no difference between increasing ITP from a basal end-expiratory level and eliminating the negative end-inspiratory ITP swings seen in spontaneous ventilation. However, removing negative swings in ITP may be more clinically relevant because:

- Many pulmonary diseases are associated with exaggerated decreases in ITP during inspiration. In restrictive lung disease states, such as interstitial fibrosis or acute hypoxemic respiratory failure, ITP must decrease greatly to generate a large enough transpulmonary pressure to ventilate the alveoli. Similarly, in obstructive diseases, such as upper airway obstruction or asthma, large decreases in ITP occur owing to increased resistance to inspiratory airflow[5]
- Exaggerated decreases in ITP require increased respiratory efforts that increase WOB, taxing a potentially stressed circulation
- The exaggerated decreases in ITP can only increase venous blood flow so much before venous collapse limits blood flow. The level to which ITP must decrease to induce venous flow limitation is different in different circulatory conditions but occurs in most patients below an ITP of $-10cmH_2O$. Further decreases in ITP, therefore, will further increase only LV afterload without increasing venous return.

Thus, eliminating the negative end-inspiratory ITP swings seen in spontaneous ventilation will reduce LV afterload without reducing venous return. This can reverse pulmonary oedema and improve gas exchange.[5] These concepts of a differential effect of increasing and decreasing ITP on cardiac function are illustrated for both normal and failing hearts in Figs 5.19 and 5.20 using the LV pressure–volume relationship during one cardiac cycle to interpose venous return (end-diastolic volume) and afterload (end-systolic volume). Therefore, performing an endotracheal intubation in patients with obstructive breathing abolishes the markedly negative swings in ITP without reducing venous return.

Ventilation as exercise

Spontaneous ventilatory efforts are exercise and represent a metabolic load on the cardiovascular system. They require muscular activity, have a large voluntary component to their action, consume O_2, and produce CO_2. Although ventilation normally requires less than 5% of total O_2 delivery to meet its demand, in lung disease states where WOB is increased, such as pulmonary oedema or bronchospasm, the requirements for O_2 may increase to 25% or more of total O_2 delivery. If cardiac output is limited (e.g. heart failure) then spontaneous ventilation may not be possible even with additional cardiovascular support.

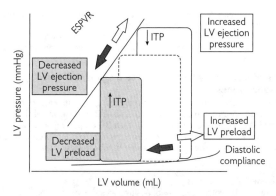

Fig. 5.19 The effect of ITP on the pressure–volume loop of the cardiac cycle. The slope of the LV end-systolic pressure–volume relationship (ESPVR) is proportional to contractility. The slope of the diastolic LV pressure–volume relationship is proportional to diastolic compliance.

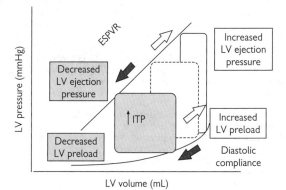

Fig. 5.20 The effect of ITP on the pressure–volume loop of the cardiac cycle in congestive cardiac failure (reduced LV contractility and expanded intravascular volume). The slope of the LV end-systolic pressure–volume relationship (ESPVR) is proportional to contractility. The slope of the diastolic LV pressure–volume relationship is proportional to diastolic compliance.

Mechanical ventilation, when adjusted to the metabolic demands of the patient, may dramatically decrease WOB, resulting in increased O_2 delivery to other vital organs and decreased serum lactic acid levels. Under conditions in which fixed right-to-left shunts exist, such as occurs in patients with pneumonia and acute lung injury, the obligatory increase in SvO_2 will result in an increase in the PaO_2, despite no change in the ratio of shunt blood flow to cardiac output.

Cardiovascular insufficiency and failure to clear airway secretions are the two most common causes of failure to wean from mechanical ventilation.

Use of heart–lung interactions to diagnose volume responsiveness

Positive pressure ventilation induces cyclic changes in the pressure gradient for venous return and so causes cyclic changes in RV filling. If the RV is responsive to these changes in filling, then RV output will also vary with the phases of the ventilatory cycle. Similarly, if LV output is responsive to changes in end-diastolic volume, then LV output will also vary.

Volume responsiveness:
- Ventricular volumes vary with positive pressure ventilation.
- If a patient is volume responsive, cardiac output will vary with these changes.
- This is best assessed by stroke volume or pulse pressure variation

Accordingly, if both ventricles are volume responsive, then positive pressure ventilation will induce cycle-specific changes in both LV stroke volume and arterial pulse pressure, as a surrogate of stroke volume. Numerous studies have documented that quantifying this stroke volume or pulse pressure variation allows one to identify those subjects who are volume responsive.[6] Threshold values around 10–15% maximal variation across the ventilatory cycle appear to be highly predictive of volume responsiveness. Since the physiological forcing function is the dynamic changes in ITP, both tidal volume and chest wall compliance will influence the degree of variation.

However, during spontaneous ventilation, ventricular interdependence-induced changes in diastolic compliance can also alter stroke volume without altering LV wall stress (preload). Thus, the clinical utility of stroke volume or pulse pressure variation to identify subjects who are volume responsive is only applicable during positive pressure breathing.

Being volume responsive does not equate to the need for fluid resuscitation, which is a clinical determination.

Summary

Detrimental heart–lung interactions can be minimized by:
- Reducing WOB
- Minimizing excessive negative pressure swings in ITP during spontaneous breathing
- Preventing hyperinflation
- Avoiding alveolar derecruitment
- Preventing volume overload during weaning.

Further reading

Pinsky MR (2007) Heart lung interactions. *Curr Opin Crit Care* **13**(5), 528–531.

1 Buda AJ, Pinsky MR, Ingels NB, *et al.* (1979) Effect of intrathoracic pressure on left ventricular performance. *N Engl J Med* **301**, 453–9.
2 Van den Berg P, Jansen JRC, and Pinsky MR (2002) The effect of positive-pressure inspiration on venous return in volume loaded post-operative cardiac surgical patients. *J Appl Physiol* **92**, 1223–31.
3 Viellard-Baron A, Schmitt J, Augarde R, *et al.* (2001) Acute cor pulmonale in acute respiratory distress syndrome submitted to protective ventilation: Incidence, clinical implications, and prognosis. *Intensive Care Med* **29**, 1551–8.
4 Taylor RR, Covell JW, Sonnenblick EH, and Ross Jr J. (1967) Dependence of ventricular distensibility on filling the opposite ventricle. *Am J Physiol* **213**, 711–8.
5 Kaneko Y, Floras JS, Usui K, *et al.* (2003) Cardiovascular effects of continuous positive airway pressure in patients with heart failure and obstructive sleep apnea. *N Engl J Med* **348**, 1233–41.
6 Michard F, Boussat S, Chemla D, *et al.* (2000) Relation between respiratory changes in arterial pulse pressure and fluid responsiveness in septic patients with acute circulatory failure. *Am J Respir Crit Care Med* **162**, 134–8.

5.10 Effects of mechanical ventilation on oxygenation

Poor oxygenation in ventilated patients is a challenging part of ICU management. Dealing effectively with this common problem requires the clinician to understand the potential interactions between the treatment instituted and the underlying pathophysiological process.

There are a limited number of therapeutic interventions available.

This chapter will concentrate primarily on the effects of mechanical ventilation (MV) on oxygenation; hypercapnia is dealt with in 📖 Hypercapnia while on a ventilator, p 296. It should be read in conjunction with 📖 Respiratory physiology and pathophysiology, p. 2 and will assume knowledge from that chapter in the discussion.

Important principles

- MV is not a treatment of the underlying disease process.
- MV allows time for medical treatment to work or for natural recovery to take place.
- The primary aim of MV is to provide acceptable gas exchange while avoiding additional lung and other organ damage.
- Improvement in gas exchange does not necessarily improve O_2 delivery.
- Improvement in gas exchange is a poor surrogate marker for important outcomes such as mortality.

Methods to improve oxygenation

We can:
- Increase FiO_2
- Increase airway pressure (peak, plateau, PEEP, or mean)
- Perform an RM
- Increase global $\dot{V}/\dot{Q}$ ratio (by increasing minute ventilation)
- Change the ventilatory mode or overall strategy completely
- Alter the inspiratory airflow pattern
- Improve SvO_2
- Reduce pulmonary oedema
- Change patient position
- Reduce asynchrony
- Consider paralysis
- Consider adjuncts.

Increase FiO_2

- Increasing FiO_2 quickly corrects hypoxaemia due to hypoventilation.
- Gas exchange abnormalities are usually due to $\dot{V}/\dot{Q}$ mismatch and shunt. As shunt fraction increases above 20%, increases in FiO_2 have less effect on PaO_2. An increase in FiO_2 will still improve blood oxygen content to some extent by increasing dissolved oxygen in those capillaries exposed to ventilation.
- High FiO_2 encourages the formation of reactive oxygen species and may worsen the pulmonary insult.

- In areas of low $\dot{V}/\dot{Q}$, high FiO_2 will predispose the patient to absorption atelectasis and increased shunt fraction.
- See 📖 Oxygen therapy, p 74.

Increase airway pressure

Traditionally, increasing mean airway pressure is associated with improved oxygenation, but it can also result in haemodynamic instability, fluid retention, and barotrauma (Table 5.10).

Table 5.10 Traditional disease response to increases in MAP

'Responsive' diseases	Unpredictable or limited response
Pulmonary oedema	Lobar consolidation
Secondary ARDS (exudative stage)	ARDS (fibroproliferative stage)
Atelectasis	Primary ARDS
	Pulmonary haemorrhage
	Pulmonary contusions
	Fibrotic lung disease

Potential benefits

- Alveolar recruitment.
  - Reduced shunt.
  - Increased $\dot{V}/\dot{Q}$.
  - Improved compliance and reduced WOB.
- Reduced LV preload and afterload in cardiogenic pulmonary oedema.
- Reduced PVR by increasing lung volumes towards normal and reversing hypoxic pulmonary vasoconstriction.

Potential harms

- Increased shunt fraction—elevating mean airway pressure will increase PVR in compliant, healthy areas of lung and divert blood to consolidated areas.
- Increased dead space—decreased blood flow to ventilated areas, especially in apical regions.
- Decreased compliance—over-distended lung on the flat upper portion of the P/V (compliance) curve.
- Increased PVR (if lung is over-distended).
- Decreased cardiac output
  - Reduced LV preload or increased PVR in normo- or hypovolaemic states.
  - Reduced cardiac output may increase $\dot{V}/\dot{Q}$, but will reduce oxygen delivery and SvO_2.

Principles

Increases in airway pressure are designed to open (or recruit) collapsed alveoli. The lung volume response to airway pressure is described by the static pressure–volume curve. In the respiratory system the same airway pressure produces different volumes depending on whether the lung is inflating (lower volumes for the same pressures) or deflating (higher volumes for the same pressures). This phenomenon is called hysteresis (Fig. 5.21).

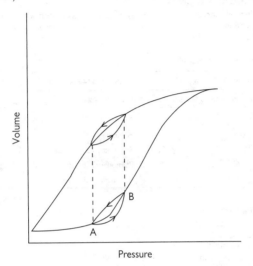

Fig. 5.21 Ventilation between pressures A and B produces different volumes, depending on lung 'history'. This is called hyteresis.

Lung hysteresis is a complex phenomenon related to the properties of surfactant, the viscosity of the alveolar lining, the law of Laplace (P = 2T/r), and the disordered sequence of alveolar reopening. It affects the relationship between mP_{aw} and oxygenation as well as influencing the relationship between mP_{aw} and haemodynamic effects.

It is easier to keep open a lung unit that has been opened than it is to open a lung unit that has been allowed to close.

In an injured lung there are pressures above which all recruitable units will open given sufficient time, and pressures below which all collapsible lung units will close. More interestingly, there is a conditional area between these values where lung unit opening will depend on the pre-existing state of the lung: if there are lots of closed lung units before airway pressure reaches the conditional zone, most will remain closed until they reach the threshold 'opening pressure'. If there are many lung units open before airway pressure drops into the conditional zone, most will remain open until they reach the threshold 'closing' pressure.

This theoretical description is a simplification of the complex behaviour produced by heterogeneous lung units, and a range of opening and closing pressures will exist within the same lung. However, it is conceptually useful to explain the different gas exchange responses produced by different approaches to raising mP_{aw} (see examples below). It also presupposes that the average threshold opening and closing pressures are known. In some circumstances they can be reasonably accurately established, for example using a decremental PEEP trial, constructing a static compliance (P–V) curve or performing the recruitment technique described by Lachmann.[1] Often the results are inconclusive. Furthermore, the threshold opening pressure may be so high that regular increases in inspiratory pressure to such a level are known to be harmful.

Interventions to increase airway pressure
Mean airway pressure can be elevated by increasing:
- Inspiratory pressure (or tidal volume in VCV modes)
- Inspiratory time as a proportion of total breath time
- PEEP
- $PEEP_i$.

Increasing inspiratory pressure
When the average opening threshold is breached by increasing inspiratory pressures inspiratory recruitment occurs, and gas exchange improves. If end expiratory collapse is then allowed to occur, VILI may be increased. If alveolae are not opened, then haemodynamics may deteriorate with no recruitment, and the resultant drop in SvO_2 will lead to deteriorating arterial oxygenation. Any increase in inspiratory pressure should provoke an assessment of current PEEP levels.

Increasing inspiratory time
Increasing inspiratory time may improve oxygenation by two methods:
- If inspiratory pressure is above threshold opening pressure, then spending longer in inspiration will improve recruitment and gas exchange. If inspiratory pressure is too low, then increasing inspiratory time may affect cardiovascular performance but not gas exchange.
- If expiratory time (Te) is short enough, $PEEP_i$ will develop.

Increasing PEEP
- The effect of PEEP is dependent on the starting position of the lung, the threshold closing pressure, and the disease process.
- When PEEP is changed in small increments without a preceding RM, response may be gauged by an assessment of oxygenation, compliance, and haemodynamics after a period of time (usually hours, sometimes minutes).
- Formal assessment of optimal PEEP is undertaken using a decremental PEEP trial or by analysing a static pressure volume curve (📖 Positive end expiratory pressure, p 119).
- The higher the PEEP, the less facility there is for a providing a reasonable driving pressure (P_{high} – PEEP) with resultant effects on overall $\dot{V}/\dot{Q}$ and CO_2 clearance.

- There is little current evidence that high PEEP makes any difference to outcome compared with moderate PEEP when used indiscriminately to treat a particular disease process in all patients.

Increasing PEEP$_i$

PEEP$_i$ is generated when expiratory time is so short that the lungs do not reach FRC before the next inspiration starts. If expiration is shorter than three times the expiratory time constant, PEEP$_i$ will develop. PEEP$_i$ is introduced by shortening expiration until the end expiratory flow does not reach zero. Classically inverse ratio ventilation is used (📖 Pressure-controlled ventilation, p 135).

There has been much discussion regarding the advantages of PEEP over PEEP$_i$ and vice versa (see text box).

Advantage of PEEP$_i$?

Some authors have argued that PEEP$_i$ may selectively allow ventilation of those areas of the lung with short time constants, while resting those with long time constants. Healthier areas of lung tend to have longer time constants, and PEEP$_i$ may therefore limit cyclic volume change in healthy units, while improving ventilation and V̇/Q̇ matching in dependent units with fast time constants. If the expiratory time is short enough, no part of the lung has time to collapse in expiration.

However, the areas with short time constants will collapse early in expiration, and it may not be possible to shorten expiration enough to prevent such collapse in diseased lungs. Areas with high resistance or compliance will develop high levels of PEEP$_i$.

Experimental work suggests a slight increase in shunt when PEEP$_i$ is compared with extrinsic PEEP.

A further problem with PEEP$_i$ is the possibility that its presence is unrecognized, and haemodynamic side effects are not considered.

Examples

In lungs with mild abnormalities, total PEEP (PEEP + PEEP$_i$) may be greater than the threshold closing pressure (little end expiratory alveolar collapse) and the inspiratory pressure may be above the threshold opening pressure. Gas exchange will be good and increases in PEEP, inspiratory time, or P$_{high}$ may not improve gas exchange and may cause haemodynamic instability.

In situations with severe gas exchange abnormalities, total PEEP may be below the threshold closing pressure (leading to end expiratory alveolar collapse) and inspiratory pressures below threshold opening pressures, limiting inspiratory recruitment (Fig. 5.22). Examples of the response to different interventions are shown in Figs 5.23 to 5.27.

Figs 5.23 and 5.24 ↑PEEP

The increase in PEEP increases P$_{high}$ (no change in P$_{set}$). Gas exchange improves significantly (inspiratory recruitment and prevention of expiratory collapse). Atelectrauma is reduced. The haemodynamic consequences of increased mean P$_{aw}$ offset by reduced PVR. Fig. 5.24 Note that if the PEEP increase does not move the curves above the opening

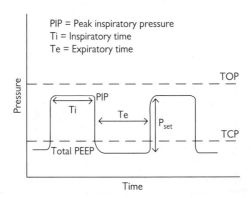

Fig. 5.22 See text for details. TOP, threshold opening pressure; TCP, threshold closing pressure; $P_{set} = P_{insp}$ = set inspiratory pressure.

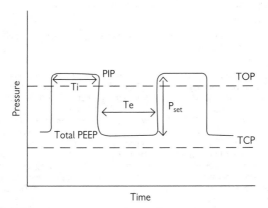

Fig. 5.23 ↑PEEP, ↔P_{set}, ↑PIP, ↑mean P_{aw}, I:E unchanged, ↑↑gas exchange, ↓↓atelectrauma, ↑ cardiovascular effects (CE), baro/volutrauma depends on pressures/volumes.

and closing pressures, there would be no gas exchange improvement, just haemodynamic consequences.

Fig. 5.25

Increase P_{set} Gas exchange will improve (inspiratory recruitment) but there is increased atelectrauma.

Fig. 5.26

Increased I:E (increased Ti, no change in Te). Te is not sufficiently short to generate PEEP$_i$. Since there is no increase in recruitment there is little

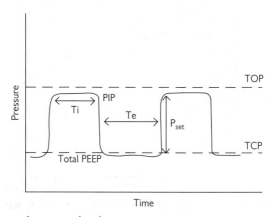

Fig. 5.24 ↑PEEP, ↔P$_{set}$, ↑PIP, ↑mean P$_{aw}$, I:E unchanged, ↔gas exchange, ↔atelectrauma, ↑CE, baro/volutrauma depends on pressures/volumes.

effect on gas exchange, but increased mean P$_{aw}$ may result in significant haemodynamic consequences.

Fig. 5.27
Increased I:E (increased Ti, no change in respiratory rate therefore reduced Te). **Increased PEEP$_i$.** 7a demonstrates the development of PEEP$_i$. This may slowly improve gas exchange, but there will also be cardiovascular effects. The tidal volume will fall (reduced driving pressure despite unchanged P$_{set}$). 7b shows **increased I:E (as in 7a)** but with increased **P$_{set}$**, resulting in inspiratory recruitment. There is a marked increase in PEEP$_i$. There will be improved gas exchange, a reduction in atelectrauma, but marked cardiovascular effects.

- The figures show theoretical examples only. They are designed to help interpret gas exchange and cardiovascular responses to interventions, and to demonstrate that increasing mean airway pressure in different ways will have different effects.
- The results of changes in real life will depend on precise respiratory mechanics and the combination of ventilatory alterations. The consequences will differ from patient to patient, and from day to day in the same patient as the pathophysiology alters.
- Achieving the ideal combination of inspiratory recruitment and prevention of expiratory collapse with minimal cardiovascular effects may not be possible within safe limits of volumes and pressures. At this stage, it is sensible to consider another ventilatory strategy.

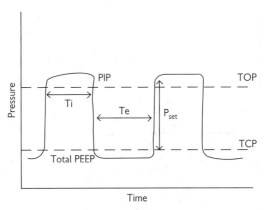

Fig. 5.25 ↔PEEP, ↑P$_{set}$, ↑PIP, ↑mean P$_{aw}$, I:E unchanged, ↑gas exchange, ↑atelectrauma, ↓CE, baro/volutrauma depends on pressures/volumes.

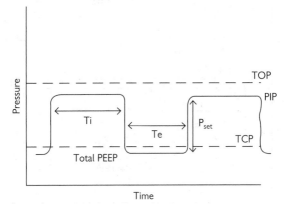

Fig. 5.26 ↔PEEP, ↔P$_{set}$, ↔PIP, ↑mean P$_{aw}$, ↑I:E (↑Ti, ↔Te, ↓respiratory rate), ↔gas exchange, ↔VILI, ↑↑CE.

Perform a recruitment manoeuvre
- RMs are also discussed in 📖 Adjuncts to ventilation, p 188. Outcome data are lacking, and there is no consensus on the method to be used or the regularity of recruitment.
- If the alveolar units are allowed to collapse after RM, any benefit will be lost. Resetting PEEP following the RM is therefore usually necessary.
- Even when PEEP is adjusted, the RMs typically require to be repeated.

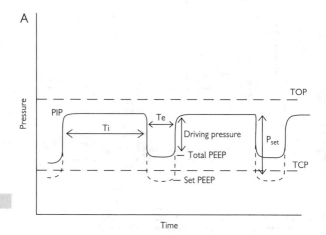

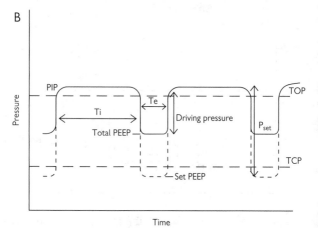

Fig. 5.27 A, ↔PEEP, ↔P$_{set}$, ↔PIP, ↑mean P$_{aw}$, ↑I:E (↑Ti, ↓Te, ↔respiratory rate; note the development of PEEP$_i$), ↑gas exchange, ↓atelectrauma, ↑CE, ↓volutrauma, ↔barotrauma. B, ↔PEEP, ↑P$_{set}$, ↑PIP, ↑mean P$_{aw}$, ↑I:E (↑Ti, ↓Te, ↔respiratory rate; note the development of PEEP$_i$, more than in A). ↑↑gas exchange, ↓atelectrauma, ↑↑CE, baro/volutrauma depends on pressures/volumes.

- Successful recruitment may allow a subsequent decrease in ventilator pressures without deterioration in gas exchange (lung hysteresis).
- Different modes of ventilation might be tried in order to recruit more slowly but in a more sustained fashion. Modes that may increase recruitment over a longer period are BIPAP, APRV, and HFOV. APRV and HFOV should be considered when recruitment should be possible, but is not sustainable within safe limits of pressure and volume.

Potential harm

The adverse effects are similar to those listed under increasing airway pressure, but are more pronounced and take place over a shorter period. They may be dramatic in susceptible patients (such as those who are hypovolaemic).

Increase global $\dot{V}/\dot{Q}$ ratio

Global $\dot{V}/\dot{Q}$ will be increased if overall MV increases or cardiac output decreases. All other things being equal, PO_2 will tend to increase and PCO_2 will tend to decrease. Be aware that other physiological changes produced by the same intervention may modify these effects, e.g an increased dead space from reduced apical perfusion may increase PCO_2; a fall in cardiac output will reduce oxygen delivery, and may decrease SvO_2 and potentially PaO_2.

Increased MV may be achieved by increasing V_t or respiratory rate. An improvement in compliance will facilitate larger V_t without the need for increased airway pressures.

Increased tidal volume
Potential benefits
- Improved recruitment.
- Decreased PVR if lung volumes increased towards normal and hypoxic pulmonary vasoconstriction reversed.

Potential harm
- Volutrauma, possibly barotrauma.
- Over-distension, with reduced compliance and increased PVR.

Increased respiratory rate
Potential benefits
- Simple way to increase alveolar ventilation.
- No increase in inspiratory pressure.

Potential harm
- Possible $PEEP_i$ with gas trapping and over-distension in volume-controlled modes or reduction of tidal volume in pressure-controlled modes.
- If tidal volume falls when using pressure-controlled modes of ventilation, there will be an increase in the proportion of dead space per breath, and therefore a reduction in alveolar ventilation if overall MV does not also increase. If the tidal volume falls by more than 25% when the respiratory rate increases, alveolar ventilation is likely to decrease despite the increased respiratory rate.

Increased compliance

In PCV, increasing compliance will increase minute ventilation if all other parameters are left unchanged. Compliance can be increased by:

- Recruitment
- Avoiding over-distension
- Addressing bronchospasm
- Treatment of pulmonary oedema (see below)
- Re-expansion of lung or lobar collapse
- Improvement in chest wall compliance (e.g. sit up, reduce intrabdominal pressure).

The effect of CO_2 on oxygenation

Increasing $\dot{V}/\dot{Q}$ >1 will reduce PCO_2 and increase PAO_2. The alveolar gas equation describes the simple displacement of O_2 molecules in the alveolus by CO_2:

$$PAO_2 = FiO_2 \times (P_B - PH_2O) - PaCO_2/R$$

where P_B = barometric pressure, PH_2O = SVP water at 37°C and R = respiratory quotient (estimated at 0.8).

This effect is generally limited, particularly because significant changes in CO_2 are difficult to achieve without substantial increases in alveolar minute ventilation. At low FiO_2, the proportionate change is greater. It is most important when oxygen therapy for chronic CO_2 retainers results in a rise in CO_2 (mechanism discussed in 📖 Oxygen therapy, p 74). When FiO_2 is subsequently reduced, the combination of low FiO_2 and high $PaCO_2$ may cause profound hypoxaemia.

Change ventilatory mode or strategy

There is very little consensus about the best mode for ventilating patients with severe gas exchange abnormalities. In choosing a mode, we want:

- Sufficient airway pressure to recruit the lung and keep it open
- Adequate CO_2 clearance
- Patient ventilator synchrony
- To minimize VILI.

Each of the many modes available has pros and cons. It is best to think in terms of interventions required and then choose a mode to deliver these interventions, rather than always use the same mode for patients who are difficult to ventilate. See the relevant chapters on individual ventilator modes, but consider PSV, APRV, BIPAP, HFOV, or changing strategy altogether: should referral for ECMO be made (📖 Extracorporeal membrane oxygenation, p 183)?

Alter inspiratory airflow pattern

Pressure-controlled modes of ventilation produce a rapid increase in inspiratory flow followed by an exponential decrease (see 📖 Pressure-controlled ventilation, p 135).

- Alveolar pressure is limited and cannot be higher than the set inspiratory pressure.

- Peak airway pressures will be lower for an equivalent tidal volume.
- For a given peak airway pressure, mean airway pressure is higher. Oxygenation may therefore be improved (but will also depend on the opening and closing pressures and PEEP).
- Improved distribution of ventilation. There is less end inspiratory gradient of pressure among regional units with heterogeneous time constants. CO_2 elimination is improved.

The incidence of VILI is unchanged and there are similar haemodynamic consequences.

If VCV is failing to produce adequate gas exchange or airway pressures are unacceptably high, PCV should be considered.

If using PCV, and inspiratory flow has not reached zero by end inspiration, an extension of inspiratory time to allow this to occur is likely to improve oxygenation and CO_2 clearance.

Increase mixed venous oxygen saturation

Increasing a low mixed venous oxygen concentration will reduce the overall effect of any shunt or areas of low $\dot{V}/\dot{Q}$ and improve oxygenation. Increased SvO_2 can be achieved by:
- Reducing oxygen consumption
- Increasing oxygen delivery.

Reduce oxygen consumption

Increased oxygen consumption is associated with hypermetabolic states: fever, sepsis, shivering, thyroid storm, malignant hyperpyrexia, and malignant neuroleptic syndrome.

The most common reason for increased oxygen consumption in patients with respiratory failure is increased WOB. This may account for up to 30% of oxygen consumption in some patients. Those patients who have an increased WOB (reduced compliance, increased resistance, rapid respiratory rate, use of accessory muscles, sweating, tachycardia, confusion) *and* who have evidence of inadequate oxygen delivery (low mixed venous oxygen saturation with a metabolic, often lactic, acidosis) may benefit from reducing WOB by instituting or increasing respiratory support.

Increase oxygen delivery

$$DO_2 = CO\ (L/min) \times 10[(Hb \times 1.34 \times SaO_2 \times 0.01) + (0.023 \times PaO_2)]^*$$

When there is evidence of inadequate oxygen delivery (above), all of these factors should be remembered.

---

* The characters within square brackets represent the oxygen content, which has traditionally been expressed per 100mL of blood. In this equation Hb is measured in g/100mL. CO = cardiac output, DO_2 = oxygen delivery.

In a patient with Hb 15g/dL, CO 5L/min and SaO_2 95%:
- A change in CO of 1L/min will alter DO_2 by 200mL/min
- A change in SpO_2 of 1% will alter DO_2 by 10mL/min
- A change in Hb of 1g/dL will alter DO_2 by 70mL/min.

If SaO_2 is improved from 90% to 95% with ventilatory manipulation, but at the same time the cardiac output falls by 1L/min, there is a reduction of 150mL/min in oxygen delivery.

Reduce pulmonary oedema

Treatment of pulmonary oedema is beneficial in LV failure, and reduces ICU length of stay in patients with ARDS.

If gas exchange is life threatening, or airway pressures or volumes are harmful, acute treatment of ARDS with diuresis or fluid removal improves oxygenation and may allow adjustment of ventilatory parameters. This strategy often produces intravascular volume depletion, increased vasoconstrictor requirement, and potentially reduces other organ function. This is sometimes a price worth paying, and may prevent further deterioration in gas exchange, allow reduction in ventilatory pressures, and prevent a vicious downward spiral towards hypoxaemic death.

Change patient position

Prone positioning has been used as a method to improve oxygenation for over 30 years. Despite often dramatic improvement in oxygenation, trial evidence is lacking to support its use for unselected patients. Subgroup analysis has identified populations of patients who may benefit (e.g. CO_2 responders), and it is still widely used both as a conventional therapy and as a rescue therapy. It is the subject of considerable debate, and is discussed in 📖 Adjuncts to ventilation, p 188.

In lobar or unilateral disease, laying the patient with the affected lung superior and the good lung inferior increases blood flow to the lung or lobe with better ventilation and may improve gas exchange.

Reduce asynchrony

This problem is dealt with in 📖 Asynchrony, p 262, and it is also discussed extensively in 📖 Pressure support ventilation, p 144.

In summary, neural inspiration and expiration should be closely matched by ventilator inspiration and expiration, and a change in patient effort should result in a change in volumes delivered by the ventilator. It is clear that these conditions are often not present, and this results in patient–ventilator asynchrony.

Causes

Agitation
Agitation is caused by pain, delirium, anxiety, and dyspnoea. Dealing with these will reduce patient–ventilator dysynchrony.

Mode
Some modes synchronize on average more successfully than others. PSV in general will cause less dysynchrony than controlled modes. NAVA potentially

is the best synchronized mode, and PAV may be beneficial. Within the controlled modes, some (such as BIPAP) will allow patient breathing at any point in the respiratory cycle. Others (such as SIMV) will allow spontaneous efforts only at set times, and breaths at other times may lead to high pressure alarms and premature termination of a breath. Clinicians should be aware of the synchronization rules of the modes on their ventilator and adjust to a better tolerated mode if dysynchrony is a problem.

Intrinsic PEEP

Not only will $PEEP_i$ increase WOB, it may decrease the efficiency of force generation by respiratory muscles and move a patient to the flat, non-compliant section of the P–V curve. $PEEP_i$ may be difficult to detect and may also be an occult cause for significant cardiovascular instability. Always consider $PEEP_i$ in the presence of bronchospasm, high respiratory rate, I:E ratios >1:2, and particularly when end expiratory flow does not reach zero.

Consider paralyisis

Paralysis is sometimes used as the option of last resort in hypoxaemia. It is assumed that fully controlling ventilation will allow an increased ability for the clinician to accurately manipulate precise physiological variables such as ventilatory pressures and I:E ratio. It will improve the cosmetic appearance of the patient and the ventilator pressure/flow/volume curves. In addition:

- It may improve chest wall compliance and therefore allow improved ventilation at lower pressures.
- It eliminates dysynchrony.
- If WOB is high, it will reduce oxygen consumption and therefore may increase SvO_2 and PaO_2.

It often fails to improve gas exchange and more often will allow basal alveolar derecruitment and increase the shunt fraction. Ventilator-induced diaphragmatic dysfunction has been demonstrated after only a few hours in animal models and some human studies. Diaphragmatic activity serves to maintain basal ventilation, and generally improves $\dot{V}/\dot{Q}$ matching, even when it appears to be dysynchronous.

In general, it is usually better to allow and even encourage spontaneous ventilation and to focus on reducing dysynchrony.

When oxygenation is problematic, a mixed mode such as BIPAP or APRV will provide the necessary high mean airway pressure while allowing spontaneous ventilation.

If CO_2 is the main concern, unless the patient is oversedated or minute ventilation is very low, it is usually easier to increase minute ventilation with spontaneous rather than controlled breaths (because of higher respiratory system compliance, see 📖 Pressure support ventilation, p 144).

Consider adjuncts

See 📖 Adjuncts, p 188.

---

1 Lachmann B (1992) Open up the lung and keep the lung open, *Intensive Care Med* **18**, 319–21.

5.11 Hypercapnia while on a ventilator

A rise in CO_2 is a common problem in ICU. It may occur as part of the disease process or because of the ventilatory strategy. Although we have become used to tolerating elevated $PaCO_2$ levels in protective ventilation strategies, this tolerance should not mean we become blinkered to the hypercapnia.

However, attempting to normalize blood gas results just makes the blood gas results better. It does not result in improved survival, and may lead to a worse outcome.

Assessment of hypercapnia

Assessment of hypercapnia requires more than a sardonic shrug and a request to increase the respiratory rate. It requires a systematic approach and constant reassessment to revisit your initial decisions.

- Identify the underlying cause.
- What are the physiological consequences?
- Should I correct the hypercapnia?
- Should I buffer the acidosis?
- What levels am I prepared to accept?
- Do I need to switch strategy completely?

Causes

Hypercapnia is caused by either increased CO_2 production or inadequate CO_2 clearance.

Increased production

CO_2 production increases in hypermetabolic states, including:

- Fever
- Sepsis
- Shivering
- Thyroid storm
- Malignant hyperpyrexia (MH)
- Malignant neuroleptic syndrome.

These conditions should be actively searched for and addressed as appropriate. The treatment of high temperatures associated with infection is controversial. There are presumed evolutionary benefits associated with a temperature rise during infection (e.g. neutrophils function more effectively at higher temperatures), so treatment should be reserved for the most extreme end of the spectrum.

Reduced clearance

Reduced minute ventilation

Normal minute ventilation (MV) for an adult is 100mL/kg/min (7L/min for a 70kg adult). This is the MV required to clear normal CO_2 production with normal $\dot{V}/\dot{Q}$ matching.

Adequate MV should be thought of as a process requiring an intact chain from the brainstem signal generation to unobstructed airways, allowing free passage of gas into the lungs. Anything interrupting this process may result in reduced MV:

- Chemoreceptor insensitivity.
- Brainstem dysfunction.
- Spinal cord lesion.
- Peripheral neuropathies.
- Neuromuscular junction disease.

- Myopathy.
- Chest wall abnormalities.
- Decreased respiratory system compliance.
- Upper airway obstruction.
- Increased airway resistance.
- Protective ventilatory strategies.

Increased dead space

If the minute ventilation is adequate and CO_2 production is not increased, then hypercapnia has to be as a result of increased dead space. This can be due to increased anatomical dead space:

- Increased equipment dead space (i.e. equipment, including HMEs, between the 'Y' piece and the ETT)—this is relatively important when low tidal volumes are being used
- Very low tidal volume ventilation, where the proportion of dead space in each breath is high.

However, it is more commonly due to increased alveolar dead space caused by:

- Alveolar destruction in COPD
- Pulmonary vascular abnormalities:
  - Early ARDS—widespread pulmonary microvascular thrombosis
  - Fibrotic stage ARDS—pulmonary arterial changes such as hyperplasia reduce perfusion to ventilated alveoli
- PEEP—will divert blood away from poorly perfused alveoli. This effect is more pronounced with high PEEP, but is also seen at moderate levels.
- Low cardiac output—apical alveoli are poorly perfused
- Pulmonary emboli
- Over-distension.

Physiological consequences

Hypercapnia and the associated respiratory acidosis have important physiological effects, which are listed in Tables 5.11–5.14. Since many of the physiological effects are directly opposing, the final result in an individual patient will be difficult to predict. For example, if sympathetic tone is already maximal, the direct effects on myocardium and vascular smooth muscle are likely to predominate.

A strategy that produces hypercapnia may also result in other physiological effects (e.g. low tidal volume strategy may predispose patient to atelectasis and increased shunt with lower PO_2).

Should I correct the hypercapnia?

Balancing risk and benefit is the great art of intensive care medicine. It is often difficult even when the risks and benefits are relatively well known and becomes very challenging when there is a degree of conjecture regarding these risks and benefits.

The arguments about correction of hypercapnia and acidosis often rest on the premise that the hypercapnia and acidosis are definitely harmful. This has never been demonstrated in terms of significant outcomes. Surrogate markers (as seen in Tables 5.11–5.14) are varied, with several physiological benefits associated with hypercapnia and acidosis.

We do know that there is a significant mortality risk associated with a strategy using high tidal volumes.[1,2] and there is a consensus that high pressures are also harmful in most circumstances.

When deciding to intervene for hypercapnia and acidosis, therefore, we should be clear that treatment involving unsafe ventilatory pressures and volumes should *not* be undertaken unless acutely lifesaving. See box for further details.

Management of hypercapnia

- *Identify causes of increased CO_2 production.* Treat if possible.
- *Reduce sedation.* This will reduce brainstem dysfunction and may increase cardiac output.
- *Remove excessive equipment deadspace.*
- *Increase ventilatory pressures and/or volumes* when these are within acceptable ranges. Safe values are tidal volume of 6–8mL/kg and plateau pressure of ≤30cmH₂O in the absence of diseases that reduce chest wall compliance.
- *PCV* clears CO_2 slightly more effectively than VCV using similar pressures. When using PCV, inspiration should be long enough that inspiratory flow reaches zero.
- *Increase respiratory rate.* This is a simple solution in many circumstances but there are potential side-effects, e.g. it may produce asynchrony. In PCV, the tidal volume may fall because of shorter inspiratory time or the development of PEEP$_i$ (if the tidal volume falls by more than 25% when the respiratory rate increases, alveolar ventilation is very likely to decrease despite the increased respiratory rate). In VCV, inspiratory airway pressures may rise and PEEP$_i$ develop.
- Consider changing to a *spontaneous ventilation mode.*
  - Improved respiratory system compliance.
  - Combined modes with some spontaneous breathing or a fully spontaneous mode will *usually* produce better MV for the same inspiratory pressures.
  - Allows sedation to be reduced.
  - Watch for signs of relative hypoventilation or derecruitment.
- *Improve respiratory system compliance*
  - Reduce bronchospasm.
  - Treat pulmonary oedema.
  - Increase chest wall compliance (sit up, reduce intra-abdominal pressures if possible).
  - Treat lung or lobar collapse with physiotherapy or bronchoscopy.
  - Assess the volume state of the lung. Is there over-distension or is recruitment required?
- Consider *PE* or decreased *RV* output.

Buffering the acidosis?

Acidosis is often the abnormality that causes most worry to clinicians. *Intracellular* acidosis from hypercapnia may be reversed within hours (active buffering, swapping Na^+ for H^+ at the cell membrane). Full renal compensation takes days and even then may be impaired because of coexisting renal dysfunction.

However, acidosis is the component of hypercapnia that seems to be associated with many of the potentially beneficial physiological effects, e.g. buffering of acidosis abolishes the favourable consequences of hypercapnia in models of lung ischaemia reperfusion. This is consistent with the often disappointing physiological effect of buffering acidosis (metabolic or respiratory) in critically ill patients.

If buffering is undertaken there are theoretical advantages for tris-hydroxymethyl aminomethane (THAM) or carbicarb (equimolar mixture of sodium bicarbonate and sodium carbonate) over sodium bicarbonate.
- Because bicarbonate does not enter cells but CO_2 does, bicarbonate may worsen intracellular acidosis.

Table 5.11 Effects of CO_2 on gas exchange

Effect on gas exchange	Mechanism
Reduced PaO_2	Increased alveolar CO_2 (alveolar gas equation)
Reduced PaO_2	Increased shunt fraction due to increased cardiac output
Increased PaO_2	Augments hypoxic pulmonary vasoconstriction (via acidosis)
Increased PaO_2	Increased mixed venous PO_2 from cardiac output increase
Increased compliance	Unclear. Improves surfactant function

Table 5.12 Effects of CO_2 on the cardiovascular system

Cardiovascular effects	Mechanism
Increased cardiac output	Increased sympathetic tone
Decreased cardiac output	Direct effect on myocardial contractility
Peripheral vasoconstriction	Increased sympathetic tone
Peripheral vasodilation	Direct effect on smooth muscle contractility
Improved peripheral O_2 delivery	Right shift of O_2Hb dissociation curve
Increased pulmonary vascular resistance	Direct effect of acidosis

Table 5.13 Effects of CO_2 on the central and peripheral nervous system

Neurological effects	Mechanism
Cerebral vasodilation	Various proposed mechanisms
Raises intracranial pressure	Increased cerebral blood volume
Increased cerebral tissue PO_2	Increased PaO_2 and cerebral blood flow
Protective for hypoxic – ischaemic injury in brain	Better glucose utilization and oxidative metabolism, lower glutamate, inhibits free radicals
Impairs neuromuscular function	

Table 5.14 Miscellaneous effects of CO_2

Miscellaneous effects	Mechanism
Protects against ischaemia reperfusion injury to the lung and heart	May reduce CA^{++} influx, or increase coronary flow
Mild immunosuppression	Reduced phagocytosis, nitric oxide production and release of cytokines
Protects hepatocytes from cell death	
May reduce Glomerular Filtration Rate	Sympathetic stimulation plus hypoxia can cause renal vasoconstriction
Attenuates free radical mediated lung injury	Reduced xanthine oxidase activity

- Bicarbonate will add to the CO_2 load, which will require an increase in alveolar ventilation (at a point where alveolar ventilation may already be a problem) to prevent further increases in CO_2.
- THAM, in contrast, can easily enter cells and does not require increased CO_2 elimination to exert its effect.
- Carbicarb also corrects intracellular acidosis and does not raise CO_2.

What levels am I prepared to accept?

There are numerous case reports of unimpaired survival following exposure to very high levels of CO_2. Clinicians will have different tolerances of hypercapnia and acidosis, and clinical circumstances will demand different tolerances in CO_2 levels, for example:

- Limits will be lower in patients with pulmonary hypertension or in those with a co-existing metabolic acidosis
- Raised ICP is an absolute contraindication to any increase in $PaCO_2$.

Our practice is outlined below, but the overall approach to hypercapnia is valid no matter the precise levels individuals choose. In an ideal world, we would only intervene if there were physiological problems associated with hypercapnia. In the real world of very unwell patients with several diagnoses and comorbidities, attributing physiological changes to hypercapnia is well nigh impossible.

Our current practice is:

- Identify contraindications to hypercapnia.
- Work through the treatment algorithm (see box).
- Consider a complete change in strategy if $PaCO_2$ >15kPa (see below). In most cases high PCO_2 (even >20kPa) is acceptable because the known risks of treatment outweigh the known risks of the condition.
- This level of hypercapnia is often associated with a pH of 7.05–7.10. We do not buffer this acidosis.

Should I change strategy?

If, despite efforts to reduce it safely, CO_2 remains above the limits acceptable to the clinician, or is causing physiological harm, consider extracorporeal removal of CO_2 using ECMO or artero-venous carbon dioxide removal ($AVCO_2R$), as discussed in 📖 Extracorporeal membrane oxygenation, p 183. Unresponsive hypercapnia is most often accompanied by significant oxygenation difficulty.

Tracheal gas insufflation is discussed in 📖 Adjuncts, p 188.

Summary

- Hypercapnia and associated acidosis are present in many ICU patients.
- The incidence is increasing because many ventilatory strategies now include permissive hypercapnia.
- When deciding what interventions, if any, are necessary thought must be given to the risks and benefits of the hypercapnia, the acidosis (and the strategy that has produced these two abnormalities if relevant), and the risks and benefits of the intervention proposed.
- The clinician must balance these effects in each patient to develop a ventilatory strategy designed to produce the best outcome and not simply improved blood gas results.

1 Darioli R and Perret C (1984) Mechanical controlled hypoventilation in status asthmaticus. *Am Rev Resp Dis* **129**(3), 385–7.

2 The National Heart, Lung and Blood Institute Acute Respiratory Distress Syndrome (ARDS) clinical trials network (2000) Ventilation with lower tidal volumes as compared with traditional tidal volumes for acute lung injury and the acute respiratory distress syndrome. *New Engl J Med* **342**(18), 1301–8.

5.12 Sudden deterioration on a ventilator

Despite our best efforts, patients sometimes deteriorate catastrophically, often without warning. When this happens, noise, fluster, and anxiety are prominent.

It is useful to have a systematic approach to this emergency committed to midbrain, thereby freeing up your cortices to think about what is actually going on. This chapter will deal with sudden respiratory deterioration, although in practice the respiratory and cardiovascular systems are inextricably linked.

Oxygen cascade

There has been an interruption in the delivery of oxygen from the hospital supply to the patient's cells. The oxygen cascade in the ICU starts at the ventilator (in reality it starts at the Schraeder valve, but the ventilator will alert you to a failure in oxygen supply immediately).

The extended oxygen cascade consists of:

Ventilator — set correctly and not currently alarming
↓
Ventilator tubing and catheter mount — patent and connected
(including humidification system)
↓
ETT — patent and correctly positioned
↓
Airways — patent and allowing free passage of gas
↓
$\dot{V}/\dot{Q}$ matching — appropriate
↓
Cardiac output and oxygen delivery — adequate

As you approach the bedspace

- Ask someone to draw up emergency drugs, drugs for intubation, and drugs for circulatory support.
- Ask for the resuscitation trolley.
- Look at the patient — from the end of the bed is their appearance consistent with the monitors. Do they appear to be very unwell?
- Is there a good and reliable pulse-oximetry trace?
- Do you need to start immediate cardiovascular resuscitation including CPR?
- Look at ventilator screen:
  - Is it the mode you expect?
  - Is FiO_2 set at 1.0?
  - Is it alarming (oxygen failure, peak airway pressure, minute volume)?
  - Are expiratory tidal volumes similar to inspiratory?
  - Is the expiratory flow trace returning to baseline?
- Can you hear or see airway leak?
- Do both sides of the chest move?
- Is the ECG trace ischaemic or irritable?

At the bedside
- Are both sides of chest moving? Is there hyperexpansion?
- Percussion (dull or hyperresonant).
- Auscultation (air entry, wheeze, crepitations, prolonged expiratory phase, murmurs, added heart sounds).
- Mapleson C circuit or AMBU bag—how does it feel?
  - Bouncing—tube blocked obstruction or bronchospasm.
  - Tight—bronchospasm, tube inspissation.
  - Normal—mucous plug, pulmonary oedema, PE, fat emboli.
- Check cardiovascular status.

Hand ventilation

Diagnostic information

Hand ventilation will provide diagnostic information. Is the ETT blocked? Is there increased resistance or reduced compliance? Does the chest wall move as expected and symmetrically?

Therapeutic benefit

Often hand ventilation will temporarily resolve hypoxaemia. You are no better at ventilating the lung than the machine. The therapeutic advantage of hand ventilation is the delivery of tidal volumes and airway pressures that in normal circumstances would be inappropriate, and that you would never set on a ventilator. These pressures are usually delivered with no real monitoring (next time you hand ventilate a patient use a flow meter/pressure gauge and measure what you are doing: you will be surprised!).

In the short term this will rarely do harm, but beware unilateral chest movement: it is possible to quickly convert a pneumothorax to a life — threatening tension pneumothorax with these pressures.

Establish cause

Perform a full examination, arrange for CXR, ABGs, ECG, and if possible echocardiography. Management is covered in the relevant chapters.

Ventilator and circuit
- Check the ventilator monitors, particularly airway pressure and expiratory tidal volume.
- Physically check all connections.

Endotracheal tube
- Endobronchial intubation (may be intermittent).
  - Unilateral air entry (usually the right side).
  - Reduced compliance.
  - Check tube position (at teeth and with direct laryngoscopy).
  - Review position on most recent CXR.
- Dislodged
  - Audible or visible leak.
  - Check tube position (at teeth and with direct laryngoscopy).

- Blocked
  - Distinctive character on hand ventilation ('bouncing').
  - Unable to pass suction catheter.
  - If in doubt look with a flexible laryngoscope.
  - There may have been large negative pressure swings to trigger inspiration because of a previous partial blockage.

Mucous plug
- Copious or thick secretions.
- Reduced air entry or evidence of new collapse.
- Sudden deteriorations without other explanations, which improve relatively quickly with hand bagging.

Bronchospasm
In acute severe asthma there will usually be some air entry with associated wheeze and prolonged expiration, but sometimes the bronchospasm is so severe that it is nearly impossible to move air into the chest and the chest is silent.
- Distinctive feeling on hand ventilation. Prolonged expiratory phase. Allow expiration to be as full as possible, even if that means disconnecting after every breath.
- Make sure the tube is not abutting the carina.
- Look for pneumothorax.

Anaphylaxis
- Hypotension is the most common isolated presentation.
- Temporal association with drug administration.
- May be wheezy but usually mild unless asthmatic.
- Flushing, urticaria, or facial or airway swelling may point to the diagnosis.

Pneumothorax
- Unilateral chest movement and hyper-resonance.
- If it is under tension—tracheal shift, increased CVP/engorged central veins, hypotension, tachycardia, and cold peripheries.

Emboli
- Emboli causing sudden deterioration will present with signs of right-sided cardiac failure and reduced cardiac output: increased CVP/engorged central veins, hypotension (may be normo- or hypertensive but still shocked), tachycardia, and cold peripheries.
- There may be a sudden loss of the end tidal CO_2 trace.
- Urgent echocardiography may be helpful in diagnosis.

Thromboembolism
- Previous unexplained stepwise deteriorations.
- Haemoptysis or signs of peripheral thrombus (DVT).

Fat
- Following a long bone or pelvic fracture.
- Often a petechial rash, particularly in conjunctiva.

Air
- In ICU, most commonly from central lines, particularly during removal.
- Occurs when atmospheric pressure greater than intravascular pressure and air enters at >0.5mL/kg/min.
- Millwheel murmur.

Myocardial infarction/pulmonary oedema
- ECG abnormalities, arrhythmias, hypotension (may be normo- or hypertensive and still shocked), tachycardia and cold peripheries, gallop rhythm, bilateral end inspiratory crepitations.
- May present as wheeze: can be difficult to differentiate from brochospasm. As well as the clinical signs above, expiratory times are usually shorter and the characteristic shape of the flow volume loop seen in bronchspasm is missing. Patients may appear to be more unwell than the degree of wheeze would suggest.
- Pulmonary oedema on suction.
- Listen for new loud pan systolic murmur (papillary muscle rupture or ischaemic ventricular septal defect (VSD)).
- 12-lead ECG and echocardiography.

Malignant arrhythmias
- The cardiovascular response to arrhythmias depends on the type of arrhythmia, the ventricular rate, and pre-existing cardiac disease.
- Hypotension is often a more pronounced feature than pulmonary oedema.
- External chest compressions may be necessary.
- Check 12-lead ECG and rhythm strip (if time).
- Check and correct electrolytes (particularly Mg^{++} and K^+).

5.13 Sedation

Sedation is the reduction of conscious level by administration of drugs. A categorization of reasons for sedating patients in ICU is shown in Table 5.15. As with any treatment, sedation has potential risks as well as benefits. Sedation requirements vary widely between patients and within individual patients at different stages of their critical illness. A systematic assessment of the needs of each patient is required to achieve optimum sedation where patient comfort is achieved without exposing them to the adverse effects of excessive sedation.

Table 5.15 Reasons for sedating patients and providing analgesia in the intensive care unit

Reason	Main requirement	Commonly used drugs	Comment
Anxiety	Hypnosis and anxiolysis	Benzodiazepines (midazolam, lorazepam) Propofol	Anxiety from fear concerning the underlying condition; anxiety associated with ongoing treatments (especially invasive procedures such as mechanical ventilation)
Amnesia	Hypnotics with amnesic properties	Benzodiazepines Propofol	Inducing amnesia is controversial Emerging evidence suggests prolonged amnesia during ICU care is associated with a higher prevalence of long-term psychological problems (especially post-traumatic stress disorder)
Endotracheal intubation	Tolerance of ETTs (decreased cough and gag reflexes)	Opiates (alfentanil, fentanyl, morphine) Sedatives (propofol, benzodiazepines)	ETT tolerance is highly variable Older patients often tolerate with little sedation, but individual assessment is needed
Mechanical ventilation	Decreased respiratory drive, synchronization with ventilator	Opioids and sedatives	Modern ventilators have modes to synchronize well with individual patient breathing patterns Patient–ventilator dys-synchrony requires careful optimization of both ventilator settings and sedation
Wound pain or other painful conditions	Analgesia	Opioids Regional anaesthetic techniques are valuable, especially after surgery or trauma	Ensuring adequate analgesia in patients with reduced conscious level from underlying condition or sedation is essential

(Continued)

Table 5.15 (Cont'd)

Reason	Main requirement	Commonly used drugs	Comment
Physiotherapy	Analgesia, anxiolysis, and anti-nociception	Opioids and hypnotics Often best given as boluses during treatments	Physiotherapy, especially chest physiotherapy, is highly stimulating and can cause intense sympathetic activation via stimulation of intrapulmonary receptors
Drug withdrawal	Control of withdrawal syndromes	Alcohol (benzodiazepines) Nicotine (nicotine patches) Heroin/methadone (opioids)	Drug withdrawal syndromes are common in patients requiring critical care Specific treatment should be considered, particularly for patients not receiving sedation for other reasons

Optimizing sedation

Optimum sedation state

No single level or prescription for sedation is suitable for all patients in the ICU because requirements frequently change and need regular re-evaluation.

For example, early during critical illness requirements may be high because patients require tracheal intubation, controlled mechanical ventilation, analgesia for underlying conditions, and anxiolysis. If advanced ventilatory strategies are required, there may be patient–ventilator asynchrony, especially if there is a high respiratory drive as a result of hypercapnia or hypoxaemia. Under these circumstances optimum sedation may be complete unconsciousness for many patients.

In contrast, a patient who has a tracheostomy after prolonged ICU stay may not require any sedation except for boluses during physiotherapy or other painful procedures.

Optimum sedation is therefore the most appropriate level of sedation for an individual at the time of assessment. The challenge during routine management is to recognize *changing* sedation requirements, especially the transition to greater tolerance of consciousness. This requires a systematic, embedded culture of assessing sedation on a frequent basis by the ICU team. It is best achieved by incorporating sedation assessments in routine management and enabling multiple members of the multidisciplinary team to alter the level of sedation within agreed guidelines. Recent studies show that sedation is still poorly managed in many ICUs, with a tendency to excessive sedation of many patients.

Relationship between sedation practice and outcome

Significant heterogeneity exists in trial design, trial quality, the population studied, the control group practice, and the interventions employed in trials of sedation practice and outcome. Overall, however, these trials provide strong evidence that optimizing sedation practice improves patient outcomes (Table 5.16).

Table 5.16 Summary of findings from trials of strategies to improve sedation practice in ICUs

Outcome	Evidence from sedation trials
Duration of mechanical ventilation	Convincing evidence from RCTs and before–after studies that systematic approaches using clinical sedation scales, decision-making protocols, and daily sedation holds can significantly reduce the duration of mechanical ventilation
ICU and hospital stay	Convincing evidence that systematic approaches reduce ICU stay and possibly hospital stay
Mortality	Some evidence that systematic approaches may decrease mortality
ICU complications	Systematic approaches to avoid over-sedation, including sedation breaks, may increase extubation rates, but do not appear to increase re-intubations, suggesting patients were ready for weaning Some evidence that systematic approaches decrease rates of investigation for unconsciousness (e.g. CT scanning) Some evidence that systematic approaches decrease rates of VAP
Delirium	Choice of sedation agent associated with prevalence of delirium: benzodiazepines increase prevalence; dexmedetomidine decreases prevalence
Psychological outcomes	Some evidence that avoiding or reducing time in deep sedation may decrease long-term psychological morbidity (post-traumatic stress disorder, anxiety, depression)
Illness cost	Reducing ventilation times, ICU, and hospital length of stay significantly reduces illness cost

Assessing sedation and analgesia requirements

Assessment of sedation and analgesia requirements should consider pre-morbid patient characteristics and acute illness related factors (Fig. 5.28).

	Factors associated with greater sedation requirements	Factors associated with lesser sedation requirements
Pre-illness status	Younger age Higher BMI Male gender High alcohol intake	Advanced age Malnutrition Significant co-morbidity, especially neurological disease
Acute illness-related factors	Need for controlled ventilation or advanced respiratory support Painful conditions, e.g. burns, multiple trauma Cerebral oedema	Encephalopathy (e.g. hepatic) Hepatic or renal failure Shock Hypothermia Low illness severity

Fig. 5.28 Some factors that may influence sedation requirements during critical illness.

From these a prediction of whether requirements will be generally high or low can be made, and sedation and analgesia initiated.

Richmond Agitation–Sedation Scale

The GCS is designed to assess non-sedated patients with brain injury and is not suited to routine sedation assessment.

A clinical sedation scale that uses patient responses to simple stimuli should be used to categorize a patient's level of sedation at regular intervals. Many sedation scales exist, but the Richmond Agitation-Sedation Scale (RASS) is the most widely validated. Assessment starts with observation and progresses through non-physical and then physical stimuli.

- Observe the patient – are they alert, restless or agitated? If so, the score is 0 to +4: 0, Alert and calm; +1 Restless (anxious but movements not aggressive or agitated); +2, agitated (frequent non purposeful movements, fighting the ventilator); +3 Very Agitated (pulls or removes tubes or catheters, aggressive); +4 Combative (overtly combative, violent, immediate danger to staff).
- Address the patient and ask them to look at you. They may be –1, Drowsy (opens eyes and sustains eye contact for >10 seconds); –2, Lightly Sedated (non sustained eye opening and eye contact < 10seconds); –3 Moderately Sedated (moves or has eye opening, but no eye contact).
- If there is no response to voice, shake the shoulder or rub the sternum. They may be –4, Deeply Sedated (moves or opens eyes); –5, Unarousable (no response).
- Low levels of inter – and intra-rater variability.
- Assessments are quick and require no specific equipment.
- Includes discrimination for different levels of agitation as well as reduced consciousness.

There is no universally agreed frequency at which clinical sedation scoring should be undertaken, and this is best determined by individual ICU protocols. Regular recording of clinical sedation scores on patient charts at pre-agreed intervals is a useful method of ensuring regular assessment.

Assessing pain

There are many potential sources of pain in ICU patients. Some of these relate to the underlying diagnosis (e.g. burns, pancreatitis), or initial treatment (e.g. surgery). In addition, many ICU interventions cause stimulation that results in nociceptive responses, notably hypertension, tachycardia, and facial grimacing, even when patients appear otherwise adequately sedated.

A common pattern in ICU patients is for staff to progressively increase sedation and analgesia dose in response to *intermittent* nociceptive responses, for example after tracheal suctioning. This approach can result in significant over-sedation because it fails to distinguish continuous from intermittent requirements.

Recognizing pain in sedated ICU patients and distinguishing analgesia from sedation requirements is difficult. In conscious patients visual analogue scales or rating scales can be used, but this is not possible in unconscious or delirious patients.

The Behavioural Pain Score

The Behavioural Pain Score (BPS) has been validated as an assessment of pain in awake and unconscious ICU patients (Table 5.17). A score of >6 is indicative of significant pain.

Systematic use of this scale during procedures such as physiotherapy is well-suited to guiding boluses of sedation or analgesia.

Table 5.17 The Behavioural Pain Score—a score >6 is considered to indicate pain

Item	Description	Score
Facial expression	Relaxed	1
	Partially tightened	2
	Fully tightened	3
	Grimacing	4
Upper limbs	No movements	1
	Partially bent	2
	Fully bent with finger flexion	3
	Permanently retracted	4
Compliance with ventilation	Tolerating movement	1
	Coughing, but tolerating ventilation for most of the time	2
	Fighting ventilator	3
	Unable to control ventilation	4

Sedative drugs
Ideal drug characteristics
Pharmacokinetics and pharmacodynamics
The ideal sedative drug would always have predictable pharmacokinetics and pharmacodynamics, especially in patients with multiple organ failure. The pharmacokinetics and pharmacodynamics of sedative drugs are complex in critically ill patients and depend on factors such as:
• Rate of drug elimination
• Context sensitive half times (CSHTs)
• Active metabolites.

Rate of drug elimination
The elimination of most sedative drugs is an exponential process described by the equation of first-order metabolism:

$$C_t = C_0 e^{-kt}$$

where C_t = concentration at time t, C_0 = initial concentration, and k = rate constant.

The elimination rate constant is the fraction of the total amount of drug in the body that is removed per unit time. It depends on volume of distribution and clearance (altered by protein binding, and renal and hepatic function).

Context sensitive half times
- The clinical effects of sedative drugs relate to the effect site concentration.
- When many short-acting sedative agents are given by bolus, effect site concentration reduces rapidly due to redistribution between pharmacokinetic body compartments (short plasma half-life).
- When these drugs are given by infusion, the pharmacokinetic compartments have all equilibrated, and the reduction in effect site concentration is determined by the slower elimination half-life.
- This change in plasma half-life depending on the dose and duration of administration of a drug is known as the CSHT.
- CSHT will influence the time taken to recover consciousness.
- Some agents (e.g. remifentanil) have a constant CSHT.

Active metabolites
Accumulation of active metabolites is also important, especially if their elimination is unpredictable.

Side effect profiles
- Cardiovascular instability is of particular relevance in critically ill patients because of the high prevalence of shock.
- The risk of neurological dysfunction, especially delirium, is increasingly recognized as class specific (see below).

Cost
Sedative agents account for a significant proportion of total drug cost in intensive care. However, when assessing cost effectiveness, factors such as reduced duration of ventilation and ICU length of stay have to be included in the analysis because these have been shown to be influenced by sedation practice.

Sedative drugs
The relevant properties of commonly used classes of sedative agents are described below and summarized in Table 5.18.

Table 5.18 Important properties and characteristics of commonly used sedative agents

Drug	Main effects	Elimination half-life	CSHT	Side-effects	Comments
Midazolam	Hypnosis, amnesia, anxiolysis	1–3h	Significant changes in CSHT with duration of infusion Typically 60–80min after 5h of infusion	Mild hypotension Respiratory depression	Can accumulate with multiple dosing or continuous infusion, especially in the presence of renal and hepatic dysfunction Active metabolite (hydroxymidazolam) with impaired clearance in renal failure Inexpensive drug
Lorazepam	Hypnosis, amnesia, anxiolysis	11–22h	Significant changes with duration of infusion Can be very prolonged during infusion, so usually used by intermittent bolus	Respiratory depression	Potential for accumulation, especially in renal or hepatic failure No active metabolite Infusions should be avoided; usually used as intermittent bolus Inexpensive drug
Propofol	Hypnosis, anxiolysis	5–12h	Increases during first hour of infusion but then tends to plateau with maximum values of 20–30min	Hypotension Respiratory depression	Low probability of accumulation No active metabolites Intermediate cost

Drug	Action		CSHT	Side effects	Comments
Dexmedetomidine	Hypnosis, analgesia, sympatholytic action	2–8h	CSHT increases significantly with duration of infusion ranging from 4min after 10min of infusion to 250min after 8h	Bradycardia Hypotension	Low probability of accumulation No active metabolites Currently only licensed for short-term sedation Relatively expensive
Alfentanil	Analgesia	1–2h	CSHT typically increases over first hour and then remains stable at about 40–50min	Bradycardia	Low probability of accumulation Intermediate cost
Remifentanil	Analgesia, hypnosis	10–20min	Metabolism relies on plasma esterases CSHT remains very short and predictable even after prolonged infusion (typically <5min)	Bradycardia Hypotension	Very predictable on/off effects with very low probability of accumulation 'Analgesia-based' sedation regimens use this agent alone to titrate to desired clinical effect Relatively expensive
Fentanyl	Analgesia	6–9h	Significant increases in CSHT with duration of infusion, which can typically reach 200min after 5h of infusion	Bradycardia Muscle rigidity in high dose or accumulation	High potential for accumulation and prolonged clinical effects due to long CSHT during continuous infusion

Benzodiazepines

Benzodiazepines act via γ-amino butyrate (GABA) receptors and are recommended in many guidelines as a first-line sedative agents. They can be given by intermittent bolus (lorazepam) or by continuous infusion (midazolam). Advantages include low cost and cardiovascular stability. Recently, several studies have highlighted the potential adverse effects of these agents:

• Unpredictable kinetics in patients with renal and hepatic dysfunction.
• Increased risk of delirium.
• Reduced respiratory muscle function, resulting in delayed weaning.
• Several RCTs have shown longer ventilation times with benzodiazepine-based sedation when compared with propofol and newer agents such as dexmedetomidine, even when evidence-based sedation protocols are used.

Propofol

Propofol also acts via GABA receptors and is widely used for ICU sedation. It has the advantage of more predictable kinetics even in the presence of organ dysfunction, and a lack of active metabolites. However it is associated with more hypotension and cardiovascular instability, especially when administered in bolus dose.

High propofol doses (>4mg/kg/h) for prolonged periods have been associated with rhabdomyolysis, cardiovascular collapse, hepatic dysfunction, and renal failure—the 'propofol infusion syndrome'. Most cases have been described in children and as a result propofol is not used for continuous sedation in this group. It is very rare in adults with commonly used dosing.

Clonidine and dexmedetomidine

These drugs are central α2-agonists. Reported advantages include:

• A dose dependent hypnotic effect
• Some analgesic properties
• Sympatholysis, resulting in less 'swings' in blood pressure and heart rate
• Predictable pharmacokinetics and a short duration of action in patients without renal and hepatic impairment. Fewer data are available in patients with organ dysfunction.

Clonidine has more generalized central and peripheral activity, whereas dexmedetomidine is primary centrally acting and has been developed primarily for sedation. Dexmedetomidine is licensed in North America for short-term sedation (<24h) in ICU patients, but is currently unlicensed in Europe.

Dexmedetomidine has been studied in several recent RCTs with favourable outcomes compared to benzodiazepines. Duration of mechanical ventilation was reduced compared with midazolam despite both trial groups achieving similar high levels of optimum sedation. Another consistent finding is clinically important decreases in rates of delirium. These data suggest that dexmedetomidine may have class-specific advantages over existing agents, although licensing approval for routine use is awaited.

Opioids
Opioid drugs act at central and peripheral opioid receptors and are primarily used as analgesic and antinociceptive agents in the critically ill. The most commonly used agents are morphine, fentanyl, alfentanil, and remifentanil. Pharmacokinetics are an important consideration, as for hypnotic agents.

Morphine
- Morphine has the least predictable kinetics.
- Relatively long elimination half-life.
- Active metabolite (morphine-6-glucuronide), which accumulates in renal dysfunction.

Fentanyl and alfentanil
These drugs have short initial plasma half-lives, but when given by infusion their CSHT prolongs (particularly fentanyl). Metabolism is predominantly hepatic, and their clearance is not dependent on renal function.

Remifentanil
- Remifentanil is an ultra-short-acting agent with highly predictable kinetics even in the presence of organ failure.
- Constant CSHT of 2–3min as a result of metabolism by plasma and tissue esterases.
- Significant sedative properties.
- May be used as a single agent for analgosedation in the ICU, although it is relatively expensive.
- A recent meta-analysis of published trials suggested remifentanil may decrease the time to awakening and extubation after discontinuing treatment, but did not find clinically important treatment effects on duration of ventilation or ICU stay compared with more conventional agents. The overall quality of trials was low, making firm recommendations about the benefit of remifentanil difficult.

Practical aspects of managing sedation
Sedation protocols
- ICUs should have a protocol that summarizes the agreed approach to managing sedation in the unit.
- Protocols usually define the type and frequency of clinical sedation scoring that nursing staff should carry out.
- A default target level, e.g. RASS of −2 to +1, for all patients should be agreed, which can be modified in individual cases.

Effective protocols empower nursing staff to adjust doses of sedative and analgesic drugs in response to clinical sedation scores to achieve the target sedation level. Simple checklists can define patients in whom nurses can reduce sedation and commence weaning trials (see box). The introduction of nurse-led 'wake and wean' strategies is central to many patient safety quality improvement programmes in ITU.

Example of a checklist of patients in whom sedation can often be safely reduced by nurses or trainee doctors without senior medical review

FiO_2 <0.5.

Patient established on a spontaneously triggered ventilation mode (e.g. PSV, assisted spontaneous breathing).

PEEP <10cmH$_2$O.

No or minor requirement for cardiovascular support with vasopressors or inotropic drugs.

No evidence of ongoing haemorrhage or hypovolaemia.

Not experiencing uncontrolled hypertension, myocardial ischaemia, or arrhythmias.

No problems with intracranial pressure.

No unstable fractures or cervical spine injury.

Cooperative non-agitated patient.

Adequate pain control.

Implementing protocols

Implementing and maintaining practice change requires planning, education, and regular audit. Several successful systems for ICU practice change have been described, notably from the Institute of Healthcare Improvement Patients Safety programmes (www.IHI.org).

Sedation holds

- A sedation hold is a period during which continuous sedation is stopped, usually until the patient regains consciousness.
- Sedation is only reintroduced if necessary.
- If sedatives are required, infusion is restarted at half the previous dose.
- Sedation breaks are best linked to assessment of ventilation and potential for weaning.
- Several RCTs have shown that a daily sedation hold can decrease the duration of coma and mechanical ventilation, and improve a range of patient outcomes. This approach is particularly valuable in patients with organ dysfunction.

Sedation monitors

Sedation monitors are devices which attempt to measure conscious level by analysing cortical electrical activity. Most devices, such as the BIS, were developed for depth of anaesthesia monitoring rather than use in the ICU. Although the output from these devices correlates with sedation state, they have poor discrimination for different sedation states and are not widely used. There is no evidence at present that these monitors are more effective than clinical protocols.

Sedation withdrawal

Some common problems encountered during sedation withdrawal are listed in Table 5.19. For most ITU patients stopping sedation does not cause a physiological 'withdrawal syndrome'. It can occur in patients who have required large doses of sedative and analgesic drugs, especially for prolonged periods. Sedation withdrawal syndromes typically include tachycardia, hypertension, sweating, and agitation. If this occurs drugs require gradual withdrawal. Different drug classes, especially α2-agonists such as clonidine, are sometimes effective during withdrawal syndromes.

Table 5.19 Common problems associated with sedation withdrawal

Problem	Possible causes	Solution
Agitated patient	Pain	Ensure adequate analgesia
	Delirium	Haloperidol; minimize precipitating factors
	Physiological withdrawal syndrome	Staged drug withdrawal; adjuvant drugs, e.g. α2-agonists
	Inadequate oxygenation/ ventilation	Review ventilator settings; ensure patient–ventilator synchronization; ensure adequate FiO_2 and mechanical support
Failure to regain consciousness	Accumulation of sedative drugs/active metabolites	Sedation hold until conscious level improves
	Encephalopathy (septic; metabolic; hepatic etc.)	Treat underlying condition; sedation hold; EEG if delayed recovery
	Undiagnosed neuropathology (e.g. cerebrovascular event)	Brain imaging (CT scan); treat appropriately

Some common vicious cycles relating to sedation in ICU

Scenarios describing four common vicious cycles are summarized in Table 5.20, together with suggested clinical approaches to managing the patient.

Table 5.20 Some common sedation-related vicious cycles in ICU

Clinical scenario	Typical clinical scenario	Suggested solution
The sedation-ventilator dyssynchrony cycle	Patient in acute stages of ARDS requiring controlled ventilation with high levels of PEEP and permissive hypercapnia Sedation dose escalating; patient unresponsive, but coughing and 'fighting' the ventilator, especially during suctioning and turning	Formally assess sedation state using RASS score Patient likely to be unconscious (RASS -4 to -5), but exhibiting intermittent nociceptive responses (coughing) or high respiratory drive due to hypercapnia (failure to synchronize) Potential solutions include: • Changing ventilation mode. The patient may be better on a patient-triggered mode, which may enable decreased sedation dose. Pressure-controlled modes may be better tolerated than volume-controlled modes. • Increase opioid rather than hypnotic to decrease respiratory drive and coughing. • Encourage bolus therapy prior to suctioning or other nociceptive stimulus, and titration of continuous sedation infusion to RASS score of -2 at other times.
The sedation-agitation cycle	Older patient with resolving multiple organ failure undergoing sedation hold on day 5 of ICU admission Septic shock and acute lung injury resolved; ongoing acute renal failure Previously sedated with propofol and alfentanil Patient hypertensive, tachycardic, and agitated when regaining consciousness Not obeying simple commands Nurse has re-sedated for similar picture several times	The key issue here is to assess whether or not pain is adequately controlled and agitation is due to delirium Potential solutions include: • Assess likely analgesia requirements based on history, procedures, and current status. Adjust analgesia if appropriate. • Perform a CAM-ICU to assess whether or not the patient is delirious. This is the most likely cause of agitation at this stage. • If delirium is present, control agitation with haloperidol boluses and prescribe regular haloperidol to ensure the patient receives a maintenance dose. • Check the usual pre-illness medication. Re-introduce antihypertensives and/or therapy for ischaemic heart disease, preferably via the nasogastric route. • Agree a staged reduction strategy in sedative drug dose over the next 24-48h. • Monitor frequently for delirium and adjust haloperidol dose accordingly.

The sedation withdrawal cycle	Young male trauma patient (without head injury) who required high doses of sedation and analgesia (midazolam, propofol, and morphine) during the acute phase of illness, which included ARDS Now in the recovery phase, but tachycardic, hypertensive, sweaty, and agitated during sedation withdrawal	This is probably predominantly a sedation withdrawal syndrome A rationale approach would be: • Check for the presence of delirium and treat with haloperidol if present. • Ensure adequate analgesia, especially in view of history. • Plan a gradual reduction in sedation over several days, preferably starting with midazolam, and document this clearly. • Consider an α2-agonist (clonidine) as an agent to facilitate withdrawal of other drugs and reduce hypertension and tachycardia. • Consider temporary pharmacologic control of cardiovascular responses (e.g. β-blockade).
The sedation for insomnia cycle	Elderly patient recovering from pneumonia with delayed weaning via tracheostomy No daytime sedation, but nurses administering midazolam boluses at night to 'help sleep' and requesting propofol infusion Patient confused and agitated at night	Drugs are likely to worsen this cycle not improve it. • Explain nature of sleep disturbance to staff, and potential pro-delirium effects of benzodiazepines. • Minimize light and noise at night (consider move to quiet part of ward if feasible; modify alarms). • Minimize nursing procedures at night. • Ensure night-time ventilator settings maximize synchronization with patient effort, and achieve appropriate morning blood gases. • Consider haloperidol at night for agitation.

Delirium

Delirium is an acute fluctuating change in mental status characterized by sensory inattention and altered conscious level.

- It has been estimated to occur in up to 80% of ICU patients.
- It often only becomes clinically apparent when sedative drugs are reduced or stopped.
- <10% have an agitated delirium, which is relatively easy to recognize.
- The majority (>80%) have hypoactive delirium, which is frequently unrecognized.

Some risk factors for delirium are listed in Table 5.21. Interest in the prevalence, pathogenesis, prevention, and treatment of delirium has increased significantly in recent years because it is independently associated with prolonged hospitalization, higher short- and long-term mortality, and poorer long-term cognitive function after critical illness.

Table 5.21 Some factors increasing the risk of delirium

Drugs	Benzodiazepines, anticholinergics, antihistamines, steroids, metoclopramide
Infection	Sepsis syndrome, hospital-acquired infections, CNS infections
Metabolic disturbances	Electrolyte disturbances, hypo/hyper-glycaemia, renal failure, hepatic failure
Age	Older age (especially >70 years)
Drug withdrawal	Alcohol, opioids, sedative drugs, nicotine
Known neuropathology	Cerebrovascular disease, dementia
Sleep disturbance	Sleep deprivation
Environment	Lack of natural light, poor lighting, loss of day/night discrimination, excessive environmental noise

Diagnosis

A common barrier to diagnosing delirium, especially hypoactive delirium, is the presence of mechanical ventilation and/or sedative drugs. This can make assessment of cognition difficult. The confusion assessment method for ICU (CAM-ICU) is a validated tool that can identify delirium within 1–2min even in intubated patients. This method has low intra- and inter-rater variability and is the method of choice in mechanically ventilated patients. The CAM-ICU is usually linked to the RASS score to form a simultaneous assessment of sedation state and delirium status (Fig 5.28 and 5.29).

A General approach to delirium assessment

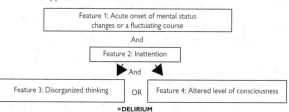

Feature 1: Acute onset of mental status changes or a fluctuating course

And

Feature 2: Inattention

And

| Feature 3: Disorganized thinking | OR | Feature 4: Altered level of consciousness |

=DELIRIUM

B CAM-ICU assessment

Feature 1: Acute onset or fluctuating course	Positive	Negative
Positive if you answer 'yes' to either 1A or 1B		
1A: Is the pt different than his/her baseline mental status? Or **1B:** Has the patient had any fluctuation in mental status in the past 24 hours as evidenced by fluctuation on a sedation scale (e.g. RASS), GCS, or previous delirium assessment?	Yes	No
Feature 2: Inattention	**Positive**	**Negative**
Positive if either score for 2A or 2B is less than 8. Attempt the ASE letters first. If it is able to perform this test and the score is clear, record this score and move to Feature 3. If pt is unable to perform this test or the score is unclear, then perform the ASE Pictures. If you perform both tests, use the ASE Pictures' results to score the Feature.		
2A: ASE Letters: record score (enter NT for not tested) <u>Directions:</u> Say to the patient, "I am going to read you a series of 10 letters. Whenever you hear the letter 'A', indicate by squeezing my hand." Read letters from the following letter list in a normal tone. **SAVEAHAART** Scoring: Errors are counted when patient fails to squeeze on the letter "A" and when the patient squeezes on any letter other than "A."	Score (out of 10): ____	
2B: ASE Pictures: record score (enter NT for not tested) Directions are included on the picture packets.	Score (out of 10): ____	
Feature 3: Disorganized thinking	**Positive**	**Negative**
Positive if the combined score is less than 4		
3A: Yes/No Questions (Use either Set A or Set B, alternate on consecutive days if necessary): Set A — Set B 1. Will a stone float on water? / 1. Will a leaf float on water? 2. Are there fish in the sea? / 2. Are there elephants in the sea? 3. Does one pound weigh more than two pounds? / 3. Do two pounds weigh more than one pound? 4. Can you use a hammer to pound a nail? / 4. Can you use a hammer to cut wood? Score___(Patient earns 1 point for each correct answer out of 4) **3B: Command** Say to patient: "Hold up this many fingers" (Examiner holds two fingers in front of patient) "Now do the same thing with the other hand" (Not repeating the number of fingers). *If pt is unable to move both arms, for the second part of the command ask patient "Add one more finger") Score___(Patient earns 1 point if able to successfully complete the entire command)	Combined score (3A+3B): ——— (out of 5)	
Feature 4: Altered level of consciousness	**Positive**	**Negative**
Positive if the actual RASS score is anything other than "0" (zero)		
Overall CAM-ICU (Features 1 and 2 and either Feature 3 or 4):	**Positive**	**Negative**

Fig. 5.29 The confusion–agitation method for assessing the presence of delirium in critically ill patients. A, General approach to the diagnosis of delirium; B, CAM-ICU assessment.

Management

Delirium can be logically managed using the flowchart shown in Fig. 5.30. A key issue is to stop or avoid factors that perpetuate or exacerbate delirium, correct reversible factors that could be contributing, and switch to using antipsychotics for agitation. The safest and most clinically effective pharmacologic therapy for delirium in the ICU setting is uncertain, and there is a requirement for high-quality trials. Most guidelines recommend 'typical' antipsychotics, usually haloperidol in small (1.25–2.5mg) escalating boluses for management of agitated delirium. The effectiveness and safety of newer 'atypical' antipsychotics, such as olanzapine, is unknown. At present it is unclear whether patients with hypoactive delirium benefit from antipsychotic treatment.

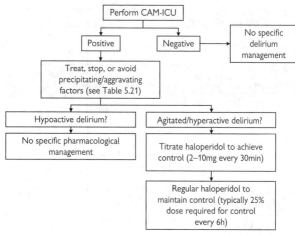

Fig. 5.30 A stepwise approach to assessing and managing the delirious patient in the ICU.

Sleep in the ICU

Sleep disturbance in the ICU is common. This is often due to:
- Factors relating to the underlying illness:
  - Stress response
  - Pain
  - Inflammation
  - Encephalopathy.
- Factors relating to the environment:
  - Excessive noise
  - Lighting
  - Diagnostic and patient care activities.

Typically there is sleep fragmentation, an increase in stage 1 and 2 sleep, and a decrease in stage 3, stage 4, and REM sleep. Circadian sleep rhythms are disturbed.

Optimizing sleep in ICU
- Minimize environmental contributing factors such as noise, lighting, and physical disturbances.
- Optimize patient–ventilator synchrony. This will decrease sleep disturbance, and several novel ventilatory modes, such as PAV, have been claimed to improve sleep.
- Benzodiazepines and other sedative drugs may prolong or increase sleep disturbance, and there is no evidence to support induction of night-time 'sleep' with sedative infusions.
- Newer non-benzodiazepine agents, such as zopiclone, may disrupt normal sleep patterns less, but there are few high-quality trials in this area.
- The role of melatonin for establishing normal sleep patterns is currently uncertain.

Conclusion

Sedation is one of the most common ICU interventions. There is strong evidence that a systematic method for assessing and managing sedation using clinical tools and protocols can improve patient outcomes and quality of care. Avoiding unnecessary over-sedation is particularly important to improve patient outcomes and reduce illness costs. Distinguishing the need for sedative drugs from the presence of delirium is increasingly recognized as important for avoiding unnecessarily prolonged sedation in the ICU.

Further reading

Ely EW, Truman B, Shintani A, et al. (2003) Monitoring sedation status over time in ICU patients—Reliability and validity of the Richmond Agitation-Sedation Scale (RASS). *JAMA* **289**, 2983–2991.

Ely EW, Inouye SK, Bernard GR, et al. (2001) Delirium in mechanically ventilated patients: validity and reliability of the confusion assessment method for the intensive care unit (CAM-ICU). *JAMA* **286**, 2703–2710.

Friese RS (2008) Sleep and recovery from critical illness and injury: A review of theory, current practice, and future directions. *Crit Care Med* **36**, 697–705.

Girard TD, Kress JP, Fuchs BD, et al. (2008) Efficacy and safety of a paired sedation and ventilator weaning protocol for mechanically ventilated patients in intensive care (Awakening and Breathing Controlled trial): a randomised controlled trial. *Lancet* **371**, 126–134.

Sessler CN and Varney K (2008) Patient-focussed sedation and analgesia in the ICU. *Chest* **133**, 522–565.

5.14 Ventilation outside the intensive care unit

Patient transfers
During inter-and intra-hospital transport there is potential for patients to become unstable and for adverse events to occur, perhaps even more so than in ICU. Risk of transfer must therefore be weighed against the benefit to the patient and the decision to transfer should involve a senior experienced doctor.

The keys to safe patient transfer are:
- Thorough assessment
- Preparation for both expected and unexpected situations
- Good communication.

Reasons for inter-hospital transfer
- Specialist investigations/treatment (e.g. burns, neurological, liver, paediatric, spinal injury).
- Upgrade care for organ support (e.g. ECMO).
- Move nearer home and family (repatriation).
- Lack of an available critical care bed.

Problems particular to patient transfer
Environmental
- Isolated.
- Limited space.
- Lighting may be poor.
- Difficulties instituting treatment in a moving vehicle.
- Noise and vibration.
- Temperature extremes.
- Potential hazards (e.g. helicopter flight, poor weather conditions).

Staffing
Specialist transfer teams are recommended, but the referring hospital often provides staff for the transfer. As the transfer team works with no immediate support the team members should be suitably experienced.

Equipment
- Limited.
- May be unfamiliar.

Potential adverse events during transfer
Although there is limited information on the rates of adverse events during patient transfer, they may be potentially catastrophic.

Airway
- Accidental extubation.
- Endobronchial intubation.
- Increased ETT cuff pressure leading to tracheal mucosal damage (pressures >30cmH$_2$O are associated with ischaemic injury).

Breathing
- Disconnection from ventilatory circuit.
- Hyper or hypoventilation.

- Deterioration requiring increased ventilatory support.
- Pneumothorax.

Circulation
- Line dislodgement.
- Cardiovascular instability due to acceleration/deceleration.
- Dysrhythmias.
- Haemorrhage (due to movement of fractures or disturbance of clot).

Equipment
- Equipment failure.
- Exhaustion of oxygen supplies.
- Battery or power failure.
- Transport breakdown or failure.

Communication
- Ensure good communication within the team: understand everyone's roles, skills, and limitations.
- Confirm receiving unit ready for patient prior to departure.
- Keep accurate documentation during transfer. Transfer team should keep a duplicate record.
- Ensure patient's family/next of kin is informed.
- Relatives should not travel with patients. Alternative travel arrangements should be made.
- Any adverse events should be reported and discussed.
- Staff should ensure adequate insurance cover.
- On arrival, there should be a comprehensive formal handover from the transfer team to the receiving team.

Infection control considerations
Universal precautions should be followed, as in ICU. The receiving hospital should be informed of any infection risk. The transport equipment should be cleaned after each transfer and HME filters changed between every patient.

Ventilator-associated pneumonia
Intra-hospital transport has been identified by some studies as a risk factor for VAP. This may be due to a lengthy period of being supine, frequent ventilator circuit manipulation, and inadequate airway suctioning.
    When possible the patient should be transferred in a 30° head-up position.
- Suction and discontinue nasogastric feeding before moving.

How to avoid problems during transfer
Patient assessment prior to transfer
Thorough assessment and stabilization prior to transfer will minimize the need for interventions *en route*. Familiarity with the patient's clinical condition will help rapid identification of changes.

History
A complete medical history should be obtained.

Examination

Carry out a full examination, paying particular attention to:

- Airway:
  - Check tube is secured
  - Position of tube at teeth/mouth
- Breathing:
  - Clinical examination
  - Current ventilator settings
  - Chest drain: Are drains working correctly? Have a low threshold for insertion of new chest drains prior to departure
- Cardiovascular:
  - Clinical examination
  - Current intravenous access adequate?
  - Haemorrhage should be stabilized and septic source controlled if possible (unless transfer is for definitive treatment)
- Neuro (examination may be limited due to sedation):
  - GCS—currently and prior to intubation
  - Extent of any neurological injury
  - Pupils
  - Pain and sedation assessment
- Abdomen and NGT placement (on free drainage)
- Urine output
- Presence and appearance of wounds
- Take note of intravenous access, drains, catheters.

Investigations

- Blood gases.
- Electrolytes, full blood count (FBC) and coagulation.
- CXR, ECG, other relevant investigations (e.g. echocardiography and imaging).

The transfer

Preparation is the key to success. Although some unstable patients need to be transferred for definitive management (e.g. ruptured abdominal aortic aneurysm (AAA)), generally a transfer should only be started once the patient is stable. A safe transfer is time-consuming.

Environmental

- Familiarize yourself with the transport surroundings if possible.
- Remain seated and wear seatbelts when travelling in the ambulance.
- If any intervention is necessary, stop the ambulance.
- Drive smoothly. Most transfers do not necessitate high-speed travel.
- Ambulance lights and sirens should only be used to aid a smooth, rapid transfer with minimal acceleration and deceleration.
- Directions: if in any doubt and transfer is urgent, request a police escort.
- Ensure adequate temperature control.

Staff

- There should be at least two people: a critical care nurse and a doctor.
- Have appropriate clothing (high visibility and warm), food, money, and a mobile phone.
- Plan for the return journey.

Patient
- Non-intubated critically ill patients have a high adverse incident rate and consideration should be given to intubation prior to departure.
- Secure head using bolsters or a rolled-up blanket either side of the head and tape across forehead (over a swab).
- Tape eyes.
- Check ABG 20min after putting the patient on the transport ventilator to ensure that gas exchange is adequate.
- Nasogastric on free drainage.
- Use a five-point harness to secure the patient to the trolley.
- Protect pressure areas and ensure monitors are not resting on patient.
- Patient positioned in ambulance head first (to minimize venous pooling during deceleration).

Monitoring
Appropriate dedicated transport equipment should be available. Minimum monitoring standards recommended by the Association of Anaesthetists of Great Britain and Ireland (2007) are:
- Pulse oximeter (due to vibration or cold peripheries, an ear probe may be more reliable)
- Invasive blood pressure monitoring is more accurate than NIBP as cuffs may malfunction due to vibration; NIBP also uses up battery power fairly quickly
- ECG
- Airway pressure, tidal volume, and respiratory rate
- Airway gases: FiO_2, end tidal CO_2.

Necessary equipment
- Specialized or adapted transfer trolley—check patient weight threshold if patient is obese (usually 180kg for ambulance, 150kg for aero medical transfers).
- Airway management equipment, including mask and self-inflating bag.
- Sufficient oxygen supplies (check ambulance reserves).
- Portable ventilator.
- Suction.
- Defibrillator.
- Infusion pumps (position below the level of the patient).
- Resuscitation drugs.
- Intravenous fluids (via a pressure bag/infusion pump).
- Vacuum mattress immobilization is useful for patient stabilization (e.g. spinal/pelvic fractures).
- Equipment cables can be contained in 22cm diameter corrugated tubing cut down its length or secured using Velcro clips.
- Drugs—all required medications will have to be brought with you. Delays and changing clinical state must be anticipated.
  - Sedation, neuromuscular blockade, analgesia—calculate requirements for journey at current infusion rate. Bring double.
  - Inotropes/vasopressors—as above, but factor in the increased requirement caused by movement or clinical deterioration.
  - Emergency drugs for treating cardiovascular instability.
  - Saline flushes.
  - Other drugs such as antiarrhythmics, mannitol, or anticonvulsants as indicated.
- Alarms should be readily visible and audible (settings to maximum).

Transfer of blood components

Call the Blood Transfusion Service in advance in order for products to be packaged appropriately according to local protocols.

Products that are required to be kept cool (e.g. red cells or fresh frozen plasma (FFP))are transported in a container validated to maintain an internal temperature of 4°C for up to 5h (e.g. a Versapak Transport Box). Once the box is opened, the contents must be used within 30min.

Platelets are transported in a cardboard box at room temperature.

The blood bank will issue appropriate documentation which must be completed at the receiving hospital so that the 'cold chain' can be fully audited.

It is not acceptable to simply repackage blood/components that have already been delivered to the clinical area.

Aeromedical transfer

Air transfer should be considered if transfer times are estimated to take longer than 90min or the distance is greater than 50 miles. Staff require additional training for air transfers (e.g. safety training, evacuation procedures, onboard communication skills). In fixed-wing aircraft, the cabin is pressurized to resemble altitudes between 1500 and 2500m (normal PaO_2 at 1500m is 10kPa). Helicopter cabins are not pressurized. Patients with respiratory failure are particularly difficult to manage in this hypobaric environment.

Problems particular to aeromedical transfers

- Decreased cabin pressure leads to increased volume of gases and gas-filled cavities expand (e.g. pneumothorax, eye injury, inner ear problems). Gaseous expansion of intestines or abdominal capacity can occur, even enough to compromise ventilation.
- At cabin pressure, gas inside the ETT cuff expands and may compromise tracheal mucosal perfusion. Gas should be partially removed during ascent and refilled during descent, and cuff pressures should be monitored. Alternatively, the cuff can be filled with saline rather than air.
- Low light levels and visibility.
- Low temperatures.
- Vibration and noise.
- Acceleration and deceleration.
- Radio communication may be required.
- Unfamiliar environment for many staff.
- Intra-aortic balloon pumps should be set to the 'auto fill' mode, which will automatically compensate for altitude changes to avoid overfilling of the helium balloon.
- Check weight limitations (of patient and equipment).
- Tissues can swell and so plaster casts should be split.

Ventilation during aeromedical transfer

- Lower barometric pressure of oxygen leads to a fall in alveolar oxygen tension. Increase FiO_2 and/or PEEP.
- Tidal volume increases as cabin pressure decreases, and so should be constantly measured to avoid VILI.
- For lengthy journeys, low-pressure liquid oxygen provides three times more gaseous oxygen compared to a similarly sized cylinder.

Patients on ECMO

Safe transfer on ECMO is possible but difficult, and ideally patients are transferred by dedicated ECMO teams from the receiving specialist units.

Checklist prior to transfer

Transfer details
- Name of referring and receiving hospitals.
- Names and direct numbers of referring and receiving trainee and consultant staff.

Patient
- Is he/she as stable as possible?

Communication
- Referral letter written, all documentation and results available.
- Admitting hospital aware and bed available.
- If awake, patient aware of transfer plan.
- Family/next of kin aware of transfer and have travel arrangements/ directions and contact details of the receiving unit.
- Driver clear of route to hospital (if not, take advice from ambulance control or request a police escort in emergency situations).

Examination and investigations
- A:
  - Are they intubated? Grade of intubation?
  - Note ETT position and check it is secure.
- B:
  - Ventilator settings and gas exchange.
  - Recent CXR.
  - Any drains *in situ*? If so, have Heimlich valves been attached? Are chest drains functioning?
- C:
  - Blood pressure, heart rate, CVP, perfusion.
  - What vascular access do they have? Two wide-bore cannulae and a central line best (check post central line CXR).
  - Inotrope concentration and dose.
  - Get blood products packaged.
- D:
  - Current GCS and GCS prior to intubation.
  - Current sedation.
- Bloods (results and correction of abnormalities if required).
- Renal:
  - Catheter and urine output.
- Gastro
  - NGT in situ? On free drainage.
- Equipment and drugs
  - Have these been checked? This should be done daily.
  - Adequate oxygen available.
  - Equipment plugged into ambulance electrical supply.
- Staff personal preparation
  - Warm visible clothing, money, mobile phone, food.
- Plans for the return journey

Portable transport ventilators

Portable ventilators allow more reliable and consistent ventilation than manual ventilation and are hands-free. They use less gas and electricity than ICU ventilators and are increasingly sophisticated, with an expanding repertoire of available ventilation modes.

- Although many transport ventilators now have spontaneous ventilation modes, it is often more appropriate to sedate, paralyse, and ventilate the patient with a mandatory mode.
- Most portable ventilators use a pressurized gas source to power the ventilator pneumatically.
- The oxygen concentrations selected by the operator are often displayed, rather than the measured FiO_2.
- The battery life is variable depending on settings, lung compliance, and ventilator characteristics.

Minimum transport ventilator requirements

- Disconnection and high-pressure alarms.
- PEEP.
- Ability to alter FiO_2, respiratory rate, tidal volume, and I:E ratio.

Desirable features

- Lightweight and robust.
- Use only a small amount of gas and electricity.
- Ability to deliver PCV, PSV and CPAP.

Calculating the oxygen requirements for a transfer

Oxygen requirements are calculated using the equation:

$$FiO_2 \times (MV + \text{driving gas*}) \times \text{transfer time} = O_2 \text{ needed (L)}$$

There should be an additional 50% added to the total to allow for unforeseen delays.

The capacities of commonly used cylinders are:
size D/CD = 340L
size E = 680L
size F/HX = 1360L

Ambulances usually carry two size F or HX (2300L) oxygen cylinders and two size D or CD (460L) cylinders.

*The quantity of driving gas varies considerably between ventilators (e.g. the Oxylog 3000 uses 0.5L/min, the VentiPAC 200D uses 20mL/cycle, and the LTV-1000 uses 10L/min).

Commonly used portable ventilators

Dräger Oxylog 2000/3000/3000 plus

- Pressure or volume controlled, patient-triggered modes.
- A bias flow (background O_2 flow) continues during expiration, which minimizes WOB.
- A continuous range of oxygen concentration is possible due to solenoid valves adjusting the entrainment ratio.

- Integrated mainstream capnography.
- The Oxylog 3000 has an altitude compensation function.

VentiPAC
- Flow controller, time cycled, volume preset, pressure limited.
- MRI compatible.
- Frequency is set by selecting inspiratory and expiratory times. Tidal volume is set by selecting inspiratory time and gas flow rate.
- Not best suited to spontaneous ventilation since it does not provide ventilatory assistance following inspiration, and so does not reduce WOB.
- Attach a manual PEEP valve (up to 20cmH$_2$O) if required.
- Ambient air is entrained into the high-pressure oxygen supply using a Venturi inside the ventilator. Switching to 'air mix' sets FiO$_2$ to 0.45 but if the entrainment port is switched off, FiO$_2$ is 1.0. *Note*: selecting 'airmix' may lead to decreased tidal volumes due to back-pressure on the internal Venturi.

LTV 1000
- Shorter battery life than other models.
- A manually adjustable PEEP valve for use within a 'T' piece is used but this can compromise the patient-triggering function.

Ventilation in specific areas
Radiology
- Space often limited.
- Harmful ionizing radiation during CT, so either stay outside the scan room or wear lead coats and thyroid protectors.
- Check how much the table will move during the scan to ensure that lines and breathing tubing will not be pulled.
- Monitors should be visible from the control room.
- If radioiodine is used during CT be aware of the potential for allergic reactions.
- Abdominal or thoracic scans may require 'breath holds' to reduce artifacts caused by respiration.
- An anaesthetic assistant or ICU nurse should accompany the doctor.

MRI
- The magnetic field means that ferromagnetic equipment (e.g. cylinders, laryngoscopes, stethoscopes, some artificial heart valves, pacemakers) can become projectiles near the scanner (where the magnetic force is greater than 5mT) or cause tissue damage. It is safe beyond the 0.5mT boundary.
- Patient and staff must undergo safety checks prior to entry.
- MRI-compatible equipment is available. Alternatively, conventional equipment can be used at a safe distance from the scanner (in the control room).
- Syringe driver motors may cease to work or become unreliable.
- Heating of electrical conductors (e.g. ECG leads) may cause burns.
- Noise: ear protectors are required in scan room.
- MRI interferes with ECG and can mimic dysrhythmias.
- ECG electrodes and leads should be MRI compatible.

- Use a south-facing preformed ETT for MRI head scans since this allows ventilator tubing to stay clear of the head coil.
- Taping the pilot tube of the ETT or laryngeal mask airway down and away from the area to be scanned prevents the metal spring in the pilot balloon from distorting the images.
- In the event of a cardiac arrest, start basic life support with a bag and mask and chest compressions, but transfer patient immediately outside the 0.5mT line.

Ventilation during MRI scanning

- Long ventilator tubing increases gas and agent sampling time (by approximately 5–10s).
- 'T' pieces are the most suitable breathing circuits (Mapleson D or E) since the length does not affect the dead space (e.g. Ayres or Bain).
- The airway pressures measured near the ventilator may not correlate to tracheal pressures because of the long tubing.
- Because of compression of the gas in the long tubing, programmed tidal volumes may not be achieved.

Emergency department

Emergency departments (EDs) are busy, noisy places, often with many patients needing immediate attention. Impulse decisions are therefore more frequent than on the ICU.

- The patient may have been intubated by ED staff or paramedics—check tube position, ventilator settings, and sedation.
- Good communication with unfamiliar ED staff is vital.
- Appropriately skilled personnel are not always available—if unsure about the skill mix, bring help from ICU or outreach with you.
- Patients are often exposed and hypothermia is common.
- Line or drain insertion should be performed as aseptically as possible.
- Be prepared to look after the patient on your own, but be assertive about the help you require and identify an ED doctor to remain assisting you.
- Caring for a patient in the ED may keep an ICU doctor away from ICU for an extended period.
- Have a plan for patients who require urgent surgical intervention in the ED (e.g. thoracotomy).
- It is important but difficult to keep accurate records of medical care in the ED.

Further reading

AAGBI (2009) AAGBI Safety Guideline. Interhospital Transfer. Association of Anaesthetists of Great Britain and Ireland, London.

Intensive Care Society (2002) Guidelines for the transport of the critically ill adult http://www.ics.ac.uk/intensive_care_professional/standards_and_guidelines/transport_of_the_critically_ill_2002.

Lutman D and Petros AJ (2005) How many oxygen cylinders do you need to take on transport? A nomogram for cylinder size and duration. *Emerg Med J* **23**, 703–704.

5.15 Weaning from mechanical ventilation

Weaning from mechanical ventilation is a process that ultimately should lead to liberation from mechanical ventilation. It remains an area of ongoing controversy, from definitions to the most effective and rapid means of weaning.

The largest review of the evidence was published in 2001 by a task force representing the American College of Chest Physicians, the American Association for Respiratory Care, and the Society of Critical Care Medicine. Currently, these definitions and recommendations have not been challenged and remain the most up-to-date consensus.

Definitions

Discontinuation of mechanical ventilation

The task force has proposed 'discontinuation of mechanical ventilation' to replace the term 'weaning'. The phrase better describes the ultimate goal and the process directly aimed at liberating a patient from ventilation. The term 'weaning' has become associated with a protracted process. However, it need not be a slow process. Indeed, many people have ventilation rapidly discontinued, for example in post-operative patients.

Ventilator dependency

Ventilator dependency has been defined as a requirement for >24h of ventilation in a patient despite attempts at discontinuation of ventilation.

How fast to wean?

Recognized patient factors that will prolong weaning from ventilation are:
• Age
• Duration of mechanical ventilation
• Chronic respiratory disease
• Chest wall disorders
• Neuromuscular disease
• Severity of acute disease
• Lowered conscious level.

Further delays are caused by a failure to recognize the potential to discontinue ventilation in some patients. Unnecessary prolongation of ventilation increases costs and potential harm to patients.
• Increased cost was estimated at $5000 per patient in 1996, and may be further increased if the patient develops a complication such as VAP.
• Each additional day on ventilation is associated with a cumulative risk of developing VAP, which has an attributable mortality and increases length of stay. Strategies to reduce days on ventilation have been associated with reduced VAP rates.
• Prolonging ventilation further exposes patients to prolonged sedative use with increased risk of delayed wake up and delirium.

However, an overly aggressive approach to weaning will increase the failed extubation rate. Failed extubation is associated with:
• An eight-fold increase in the incidence of VAP

- A six- to twelve-fold increase in mortality. This is probably not all directly attributable to the failed extubation, but rather that the failed extubation may serve as an indicator of severity of illness.

A balance clearly needs to be sought. The failed extubation rate has been used as a marker for over- or under-aggressive approaches to weaning.

Accepted failed extubation rates range from 5 to 15%. A figure below this reflects an overly conservative approach, and above this an overly aggressive approach.

Approach to weaning

The traditional approach to weaning had been a gradual reduction in the level of ventilatory support until the patient was able to breathe independently from the ventilator. This still has a role in chronic weaning and difficult to wean patients, but in the majority of ICU patients the evidence favours a structured approach once the underlying cause of respiratory failure has resolved (Fig. 5.31).

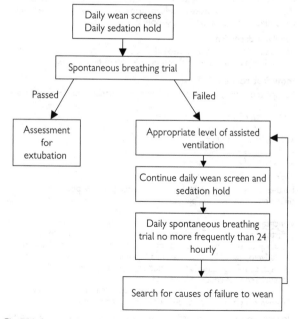

Fig. 5.31 Approach to weaning.

Respiratory capacity and loading

The balance between capacity of breathing and the load placed on that system determines the patient's ability to breathe spontaneously or require ventilatory support. A patient's capacity to breathe is dependent on neurological, respiratory, cardiovascular, and psychological factors.

Capacity
CNS

Responsible for the drive of spontaneous ventilation but also for the generation of its rhythm and pattern. This can be altered by structural lesions of the brainstem and by metabolic disorders, which include drugs, poisons, and hypercapnia.

Peripheral nervous system

Neuropathy and myopathy may affect the transmission of the signal to the muscles, e.g. Guillain–Barré or critical illness polyneuropathy/myopathy.

Respiratory muscles

'Ventilatory pump' performance can be affected by:
- Direct injury, e.g. myopathy, disuse atrophy, muscle catabolism, and fatigue.
- Metabolic derangement, e.g. hypophosphataemia, hypocalcaemia, or hypomagnesaemia.
- Pre-existing muscle disease, possibly undiagnosed.

Mechanical

- The efficiency of the ventilatory pump may be compromised by chronic chest wall problems such as kyphoscoliosis or acute hyperinflation.
- Reversible hyperinflation may be overlooked in COPD or where a high PEEP has been utilized for oxygenation and has not been decreased. The muscles operate on the least compliant part of the pressure–volume curve.
- Abdominal splinting reduces diaphragmatic descent, reduces chest wall compliance, and increases WOB.

Respiratory loading
Ventilation load

Alveolar ventilation (V_A) places a load on this system, which is determined by the oxygen consumption (VO_2). It is increased in SIRS and sepsis. Carbon dioxide production (VCO_2) is increased by carbohydrate-rich feeding and elimination of CO_2 is reduced if dead space is increased. Minute ventilation (MV) may need to be increased.

Compliance

Respiratory system compliance should be calculated. Normal compliance in the ventilated patient is in the range 50–100mL/cmH$_2$O. Chest wall and lung compliance should be considered separately. Factors affecting chest wall compliance include pleural disease, musculoskeletal diseases of the thoracic cage, obesity, restrictive dressings or scarring, and intra-abdominal pressure. Lung compliance is altered by atelectasis, interstitial and alveolar oedema, fibrosis, bronchoconstriction, posture, and changes in lung volume. Most respiratory diseases will alter compliance by impairing surfactant function or lung tissue elasticity.

Resistance
Resistance to flow in healthy airways is 5–15cmH$_2$O/L/s. Pathological conditions such as bronchoconstriction, inflammation, secretions, enlarged lymph nodes, and tumour increase the resistance and the load.

Imposed load
The presence of a long narrow tracheal tube will further increase resistance and is a potentially remediable imposed load. Inefficient ventilator triggering or other patient ventilator dysynchrony (see 📖, Patient–ventilator asynchrony, p 262) may also unnecessarily raise ventilatory load.

Capacity–load imbalance
In health, respiratory capacity greatly exceeds respiratory load, allowing normal spontaneous breathing. However, if WOB is increased or respiratory capacity is decreased, ventilatory support may be required. Reducing ventilatory support increases WOB and may create a capacity–load imbalance. This is generally exhibited as rapid shallow breathing, which is the most energy efficient breathing in this situation (see Otis' minimum WOB concept, 📖 Adaptive support ventilation, p 170). However, this breathing pattern will cause increased dead space and reduced CO$_2$ clearance.

Titration of respiratory support
Ventilation is a supportive measure and is not a treatment of the underlying cause of respiratory failure. While the patient is ventilated the underlying cause must be sought and treated.

Support with ventilation may require the use of high concentrations of oxygen, high levels of PEEP, and fully mandatory modes of ventilation, which would exclude the patient, by the wean screen, from progressing to a spontaneous breathing trial (SBT).

Some authors suggest weaning should start from the time of initiation of mechanical ventilation. This confuses the process aimed at discontinuation of ventilation with the process of titration of ventilation to match increased WOB, and changes in compliance, resistance, and inspired oxygen requirement. Progress from high levels of support towards a position where an SBT is appropriate is part of the routine management of ventilation. Once acceptable gas exchange is achieved, and the increased WOB addressed, the support should be reduced as the patient tolerates it.

Within the accepted limits of pressure, volume, and FiO$_2$ (see 📖 Ventilatory-induced lung injury, p 244), for each patient on each day, acceptable SaO$_2$, respiratory rate, tidal volume, and number of mandatory breaths should be chosen. Consider the support required for gas exchange (airway pressure and FiO$_2$) separately from the support required for WOB (inspiratory assistance).

FiO$_2$ requirement and PEEP
As the underlying condition resolves, oxygen requirements will fall, and accordingly should be titrated down to achieve the wean screen target of a P:F ratio >25kPa. Periods on high concentrations of oxygen (FiO$_2$ >0.6) should be minimized, therefore the concentration of inspired oxygen should usually be less than 60% before PEEP is reduced. PEEP will be set differently for different diseases, and the rate at which it can be reduced will differ according to the underlying pathology. PEEP levels should be regularly reviewed, as requirements will change with alterations in lung compliance.

FiO_2 and PEEP should be predominantly titrated against SaO_2 rather than PaO_2. Not only does SaO_2 reflect the O_2 carrying capacity, it is also monitored continuously in ventilated patients. Targeting SaO_2 levels >90% achieves a compromise between reducing inspired O_2 concentrations while retaining adequate O_2 carriage.

Initiating a respiratory effort
Transition to a spontaneous breathing mode is best achieved by reducing mandatory breaths, allowing increased CO_2 to stimulate respiratory effort. This process prevents a period of apnoea causing desaturation or backup apnoea ventilation and may be aided by a sedation hold or a review of the current level of sedation.

Inspiratory pressures
As pulmonary compliance improves, the pressures required to deliver a mandatory tidal volume will reduce. For spontaneously breathing patients, the inspired pressure support can be titrated against clinical indicators (respiratory rate, heart rate, accessory muscle use) and ventilator parameters (tidal volume, rapid shallow breathing index (RSBI), $P_{0.1}$; see below).

Considerations prior to weaning
Disease resolution
The success of the weaning process can be improved if resolution of the underlying disease and factors affecting that patient's capacity to breathe are optimized. Understanding the underlying disease aids in recognizing when that disease has resolved sufficiently to allow mechanical ventilation to be discontinued.

Weaning before the underlying cause of respiratory failure has resolved is likely to delay discontinuation of ventilation due to muscle fatigue. The following factors should be considered.

Pulmonary
- Pneumonia—improved oxygenation and lower PEEP requirement should be apparent before weaning is likely to be successful. A reduction in secretion load can signal an appropriate time to discontinue mechanical ventilation.
- ARDS—in addition to oxygenation, pulmonary compliance and CO_2 clearance should be taken into account before weaning is commenced.
- SIRS/sepsis place a high demand on the respiratory system with increased minute ventilation due to a raised VO_2 and V/Q mismatch. Weaning during active sepsis is unlikely to be successful. Indicators of resolution include a reduced requirement for inotropes and vasopressor, resolution of tachycardia and fever.
- COPD—resolution of exacerbation with reduced airway resistance, reduced intrinsic PEEP, and improvement in any underlying infection. No respiratory acidosis.

Cardiac
- Causes of myocardial ischaemia have been resolved.
- Toxic/myocardial depressants removed.
- Fluid overload corrected.
- Appropriate medical therapy instituted.

Neurological
- Improved conscious level.
- Improved neuromuscular function with recovering VC.

Gastrointestinal
- Resolving hepatic encephalopathy.
- Gut oedema/distension resolved.

The assessment of disease reversal is a subjective process. Objective screening tools (see box) have been developed to overcome this subjectivity.

> **Wean screen**
>
> A range of criteria has been used in weaning studies to determine when respiratory failure has resolved sufficiently to proceed to weaning attempts. It is not an exhaustive list of exclusions, but it acts as a simple gateway to the process of discontinuation of ventilation. It allows patients to be further assessed with an SBT and an assessment of extubation who may otherwise be overlooked.
>
> Daily wean screens have been shown to be simple to perform and in combination with SBTs have reduced days on mechanical ventilation.[1]
>
> **Daily wean screen criteria for assessing potential to wean**
>
> | | |
> |---|---|
> | 1. Evidence of reversal of the underlying cause for respiratory failure | |
> | 2. Adequate oxygenation | PaO_2/FiO_2 ratio greater than 20–25kPa |
> | | PEEP less than or equal to 5–8 |
> | 3. Haemodynamic stability | No myocardial ischaemia |
> | | Low dose or no vasopressors or inotropes |
> | 4. Capable of initiating a respiratory effort | |

Predicting successful liberation from ventilation

A survey of intensivists revealed that though we may be relatively good at spotting patients who will fail off ventilation with a specificity of 79% our sensitivity (i.e. our ability to recognize who will successfully extubate) is low at 35%.

Clinical assessment
- Subjective dyspnoea.
- Accessory muscle use.
- Abdominal paradox (see-saw motion of the abdomen and chest wall).
- Diaphoresis.
- Tachycardia.
- Subjective comfort.

Measurements
Simple
- Minute ventilation.
- Vital capacity.
- RSBI—frequency (breaths per minute)/tidal volume (litres).

Ventilator enabled
- Maximal inspiratory pressure (MIP, sometimes called PI_{max}) against a closed inspiratory valve for 20s.
- P0.1 measures the negative pressure generated against an occlusion for 100ms. The normal value of P0.1 is between -3 and $-4cmH_2O$. The occlusion time is sufficiently short to be undetectable by the patient's respiratory control centres, preventing any increase in effort. High loading is detected by an increased negative pressure. Levels of $-6cmH_2O$ are predictive of weaning failure.

Specific device required
- Oesophageal pressure (P_{ES}) is an estimate of pleural pressure.
- $WOB = P_{ES} \times V_t$.
- Pressure time index (P_{TI}) = $(P_{ES}/PI_{max})(T_i/T_T)$. P_{TI} is a measure of respiratory muscle loading and is predictive of fatigue if greater than 0.15. T_i = inspired time, T_{tot} = total breath time.

Integrated factors
- $P_{0.1}/PI_{max}$ ratio.
- Compliance respiratory rate oxygenation and pressure (CROP):
$$\frac{(\text{dynamic compliance} \times PaO_2)/(\text{alveolar } PO_2 \times PI_{max})}{\text{respiratory rate}}$$

Table 5.22 Measurements whilst either receiving ventilatory support or during an SBT which have been shown to have a positive likelihood ratio (LR) on ventilation discontinuation in more than one study[1]

Parameter	Threshold values	Positive LR value
Measured on ventilator		
MV	10–15L	0.81–2.37
MIP	−20 to −30cmH$_2$O	0.23–2.45
P$_{0.1}$/PI$_{max}$	0.3	2.14–25.3
CROP	13	1.05–19.74
Measured during SBT		
Respiratory rate	30–38 breaths/min	1.00–3.89
V$_T$	325–400mL (4–6mL/kg)	0.71–3.83
RSBI (f/V$_t$ ratio)	60–105	0.84–4.67

Clinical applicability
When applied individually these measures do not have an LR great enough to clinically outperform the SBT as a useful predictor of successful liberation from ventilation (Table 5.22).

LR incorporates both the sensitivity and specificity of a test, providing an estimate of how much a test will alter the pre-test odds of identifying success or failure.

LR >1: increased likelihood of successful weaning
LR <1: decreased probability of successful weaning
LR 1–2 or 0.5–1: minimally alters the pre-test probability
LR 2–5 or 0.3–0.5: small changes in pre-test probability
LR 5–10 or 0.1–0.3: moderate changes in pre-test probability
LR >10 or LR <0.1: a large and conclusive difference

Spontaneous breathing trials

An SBT is currently the best predictor for successful liberation from ventilation. It allows assessment of load capacity imbalance under a situation of full respiratory loading. In simpler terms, to assess if a patient can breathe independently from a ventilator, the best test is to try the patient breathing without the ventilator.

- At least 77% of patients passing an SBT will go on to successful extubation.
- The remainder are either not extubated when assessed on extubation screening or are true failed extubations within 48h with reported rates in the range of 15–17%. This relatively high rate of failed extubation may be a consequence of aggressive protocolized weaning. Since weaning protocols shorten overall ICU stay without increasing mortality, this may be an acceptable price to pay.
- The number of false negatives (failure predicted incorrectly) is unknown.
- The SBT does not take into account oxygenation and secretion load, and therefore these must be considered separately and should be included in the initial screening checklist.
- Passing an SBT should instigate an assessment for extubation.

Patients should be considered for an SBT if they fulfill the criteria of the weaning screen and have the capacity to initiate spontaneous breaths.

The patient should be screened for the first few minutes of the breathing trial using the criteria shown in Table 5.23. This should recognize early failure and allow a patient who will clearly fail to be returned to ventilatory support. If the screening phase is passed the patient should continue on to the full SBT.

Duration
- The 'task force' has recommended an SBT of between 30min and 2h.
- A single RCT has found that a 2-h SBT is no more predictive than a 30-min test.
- A 30-min SBT may be favourable due to speed and simplicity.

Frequency
- 35% of patients will fail the first SBT and will therefore require further SBT.
- SBTs should generally be conducted no more frequently than every 24h to avoid respiratory muscle fatigue.

Conducting the trial

The SBT was designed to standardize the approach to discontinuation of ventilation and function as a tool to reduce days on ventilation. As such it is a 'best fit' for the majority of patients. Not all patients passing the test are successfully extubated and in certain patients, particularly in those with LV dysfunction, further assessment is warranted (review of medical treatment and withdrawal of PEEP). The original description of the SBT specified spontaneous breathing through a 'T' piece. This essentially represents a supraphysiological challenge due to:

• Zero end expiratory pressure from the 'T' piece. (However, this may be a useful test in itself of withdrawal of the left ventricular support afforded by positive pressure ventilation).

• No compensation for imposed load of resistance from the tracheal tube.

A system to deliver CPAP in the range of 5 cmH$_2$O may be used to maintain alveolar recruitment during the trial, but this does not compensate for any imposed load of resistance.

• The addition of 5 to 7 cmH$_2$O pressure support is said to overcome the resistance of the tracheal tube and the ventilator circuit. A low level of pressure support has been shown to increase the likelihood of a patient passing the SBT but does not increase the number of false positives (those passing SBT but who fail to tolerate extubation).

• If the ventilator is equipped with a form of automatic tube compensation this can be used to provide a level of pressure support dependent on flow and the internal diameter of the airway, producing what has been described as electronic extubation.

None of the methods described above can predict the effects of upper airway oedema when patients are extubated, and this may account for a proportion of the false positives.

Table 5.23 Criteria for discontinuing SBT (adapted from ref 1)

Objective measurements		
Gas exchange	PaO$_2$/FiO$_2$	<25
Haemodynamic stability	Heart rate	>120 to 140 or greater than 20% change in heart rate
	Systolic BP	>180mmHg or <90mmHg
Ventilatory pattern	Respiratory rate	>35 breaths/min or a change >50%
Subjective clinical assessments		
Mental status	Somnolence, coma, agitation, or anxiety	
	Discomfort	
	Diaphoresis	
Signs of WOB	Use of accessory muscles of respiration, thoracoabdominal paradox	

The Awakening and Breathing Controlled trial[2] studied the effect of combining sedation holds and SBTs. It demonstrated a 14% absolute reduction in mortality and a 3-day reduction in duration of mechanical ventilation.

Management between spontaneous breathing trials
If a patient fails an SBT, how should we manage ventilation until the next attempt (usually in 24h)? Should we increase the support, leave it unchanged, or try to reduce the support between daily SBTs?
• Too little support will lead to fatigue and respiratory muscle injury.
• Too much support will retard muscle reconditioning and recovery.
• An appropriate level of support leaves the patient with normal WOB.

Reducing support may improve respiratory muscle function and ease the transition to an SBT. Stable support reduces the chance of muscle fatigue. There is no evidence available to guide us, and a sensible compromise may be to provide adequate support in order that the patient's WOB is not excessive. Reassessment of the support provided may allow a reduction during the period between SBTs if support is clearly excessive. Changes in the patient's condition may mandate an alteration to this strategy.
• The level of support is best guided by measures of respiratory capacity load imbalance.
• A RSBI < 65 breaths/min/L indicates comfortable breathing and had a predictive power of successful weaning of 90% in a small study of stepwise reductions in ventilatory support.

There is reasonable consensus that assisted modes of ventilation are more suitable than controlled modes, unless mandatory breaths are required.

Considerations
• An ongoing search should continue for causes of weaning failure (see above).
• Address any ventilator–patient dysynchrony, which can further worsen muscle injury. This is better achieved by using a mode of partially assisted ventilation such as PSV (see 📖 Patient ventilator asynchrony p 262 and Pressure support ventilation, p 144).
• Ventilation pressures and volume should be set to avoid/minimize VALI from ongoing ventilation.
• Care must be taken in the early weaning of patients with recovering ARDS.
  • ARDS affects the lungs in a heterogeneous fashion, which remains the case during recovery.
  • The lungs will have areas of varying compliance that are at risk of over-distension with the risk of barotrauma and pneumothoraces.
  • Patients with resolving ARDS often have a large dead space and minute ventilation requirement. This is normally best delivered with a spontaneous mode of ventilation because the respiratory system compliance is increased compared with controlled ventilation, and high minute ventilation is more easily and safely achieved. However, a balance must be sought between high levels of pressure

support and tachypnoea. If this is not possible, it may signal that the patient is not suitable for weaning and may be better supported by controlled ventilation with close control of volumes and pressures.

Weaning protocols

A weaning screen, sedation hold, and an SBT represent a protocol for weaning that can be nurse-led. There are many studies comparing such a weaning protocol against 'standard' physician-led weaning. Most demonstrate benefit from protocols as defined by shorter weaning periods and a higher percentage of successful weans.

Some studies address the concern that protocols may only lead to improvement in those units with low medical and nursing staffing levels. For example, in a unit with a doctor to patient ratio of 1:1.2, protocolized weaning was equivalent to physician-led weaning.

Vitacca[3] compared SBT and PSV in difficult-to-wean COPD patients and found no difference. However, the protocolized weaning of patients with either SBT or PSV was found to be quicker than in historical controls.

- A protocol for weaning is suitable for the majority of patients.
  A weaning guide should be in place to deliver a degree of automation to the weaning process. This frees up staff time for the more complex weaning patients.
- Straightforward weaning should be able to take place with early identification of those suitable for weaning and extubation.
- A protocol will not be successful in some patients and as such identifies them as more difficult to wean.
- Difficult-to-wean patients should have regularly reviewed individualized weaning plans.

Weaning modes

Several modes are available to deliver partial respiratory support between SBTs. Ideally these modes should be chosen to maximize patient comfort and reduce imposed loads. When choosing a ventilator mode, the following should be considered:
- Allow spontaneous breathing
  - Reduced muscle atrophy
  - Reduced sedation requirement
  - Spontaneous modes may allow easier sleep but may also be associated with an increased incidence of apnoeic spells and arousal.
- Most modern ventilators default to flow triggering, which is more sensitive and decreases WOB when compared to pressure triggering.
- Avoid gas trapping and breath stacking when the patient has insufficient time to exhale fully. If expiratory flow does not return to baseline, there is insufficient time for the volume delivered to be exhaled.
  This may be problematic on high levels of pressure support or in a proportional assist mode.

Synchronized intermittent mandatory ventilation
- As a means of weaning SIMV is limited. Several studies have found SIMV breath rate reductions to be the slowest method of weaning when compared to PSV or SBT.

Pressure support ventilation
- Gradual reductions in PSV, although effective in weaning, have been found to be slower at discontinuing ventilation than daily SBTs.
- However, gradual reduction of PSV combined with daily SBTs has not been studied.

Proportional assist ventilation
- See 📖 Proportional assist ventilation, p 174.
- Compared with other weaning modes it has been found to:
  • Decrease triggering delay
  • Decrease the likelihood of ineffective efforts
  • Decrease expiratory asynchrony
  • Increase sleep efficiency.
- Duration of mechanical ventilation is unchanged.

Automated weaning modes
These are essentially closed-loop weaning protocols driven by the ventilator with many human factors removed.

Knowledge base (Smartcare®)
This system is based on a fuzzy logic controller, which aims to reduce the level of pressure support stepwise in increments of 2–4cmH$_2$O. It uses parameters of respiratory capacity load balance.
- Respiratory rate <30 breaths/min (<34 breaths/min in neurological disease).
- Tidal volume >300mL (>250mL if patient weight <55kg).
- End-tidal CO$_2$ <7.3kPa (8.6kPa in COPD patients). (End-tidal CO$_2$ should be used with caution as it may not adequately represent PaCO$_2$).

Initial studies were positive: a reduction in time to discontinuation of ventilation by 33%. This improvement was probably due to the fact that the computer strictly adheres to the protocol. A more recent study comparing Smartcare to nurse-led weaning has shown no benefit.

Adaptive support ventilation
See 📖 Adaptive support ventilation, p 170. Earlier extubation after cardiac surgery has been reported with ASV. However, this was in comparison to SIMV.

Non-invasive ventilation
The use of NIV as an adjunct to weaning has been studied in three main situations: electively post extubation to continue the weaning process, electively post extubation to prevent extubation failure, and in the event of extubation failure.
- NIV may be used electively, i.e. extubate to NIV, then progressively wean on NIV. This is particularly successful in COPD patients but may also be of benefit in neuromuscular disease.
- NIV as an adjunct in COPD patients resulted in fewer invasive ventilator days, shorter length of stay in ICU, and reduced incidence of VAP.

- COPD patients who are at high risk of reintubation will benefit from NIV.
- In a recent study patients with chronic respiratory disease who had hypercapnia after an SBT had lower mortality and lower rates of respiratory failure when supported electively with NIV.
- Additionally, a recent meta-analysis demonstrated reduced mortality and VAP with NIV compared to invasive weaning. The majority of patients in the 12 identified studies had underlying COPD.
- COPD patients probably benefit the most as they are at higher risk of VAP and will often require ventilatory support for less severity of illness than a previously fit patient.

- The use of NIV in unselected patients failing within 48h of extubation, compared to standard medical management, did not reduce the need for reintubation but increased the ICU mortality with a relative risk of 1.78.

NIV in this situation is potentially dangerous as it may delay reintubation.

Weaning failure

Even with the appropriate application of screening, SBTs, and a weaning protocol, some patients will fail to wean. The Department of Health has defined a delayed wean as ventilator dependency greater than 14 days in the absence of any non-respiratory factors and a failed wean as ventilator dependency greater than 21 days.

An important part of the weaning process in a patient failing an SBT is the ongoing search to identify a reason for weaning failure.

- Sufficient resolution of the underlying cause of respiratory failure?
- Previously unrecognized chronic lung, cardiac, or neuromuscular condition?
- Increased respiratory loading or decreased ventilator pump capacity?
- Impaired cardiac function?

Review the history

When weaning delay or failure occurs, a repeat history from patient or family may bring to light previously unrecognized chronic disease, for example:
- Lung:
  - COPD
  - Interstitial lung disease
- Cardiac:
  - Ischaemic heart disease
  - Cardiomyopathy
- Neuromuscular
  - Motor neurone disease
  - Myasthenia
  - Myotonic dystrophy.

Increased respiratory loading
Increased respiratory demand
This can be due to increased CO_2 production as a result of:
- SIRS/sepsis
- Burns
- Shivering
- Agitation
- Excess carbohydrate

or because of reduced clearance secondary to:
- $\dot{V}/\dot{Q}$ mismatch, e.g. COPD or ARDS
- Excessive equipment dead space.

Resistive loads
- Bronchospasm, airway oedema, and secretions.

Imposed loads
- Narrow ETT and ventilator circuit resistance.
- Poorly set triggering.

Decreased chest wall compliance
- Pleural effusion.
- Pneumothorax.
- Obesity may reflect obesity hypoventilation syndrome.
- Abdominal distention; ascites or dilated bowel.
- Chest and abdominal wall oedema.

Decreased lung compliance
- Pulmonary oedema.
- Pulmonary fibrosis.
- Infection.
- ARDS.

Decreased ventilator pump capacity
Respiratory drive failure
- Opiate and sedative drugs with respiratory depressant effect.
- Brainstem lesion.
- Metabolic alkalosis.
- Chronic hypercapnia, with metabolic compensation.

Neurological disease
- Spinal cord lesion or direct phrenic nerve injury.
- Critical illness polyneuropathy.
- Guillain-Barré.
- Persistent neuromuscular blockade.
- Myasthenia gravis, which may be exacerbated by drugs such as aminoglycosides.
- Motor neuropathy, e.g. motor neuron disease.

Muscle weakness
- Disuse atrophy.
- Fatigue injury.
- Malnutrition.
- Myopathy, including steroid and neuromuscular blockade induced.

- Hyperinflation creates a mechanical disadvantage with the muscles operating on the least compliant part of the pressure–volume curve.
- Electrolyte derangement, in particular hypophosphataemia.
- Pre-exisiting myopathy, e.g. muscular dystrophy.

Myocardial disease

Myocardial dysfunction is an often overlooked cause of weaning failure, as the signs are similar to weaning failure from capacity load imbalance. It is important to recognize as it is amenable to treatment. Elevated pulmonary artery occlusion pressures were demonstrated in a group of patients failing to wean. However, 60% successfully weaned after a period of diuresis.

A return to spontaneous breathing loads the cardiovascular system in several ways.

Reversal of positive to negative intrathoracic pressure

- Increased venous return.
- Increased LV afterload.
- Increased cardiac transmural pressure gradient, which equates to increased cardiac work.

Increased respiratory muscle demand

- Increased cardiac output.
- Increased circulating catecholamines.

Management of weaning failure

A fresh approach is required in initiating the management of the weaning failure patient.

All the potential factors that may have been the cause of weaning failure must be evaluated, and potential areas to treat identified.

Respiratory

Respiratory management is best guided with recent chest radiology. CT thorax is useful to assess the extent of chronic lung disease and to investigate acquired conditions such as ARDS, fibrosis, effusions, or empyema.

- Treat any persisting infection.
- Drain pleural effusions.
- Treat bronchospasm.
- Reduce FiO_2 as tolerated and normalize $PaCO_2$ if possible.

Bronchoscopy may help to re-expand lobar or segmental collapse and establish microbiological diagnoses with bronchoalveoloar lavage.

Cardiovascular

- LV function should be assessed with echocardiography. However, this gives a snapshot of the current level of positive pressure ventilation and any inotropic support. More dynamic measurements with echocardiography or pulmonary artery measurements of SvO_2 may expose cardiac decompensation associated with weaning attempts.
- Treat any myocardial dysfunction.
- Maintain cardiovascular support during the weaning process in patients with identified LV failure.
- Correct dysrhythmias.
- Treat and prevent cardiac ischaemia.

- Clear oedema rigorously with diuretics and maintain careful fluid balance.

Central nervous system
- Avoid oversedation.
- Ensure sleep, normalize wake and sleep patterns.

Metabolic
- Correct hypophosphataemia.
- Optimize nutrition.

Acid/base status
Metabolic alkalosis in the failing to wean patient should be normalized if secondary to:
- Prolonged periods of hypoventilation during weaning attempts
- Permissive hypercapnia
- Diuretic use.

However, patients with chronic hypercapnia due to underlying lung disease will have insufficient respiratory capacity to cope with this increased drive and should be corrected close to their normal level of metabolic compensation.
- Acetazolamide may be used to correct metabolic alkalosis. It is most effective in normal renal function and when combined with normalization of arterial CO_2 with adequate ventilation.
- Up to 4 days of enteral acetazolamide 250mg twice daily may be required but the duration of the course should be titrated to bicarbonate correction.

Approach in the delayed wean
As well as the specific issues outlined above, an individual plan must be drawn up for the patient encompassing the whole environment, the structure of the day, and the ethos of the medical and nursing care.

Weaning pattern
Weaning and periods of increased work for the slow-weaning patient should be conducted during daylight hours, including:
- Reductions in pressure support
- Increasing periods of time off ventilatory support.

The overnight period should focus on:
- Rest
- Ensuring sleep
- Correction of hypercapnia
- Re-recruitment of alveoli.

Respiratory failure is associated with increased periods of apnoea during sleep. It is particularly distressing to the weaning patient to be repeatedly woken from sleep by ventilator alarms. A ventilator with a mandatory back-up rate to prevent apnoeas during sleep is helpful.

General care
- Normalize care as far as possible: access to TV, reading materials, and items from home, including normal clothes, all help to de-medicalize the environment and improve the psychological well-being of the patient.
- Sitting the patient out of bed optimizes the position for weaning and improves their interaction with their environment.
- Encourage eating and drinking.
- Tracheotomy cuff deflation and use of a one-way 'speaking' valve improves patient morale and vocal cord function, particularly adduction to aid coughing.

Some patients, particularly those with a chronic neuromuscular or chest wall disorder, will never be fully weaned from ventilatory support, but may be stabilized on NIV for the longer term (see 📖 Long-term (home) ventilation, p 354).

1 MacIntyre NR (2001) Evidence-based guidelines for weaning and discontinuing ventilatory support. *Chest* **120**, 375S–395S.
2 Girard TD, Kress JP, Fuchs BD, *et al.* (2008) Efficacy and safety of a paired sedation and ventilator weaning protocol for mechanically ventilated patients in intensive care (Awakening and Breathing Controlled trial): a randomised controlled trial. *Lancet* **371**, 126–34.
3 Vitacca M, Vianello A, Colombo D, *et al.* (2001) Comparison of two methods for weaning patients with chronic obstructive pulmonary disease requiring mechanical ventilation for more than 15 days. *Am J Resp Crit Care Med* **164**(2), 186–7.

5.16 Extubation

Following a successful wean from ventilation, a decision to remove the ETT is made (extubation).

Extubation may be carried out before weaning is complete if the patient is being considered for NIV. This approach is increasingly used in patients with acute exacerbation of COPD and in those with neuromuscular disease (nocturnal NIV).

Pre-conditions for extubation

- Stable spontaneous ventilation.
- Successful SBT (see 📖 Weaning, p 333).
  - 30–120min in uncomplicated patients.
  - Up to 24h may be appropriate following prolonged ventilation.
- Adequate oxygenation (PaO_2:FiO_2 ratio >25kPa).
- Normal $PaCO_2$ (except in those known to be chronically hypercarbic).
- Adequate level of consciousness: in general the ability to obey commands (GCS M6) is necessary to allow co-operation, clear secretions, and maintain an airway.
- Intact cough and bulbar function. Cough strength is generally assessed clinically and is very subjective. Stronger cough required with thick or viscous secretions. Peak cough expiratory flow >60L/min is only a useful measure of cough strength in extubated patients.
- Adequate respiratory muscle strength. This can be assessed at the bedside using VC measurements. A VC of 12–15mL/kg is generally required to successfully extubate an average patient.
- Adequate cuff leak.

Laryngeal oedema

Laryngeal oedema may cause extubation failure and post-extubation stridor. An indirect assessment of laryngeal oedema can be made by measuring the leak around the deflated cuff of the ETT. The leak is inversely proportional to the extent of laryngeal oedema. It is of no value in patients who have been ventilated for <24h.

Cuff leak test

In a formal cuff leak test, the patient should be ventilated on a mandatory mode with a low respiratory rate (8 breaths/min) and 8–10mL/kg tidal volume. Inspiratory and expiratory volumes are measured before and after cuff deflation. Several measures have been described:

- Auscultation
  - No leak audible
  - Audible on auscultation of neck
  - Audible at bedside
- Absolute volume leak <110mL is predictive of post-extubation stridor
- Percentage volume leak (pre vs post cuff deflation) <18% is predictive of post-extubation stridor.

Limitations

- Although the cuff leak test is good for predicting post-extubation stridor, it is less able to predict the need for reintubation.

- Ventilating the patient using a mandatory mode when they have just been weaned often presents a problem.
- A non-evidence-based alternative is to perform an 'auscultation' leak test (above) with 10cmH$_2$O of PEEP or CPAP.

Steroids for laryngeal oedema

Laryngeal oedema and post-extubation stridor may be reduced with the administration of corticosteroids. A recent meta-analysis looking specifically at re-intubation attributable to laryngeal oedema showed benefit with intravenous corticosteroids prior to extubation in those at risk of laryngeal oedema.[1]

Our current practice is dexamethasone 4mg four times daily for 48h in those who are suspected of having laryngeal oedema before extubation or for those who have developed post-extubation stridor.

Process of extubation

Extubation should be a simple smooth process if the pre-conditions have been satisfied and adequate preparations have been made.

Preparation

- Drugs and equipment for reintubation should be immediately available, including bag valve mask and airway adjuncts.
- An oxygen mask and a system capable of delivering humidified oxygen.
- Suction equipment and catheters.

Process

- Inform the patient.
- Stop enteral feed (preferably for 4h).
- Aspirate NGT.
- Sit patient up.
- Suction mouth and oropharynx, and aspirate sub-glottic port if present.
- Cut or undo tube ties.
- Deflate cuff with suction catheter passed through tube to withdraw secretions present above cuff, which would otherwise fall into airway.
- Withdraw the ETT with constant aspiration of the suction catheter.
- Apply oxygen mask and observe for any immediate stridor.

Extubation failure

Post-extubation respiratory distress requiring re-intubation is associated with a marked increase in mortality and ICU length of stay. This may be because of the direct complications of re-intubation, an association of re-intubation with unidentified patient factors leading to a worse outcome (the patients who are re-intubated are more unwell), or the development of a new complication post extubation. It is manifested by:

- Dyspnoea
- Tachypnoea
- Tachycardia
- Hypoxaemia: reduced saturations or increased oxygen requirement
- Stridor
- Wheeze
- Noisy or retained secretions.

Early extubation failure (within 4h) in a patient deemed suitable for extubation is usually due to post-extubation stridor or inadequately treated/unrecognized LV dysfunction.

Stridor

Post-extubation stridor occurs in 2–16% of patients extubated after more than 24h of ventilation and accounts for up to 38% of early re-intubations. Factors associated with the development of post-extubation stridor include long-term mechanical ventilation, high cuff pressure, difficult or traumatic intubation, periods of 'fighting the ventilator', and female sex. The most common causes of post-extubation stridor are:
- Laryngospasm—generally clears with 100% oxygen, CPAP, and time
- Laryngeal oedema—a common consequence of endotracheal intubation, but the cuff leak test should identify those at high risk
- Excessive dynamic airway collapse and tracheobronchomalacia—these conditions are considered in 🕮 Chronic obstructive pulmonary disease, p 427. Their significance is unclear.

Management of upper airway oedema

If it is possible to examine the airway with a fibreoptic laryngoscope, it allows a dynamic assessment of the cause of stridor. Patient distress and the emergent situation often preclude such examination.
- Nebulized adrenaline 5mL of 1:1000 repeated 4 hourly. Adrenaline is traditionally the *levo*-isomer, although evidence for increased efficacy or reduced side-effects compared with racemic adrenaline is weak.
- Dexamethasone 4mg four times daily for 48h.
- If the laryngeal oedema persists with a fall in PaO_2, the patient requires re-intubation and a further extubation trial 24–48h later.

Left ventricular failure

Certain factors predispose to LV failure, even when there was no evidence of myocardial dysfunction pre extubation.
- Removal of positive ITP leads to increased preload and afterload.
- If minute ventilation increases after extubation, oxygen demand will increase.
- Patients may find liberation from the ventilator stressful and increase sympathetic output.

If possible, perform a full examination, CXR, ECG, echocardiogram, and SvO_2 before re-intubation in order to guide further therapy.

Respiratory dysfunction

- Atelectasis related to loss of positive airway pressure may increase WOB and cause a failure of gas exchange. Physiotherapy may be valuable in prevention.
- Muscle weakness may contribute to failure of secretion clearance, alveolar hypoventilation, and atelectasis. This combination leads to exhaustion and gas exchange failure.

- Secretion retention is a common cause of failed extubation. An inadequate cough, very large volumes of secretions, or very thick secretions leads to hypoventilation, consolidation, and increased WOB.
- Bronchospasm is common in asthma or COPD. Consider cardiac cause.

Inadequate assessment

Inevitably some patients will be extubated when the assessment of the pre-extubation conditions (above) has been incorrect. The most common causes of extubation failure in this situation are:
- Neurological failure (and failure to keep the airway patent/protected)
- Respiratory muscle weakness
- Poor cough with secretion retention
- Inadequate resolution of underlying pathology.

Management of extubation failure

If possible perform a full examination, CXR, ECG, echocardiogram, and SvO_2 before re-intubation to ascertain cause. Consider fibreoptic laryngoscopy for stridor. The clinical priority of treating the respiratory distress often takes precedence. Depending on the aetiology, consider:
- Nebulized adrenaline for laryngeal oedema
- Bronchodilators for bronchospasm
- Diuretics and ACE inhibition for LV dysfunction
- Physiotherapy
- Access for tracheal suction
  - Nasopharyngeal airway to facilitate suction
  - Mini-tracheostomy may help by facilitating airway toilet and by stimulating a strong cough. Often useful in weak patients, although the only published evidence is for post-thoracic surgical patients.

Non-invasive ventilation

Patients who have respiratory distress post extubation generally need re-intubation rather than NIV. When used as a rescue therapy in unselected patients, NIV has been shown to increase mortality.

When used as a planned therapy (i.e. extubate onto NIV in suitable patients), NIV has been shown to reduce the failed extubation rate.

Re-intubation

This should not be unduly delayed while a cause is found and intubation equipment should be immediately available when any patient is extubated. Consideration should be given to the choice of muscle relaxant as life-threatening hyperkalaemia has been described with the use of suxamethonium in patients with critical illness polyneuropathy requiring reintubation.

1 Fan T, Wang G, Mao B, et al. (2008) Prophylactic administration of parenteral steroids for preventing airway complications after extubation in adults: meta-analysis of randomised placebo controlled trials. *Br Med J* **337**, 1088–91.

5.17 Long-term (home) ventilation

Long-term ventilation (LTV) refers to ventilatory support that is provided for specific periods on a recurring daily basis. It ranges from nocturnal NIV to 24-h continuous tracheostomy ventilation. It can be delivered in the non-hospital environment and is the fastest growing sector of the 'home care' economy, with an estimated prevalence of 6 patients per 100,000 population across Europe. Greater provision of LTV services will be required in the future due to increased survival of patients with congenital disorders resulting in respiratory failure, and increased expectations of survival in patients with critical illness.

LTV allows patients to be discharged from hospital and reduces the frequency of readmission, thereby increasing the efficiency of healthcare resource use. In certain patient groups, such as motor neurone disease, it improves survival and enhances quality of life. In other circumstances it may be used as a bridge to definitive treatment, such as heart–lung transplantation.

Indications

Chest wall disorders
- Kyphoscoliosis,
- Post thoracoplasty (TB treatment).
- Obesity hypoventilation syndrome.
- Ankylosing spondylitis.

Neuromuscular disorders
- Muscular dystrophies: Duchenne, Becker's, limb girdle, Facioscapulohumeral (FSH).
- Myotonic dystrophy.
- Motor neurone disease/amyotrophic lateral sclerosis.
- Spinal muscular atrophy.
- Demyelinating polyneuropathies: Guillain–Barré.
- Cervical spinal cord injury: Chiari malformation, syringomyelia, post-traumatic.

Lung disease
- COPD.
- Brochiectasis.
- Cystic fibrosis.

Central neurological disorders
- Congenital: central hypoventilation syndrome.
- Acquired: brain stem disease, e.g. stroke, tumour.

Other
- Obstructive sleep apnoea hypopnoea syndrome.
- Heart failure when complicated by nocturnal breathing disorders or secondary to respiratory failure from another cause or occurring as a co-morbidity in chronic neuromuscular disorders, e.g. cardiomyopathy in Duchenne muscular dystrophy.
- Failure to wean from acute ventilation following critical illness.

Presentation

Patients who may benefit from LTV may present as:

- An emergency with acute de-compensation in the context of potentially undiagnosed chronic respiratory failure
- A consequence of underlying disease progression
- Failure to wean from 'acute' ventilation.

The principal pathophysiological problem is that of alveolar hypoventilation leading to hypercapnic respiratory failure, but it may be compounded by a loss of respiratory drive secondary to chronic hypercapnia. The symptoms and signs of type II respiratory failure and the investigations required are covered in detail in ☐ Extrapulmonary causes of respiratory failure, p 444.

Patient selection

Patient understanding, family support, pre-existing quality of life, personal care needs, and financial provision are all important factors in deciding whether LTV can usefully be provided.

Evidence of daytime hypercapnia with significant symptom burden is almost always an indication to offer LTV.

In other circumstances the decision to instigate LTV is made by considering the underlying disease, its expected rate of progression, current symptomatology, and degree of abnormal physiology. There are no absolute values which mean that LTV should be instigated.

In general

- Symptoms of respiratory or sleep associated problems
  plus
- Evidence of respiratory muscle or lung disorder (low VC)
  plus
- Evidence of disordered gas exchange (low overnight SpO_2, elevated transcutaneous CO_2 ($tcCO_2$), hypoxia or hypercapnia on ABG, metabolic compensation for chronic hypercapnia)

Specific

- Restrictive conditions—an awake $PaCO_2 > 6.5kPa$ and $PaO_2 < 8.0kPa$.
- Neuromuscular conditions—awake $PaCO_2 > 6.0kPa$ and $PaO_2 < 9.0kPa$.

Individual diseases

- Patients with neuromuscular disorders and kyphoscoliotic patients will generally present semi-electively with significant symptoms. They are most likely to benefit from, and be compliant with, LTV due to previous experience of requiring support to live independently. Occasionally, a co-incidental event (e.g. surgery) will precipitate an ICU admission and patients will present as a 'failed wean'.
- COPD and other lung disease. There is no consensus on which patient groups benefit from NIV used as a treatment for COPD in its own right. However, patients who present acutely with type II respiratory failure will often be referred as a 'failed wean' in ICU. They should be considered for LTV when they have:
  - Weaned successfully to spontaneous (preferably non-invasive) ventilation during the day

- Developed significant hypercapnia overnight due to sleep-disordered breathing.
- Patients with obesity hypoventilation who are admitted with type II respiratory failure may benefit from LTV.

Initiation of therapy

Many patients starting NIV can be initiated either as a day case or at home if outreach nursing support is available. Patients with tracheostomies are usually those who are unable to wean from acute ventilatory support. LTV is therefore initiated in the critical care unit and the need to continue with treatment re-evaluated after weeks or months following discharge.

With PSV an inspiratory pressure of $10cmH_2O$ is the usual starting point. The response is monitored clinically in terms of subjective patient response and comfort. The pressure is titrated (see 'Aims of LTV' below) depending on response to initial settings. A pressure of $>20cmH_2O$ is seldom required. In patients with volume-supported ventilation, large preset tidal volumes are required (10–15mL/kg) to deliver adequate actual tidal volumes due to leaks. In patients in the community, the minimum monitoring required on commencing therapy is SpO_2, preferably with $tcCO_2$.

Aims of long-term ventilation

- To improve ABG to nearly normal values to prevent 'medical' complications of hypoventilation, e.g. cor pulmonale, hypertension.
- To resolve symptoms without discomfort, reduction in quality of life, or sleep disruption.
- To maximize ventilator-free time.
- To facilitate independent living.

Methods of long-term ventilation

Non-invasive ventilation

- Usually only used for nocturnal ventilation or up to ~16h per day.
- Longer periods (even up to 24-h continuous ventilation) are possible but may compromise quality of life.
- Requires intact bulbar function.

NIV interfaces

- Facemask—used in acute settings, generally less well tolerated due to discomfort, reduction in communication, and tendency to cause nasal bridge necrosis.
- Nasal mask—most common, may need chin strap/cervical soft collar to prevent mouth losses.
- Nasal pillows—fit into nostrils; increasingly effective and popular as allow extension of NIV into 'normal daytime living'.
- Mouthpiece—used during the day to supplement nocturnal NIV.

Non-invasive ventilators and modes

- The choice of ventilator is determined by the degree of dependence the patient has on this equipment.
- For ease of use, simple ventilators with few alarms are better for patients who are primarily using NIV for symptomatic control.
- Complex ventilators with a comprehensive alarm system are required for patients in whom the therapy is genuinely life supporting.

- Battery life and battery charging requirements (independent of ventilator preferable) also influence choice.
- Bilevel turbine ventilators with leak circuit (e.g. whisper valve) to allow CO_2 elimination are commonly used.
- The mode most frequently employed is PSV with back-up timed pressure control breaths (S/T mode).

Complications of long-term NIV
- Air leaks reduce the efficiency of ventilation and may cause sleep fragmentation. Treatments include chin straps, preventing neck flexion with collars, semi-recumbent positioning, decreasing peak pressures, increasing ramp time, increasing delivered volume, and changing interface.
- Nasal dryness, congestion, and rhinitis: humidification vital. HMEs are not usually effective in NIV and heated water humidifiers may be needed, depending upon patient preference. Approximately 60% of patients use humidification.
- Aerophagia may cause flatulence and abdominal distension, compromising ventilation. A didactic bowel regimen and maintaining IPAP <25cmH$_2$O helps to prevent this.
- Gastric distension may predispose to regurgitation of gastric contents so nocturnal gastrostomy feeding should be avoided.

Invasive (tracheostomy) ventilation
- Used in patients without intact bulbar function or requiring more than 16h of ventilation per day.
- May be appropriate in patients who are unable to clear secretions and require regular tracheal toilet.

Tracheostomy interface
- Generally an uncuffed tracheostomy tube is used to allow speech and facilitate swallowing.
- Should have an inner tube that can be easily changed in the event of blockage and to prevent development of potentially pathogenic biofilm.
- A siliconized (Bivona) tube, which requires changing every 5–7 days, is useful.
- Use a suction machine for secretion clearance, mucolytics (nebulized saline), and a daily routine of 'bagging'.

Invasive ventilators and modes
- Complex ventilators with comprehensive alarms are generally used in pressure-control mode to compensate for leak. If volume modes are used typically values up to 15mL/kg are required to compensate for the leak.
- Prolonged inspiratory time facilitates speech.
- Expiratory valve required to optimize CO_2 clearance.
- Bilevel pressure ventilation with a leak circuit may achieve adequate CO_2 clearance. EPAP maintains lung volume in expiration.

Complications of long-term tracheostomy ventilation
- Chronic aspiration.
- Tracheal ulceration/mucus plugging: from poor tracheal hygiene or inadequate humidification.

- Social aversion.
- Sudden death from accidental de-cannulation or disconnection or power failure.
- Granulation formation.
- Acquired suprastomal tracheomalacia.

General considerations for the long-term ventilation patient

- Patients are commonly ventilator dependent so provision for power and equipment failure must be made. Ventilators must have internal and external batteries (to allow charging and changing when out and about).
- A second ventilator is often required (one wheelchair mounted and one domestic), which will also cover equipment failure.
- Pulse oximetry is required for overnight monitoring to avoid unrecognized life-threatening equipment failure causing hypoxaemia in ventilator-dependent patients (>12h per day).
- An audible alarm system is needed to alert carers to disconnection or blockage. Carers themselves will often need to be resident or able to attend rapidly in the event of alarm.

Simple problems can have an immense impact on respiratory function. Aggressive early management may avoid these issues.

- Constipation should be treated aggressively and specific bowel protocols used.
- Cough assist devices can be extremely useful for assisting sputum expectoration in weak patients.
- Early antibiotic therapy.
- The use of anti-inflammatory/immunostimulant (e.g. azithromycin) in specifc conditions. These agents have a long history of use in cystic fibrosis and pan-bronchilolitis, where they have been shown to reduce the frequency of infective exacerbations and improve VC. Their use is not associated with a reduced microbiological load and hence is thought to improve mucosal integrity and immune response, as well as reduce inflammation. They are particularly effective in patients colonized with pseudomonas.

Long-term management of patients in the community

Ongoing monitoring of response to and efficacy of treatment can be done in the home with SpO_2 and $tcCO_2$ measurements when required. This requires a dedicated home ventilation team, including:

- A consultant with specific commitment and appropriate experience.
- Specialist nurses co-ordinating day-to-day patient management.
- A physiotherapist.

There should also be support services:

- A minimum of yearly attendance at an outpatient clinic to facilitate holistic care: clinical assessment, input from other medical specialities, equipment monitoring and update, compliance with therapy, screening for common complications of underlying disease, e.g. cardiomyopathy, progression of bulbar dysfunction.
- An on-call service for advice and an action plan for patients becoming acutely unwell.

5.18 **Outcome and follow-up**

Patient outcome from ICU treatment can be described in terms of short- and longer-term survival (mortality outcomes) and quality of life, and neuropsychological and functional status (non-mortality outcomes).

Mortality outcomes

The ICU mortality in the UK is over 20% and by the time of hospital discharge approaches 30%. Differences in case mix and staffing between ICUs in different countries make it difficult to produce meaningful international ICU mortality comparisons. France has similar overall outcomes to the UK, but Australia reports hospital mortality at around 15%.

Risk-adjusted analysis of mortality outcomes has become common, most frequently using the standardised mortality ratio. These analyses seek to control for variation in mortality rates caused by differences in severity of illness, case mix, diagnostic categories, co-morbidities, and physiological derangement at presentation. While useful as screening tools to identify areas for further investigation, significant error arises from poor-quality data, poor-quality risk-adjustment models, small population sizes, and often from misinterpretation of accurate analyses.

Kaplan–Meier survival curves for an ICU population demonstrate a very high initial mortality that gradually diminishes with time (Fig. 5.32). The survival time corresponding to any proportion of the patient cohort is easily calculated, and survival curves of different cohorts can be compared (Fig. 5.33). A large UK study demonstrated 5-year mortality amongst ICU survivors of 33.4%. Mortality was greater than that of the general population for 4 years following ICU admission. Multivariate analysis showed that the risk factors for mortality in those admitted to ICU were age, APACHE II score on admission, and diagnostic category.

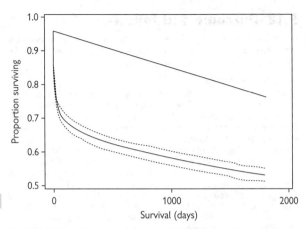

Fig. 5.32 A Kaplan–Meier survival curve model for ICU patients. The dashed lines represent the 95% CI for the survival line. The straight line represents the survival of the same cohort of patients if they were subjected to the same age- and sex-adjusted mortality rates as the normal population. Reproduced with permission from Wright JC, Plenderleith L, and Ridley SA (2003) Long-term survival following intensive care: Subgroup analysis and comparison with the general population. *Anaesthesia* **58**(7), 637–642. © John Wiley and Sons, 2003.

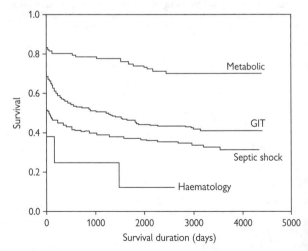

Fig. 5.33 Survival curves for different patient groups. GIT, gastrointestinal system. Reproduced with permission from Wright JC, Plenderleith L, and Ridley SA (2003). Long-term survival following intensive care: Subgroup analysis and comparison with the general population. *Anaesthesia* **58**(7), 637–642. © John Wiley and Sons, 2003.

Non-mortality outcomes

The most commonly considered non-mortality outcomes are:
- Physical impairment and disability
- Neuropsychological impairment
- Health-related quality of life.

Physical impairment

Physical recovery following critical illness can take >12 months, particularly in patients over 50 years and with longer ICU lengths of stay.

Patients often have a variety of symptoms and physical signs.

Muscle wasting

Prolonged ICU treatment is associated with a dramatic loss of muscle mass, with losses of 2% lean body mass per day reported. Functional return is dependent on regaining this muscle mass, which in turn is dependent on adequate nutrition. However, nutritional intake during the recovery period is often inadequate because of:
- Lack of appetite
- Generalized weakness
- Depression
- Breathlessness
- Swallowing difficulties
- Altered taste perception
- Dysfunction of gut-derived appetite regulatory hormones.

Critical illness polyneuromyopathy

A significant proportion of patients in the ICU develop a generalized weakness that may persist for years after hospital discharge. ICU-acquired neuromuscular disorders present as diffuse skeletal-muscle flaccid weakness and reduced or absent deep tendon reflexes. Terms adopted to define ICU acquired weakness include critical illness polyneuropathy (CIP), critical illness myopathy (CIM), and the overlap syndrome critical illness polyneuromyopathy (CIPM).

The risk factors for CIPM are:
- Sepsis
- SIRS
- Multiorgan failure
- Hyperglycaemia
- Female sex
- Drugs (corticosteriods, neuromuscular blockade, aminoglycosides).

Arthropathy

- Patients often complain of joint stiffness (commonly due to heterotropic ossification) and joint pain.

Breathlessness

Breathlessness on exertion is a common symptom reported by ICU survivors. Causes include:
- Muscle weakness
- Neuropathy
- Pulmonary fibrosis
- Progression of premorbid respiratory and cardiac disease
- Psychological factors.

Respiratory function following ICU discharge has been most extensively investigated in ARDS survivors. Although they all have abnormal pulmonary function tests in the first 3 months of recovery, this gradually improves and reaches a stable plateau over the following 12 months. Pulmonary function tests following ARDS generally demonstrate a restrictive ventilatory defect with some impairment of diffusion capacity. The most frequent persistent radiological abnormality seen in ARDS survivors is a course reticular pattern with an anterior distribution visible on a CT scan. However, the importance of these radiological changes to function remains unclear. A 5-year follow-up of young ARDS survivors demonstrated that over 70% of these patients returned to work despite some degree of functional disability. The functional disability is normally 'extrapulmonary' in origin and therefore not related to deficits in lung function.

Sexual dysfunction
See box.

Sexual dysfunction in ICU survivors

Sexual dysfunction is commonly reported in ICU survivors and specific causes include:
- Poor body image scores
  - Scars
  - Weight loss/gain
  - Surgical stomata
  - Amputations
  - Dressings
- Pre-existing medical conditions (e.g. diabetes, coronary artery disease)
- Surgery (vascular, urological, gynaecological, gastrointestinal)
- Pelvic trauma
- Medications (antidepressants, beta adrenergic antagonists, proton pump inhibitors, cardiac glycosides, diuretics, anti-hypertensives, dopamine agonists).

When a patient who has survived a period of illness is still sexually active, or wants to have a sexual relationship, it is important to openly acknowledge this as an integral part of the recovery process. Although most cases of sexual dysfunction can be treated with pharmacological or psychological interventions, at the current time medical practitioners rarely seek the presence of sexual dysfunction in ICU survivors or offer any referral or treatment.

Other physical limitations
- Small bladder syndrome.
- Sleep disturbances.
- Pain.
- Loss of taste and smell.
- Alopecia.

Psychological impairment

Delirium

Delirium is defined as a disturbance of consciousness with inattention, accompanied by a change in cognition or perceptual disturbance, that develops over a short period of time (hours to days) and fluctuates over time. Recent studies have estimated the incidence of delirium in certain cohorts of ICU patients to be as high as 80%. The hypoactive form of delirium commonly predominates, particularly in the elderly, and is often called acute encephalopathy rather than delirium. Accurate bedside assessment of delirium on the ICU remains a challenge but the recent validation of the CAM-ICU tool should prove a valuable research tool for future studies.

Aetiological factors for delirium on the ICU are summarized in the box. It is important to remember that delirium usually has more than one cause.

Delirium on the ICU is associated with prolongation of ICU and hospital stay, and long-term psychological morbidity, and is independently associated with increased mortality.

Causes of delirium on ICU

D	Drugs, drugs, drugs
E	Eyes, ears[1]
L	Low O_2 states (MI, ARDS, PE, chronic heart failure (CHF), COPD)[2]
I	Infection
R	Retention (of urine or stool), restraints
I	Ictal
U	Underhydration/undernutrition
M	Metabolic
(S)	Subdural, sleep deprivation

[1] Poor vision and hearing are considered to be more risk factors than true causes, but should be 'fixed' or improved if possible. Cerumen is a common cause of hearing impairment.

[2] 'Low O_2 states' does *not* necessarily mean hypoxia, rather it is a reminder that patients with a hypoxic insult (e.g. MI, stroke, PE) may present with mental status changes with or without other typical symptoms/signs of these diagnoses.

Anxiety and depression

Survivors of general ICU treatment have an estimated prevalence of clinically significant anxiety and depression of 30–50% following discharge, falling to 20–30% in the long term. Patients are more likely to suffer from anxiety and depression if they have no factual recall for the ICU experience. Rates of long-term clinical depression up to 67% have been reported in survivors of ARDS. There is a correlation with the number of days actively sedated.

Post-traumatic stress disorder

Prevalence rates of post-traumatic stress disorder (PTSD) and PTSD symptomatology have been reported in up to 64% of ICU survivors (extremely high relative to other medical populations).

Potential risk factors for the development of PTSD after ICU treatment include:
- Previous psychological/psychiatric history
- Delirium on ICU
- Delusional memory for ICU experience
- Traumatic memory for ICU experience
- Female gender
- Greater levels of sedation
- Younger age
- Longer duration of mechanical ventilation
- Prolonged hospital stay
- Prolonged ICU length of stay.

Cognitive dysfunction
Cognitive dysfunction affects up to 78% of ICU survivors. Follow-up of ARDS survivors has demonstrated neurocognitive impairments up to 2 years after ICU discharge. Deficits occur predominantly in memory, attention and executive function. The exact mechanisms involved remain unclear, but include neurotransmitter imbalances and brain injury following hypoxia or hypotension. Neuropsychological testing is difficult on the ICU, but can be easily performed in the ICU follow-up clinic. Screening for delirium on the ICU, sophisticated imaging techniques, and measurement of specific markers of brain injury may help identify patients at risk of prolonged cognitive dysfunction.

Other psychological impairments
- Paranoia and delusions.
- Guilt and anger.
- Recurrent nightmares.
- Reduced confidence.
- Family conflict.
- Reduced libido.
- Irritability.
- Financial difficulties.

Quality of life and heath-related quality of life
Quality of life is a subjective, multidimensional concept comprising five major domains:
- Physical status and functional abilities
- Psychological status and well-being
- Social interactions
- Economic and/or vocational status and factors
- Religious and/or spiritual status.

Healthcare researchers commonly restrict their focus to the quality of life dimensions associated with illness and treatment. This focus is termed 'health-related quality of life' (HRQL, Fig. 5.34). Many different outcome measures of HRQL have been developed (see box).

Changes in HRQL scores
Several questionnaire-based studies have estimated pre-ICU HRQL scores and compared these with scores measured after ICU discharge. These studies demonstrate:

- Overall post-ICU HRQL scores are poor and lower than population norms
- Prolonged stays in the ICU do not necessarily result in lower long-term HRQL
- Patients who enjoy a normal HRQL before ICU admission suffer significant decreases following their illness
- The 6-month HRQL scores of survivors of general ICU treatment are predominantly a function of admission diagnosis
- Patients with pre-existing morbidity show some improvement in their HRQL score 6 months after ICU admission, principally by improvements in mental health, vitality, and social functioning.

Follow-up from intensive care

The evolution and development of intensive care as a specialty has resulted in more patients surviving a period of critical illness. However, extended follow-up of survivors of critical illness has highlighted that these patients can experience longer-term physical and psychosocial complaints.

One mechanism of extended follow-up is the ICU follow-up clinic. A 2006 survey demonstrated the existence of approximately 80 of these clinics in the UK, the first being established in 1987. ICU follow-up aims to ameliorate or treat the physical and psychological burden by improving and speeding up the quality of recovery (see box). Evidence that non-mortality outcomes are improved by ICU follow up is awaited.

Objectives of extended ICU follow-up
- Explanation of critical illness and ICU-based treatments.
- Opportunity for discussion and questions.
- Identification of ICU/critical illness specific morbidity.
- Surveillance and treatment of physical and psychological morbidities.
- Opportunity for audit, research, and information gathering to aid service improvement.

A variety of instruments are available to assess non-mortality outcomes. These can be disease-specific measures (more appropriate in investigating specific symptom sets) or generic measurements. However, the majority of outcome instruments that have been used in ICU follow-up have not been rigorously validated in this setting and results must be interpreted with caution.

A brief description of the most commonly applied generic outcome measures is given in the box.

Hospital Anxiety and Depression Scale (HADS)

The HADS is a questionnaire composed of statements relevant to either generalized anxiety or depression. The HADS has been validated in a variety of settings to provide a reliable and simple tool for the measurement of mental function.

Short-Form Health Survey—36 items (SF-36)

The SF-36 is a generic, self-administered general health status survey with 36 questions aggregated into eight domains/dimensions: general health, physical functioning, role physical, role emotional, social functioning, bodily pain, vitality, and mental health. Each is scored from 0 (worst score) to 100 (best score). These dimensions can be combined to form physical and mental component scores. The SF-36 has been found to be reliable, stable over time, and valid in the ICU setting.

EuroQol five-dimensions (EQ-5D)

The EQ-5D questionnaire is a simple, standardized generic instrument designed to measure health outcome. The EQ-5D comprises two parts: the EQ-5D self-classifier, a self-reported description of health problems according to a five-dimensional classification, i.e. mobility, self-care, usual activities, pain/discomfort, and anxiety/depression, and the EQ visual analogue scale (VAS), a self-rated health status using a VAS to record perceptions of the patient's own current overall health.

Karnofsky Performance Status (KPS) and Karnofsky index

KPS is a simple, objective measure of physical functional status. The Karnofsky index ranges in units of 10 from 0 (death) to 100, where 100 = no limitations, >80 indicates the ability to carry on normal activities independently, and <80 suggests disability in physical performance. KPS has been validated and recommended as a reliable measure of physical performance in HRQL.

ICU outcome studies are often difficult to compare as they frequently include a different case mix of patients and employ a variety of outcome measures that are administered at different follow-up time points. However, extended follow-up of ICU survivors has provided a wealth of information on the common physical and psychological problems encountered during the recovery period.

Further reading

Cuthbertson BH, Scott J, Strachan M, Kilonzo M, and Vale L (2005) Quality of life before and after intensive care. *Anaesthesia* **60**(4), 332–339.

Ely EW, Shintani A, Truman B, *et al.* (2004) Delirium as a predictor of mortality in mechanically ventilated patients in the intensive care unit. *JAMA* **291**(14), 1753–1762.

Griffiths J, Fortune G, Barber V, and Young J (2007) The prevalence of post traumatic stress disorder in survivors of ICU treatment: a systematic review. *Intensive Care Med* **33**, 1506–1518.

Heyland DK, Guyatt G, Cook DJ, *et al.* (1998) Frequency and methodologic rigor of quality-of-life assessments in the critical care literature. *Crit Care Med* **26**(3), 591–598.

Treatment of specific diseases

6.1 Acute respiratory distress syndrome

Definition

Acute respiratory distress syndrome (ARDS) was first described in 1967 as a syndrome of refractory hypoxaemia. Since then a number of definitions have been used for diagnostic purposes and to identify patients for enrollment into clinical trials.

Murray Lung Injury Score

Proposed in 1988, this definition incorporates a lung injury score (Table 6.1) and includes consideration of the time course (acute or chronic) and aetiology of ARDS.

Table 6.1 Lung injury scores

Chest radiograph	Score
No alveolar consolidation	0
Alveolar consolidation confined to 1 quadrant	1
Alveolar consolidation confined to 2 quadrants	2
Alveolar consolidation confined to 3 quadrants	3
Alveolar consolidation confined to 4 quadrants	4
Hypoxaemia score	
PaO_2/FiO_2 >300mmHg	0
PaO_2/FiO_2 225–299mmHg	1
PaO_2/FiO_2 175–224mmHg	2
PaO_2/FiO_2 100–174mmHg	3
PaO_2/FiO_2 <100mmHg	4
PEEP score (when mechanically ventilated)	
<5cmH$_2$O	0
6–8cmH$_2$O	1
9–11cmH$_2$O	2
12–14cmH$_2$O	3
>15cmH$_2$O	4
Respiratory system compliance score (when available)	
>80mL/cmH$_2$O	0
60–79mL/cmH$_2$O	1
40–59mL/cmH$_2$O	2
20–39mL/cmH$_2$O	3
<19mL/cmH$_2$O	4

The score is calculated by adding the sum of each component and dividing by the number of components used.

No lung injury	0
Mild to moderate lung injury	0.1–2.5
Severe lung injury (ARDS)	>2.5

The Murray score is still used as a method of quantifying the severity of lung injury.

North American-European Consensus Conference definition[1]

The North American-European Consensus Conference (NAECC) definition was published in 1994 and proposed that ALI was a continuum, with ARDS representing the more severe form of injury.

Acute lung injury
- Acute onset.
- PaO_2/FiO_2 < 40kPa (300mmHg), regardless of PEEP.
- Bilateral infiltrates seen on frontal chest radiograph.
- Pulmonary artery occlusion pressure ≤18mmHg (when measured) or no clinical evidence of left atrial hypertension.

Acute respiratory distress syndrome
As ALI except:
- PaO_2/FiO_2 ≤27kPa (200mmHg) regardless of PEEP level.

These definitions of ALI and ARDS are the most current and have the most widespread acceptance. Despite a number of criticisms, they were not revised when the Consensus Conference met again in 2000. Criticisms include:
- Lack of definition for 'acute'
- No mention of the effect of aetiology on prognosis
- No standardized approach to interpreting the chest radiograph
- The effect of ventilatory strategy is not included
- No mention is made of likely pathological processes.

Epidemiology

The reported incidence of ARDS varies from 4.8 to 34 per 100,000 population annually (105 person·years). It is present in 5–15% of critically ill patients on ICUs while approximately 20% of mechanically ventilated ICU patients fulfill the criteria for ARDS. The incidence rises with increasing patient age and changes with the underlying clinical condition.

ALI is more common, with reported incidences of up to 78.9/105 person years. This translates to approximately 190 000 cases of ALI annually in the USA.

Aetiology

The aetiology of ARDS is important as each underlying cause requires specific management (Table 6.2). A recent meta-analysis suggests that there is no difference in mortality between pulmonary and extra-pulmonary causes of ARDS. Some diagnostic subgroups (such as trauma) appear to have a lower mortality.

Table 6.2 Causes of ARDS[2]

Cause	Frequency (%)	Cause	Frequency (%)
Pulmonary	54.7–57	Extra-pulmonary	20.4–43
Pneumonia	30–46.4	Sepsis	25.4–32
Aspiration	17	Trauma	2
Contusion	10.5–11	Transfusion-related ALI	3.3–5
Fat emboli	Rare	Pancreatitis	2
Inhalational injury	Rare	Drug overdose	0.7
Reperfusion (following lung transplantation)	Rare	Cardiopulmonary bypass	Rare

Sepsis

Sepsis, including pulmonary infections, is the most common cause of ARDS. As such it must be considered in any patient with ARDS associated with hypotension or fever.

Pneumonia

Common community and hospital-acquired organisms can lead to the development of ARDS, including:

- *Streptococcus pneumonia*
- *Legionella pneumophilia*
- *Staphylococcus aureus*
- *Pseudomonas aeruginoa*
- *Escherichia coli* and other Gram-negative rods
- *Pneumocystis jirovecii*
- Respiratory viruses.

Aspiration pneumonitis

ARDS develops in around a third of patients following aspiration of gastric contents. Aspiration of non-acidic stomach contents may be harmful to the lung, suggesting that gastric enzymes as well as stomach acid cause lung injury.

Massive blood transfusion

Massive blood transfusion itself may be a cause of ARDS or be a surrogate marker that identifies high-risk patients. Transfusion of >15 units of blood is a risk factor for subsequently developing ARDS.

Transfusion-related acute lung injury

Transfusion-related acute lung injury (TRALI) may develop following transfusion of a single unit of plasma-containing blood product which includes fresh frozen plasma, platelets, and packed red cells. Diagnosis is difficult but lung injury must develop within 6h of transfusion and there should be no alternative explanation for ARDS.

Lung transplantation

Lung injury may develop in the first few hours following lung transplantation as a result of reperfusion injury or in the first 2–3 days as a result of primary graft failure and acute rejection.

Drugs

ARDS may develop following ingestion of:

- Amiodarone
- Aspirin
- Bleomycin
- Cocaine
- Iodine (radiographic contrast media)
- Methotrexate
- Mitomycin
- Nitrofurantoin
- Opiates
- Propylthiouracil
- Tricyclic antidepressants.

See 📖 Drug-induced lung disease p 438 and www.pneumotox.com.

Patient factors

A high risk of progression to ARDS is seen in patients with:

- Sepsis
- Chronic liver disease
- History of chronic alcohol excess
- Chronic respiratory disease
- Low serum pH.

Pathophysiology

ARDS is classically described as having three phases:

- Exudative
- Proliferative
- Fibrotic.

However, there is considerable overlap between these three stages, with fibrosis, traditionally thought of as a late phenomenon, now known to start early in the evolution of ARDS.[3]

Initial insult

Following lung injury, type 1 pneumocytes become swollen, damaged and detached from their basement membrane. Pulmonary vascular endothelial cells also swell and the capillaries become occluded with fibrin thrombi.

This widespread damage disrupts the alveolar–capillary barrier and is pathologically known as DAD. Loss of integrity of this barrier allows proteinaceous fluid, mostly comprising plasma proteins such a fibrin and complement, to cross into the alveolar airspaces.

Damage also occurs to type 2 pneumocytes, resulting in decreased surfactant production.

Inflammatory activation
- Alveolar macrophages secrete IL-1, IL-6, IL-8, IL-10, and TNF-α, which attract and activate neutrophils.
- Neutrophils collect in the capillary bed before crossing into the oedema-filled alveolae. Neutrophils release a range of pro-inflammatory molecules, including proteases, leukotrienes, and platelet-activating factor. Whether neutrophilic inflammation is the cause of lung injury or occurs as a result is unclear. Neutropenic patients still develop ARDS and an increased risk of ARDS was not seen in a trial where patients with pneumonia were given granulocyte colony-stimulating factor to boost neutrophil numbers.
- Abnormal activation of the coagulation cascade and the formation of platelet-fibrin thrombi further impacts on ventilation/perfusion mismatching.

Repair and fibrosis
Following the initial injury there is expansion in the number of vascular endothelial cells and type 2 pneumocytes. Ongoing vascular damage leads to intimal proliferation, while the numbers of type 2 cells increases in an attempt to cover the basement membrane left exposed by the damaged type 1 cells.
- The fibrinous exudate becomes organized and hyaline membranes form.
- Myofibroblasts begin to enter the interstitial and alveolar spaces.
- Fibrosis occurs in both the interstitium and vessel walls, with myofibroblasts, activated by IL-8, producing collagen in both the interstitium and the alveoli.
- Type 2 pneumocyte numbers increase, with many differentiating into type 1 pneumocytes and relining the basement membrane.

Resolution
- As critical illness resolves, sodium is actively transported from the airspaces with water following the osmotic gradient out of the alveolus.
- Soluble proteins diffuse out of the alveolus while less soluble proteins, such as hyaline, are removed by epithelial cells and macrophages.
- Neutrophils undergo apoptosis and are then phagocytosed by macrophages.

Following ARDS, the lungs of some patients may show complete recovery, although this process may take many months. At its most destructive ARDS leaves patients with severe honeycombing in keeping with end-stage fibrotic lung disease.

Ventilator-associated lung injury
Mechanically ventilating a patient with ALI or ARDS can perpetuate or increase the damage to the lungs. VALI is said to occur when a patient develops acute lung injury whilst mechanically ventilated. It is distinct from VILI, which refers to ALI where the sole aetiology is injurious mechanical ventilation (see Complications of ventilation, p 244).

Because of the heterogeneous nature of the lung in ARDS, with areas of atelectasis, epithelial and endothelial damage, altered regional lung compliance, and surfactant deficiencies, mechanical ventilation, whilst unavoidable, may contribute to perpetuating lung injury. Mechanical ventilation affects the lung in multiple ways.[4]

Biotrauma
Biotrauma is the term given to the systemic inflammation produced by mechanical ventilation. Biotrauma is a risk factor for developing the multiorgan dysfunction that is responsible for the high mortality of ARDS.

Atelectrauma
The cyclical opening and closing of lung units during ventilation is referred to as atelectrauma. Alveolar trauma occurs when the alveolus snaps open with inspiration and then collapses with expiration. The recurrent cycling of adjacent alveolar units creates shear stress in the interstitium, exacerbating the inflammatory insult.

Volutrauma
Volutrauma refers to alveolar over-distension that occurs during mechanical ventilation with large tidal volumes. Animal models comparing increased or limited lung volumes with increasing airway pressure show significant lung injury with high lung volumes and high pressures but little injury with normal lung volumes and high pressures. Observational studies in humans show that increasing tidal volume, where over-distension occurs, is an independent risk factor for VALI.

With a large amount of alveolar fluid and airway collapse the area of lung available for ventilation is small—the concept of the 'baby lung'. Volutrauma may occur in established ARDS despite relatively small tidal volumes being delivered by mechanical ventilation because of a dramatic reduction in available, ventilatable lung.

Barotrauma
The use of high peak airway pressure is damaging to the lung. Over-distension of the alveolus leads to alveolar rupture, allowing air to escape into the interstitium. At its most subtle barotrauma manifests itself as pulmonary interstitial emphysema, visible on CT scans, but may also cause pneumothorax, subcutaneous emphysema, pneumopericardium, and potentially cardiorespiratory arrest.

Diagnosis
There is no specific test for the diagnosis of ARDS. Diagnosis of ARDS is made on clinical grounds in accordance with the NAECC definition. Significant differential diagnoses must be excluded (see below).

Difficulty arises around the exclusion of raised left atrial pressure with the diminishing use of pulmonary artery occlusion catheters. Additionally, patients with ARDS may have simultaneous cardiac dysfunction. Both brain natriuretic peptide (BNP) and echocardiography have been used to exclude cardiogenic pulmonary oedema.

Previous pulmonary imaging may provide information regarding pre-existing pulmonary disease. Bronchoscopy, BAL, CT scanning, and possibly open-lung biopsy are useful to help exclude other diagnosis that may mimic ARDS.

Differential diagnosis
- Multilobar pneumonia (including PCP, mycobacteria, legionella) (📖 Pneumonia, p 493).
- Viral pneumonia (📖 Pneumonia, p 493).
- Acute interstitial pneumonia (Hamman–Rich syndrome, idiopathic ARDS) (📖 Interstitial lung disease, p 468).
- Cardiogenic pulmonary oedema (📖 Cardiogenic pulmonary oedema, p 402).
- Diffuse alveolar haemorrhage (Goodpasture's, Wegener's, SLE) (📖 Alveolar haemorrhage and pulmonary vasculitis, p 388).
- Idiopathic acute eosinophilic pneumonia (📖 Pneumonia, p 493).
- Lymphangitis carcinomatosis.
- Cryptogenic organizing pneumonia (📖 Interstitial lung disease, p 468).
- Graft versus host disease (📖 The haematology patient, p 452).

Clinical picture

Typically ARDS will develop 24–48h after the initial insult but may be the presenting feature. Patients complain of progressive, severe dyspnoea and in some case a dry cough.

Examination of the patient may reveal a diminished air entry at the lung base with an area of coarse crackles reflecting the areas of consolidated and atelectatic lung. Respiratory examination, however, is often surprisingly normal. Symptoms and signs of the cause of ARDS may also be apparent on examination.

ARDS is characterized by severe and often refractory hypoxia. This is a product of ventilation/perfusion mismatch and intrapulmonary shunt due to alveolar flooding and atelectasis. There is some contribution to hypoxia from a reduction in gas diffusion.

Pulmonary compliance is reduced due to atelectasis, alveolar oedema, and fibroproliferation. Compliance is normal in relatively unaffected lung units within the heterogeneous ARDS lung. Increasing dead space due to extensive fibroproliferation in late-stage ARDS leads to significant hypercapnia.

Pulmonary hypertension occurs frequently, with resultant RV failure. This is due to hypoxic pulmonary vasoconstriction and the effect of inflammatory mediators (e.g. thromboxane A2) and may be seen in the late stages of ARDS following vascular remodelling.

ARDS is often seen as the pulmonary manifestation of a systemic inflammatory response and is therefore usually accompanied by other organ disease, including vasodilation, hypotension, and acute kidney injury. Death is usually as a result of multiorgan failure related to systemic inflammation, rather than as a result of hypoxaemic respiratory failure.

Investigation

Radiology

CXR

Although the chest radiograph appearances form part of the definition of ARDS the changes seen are rather non-specific.

- Initial appearances may be unremarkable unless ARDS is secondary to a pulmonary cause such as pneumonia. During the first 12–24h bilateral, hazy opacities develop, often described as 'ground glass'.
- Cardiomegaly, perihilar distribution of infiltrates and consolidation, septal lines, and early pleural effusion may point towards cardiogenic pulmonary oedema, but radiographic features are often indistinguishable (see 📖 Diagnosis of respiratory failure, p 22).
- Over the following days to weeks lucencies form, demonstrating the heterogeneous pulmonary changes seen in ARDS, see Fig. 6.1.
- New infiltrates that later develop may represent VAP.

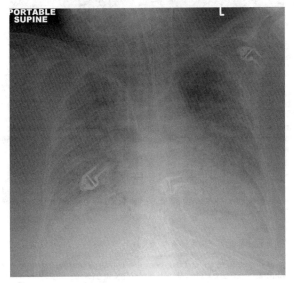

Fig. 6.1 Chest radiograph of a patient with typical ARDS. Diffuse, bilateral pulmonary opacification affecting all lung zones equally in an ICU patient with multiple tubes/lines.

Computerized tomography

Thoracic CT imaging shows a range of changes from consolidated lung, ground glass to normally aerated lung. Consolidation is predominantly seen in the dependent areas, progressing through ground glass to normally aerated lung above, see Fig. 6.2.

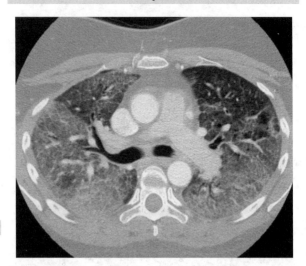

Fig. 6.2 CT of ARDS pattern with diffuse ground glass opacity bilaterally, exhibiting ventrodorsal gradient with increasing opacity posteriorly where ground glass opacity merges to consolidation.

Bronchoalveolar lavage
In the early phase of ARDS neutrophils predominate in lavage fluid but as inflammation continues a larger number of macrophages appear while the numbers of neutrophils diminish.

Lung function
Conventional pulmonary function testing cannot be performed on mechanically ventilated patients. However, re-breathing techniques used during mechanically ventilation show significant reduction of FRC and gas diffusion.

Lung biopsy
Transbronchial lung biopsy
Transbronchial lung biopsy (TBLB) in combination with BAL shows good correlation with open-lung biopsy in the investigation of new pulmonary infiltrates in mechanically ventilated critically ill patients. Studies of TBLB are limited by small sample sizes but no deaths are reported. Bleeding and pneumothorax represent the major complications. There are no specific studies of TBLB in the management of ARDS.

Open lung biopsy
Open-lung biopsy (OLB) can be used to confirm the diagnosis of ARDS in patients where pulmonary infiltrates are slow to resolve and diagnostic queries remain. Major complications (including bleeding, pneumothorax, and persistent air leak) are seen in 7% of patients, with minor complications in 40%. Mortality rates are low (<1%) and recent studies suggest that

OLB can be performed safely at the bedside in ICUs. Retrospective and prospective studies suggest the results of OLB changes patients' management in around 85% of patients with either addition of specific therapy or withdrawal of unnecessary treatment. It should be noted that the majority of these patients were immunosuppressed and the most common diagnoses included CMV pneumonits, cryptogenic organizing pneumonia, and graft versus host disease.

Management

The aim of the management of patients with ARDS is to maintain tissue oxygenation with a ventilation strategy that minimizes ongoing lung damage, while supporting other failing organs, until the lung injury resolves.

Many drug treatments have been trialled for the treatment of ARDS and were the subject of an extensive Cochrane review in 2004.[5] To date none have conferred a survival advantage.

Anti-inflammatory drugs

Corticosteroids

Steroids reduce levels of pro-inflammatory cytokines (e.g. TNF-α, IL-1β, IL-6) and arachidonic acid metabolites by suppressing transcription at a nuclear level. The use of steroids has been studied in both early (<72h) and late (7–28 days) ARDS. Steroids cause hyperglycemia and exacerbate critical illness poly(myo)neuropathy, and concern exists surrounding the potential increased risk of infection.

- The use of steroids in patients at risk of ARDS is not recommended. A recent meta-analysis in the *BMJ*[6] suggests that steroids may increase the possibility of ARDS in at-risk patients and that there is no effect on mortality.
- The use of corticosteroids for the treatment of ARDS is not currently recommended after the ARDS Network showed no change in either 60- or 180-day mortality. This result is supported by the *BMJ* meta-analysis but refuted by a separate meta-analysis performed by Meduri *et al.* (despite both analyses containing almost the same papers, including the ARDS Network data).[7] The conclusion raised by the Meduri meta-analysis, while interesting, requires validation in a large double-blind placebo-controlled trial before further clinical implementation. They were able to demonstrate an improvement in oxygenation and lung compliance but also an increase in the rate of neuromuscular weakness and hyperglycemia. There was no increase in nosocomial infection in the steroid group.

Prostaglandin E1

Endogenous prostaglandin E1 (PGE1) has anti-inflammatory action by reducing neutrophil oxygen-radical production as well as being a vasodilator and inhibitor of platelet aggregation.

It is associated with a number of side-effects, including hypotension, hypoxia, and dysrhythmias. An RCT of 100 patients with ARDS failed to show that PGE1 conferred a survival advantage in ARDS and its use is not recommended.

Ibuprofen

Non-steroidal anti-inflammatory drugs (NSAIDs) reduce the production of prostaglandins that are implicated in the pathogenesis of ARDS. Trial data suggest that the use of ibuprofen in sepsis does not reduce the incidence of ARDS or overall mortality.

Ketoconazole

Ketoconazole is an antifungal drug that inhibits production of thromboxanes and leukotrienes by pulmonary endothelial cells.

Thromboxanes cause vasoconstriction and platelet aggregation, while leukotrienes cause bronchoconstriction and are important neutrophil chemokines. Both thromboxanes and leukotrienes are implicated in the pathogenesis of ARDS.

A large RCT performed by the ARDS Network failed to show an improvement in oxygenation or mortality with ketoconazole and its use is not recommended.

N-acetylcysteine

N-acetylcysteine (NAC) is a potent antioxidant that may reduce the damage caused by reactive oxygen species. NAC is the precursor of glutathione, which has been shown to be reduced in the lungs of patients with ARDS. NAC has been shown to improve lung compliance and oxygenation but have no effect on mortality.

Pentoxifylline and lisofylline

Pentoxifylline and its metabolite lisofylline are phosphodiesterase inhibitors that exhibit an anti-inflammatory action by reducing circulating levels of free fatty acids and inhibiting free radical formation. They both reduce levels of circulating pro-inflammatory cytokines such as TNF-α, IL-1, and IL-6.

There is no clinical trial data evaluating the use of pentoxifylline in ARDS, while a single RCT of lisofylline showed no survival advantage in ALI or ARDS. Use of these agents is therefore not recommended.

Inhaled vasodilators

Vasodilatation within ventilated lung units should improve oxygenation by improving ventilation/perfusion matching. This can be achieved using short-acting inhaled vasodilators such as nitric oxide (NO) and prostacyclin. They have the additional benefit of reducing pulmonary artery pressure.

Inhaled nitric oxide

Inhaled NO is typically administered at a concentration of less than 10 parts per million. NO has been shown, in ALI, to improve oxygenation, especially in the first 24h of administration. It has no effect on duration of ventilation or mortality. NO may have some useful anti-inflammatory and anti-platelet effects, but also produces free radicals and is associated with renal dysfunction. The use of NO in ARDS is currently not recommended in standard practice.

Epoprostenol

Like NO, epoprostenol may produce beneficial effects on oxygenation and pulmonary artery pressure but these short-term improvements are not translated into mortality benefit in patients with ARDS.

Other drugs

Salbutamol (beta-agonists)

The BALTI trial was based on observations that beta-agonists appear to reduce alveolar oedema in patients with ARDS. The use of intravenous salbutamol reduced alveolar water as measured by thermodilution (PiCCO). BALTI 2 has been stopped at interim analysis for lack of efficacy.

Sildenafil

Sildenafil is a selective inhibitor of phosphodiesterase-5 that leads to relaxation of vascular smooth muscle, predominantly leading to pulmonary vasodilatation. The results of two RCTs support the use of sildenafil as an effective treatment for idiopathic pulmonary artery hypertension. Physiological studies and case reports suggest that sildenafil may have a role in the treatment of pulmonary hypertension due to ARDS.

Almitrine

Almitrine causes pulmonary vasoconstriction by stimulating peripheral chemoreceptors. By augmenting hypoxic pulmonary vasoconstriction, almitrine is thought to improve hypoxaemia. Physiological studies suggest that in combination with inhaled NO almitrine does improve hypoxaemia without causing a harmful rise in pulmonary artery pressure. However, no RCTs exist to support its use in ARDS.

Surfactant

Surfactant prevents alveolar collapse by attenuating surface tension in the alveoli. Surfactant is a mix of four different proteins (10%) and lipid (90%) that is produced by type 2 pneumocytes. Endogenous surfactant levels and functionality are significantly reduced in patients with ARDS.

Animal studies have suggested a role for surfactant in ARDS, decreasing the surface tension within the alveoli, reducing cyclical collapse, and improving oxygenation. Surfactant may have an anti-inflammatory role that reduces the harmful effects of VALI.

Exogenous surfactant may be nebulized or directly distilled into the airway via a bronchoscope. Multiple applications are often required as surfactant is dispersed by alveolar oedema.

A meta-analysis of human trials showed a non-significant improvement in oxygenation and no effect on mortality. Currently use of surfactant is not indicated in ARDS.

Fluid balance

Alveolar oedema forms as a result of increased vascular permeability and raised hydrostatic pressure. By reducing hydrostatic pressure less fluid should leak into the alveolar air spaces. Overall and persistent positive fluid balance is associated with a poor outcome. In 2006 the ARDS Network group published a study that randomized 1000 ALI or ARDS patients to 'dry' (CVP <4 mmHg or PAOP <8mmHg) or 'wet' (CVP 10–14mmHg or PAOP 14–18mmHg) regimes. Institution of the study protocol did not occur until approximately 48h to allow appropriate fluid resuscitation in the acute phase. The dry regime was associated with improved oxygenation, a reduction in the amount of time patients required ventilation and days on ICU, and no significant increase in episodes of organ failure. Sixty-day mortality remained unaltered between the two groups. As long as haemodynamic stability and organ perfusion can be adequately maintained, patients with ARDS may be better managed using a restrictive fluid regime.

Nutrition

Appropriate nutritional support is required to look after all critically ill patients. A reduction in the ratio of carbohydrate in feed ('pulmonary' feed) has been advocated as a technique to reduce carbon dioxide production. This practice is not recommended as it increases the risk of malnutrition and is not supported by an evidence base. The use of additional fish oils in enteral nutrition has recently been investigated by the ARDS Network after small studies suggested an improvement in endothelial damage and permeability. The study was stopped early for futility.

Sedation and neuromuscular blockade

For patients to tolerate the ventilation strategies used in ARDS, sedation is often required. The use of sedation also reduces the respiratory muscles' (and therefore the total) oxygen demand. In extreme circumstances there may be a need to add neuromuscular blocking drugs to heavy sedation. The effect of paralysis is unpredictable as gas exchange may be improved by reducing ventilator dyssynchrony or increasing chest wall compliance, or potentially worsened by increasing atelectasis resulting from abolishing any spontaneous breaths. Sedation and paralysis may increase the risk of CIP and CIM, which may in turn impair the recovery of patients following ARDS. The effects of the medication are difficult to disentangle from the effects of mechanical ventilation (which has been shown to cause significant and rapid atrophy of the diaphragm[8]).

Daily breaks ('holds') in sedation, or sedation scoring and very regular adjustment of sedation to maintain patients as lightly sedated as safely possible, should be used to reduce the time to waking and decrease the risk of neuromuscular complications.

Cardiovascular manipulation

Increasing O_2 delivery by addressing cardiac output and Hb concentration will increase the mixed venous oxygen saturation, and reduce the impact of intrapulmonary shunting on arterial oxygenation.

Ventilatory management

Open-lung ventilation is a strategy combining low tidal volume ventilation to reduce the incidence of VALI with enough PEEP to maintain alveolar recruitment in atelectatic lung units found in ARDS.

Tidal volume

The biggest change in ARDS management relates to the use of small tidal volumes for mechanical ventilation of patients with ARDS. The hypothesis of the ARDS Network ARMA[9] study was based on experimental studies on VILI. By using small tidal volumes it was hoped that the progressive lung injury caused by mechanical ventilation could be minimized. The ARMA study published in the *New England Journal of Medicine* in 2000 randomized 861 to conventional tidal volumes (10–12mL/kg ideal body weight) or low tidal volumes (4–6mL/kg). In the low tidal volume group plateau pressure was limited to ≤30cmH$_2$O. The low tidal volume group had a significantly lower mortality rate (31% vs 40%). Some criticism has been levelled at this trial for the relatively high tidal volumes used in the control arm, which may be injurious and are higher than are commonly used.

Permissive hypercapnia

A low tidal volume ventilation strategy will cause alveolar hypoventilation with resulting hypercapnia. This can be offset to a degree by increasing the respiratory rate (although the reduced inspiratory and expiratory times may cause a further fall in tidal volume).

Permissive hypercapnia means that, as long as the ventilation strategy has been optimized with low tidal volumes and high respiratory rate, hypercapnia is tolerated.

Hypercapnia has been reported to have a number of contradictory actions, including protecting in lung reperfusion injury, VILI, and lipopolysaccharide (LPS)-induced lung injury, while also reported to impair gas exchange, impair membrane healing, and worsen VILI and LPS injury. See also 📖 Hypercapnia while on a ventilator, p 296.

Positive end expiratory pressure

Lungs affected by ARDS have significant areas of atelectasis, some of which may be recruited for gas exchange. The recruited areas are kept open by using higher levels of PEEP. By preventing cyclical opening and closing of these units, the damaging effects of atelectrauma can be prevented.

However, PEEP may also contribute to lung injury by causing over-distension of compliant, already open lung units. It may exacerbate ventilation perfusion mismatching by increasing the physiological dead space.

The cardiovascular effects of PEEP are discussed in 📖 Heart–lung interactions, p 275, and include pulmonary hypertension, RV dysfunction, and reduced cardiac output.

The optimum level of PEEP is not known. It differs between patients and will change in the same patient with disease progression, fluid status, patient position etc. The setting of 'optimal PEEP' is discussed in 📖 Positive end expiratory pressure, p 119.

The ALVEOLI study[10] randomized 549 patients to high PEEP (13cmH$_2$O) or low PEEP (8cmH$_2$O) strategies. Using higher levels of PEEP improved oxygenation but did not affect overall mortality. The Canadian Critical Care Trial Group showed a similar improvement on oxygenation but lack of effect on mortality when they compared low tidal volumes with low tidal volumes, high PEEP, and RMs. It has been suggested that the failure to show a reduction in mortality with higher PEEP is a reflection of the heterogeneous nature of a group of patients with ALI/ARDS with the benefits of high PEEP only being seen in the most severe patients. Meta-analysis of all studies of PEEP in ARDS suggests a modest mortality advantage in favour of high PEEP.

Inspired oxygen concentration

High fractions of inspired oxygen are often required by patients with ARDS. Mechanical ventilation allows delivery of high concentrations of oxygen and has the added advantage of resting the respiratory muscles and therefore reducing oxygen demand. Oxygen delivery should also be optimized with appropriate fluid management and additional inotropy if required. Typically patients with ARDS require SaO_2 >90% and PaO_2 >8kPa. Oxygen concentrations should be reduced as quickly as possible in order to reduce the potentially toxic effects of reactive oxygen species and to help limit absorption atelectasis.

Ventilator modes

Despite the number of ventilatory modes and the plethora of published descriptions using different modes in ARDS, to date no mode has been clearly demonstrated to be superior.

Pressure- vs volume-controlled modes of ventilation

There are no trials directly comparing pressure- with volume-limited ventilation.

The decelerating flow pattern in PCV reduces the peak inspiratory pressure for a given tidal volume when compared with VCV. There are physiological differences between the modes that are more fully discussed in 📖 Pressure control ventilation, p 135. Newer ventilators can deliver volume-limited breaths with decelerating waveforms.

Practically, both the peak pressure and volume must be monitored and limited when ventilating patients with ARDS. Changes in lung compliance will affect either the airway pressure or tidal volume when using a volume-limited or pressure-limited mode of ventilation, respectively.

Inverse I:E ratio ventilation

The theory and practice of inverse ratio ventilation is discussed in 📖 Pressure-controlled ventilation, p 135. Prolonging inspiration is designed to increase total PEEP and mean airway pressure within safe limits of tidal volume and peak airway pressures. It may also improve gas flow distribution and CO_2 removal. However, a significant reduction in expiratory time (either by adjusting the I:E ratio or by increasing the overall respiratory rate) will reduce expiration to a point where CO_2 clearance is impaired and dynamic hyperinflation occurs with generation of $PEEP_i$. This is turn leads to breath stacking and potential cardiovascular compromise. Evidence that inverse I:E ration ventilation improves oxygenation in patients in ARDS is mixed.

Airway pressure release ventilation

APRV maintains the inspiratory pressure for many seconds before allowing a short period of expiration. It has the same advantages and disadvantages as inverse ratio ventilation. By holding patients at a high plateau pressure lung recruitment can be maintained as there is little time in the respiratory cycle for atelectasis to occur. See 📖 Airway pressure-release ventilation and biphasic positive airways pressure, p 151 for further detail.

BIPAR

Biphasic positive airway pressure ventilation provides a high and a low PEEP at which patients can take spontaneous breaths. If no spontaneous breaths are taken then a tidal volume is generated by cycling from one pressure to the other. By allowing the patient to take a spontaneous (but pressure-supported) breath at either the high or low PEEP it is hoped that there will be less deconditioning of the respiratory muscles. A gradual reduction in the difference between the two PEEP levels and an increase in the pressure support allows weaning to occur without a change in ventilator mode. See 📖 Airway pressure-release ventilation and biphasic positive airways pressure, p 151 for further detail.

Non-invasive ventilation

NIV can be used for patients with ALI. However, it may not be possible to maintain oxygenation with this strategy and its use may lead to potentially dangerous delays in endotracheal intubation. The most usual cause for failure of non-invasive respiratory support is the ability of the patient to tolerate the mask or hood, rather than the failure of oxygenation. There is little data to support the use of NIV in ARDS.

High frequency oscillatory ventilation

HFOV uses tidal volumes that are less than the anatomical dead space of the lung, with a respiratory rate greater than 60 breaths/min, typically 5Hz. Gas transfer occurs by diffusion rather than conventional flow. The potential benefit of HFOV is the reduction in biotrauma from VALI associated with conventional ventilation and improved ventilation/perfusion matching. Small trials suggest an improvement in oxygenation but not survival. Larger randomized trials of HFOV are currently underway. See 📖 High-frequency oscillatory ventilation, p 158 for further detail.

Adjuncts to ventilation

Adjuncts to ventilation, including prone positioning, RMs, beta 2 agonists, rotational therapy, surfactant, partial liquid ventilation, and tracheal gas insufflation are considered fully in 📖 Adjuncts to ventilation, p 188. ECMO and extracorporeal CO_2 removal are considered in 📖 Extracorporeal membrane oxygenation, p 183.

Complications

Ventilator-associated pneumonia

Approximately half of ARDS patients will develop VAP. The effect on mortality is difficult to ascertain. VAP doubles the mortality of critically ill patients when compared to a cohort who do not have VAP. VAP is often difficult to diagnose in ARDS patients who already have grossly abnormal chest radiographs and signs of systemic inflammation.

Prevention of VAP is an important aspect of the management of ARDS. Avoiding putting patients supine and regular oral decontamination with chlorhexidine are associated with a reduced rate of VAP in critically ill patients. See 📖 Complications of ventilation, p 244, for further detail.

Pneumothorax

Pneumothorax is a common (4–15%) complication of ARDS and often presents with a change in lung compliance and desaturation. Frontal chest radiographs are frequently inadequate for the detection of pneumothorax as they may be multiloculated and anterior in the chest. CT may be required for diagnosis and to assist with drain placement. Chest drain placement is always required and drains may have to be left in place until the patient has been weaned from positive pressure ventilation. See 📖 Pleural disease, p 481.

Acute kidney injury

Patients with ARDS have an increase rate of renal dysfunction. Possible mechanisms for AKI include the systemic inflammation ('biotrauma') of ARDS, reduction in cardiac output (associated with high PEEP ventilation), hypoxia, and hypercapnia.

Practical guide for managing a patient with ARDS
- Intubation and mechanical ventilation if unable to maintain adequate gas exchange with FiO_2 >60% and CPAP 10cmH$_2$O.
- Confirm diagnosis of ARDS and search for the cause.
- Increase sedation and analgesia (aim to suppress respiratory drive) and consider use of non-depolarizing muscle relaxants.
  - Aim to limit sedation as soon as feasible.
- Adopt an 'open-lung' strategy.
  - Limit tidal volume to 4–6mL/kg (ideal body weight).
  - Limit pressure to 30cmH$_2$O.
  - Set PEEP at 5–20cmH$_2$O—titrate up, monitoring response in tidal volume, oxygenation, and blood pressure.
- Consider RMs between PEEP adjustments (if blood pressure stable).
- Aim for oxygen saturations of 90–94% and PaO$_2$ >8kPa. (Consider permissive hypoxaemia if target unachievable.)
- Increase respiratory rate to limit PCO$_2$ rise (permissive hypercapnia is acceptable if PCO$_2$ cannot be controlled).
- Adjust the I:E ratio in favour of inspiratory time (monitor for signs of auto-PEEP, breath stacking, and cardiovascular instability).
- Maintain tissue perfusion with relative hypovolaemia (if possible).

Further suggestions if patient remains hypoxic
- Consider turning patient into the prone position (aim for >12h).
- Consider other modes of ventilation (bilevel, high frequency) if available.
- Address fluid management and cardiovascular performance.

Outcome

Mortality

Mortality from ARDS in the ITU varies from 36% in RCTs to 44% in observational studies.[10] However, hospital mortality is significantly higher, at nearer 60%. This mortality of ARDS in studies has not reduced since 1994, when the NAECC definition was introduced. The majority patients with ARDS die from sepsis and multi-organ failure rather than hypoxia.

In late-stage ARDS, sepsis is the leading cause of death (70%). Severe ARDS is associated with a prolonged period of ventilator dependence, which increases the rate of nosocomial infection such as VAP and catheter-related sepsis.

Morbidity

Patients surviving ARDS report significant levels of physical and psychological morbidity following discharge from ICU. Long-term disability is most commonly due to extra-pulmonary conditions such as weakness and muscle wasting.

- Neuromuscular—significant levels of critical illness polyneuropathy are seen in patients surviving ARDS. The muscle wasting associated with critical illness may take months to reverse.
- Respiratory—spirometry can show both obstructive and restrictive patterns of lung disease in ARDS survivors. Even in patients with normal spirometry, gas diffusion may be reduced. Pulmonary function tests correlate with overall health-related quality of life and lung function can continue to improve for up to 1 year.
- Psychological—depression, PTSD, and cognitive defects are common.
- Relatives/carers—carers of patients surviving ARDS have to carry a large psychological and healthcare burden during a prolonged convalescence phase.

1 Bernard GR, Artigas A, Brigham KL, et al. (1994) The American–European consensus conference on ARDS. Definitions, mechanisms, relevant outcomes, and clinical trial coordination. *Am J Respir Crit Care Med* **149**, 818–24.
2 Brun-Buisson C, Minelli C, Bertoloni G, et al. (2004) Epidemiology and outcome of acute lung injury in European intensive care units. Results from the ALIVE study. *Intensive Care Med* **30**, 51–61.
3 Bellingan GJ (2002) The pulmonary physician in critical care: The pathogenesis of ALI/ARDS. *Thorax* **57**, 540–6.
4 Pinhu L, Whitehead T, Evans T, and Griffiths M (2003) Ventilator-associated lung injury. *Lancet* **361**, 332–40.
5 Adhikari NKJ, Burns KE, and Meade MO (2004) Pharmacologic therapies for adults with acute lung injury and acute respiratory distress syndrome. *Cochrane Database of Systematic Reviews*, Issue 4.
6 Peter JV, John P, Graham PL, Morgan JL, George IA, and Bersten A (2008) Corticosteroids in the prevention and treatment of acute respiratory distress syndrome (ARDS) in adults: meta-analysis. *BMJ* **336**, 1006–9.
7 Meduri GU, Marik PE, Chrousos GP, et al. (2008) Steroid treatment in ARDS: a critical appraisal of the ARDS network trial and the recent literature. *Intensive Care Med* **34**, 61–9.
8 Levine S, Nguyen T, Taylor N, et al. (2008) Rapid disuse atrophy of diaphragm fibers in mechanically ventilated humans. *New Engl J Med* **358**, 1327–35.
9 The Acute Respiratory Distress Syndrome Network (2000) Ventilation with lower tidal volumes as compared with traditional tidal volumes for acute lung injury and the acute respiratory distress syndrome. *New Engl J Med*, **342**(18), 1301–8.
10 Brower RG, Lanken PN, MacIntyre N, et al. (2004) Higher versus lower positive end-expiratory pressures in patients with the acute respiratory distress syndrome. *New Engl J Med* **351**, 327–36.
11 Fan E, Wilcox ME, Brower RG, et al. (2008) Recruitment maneuvers for acute lung injury: a systematic review. *Am J Respir Crit Care Med* **178**(11), 1156–63.
12 Phua J, Badia JR, Adhikari NK, et al. (2009) Has mortality from acute respiratory distress syndrome decreased over time? A systematic review. *Am J Respir Crit Care Med* **179**, 220–7.

6.2 Alveolar haemorrhage and pulmonary vasculitis

Presentation

Diffuse alveolar haemorrhage is a rare clinical presentation that is likely to be misdiagnosed. If massive, then the patient may present in extremis and be at risk of asphyxiation. Alveolar haemorrhage may also be the first presentation of a potentially life-threatening systemic disease in which early diagnosis and treatment may be life saving.

The combination of alveolar haemorrhage and acute glomerulonephritis is referred to as pulmonary–renal syndrome and may lead to rapidly progressive renal failure without prompt treatment.

The diagnosis of acute alveolar haemorrhage should be considered in individuals presenting with the triad of:

• Dyspnoea
• Haemoptysis
• Alveolar infiltrates on CXR.

The degree of blood loss may render the patient anaemic. However, there may not be a clear history of haemoptysis or it may not be possible to obtain a clear history of haemoptysis in patients who present in extremis. There are no reliable, specific radiological features to differentiate alveolar haemorrhage from other causes of diffuse alveolar shadowing, but additional imaging with high resolution CT (HRCT) may provide clues to the underlying diagnosis.

Differential diagnosis

Acute or sub-acute dyspnoea with diffuse alveolar infiltrates

• Pulmonary oedema.
• Pneumonia (in the immunocompetent and immunocompromised).
• ALI/ARDS.
• Rapidly progressive interstitial lung disease.

Respiratory failure and haemoptysis

• Pulmonary oedema (especially if secondary to mitral valve disease).
• Pneumonia (especially necrotising pneumonia caused by PVL positive *Staphylococcus aureus*).
• ARDS.

Causes of pulmonary haemorrhage

Diffuse alveolar haemorrhage results from disruption of the alveolar capillary basement membrane, and the aetiology of alveolar haemorrhage can be classified by the predominant histological features (capillaritis, bland haemorrhage, or diffuse alveolar damage).

- In a patient presenting with suspected acute alveolar haemorrhage, it is essential to exclude infection, which if untreated may be life threatening.
- Alveolar haemorrhage may be the presenting symptom of a systemic vasculitis and of Goodpasture's disease. It is essential to identify those with a treatable systemic disease where intervention may be life saving or prevent chronic renal failure.
- Pulmonary haemorrhage is a recognized complication of SLE and needs to be differentiated from other causes of diffuse infiltrates in SLE, including acute lupus pneumonia and pulmonary oedema.
- Alveolar haemorrhage has also been described in rheumatoid disease, mixed connective tissue disease, systemic sclerosis, and Behcet's, and should be considered in a patient with a history of one of these conditions who presents with pulmonary infiltrates on the CXR.
- Pulmonary haemosiderosis is a disease of unknown aetiology in which there may be repeated episodes of alveolar haemorrhage. It usually occurs in childhood and is a diagnosis of exclusion.

A particular aetiology may give rise to more than one histological pattern, and it may be clinically more useful to categorize the possible causes as shown in the box.

Possible causes of diffuse alveolar haemorrhage

Vasculitic, autoimmune, and rheumatological disease:
- Wegener's granulomatosis.
- Microscopic polyangiitis.
- Anti-glomerular basement membrane (GBM) disease (Goodpasture's disease).
- SLE.
- Cryoglobulinaemia.
- Mixed connective tissue disease.
- Systemic sclerosis.
- Behcet's syndrome.
- Polymyositis.
- Henoch–Schoenlein purpura.

Infection
- Bacterial infection causing ARDS.
- Opportunistic infection in immunocompromised host.
- Viral pneumonia.
- Leptospirosis.

Drugs*
- Anticoagulant and anti-platelet therapy (IIA/IIIB inhibitors).
- Propylthiouracil.
- Amiodarone.
- Crack cocaine.

Other causes
- Mitral stenosis.
- Idiopathic pulmonary haemosiderosis.
- Idiopathic pulmonary capillaritis.
- Pulmonary veno-occlusive disease.
- Pulmonary embolism with infarction.
- Arteriovenous malformations.
- IgA nephropathy.

*Numerous other drugs have been reported. Pneumotox provides a comprehensive list (http://www.pneumotox.com/).

Pulmonary vasculitis

The vasculitides are a group of diseases characterized by the presence of leukocytes within the vessel wall, resulting in reactive damage. This can cause haemorrhage as a consequence of loss of integrity, or mural occlusion with subsequent tissue ischemia. The vasculitidies are classified as primary or secondary, and also by the size of vessel affected:

- Large vessels (Takayasu's arteritis, giant cell arteritis)
- Medium-sized vessels (polyarteritis nodosa, Kawasaki disease)
- Small vessels (Wegener's granulomatosis, microscopic polyangiitis, Churg–Strauss syndrome, Henoch–Schönlein purpura).

Pulmonary involvement is most commonly seen in small vessel vasculitis.

Wegener's granulomatosis and microscopic polyangiitis

These vasculitides are characteristically associated with anti-neutrophil cytoplasmic antibodies (ANCAs).

- Wegener's granulomatosis is associated with c-ANCA (the antigen is proteinase 3, (PR3)). 10% are antibody negative.
- Microscopic polyangiitis can be associated with either p-ANCA (the antigen is myeloperoxidase (MPO)) or c-ANCA.

Both conditions have the same histological pattern of necrotising vasculitis of small arterioles and venules, which may cause alveolar haemorrhage and crescentic glomerulonephritis.

They usually present with several weeks of prodromal illness (fever, malaise, weight loss, arthralgia, and anaemia). Both can also be associated with the involvement of multiple organ systems, and features may include any combination of:

- Renal impairment, blood/protein in the urine
- Pulmonary haemorrhage, pulmonary fibrosis
- Vasculitic rash, splinter haemorrhages, nail fold infarcts, ulceration
- Episcleritis, scleritis, retinal vasculitis
- Gastrointestinal haemorrhage, intestinal ischaemia
- Mononeuritis multiplex, peripheral neuropathy, cerebral vasculitis.

Wegener's granulomatosis is differentiated by having associated granulomatous disease of the upper and/or lower respiratory tract. This can result in chronic inflammatory change and scarring in the sinuses, ears, trachea, and bronchi, as well as proptosis and lung nodules. Collapse of the nasal bridge can cause a saddle nose deformity. The patient may describe symptoms such as:

- Rhinorrhoea, purulent, or bloody nasal discharge, nasal and/or oral ulcers
- Sinus pain
- Hearing loss and or earache
- Hoarse voice
- Stridor
- Cough
- Haemoptysis
- Dyspnoea
- Pleuritic chest pain.

Pulmonary nodules are distinct from, but may co-exist with, alveolar haemorrhage. They range in size from millimetres to several centimetres, and may be cavitating. CXR features are non-specific and include:

• Alveolar opacities
• Ground glass shadowing
• Pleural opacities.

CT scanning can be very useful in confirming pulmonary nodules and can demonstrate typical sinus soft tissue changes and bony destruction.

Other causes of small vessel disease

Churg–Strauss syndrome is most commonly associated with asthma, but has rarely been associated with alveolar haemorrhage. Characteristically there is a prominent eosinophilia and it may be associated with a p-ANCA.

Henoch–Schönlein purpura and mixed essential cryoglobulinaemia are rare but recognized causes of alveolar haemorrhage.

Anti-GBM disease

Anti-GBM disease, or Goodpasture's disease, is caused by the deposition of antibodies to the alpha 3 chain of type IV collagen along the glomerular basement membrane and alveolar basement membrane. This results in a rapidly progressive crescentic glomerulonephritis and/or pulmonary haemorrhage. Onset is usually acute and may present with:

• Fever
• Malaise
• Nausea and vomiting
• Breathlessness
• Chest pain
• Haemoptysis
• Oliguria.

Pulmonary involvement may be precipitated by exposure to toxins such as hydrocarbons, organic solvents, and tobacco smoke. Renal disease frequently leads to end-stage renal failure.

Anti-GBM antibodies are detected in peripheral blood. These may co-exist with ANCA in a small proportion of patients (these patients behave like anti-GBM disease rather than vasculitis).

Investigation of suspected diffuse alveolar haemorrhage

Investigation is aimed at confirming the diagnosis and identifying any underlying aetiology that may require urgent treatments (such as systemic vasculitis). Apart from open-lung biopsy, there is not a definitive test for alveolar haemorrhage. However, the following investigations should be undertaken (where possible):

• Full blood count, urea and electrolytes, CRP and plasma viscosity (or ESR).
• CXR—may show alveolar infiltrates (non-specific) or provide evidence of an alternative diagnosis.

- Urinalysis for blood and protein. If positive on dipstick testing, a fresh sample (the laboratory needs to know it is coming) should be sent for urgent microscopy for red cell casts. Proteinuria should be quantified with a protein/creatinine ratio.
- Blood serology for ANCA, anti-GBM, rheumatoid factor, antinuclear antibodies, and complement levels. If complement levels are low and rheumatoid factor is positive then cryoglobulins should be assessed.
- Echocardiogram to exclude mitral stenosis and left-side cardiac dysfunction.
- HRCT scan—may show dense consolidation or ground glass opacification depending on the extent of the haemorrhage. Although non-specific, it may identify alternative diagnoses and identify target areas for BAL or biopsy.
- Measurement of carbon monoxide gas transfer—the presence of haemoglobin in the alveolar spaces will increase the uptake of carbon monoxide. This may not be practical as ideally it should be performed soon after the haemorrhage and a breathless patient may not be able to perform the test.
- Fibre-optic bronchoscopy and BAL—may identify blood in the proximal airway or identify upper airway or endobronchial lesions in Wegener's granulomatosis (including airway stenosis). A BAL is essential to exclude infection (especially if high-dose immunosuppressants are contemplated). The lavage fluid itself may be heavily blood stained or contain haemosiderin-laden macrophages in alveolar haemorrhage. In the acutely unwell patient, a transbronchial biopsy may not be safe and is unlikely to provide sufficient material to enable a definitive diagnosis.
- Renal biopsy may be required to confirm a suspected diagnosis of systemic vasculitis or anti-GBM disease.

Clues to treatable systemic vasculitis

The most common cause of renal and respiratory failure in ICU is sepsis and acute tubular necrosis. There may be clues that this is not the case:

- Blood and protein in urine (common in urinary infection, but should prompt consideration of vasculitides)
- Symptoms or signs (above)
- Prolonged prodrome
- Persistently raised CRP, erythrocyte sedimentation rate (ESR)
- Platelets (down in SLE, up in vasculitis)
- Alkaline phosphatase (up in Wegener's)
- Eosinophilia and/or asthma (Churg–Strauss)
- Unexplained anaemia with respiratory infiltrates
- Unresolving 'pneumonia' with no positive microbiology.

Treatment

Treatment of pulmonary haemorrhage associated with vasculitis or anti-GBM disease should include plasma exchange acutely, using FFP or solvent/detergent-treated human plasma solution replacement if actively bleeding. Intravenous methylprednisolone can be used as an alternative if plasma exchange is not available. Additional induction treatment usually comprises high-dose oral prednisolone (1mg/kg) together with oral or intravenous cyclophosphamide. Patients should have PCP prophylaxis (co-trimoxazole first line), nystatin oral suspension, and a proton pump inhibitor. If possible and glomerular filtration rate (GFR) >30ml/min, bone protection with bisphosphonates should be used. There is limited evidence for the use of intravenous immunoglobulin in vasculitis.

Fluid overload should be avoided, as pulmonary oedema can exacerbate the pulmonary haemorrhage. If renal replacement is required, minimal anticoagulation regimes should be used. Suspected vasculitis should be discussed with a nephrologist, rheumatologist, or respiratory physician as most appropriate.

Goodpastures
- Untreated usually fatal.
- Small window to rescue renal function. Once dialysis dependent, renal recovery is rare.
- Creatinine <600: immunosuppression.
- Pulmonary haemorrhage: immunosuppression.
- Creatinine >600, no pulmonary haemorrhage: rationale for immunosupression less clear.
- 90% survival, 40% renal recovery.

Wegener's granulomatosis and microscopic polyangiitis
- Untreated usually fatal.
- 90% remission, 80% 1-year survival, 60% 5-year survival.
- 70% renal recovery post dialysis.

6.3 Asthma

Pathophysiology

Asthma is a chronic disease characterized by the development of acute episodes. These may be triggered by a number of factors (see box) or appear with no identifiable precipitant. The underlying process is inflammation within the small airways, which results in mucosal oedema, excessive production of luminal mucus, and bronchoconstriction due to bronchial smooth muscle contraction. There is an imbalance between the ease of inflation of the lungs during inspiration and deflation of the lungs during expiration caused by partial collapse of airways during expiration. The turbulent air flow caused by this collapse results in expiratory wheeze and the resultant trapping of gas leads to increase residual volume and increased WOB. Dynamic hyperinflation results in raised ITP and in severe acute asthma reduced venous return.

Hypoxaemia mainly results from V/Q mismatch. Ventilation to lung units is severely reduced because of airway constriction, oedema, inflammation, and mucous plugs. Perfusion of these under-ventilated lung units results in shunting and hypoxaemia. Hypercapnia, which occurs during prolonged severe acute asthma, is mostly due to relative alveolar hypoventilation caused by muscle fatigue.

The hypoxaemia is initially attenuated by an increase in cardiac output (and SvO_2), but as the attack progresses cardiac output and oxygen delivery may fall while oxygen consumption by respiratory muscles increases. The resultant fall in SvO_2 will exaggerate any effect of low V/Q ratios and shunt. The reduced cardiac output triggers a release of endogenous catecholamines, causing tachycardia and vasoconstriction.

Factors triggering asthma exacerbations

Inhaled allergens
- House dust mite.
- Animal danders.
- Grass and tree pollens.

Air pollutants
- Tobacco smoke.

Respiratory infection
- Viral.
- Small bacterial, e.g. mycoplasma.

Occupational exposure
- Flour dust—bakers.
- Isocyanates—paint sprayers.

Cold air
- Exercise.

Emotion

Epidemiology

The prevalence of asthma is around 7.2% of the world population (about 100 million individuals), affecting about 6% of adults and 10% of children. In the UK 1.1 million children and 4.1 million adults are currently being treated for asthma. Approximately 40,000 deaths (1 in 250) per year worldwide can be attributed to asthma. In the UK asthma is reported to kill 1400 people per year or one individual every 7h.

Clinical presentation

Most severe asthma attacks develop relatively slowly (one study reported worsening symptoms for 48h prior to presentation in >80% of patients). The most common symptoms are wheeze, cough, and breathlessness.

The combination of a life-threatening illness, endogenous catecholamines, and therapeutic interventions such as salbutamol, adrenaline, and theophyllines mean that anxiety is a major component of many patients' presentation. This anxiety is part of the physiological process and should not be seen as failure to cope.

Initial investigations should include arterial blood gases, CXR (to exclude pneumothorax) and peak expiratory flow (PEF).

Assessment of severity

Definitions of the levels of severity of acute asthma exacerbations are given in Table 6.3 (BTS table). Most cases fall into the moderate exacerbation category and will respond well to standard therapy with oxygen, nebulized bronchodilators, and oral or intravenous steroids.

In severe cases, the patient will be pale and sweaty, tachypnoeic, and tachycardic, with increased WOB driven by the increased respiratory rate, use of accessory muscles, and the necessity to expend muscular energy throughout the whole ventilatory cycle. As the patient deteriorates, bradypnoea and feeble ventilatory efforts ensue; bradycardia and obtunded conscious level herald imminent respiratory arrest.

Referral to ICU

An understanding of the natural history of acute asthma should help clinicians identify the sick patient at a point where appropriate support and intervention should prevent decline into respiratory arrest.

In the initial stages of an acute asthma attack there is an increase in minute ventilation. As the attack intensifies, peak minute ventilation of 20–25L/min may be achieved, resulting in a significant fall in arterial $PaCO_2$. This hyperventilation may benefit arterial oxygenation as the lower the alveolar $PaCO_2$ the higher the PAO_2 and PaO_2.

The respiratory muscles cannot maintain the sustained additional WOB indefinitely. Minute ventilation begins to drop and the arterial $PaCO_2$ starts to rise. By the time the $PaCO_2$ has returned to a normal value the patient may have developed features of life-threatening asthma. Lactate may be high, although the presence of a normal lactate does not rule out significant tissue hypoxia. Exhaustion and falling conscious level result in worsening hypoxia, causing bradycardia and eventual respiratory arrest followed by cardiac arrest.

Patients with the following features should be referred to ICU:
• Exhibiting any 'severe' or 'life-threatening' features (Table 6.3)

Table 6.3 Levels of severity of acute asthma exacerbations (adapted from BTS guidelines 2010). Note patients with life threatening asthma may not be able to perform a peak flow

Near fatal asthma	Raised $PaCO_2$ and/or requiring mechanical ventilation with high inflation pressures	
Life threatening asthma	Clinical signs:	Measurements:
	Poor inspiratory effort	SpO_2 <92%
	Cyanosis	PaO_2 < 8kPa
	Silent chest	'Normal' $PaCO_2$ (4.6–6.0 kPa)
	Arrhythmia	PEF <33% best or predicted
	Hypotension	
	Exhaustion	
	Altered conscious level	
Acute severe asthma	Any one of:	
	PEF 33–50% best of predicted	
	Respiratory rate ≥ 110/min	
	Inability to complete sentences in one breath	
Moderate exacerbation	Increasing symptoms	
	PEF 50–75% best or predicted	
	No features of acute severe asthma	

- Worsening hypoxia
- Rising $PaCO_2$
- Increasing acidosis.

Differential diagnosis

- Acute anaphylaxis—multi-system involvement possibly including stridor, pulmonary oedema, skin rashes, and abdominal symptoms.
- Acute exacerbation of COPD—past history, radiological and ECG appearances.
- Acute LV failure—'cardiac asthma': cardiac history, orthopnoea, paroxysmal nocturnal dyspnoea (PND), examination findings of added heart sounds (gallop rhythm), presence of crackles on auscultation of chest, typical CXR changes.
- Aspiration or inhalation of toxic substances.
- Acute upper airway obstruction (stridor rather than wheeze).

Treatment

Oxygen

Patients with severe acute asthma are hypoxic. High concentration supplemental oxygen should be delivered urgently using a face mask and should be adjusted as necessary to maintain SpO_2 of 94–98%.

β-agonist bronchodilators

As acute asthma deteriorates β-adrenergic receptors within the airways are down-regulated. Patients should therefore be taught that worsening symptoms and lack of improvement after using their usual relief inhaler may indicate developing severe acute asthma. In acute asthma without life-threatening features, a pressurized metered dose inhaler (pMDI) with a large volume spacer is an effective way of delivering inhaled β-agonist.

In acute asthma with life-threatening features oxygen-driven nebulizers should be used. If there is inadequate response to initial treatment, repeat the dose at 15–30min intervals. Continuous nebulization using an appropriate nebulizer has been shown to be as effective as bolus nebulization. Intravenous β-agonist therapy is rarely used. It is occasionally added if air entry is extremely poor, although these patients should be urgently referred to ICU. Intravenous salbutamol causes significant tachycardia and hypokalaemia.

Ipratropium bromide

Combining nebulized ipratropium bromide with a nebulized β-agonist produces significantly greater bronchodilatation than β-agonist alone. This should be used in those with life-threatening features or with poor initial response to β-agonist therapy.

Steroid therapy

Steroids reduce mortality, relapses, subsequent hospital admission, and requirement for β-agonist therapy. They should be administered early as there is a lag time before their full effect is realized.

In life-threatening asthma, gastric emptying is often delayed and absorption is not guaranteed because sympathetic tone is high. The intravenous route is preferred in these circumstances. Likewise, the intravenous route should be used in intubated patients until enteral feeding is established (i.e. gut absorptive function is secured).

In less ill patients steroid tablets are as effective as intravenous hydrocortisone. Prednisolone 40–50mg daily or parenteral hydrocortisone 100mg 6-hourly for 5 days are commonly used in adults. There is no need for gradual dose reduction.

Antibiotics

Even if infection is the precipitant for the attack, most will be viral. Many patients with acute asthma will have a cough productive of small amounts of yellow sputum caused by eosinophils rather than neutrophils. Routine prescription of antibiotics is therefore not indicated in acute asthma. Some ICU clinicians add antibiotics empirically in the very small subgroup with near-fatal asthma and some indication of infection.

Magnesium sulphate

Magnesium is a bronchial smooth muscle relaxant and there is some evidence that, in adults, it has a bronchodilating effect. A dose of 1.2–2g intravenous infusion given over 20min may improve lung function, especially in those with severe asthma. Significant hypotension does occur, particularly in patients with coexisting cardiovascular compromise. There is no evidence for repeated doses.

Intravenous aminophylline

There are some patients with life-threatening asthma who appear to gain significant benefit from aminophylline and it should be considered as a rescue therapy in patients who continue to deteriorate despite best standard treatment. It is synergistic with salbutamol. Aminophylline is a chronotrope, inotrope, and diuretic with a narrow therapeutic index, and serum levels need to be monitored. It can cause life-threatening arrhythmias. A loading dose should be omitted in the presence of major tachycardias or if the patient has taken oral theophyllines. Aminophylline should only be used after consultation with senior staff.

Heliox

This low-density gas should reduce WOB, but a systematic review of 554 adults with acute asthma failed to show any improvement in lung function or other outcomes. Delivery of heliox requires the use of specifically designed or modified breathing circuits and ventilators.

Non-invasive ventilation

Hypercapnic respiratory failure during acute asthma is an indication for urgent ITU referral, and NIV should not be used to delay such referral. There is currently no indication for NIV outside the ITU, and little indication at all, except as a temporizing measure while preparing for intubation.

Sedation

In patients with significant anxiety, benzodiazepines may reduce the respiratory rate and gas trapping, and occasionally avoid the need for ventilation. This is high-risk practice and should only be done by senior clinicians where there is potential to quickly proceed to intubation, or where there is a known history of previous improvement with such treatment.

Mechanical ventilation

With asthma the clinical situation may deteriorate markedly after anaesthesia and institution of mechanical ventilation. Reasons for this include:
- Drugs causing histamine release and worsening bronchospasm
- Reflex bronchoconstriction due to direct physical stimulation when the trachea is intubated
- Positive pressure ventilation may result in dynamic hyperinflation with cardiorespiratory compromise
- Positive pressure ventilation may uncover and enlarge a pre-existing pneumothorax
- Positive pressure ventilation may cause *de novo* barotrauma
- Cardiovascular instability—positive pressure ventilation, anaesthesia, and hypovolaemia often result in significant hypotension.

In addition to adequate intravenous access, if possible an arterial line should be sited prior to intubation. Full resuscitation equipment, including the facility to insert pleural drains, must be immediately to hand. One in 100,000 adrenaline (10mcg/mL) can be used for severe bronchospasm and in the treatment of hypotension.

It may be necessary to hand-ventilate the patient for a significant time.

The aim of mechanical ventilation is to keep the patient alive, and to limit iatrogenic damage, until the bronchospasm improves. When aggressive blood gas correction was the normal policy, ICU mortality approached 25%. The first description of permissive hypercapnia was in 1984, in a cohort of asthmatic patients. Since then reported mortality for asthmatics in ICU has been very low.

Avoid high pressure and dynamic hyperinflation as far as possible. Hyperinflation is the best predictor of complications in asthma. Because hyperinflation reduces lung compliance, end inspiratory plateau pressure is a good marker of dynamic hyperinflation in asthma. Use slow ventilatory rates, small tidal volumes, and a prolonged expiratory phase. Hypercapnia is inevitable.

Volume-controlled vs pressure-controlled

VCV ensures adequate tidal volume delivery, but is more likely to result in dynamic hyperinflation. Peak pressure will be significantly higher than plateau pressure, reflecting the high airway resistance. In order to shorten inspiration as much as possible, high inspiratory flows (80–100L/min) should be used. This will further increase the peak airway pressure (but not the plateau pressure).

PCV limits airway pressure and reduces the occurrence of dynamic hyperinflation because if bronchospasm develops or worsens, tidal volumes reduce. However, these dramatically reduced tidal volumes can also be life threatening. In order to shorten inspiration, the pressure ramp speed should be shortened to 25ms.

Whatever strategy is chosen, careful setting of the ventilator and the ventilator alarms is vital. A low tidal volume alarm is mandatory if PCV is used.

A target sheet for respiratory variables should be left at the bedspace, and significant deviation from these parameters mandates a complete reassessment of the patient, the medical treatment, and the ventilatory strategy.

Positive end expiratory pressure

In the presence of severe bronchospasm, and if the patient is fully ventilated, $PEEP_i$ will be significant and there is no necessity for extrinsic PEEP. In contrast to COPD, dynamic airway compression is less common in asthma, and there is a higher chance that extrinsic PEEP will worsen hyperinflation. Any additional hyperinflation will reduce compliance: plateau pressure will increase (if VCV is used) or tidal volume will reduce (if PCV is used).

However, there is a concern that if zero end expiratory pressure is set, when the bronchospasm resolves significant atelectrauma may occur.

A sensible approach is to set low level PEEP (5cmH$_2$O), making sure that there is no sign of reduced compliance (increased pressures or reduced tidal volumes). If airway pressures or compliance are problematic, consider whether extrinsic PEEP is contributing to the problem—does removal improve compliance?

If there is ongoing bronchospasm when the patient is breathing spontaneously, extrinsic PEEP will reduce the threshold WOB caused by $PEEP_i$ (see 📖 Positive end expiratory pressure, p 119).

Practicalities

The aim is to keep the patient alive, not to normalize blood gases.

- Initial tidal volume target of 4–6mL/kg, respiratory rate of 8 and I:E ratio of 1:6. Inspiratory flow rate 80–100L/min or ramp speed 25ms.
- End expiratory flow should reach as close to zero as possible. Adjust respiratory rate and I:E ratio to prolong expiratory time if necessary.
- Aim for plateau pressure below $30cmH_2O$. In VCV peak pressures may be significantly higher.
- Intermittently disconnect the ventilator at end expiration and listen to the breath sounds. The length of ongoing expiration will allow assessment of expiratory emptying.
- Ignore the CO_2.
- Occasionally, unrecognized dynamic hyperinflation will produce life-threatening cardiovascular collapse. If the blood pressure falls precipitously in an asthmatic patient, consider ventilator disconnection. This may be life saving if there has been significant breath stacking. Mechanical manoeuvres (manual chest deflation) may be tried in extremis. Disconnect the ETT and perform side-to-side pressure on the chest in an attempt to push out trapped gas.

The ventilatory management of severe asthmatics can be very challenging. It requires constant presence at the bedside. The effect of small adjustments of respiratory parameters should be assessed in terms of the therapeutic targets: high pressure and hyperinflation are the dangers to the patient.

Rescue therapies

- Volatile anaesthetics. Once intubated with persisting severe bronchospasm and difficulty in ventilating, inhaled volatile anaesthetic agents (e.g. sevoflurane or isoflurane) may be highly effective. Low doses are used but there are issues over scavenging of anaesthetic gases in the ICU setting.
- Adrenaline is a highly effective bronchodilator and a low dose intravenous infusion may be effective in this context.
- Ketamine also has significant bronchodilator effects.
- Bronchoscopy and lavage of mucus plugs may also be beneficial but is potentially hazardous.
- The use of ECMO has been described but will rely on local availability and expertise.

Further reading

British Thoracic Society/Scottish Intercollegiate Guideline Network. British Guideline on the Management of Asthma (2008) *Thorax* **63**(suppl IV), p1–121. Available at: http://www.brit-thoracic.org.uk and http://www.sign.ac.uk.

Fisher MM, Whaley AP, and Pye RR (2001) External chest compression in the management of acute severe asthma. *Prehosp Disaster Med* **16**(3) 83–86.

6.4 Cardiogenic pulmonary oedema

Cardiogenic pulmonary oedema is a common end result of a spectrum of acute and chronic pathologies that compromise left heart function. In the developed world cardiogenic pulmonary oedema is predominantly due to coronary artery disease or its complications.

Acute heart failure is graded in severity using the Killip scoring system (see box). This is a powerful prognostic tool with studies demonstrating more than double the mortality rate in class III/IV compared to class I. Cardiogenic shock is officially defined as hypotension and inadequate organ perfusion due to cardiac dysfunction. However, shock states (defined as tissue hypoperfusion) due to myocardial dysfunction may exist in the absence of hypotension.

The publication of large registries has given useful epidemiological information about acute heart failure. In the UK, it is more common in the elderly (>70 years) and in those with a history of chronic heart failure. The sexes are equally represented, but women are usually older at presentation and are more likely to have preserved LV systolic function.

In-hospital mortality is around 15% but is much higher in the setting of acute myocardial infarction, and higher still in the presence of cardiogenic shock. Indicators of a poor outcome are increasing age, renal dysfunction, and cardiogenic shock.

Killip classification of acute heart failure

I   No signs of heart failure
II Heart failure with bibasal crepitations/S3 gallop
III Severe heart failure with clinical florid pulmonaryoedema
IV Cardiogenic shock

Aetiology

Ischaemic causes

Coronary artery disease is characterized by the development of atherosclerotic plaques on the luminal surface of the coronary arteries. Many patients are asymptomatic until the lesions become large enough to impede coronary flow, at which point they develop exertional angina. Rupture of these atherosclerotic plaques leads to platelet aggregation and thrombus formation, which can cause total, transient, or sub-total arterial occlusion and subsequent myocardial infarction. Current guidelines divide such events according to the accompanying ECG changes, i.e. ST-segment elevation (STEMI) or non-ST-elevation myocardial infarction (NSTEMI).

Myocardial infarction

Pulmonary oedema due to LV pump failure is common in the setting of a large acute myocardial infarction. If occurring shortly after the index infarct, acute mitral regurgitation due to papillary muscle rupture or ventricular septal rupture must be excluded.

Myocardial ischaemia
Severe ischaemia causing transient LV systolic and diastolic dysfunction is most commonly seen in patients with severe coronary artery disease, e.g. left main stem or triple vessel disease.

Decompensation of chronic heart failure
The cause of this is commonly unclear, but includes sepsis, anaemia, poor compliance with medication, excess fluid or sodium intake, or the development of arrhythmias.

Non-ischaemic causes of cardiogenic pulmonary oedema
Acute
- Sepsis-induced myocardial dysfunction. This is seen in severe systemic sepsis or inflammation and is usually associated with global LV depression. It is thought to be predominantly due to the negative inotropic effects of pro-inflammatory cytokines on the myocardium.
- Acute cardiomyopathies.
  - Viral.
  - Peri-partum.
  - Tako-Tsubo (catecholamine induced).
- Poorly tolerated tachy-arrhythmias, e.g. atrial fibrillation (AF) with a fast ventricular rate in a patient with significant mitral stenosis or LV systolic dysfunction. Patients with impaired early ventricular filling (such as those with LV hypertrophy) are more dependent on atrial contraction to maintain cardiac output and atrial fibrillation is poorly tolerated.
- Bacterial endocarditis causing acute valvular insufficiency.

Acute on chronic
- Decompensation of pre-existing chronic conditions.
  - Dilated cardiomyopathy.
  - Hypertropic cardiomyopathy.
  - Restrictive cardiomyopathy.
  - Congenital heart disease.
  - Valvular disease.

Non-cardiogenic causes of pulmonary oedema
- Phaeochromocytoma—probably due to the vasoconstricting and direct toxic effects of chronically raised plasma catecholamine levels on the myocardium, which can result in a dilated cardiomyopathy.
- 'Flash' pulmonary oedema due to bilateral renal artery stenosis. Thought to be due to reflex hyperactivation of the renin–angiotensin system and subsequent fluid retention due to reduced renal perfusion.
- ARDS (see 🕮, Acute respiratory distress syndrome, p 370).

Pathophysiology
The mechanism underpinning cardiogenic pulmonary oedema is increased intravascular pulmonary pressures with transudation of protein-depleted plasma down a pressure gradient into the pulmonary interstitium and alveoli. The pressure required to produce pulmonary oedema is reduced in the presence of capillary leak and hypoalbuminaemia. This results in significant impairment of gas exchange and respiratory failure.

- In the setting of acute myocardial dysfunction this is primarily due to LV systolic dysfunction with resultant back-pressure in the pulmonary vasculature.
- In patients with pre-existing chronic heart failure this is compounded by up-regulation of the sympathetic and renin–angiotensin–aldosterone systems, which promotes renal retention of sodium and water, chronically raised pulmonary venous pressure +/− hypoalbuminaemia.

Diagnosis

Clinical presentation

The symptoms reflect hypoxia and reflex-increased sympathetic drive. The time course of these symptoms depends on the underlying cause, i.e. the chronic heart failure patient with a decompensation may become gradually unwell over a period of days whereas a post-MI patient with an acute papillary muscle rupture will develop symptoms and signs extremely rapidly. Symptoms include:

- Dyspnoea at rest
- Orthopnoea
- Paroxysmal nocturnal dyspnoea
- Cough productive of frothy (occasionally blood stained) sputum.

Other symptoms depend on the underlying cause, e.g. chest pain, palpitations, cardiac arrest etc.

Clinical assessment

Effective clinical examination and basic bedside investigations can confirm the diagnosis of cardiogenic pulmonary oedema and the presence of coexisting cardiogenic shock, and help ascertain the underlying cause.

General signs

The signs of cardiogenic and non-cardiogenic pulmonary oedema are very similar. Signs reflecting fluid retention or cardiac pressure or volume overload are more specific for a cardiogenic cause. General signs include:

- Anxiety
- Diaphoresis
- Tachypnoea
- Tachycardia (or, less commonly, bradycardia)—the underlying rhythm needs to be determined
- Raised jugular venous pressure (JVP) due to fluid retention or predominant right heart failure
- Auscultation of the heart
  - Gallop rhythm—this sign is specific but not very sensitive for cardiogenic pulmonary oedema and is caused by added heart sounds in diastole reflecting volume overload (S3, due to rapid ventricular filling in early diastole) or pressure overload (S4, due to accentuated atrial contraction in late diastole)
  - Murmur—remember to ascertain if murmurs have been noted before or if they are new, e.g. in the case of evolving bacterial endocarditis or papillary muscle rupture post MI
- Auscultation of the lungs—post tussive bilateral lung field crepitations. Coexisting pleural effusion(s) in chronic heart failure patients may mask underlying crepitations so correlate clinical finding with the CXR
- Peripheral oedema—may be present in chronic heart failure patients.

Signs suggestive of cardiogenic shock
- Hypotension (systolic blood pressure <90mmHg).
- Poor peripheral perfusion.
- Pallor/skin mottling.
- Oliguria/anuria.
- Confusion/agitation indicative of hypoxia and/or hypercapnia.

Investigations

- Arterial blood gases may exhibit profound hypoxaemia (i.e. type I respiratory failure). In more severe cases type II respiratory failure may be seen. A metabolic acidosis secondary to elevated lactate may also occur when tissue perfusion is markedly reduced.
- ECG identifies arrhythmic and/or ischaemic aetiologies (e.g. ST depression/elevation, new left bundle branch block). Compare to older ECGs if available. Occasionally subtle ECG changes are seen in situations of global severe ischaemia such as a left main stem lesion. A common feature of such a lesion is ST elevation in lead aVR, with sometimes minimal global ST depression.
- CXR identifies pulmonary congestion, septal lines, peri-bronchial cuffing, and pleural effusions. A normal cardiothoracic ratio does not exclude LV systolic dysfunction.
- Echocardiography allows a comprehensive bedside assessment of cardiac structure and function, especially ventricular and valvular function. Trans-thoracic windows are often very poor in ventilated patients and trans-oesophageal echocardiography may be necessary. Positive ITP will flatter LV performance as the transmyocardial pressure gradient, preload, and afterload are reduced.
- Routine haematology and biochemistry can help identify underlying causes such as anaemia and infection as well as identifying coexisting renal or hepatic dysfunction (especially albumin). If these are deranged always remember to compare to baseline levels.
- Thyroid function should be ascertained in patients with a new presentation of cardiomyopathy and those with arrhythmias, especially AF.
- Cardiac troponins T and I are specific for cardiac muscle and detectable serum levels will confirm myocyte necrosis. It must be remembered that this simply signifies a disturbance of cardiomyocyte integrity, which has multiple causes, not just myocardial infarction due to atherosclerotic plaque rupture. These can largely be classified into conditions causing myocardial overload/stretch (e.g. acute decompensation of chronic heart failure, tachyarrhythmia) or reduced coronary perfusion (e.g. systemic sepsis). The magnitude of the troponin release directly correlates with risk of subsequent mortality. Troponin levels may be elevated in renal failure in the absence of myocardial disease.
- Obtain plasma B-type natriuretic peptide (BNP) levels if possible. BNP is secreted by the ventricular myocardium predominantly in response to stretch or overload. Current European Society of Cardiology guidelines endorse the use of BNP in the diagnosis (and prognostication—plasma levels predict subsequent mortality in these patients) of heart failure in the acutely breathless patient.

- Right heart (Swan–Ganz) catheterization delineates LV filling pressures and may help guide management. Can also differentiate between cardiogenic pulmonary oedema (high pulmonary artery wedge pressure) and ARDS (not elevated). No overall outcome benefit from pulmonary artery catheterization has been demonstrated, and there is a worry that use of such invasive monitors may lead to overly aggressive therapy.
- A 'cardiomyopathy screen' should be undertaken in new cases of non-ischaemic heart failure, including ferritin, autoantibody screen, and viral serology, including CMV, coxsackie, HIV, and hepatitis B and C.

Treatment modalities

Diuretics and fluid removal

Intravenous furosemide 50–80mg has a venodilator as well as a diuretic action.

Patients with chronic LV impairment will have some degree of fluid retention due to the activation of the renin–angiotensin–aldosterone system. In contrast, patients who have had acute onset LVF will not usually be fluid overloaded; the fluid is merely in the wrong place. These patients may still benefit from diuresis to reduce LV preload, but it must be remembered that in doing so this may increase peripheral vasoconstriction and LV afterload.

Some patients may require ultrafiltration if there is a poor response to diuretic due to poor renal perfusion and/or pre-existing chronic renal impairment.

Nitrates

Start intravenous glyceryl trinitrate (GTN) at 1mg/h and titrate to a systolic blood pressure of 100–110mmHg. GTN is predominantly a venodilator-reducing preload. It will also cause hypotension and reduce afterload, and in reducing LV end diastolic pressure will improve diastolic myocardial blood flow.

Opiates

Patients with cardiogenic pulmonary oedema are often anxious and distressed, and opiates should be administered if possible. Intravenous morphine 2.5–10mg has a vasodilator action (remember antiemetic).

Pharmacological inotropic therapy

Agents of choice differ between centres as no robust evidence base exists. Inotropes represent rescue therapy. Their use when other organ perfusion is compromised is justified if there are reversible features or if interventions (surgery, percutaneous coronary intervention (PCI)) are planned. Although myocardial oxygen consumption is increased by increased contractility, heart rate, or tachyarrhythmias, it will be lowered by reduced ventricular volumes and wall stress. Increased blood pressure and cardiac output may also improve myocardial oxygen delivery.

In the setting of LV dysfunction, inodilators are the preferred option, but their use may be limited by the development of hypotension.

Dobutamine

This is a synthetic catecholamine that has an inodilating effect due to its actions on β1- and β2-adrenoreceptors. Dose 5–20mcg/kg/min.

Adverse effects include tachycardia and hypotension. Use with caution in diastolic dysfunction.

Adrenaline
A naturally occurring catecholamine with effects on β- (lower dose) and α- (higher dose) adrenoreceptors. It is positively inotropic and causes peripheral vasoconstriction. Dose 0.05–0.5mcg/kg/min. Adverse effects include tachydysrhythmias, vasoconstriction, hyperglycaemia, acidaemia hypokalaemia, and hyperlactataemia.

Noradrenaline
A naturally occurring catecholamine that is predominantly an agonist at α adrenoreceptors, with minor β activity. It causes vasoconstriction with some positive inotropy. Dose 0.05–0.5mcg/kg/min. Adverse effects include increased afterload with peripheral vasoconstriction. It should be used with caution in the treatment of LVF and use as a sole agent is not normally advised.

Phosphodiesterase inhibitors
This group of drugs are inodilatory and includes amrinone, milrinone, and enoximone. They are associated with less tachycardia than catecholamines, and have the advantage of increasing the rate of diastolic relaxation (lusitropy). Pulmonary vascular resistance is not increased. Hypotension is often a problem, especially when loading doses are administered.

Calcium sensitisers
There has been considerable interest in levosimendan, which is reported to increase contractility without increasing myocardial oxygen demand. It is an inodilator. Some studies have shown it to improve outcome in patients with acute decompensated heart failure without cardiogenic shock when compared to placebo or dobutamine. It is given as a loading dose of 24mcg/kg over 10min followed by an infusion of 0.1mcg/kg/min for 24h. In practice, the loading dose may cause hypotension and is sometimes incorporated in the 24h infusion. The inotropic effects persist beyond the period of infusion.

CPAP
The role of CPAP in LV dysfunction is discussed in 📖 Continuous positive airway pressure, p 95.

Intra-aortic balloon pumps
Intra-aortic balloon pumps (IABPs) increase diastolic pressure and coronary perfusion while reducing LV afterload. As such they are useful in the advanced management of LVF. They are commonly placed in shocked patients during/following PCI as a bridge to recovery or to further definitive treatment (see below). There is no evidence that they reduce mortality.
- Inserted via femoral artery.
- Balloon positioned in the descending thoracic aorta just distal to the subclavian artery.
- Synchronized with the ECG tracing to inflate during diastole only.
- Improve coronary flow and resultant myocardial perfusion.
- Augment ventricular performance as deflation in late diastole reduces afterload.

- Indications—all patients should have an identifiable 'exit strategy', i.e. be suitable for revascularization or transplant:
  - Cardiogenic shock secondary to LV systolic dysfunction
  - Acute mitral regurgitation/ventricular septal rupture
  - Refractory ischaemia in patients awaiting CABG.
- Contra-indications:
  - Severe aortic regurgitation
  - Aortic aneurysm/dissection.

Left ventricular assist device

Certain patients not responding to the above measures may be suitable for left ventricular assist device (LVAD) and/or cardiac transplantation. In the UK LVADs are licensed only for use as a bridge to transplant (i.e. to support an advanced heart failure patient who is awaiting transplant) or recovery (a patient in whom ventricular function may recover, e.g. myocarditis, peripartum cardiomyopathy).

Management

See Fig. 6.3. The aim of treatment is to:
- Improve cardiac function by addressing preload, afterload, and contractility
- Improve respiratory function and gas exchange
- Address any underlying cause or precipitant.

DVT prophylaxis should given to all patients.

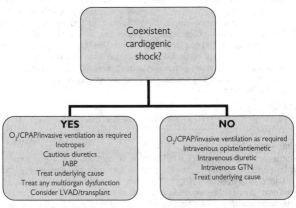

Fig. 6.3 Management of confirmed cardiogenic pulmonary oedema.

Non-shocked and well perfused ('wet and warm')

- Sit up.
- High flow O_2/CPAP/invasive ventilation as required to correct hypoxaemia.
- Morphine 2.5–10mg.
- Intravenous furosemide 50–80mg.

- Intravenous GTN 1mg/h, then titrated to blood pressure.
- Identify and treat cause.

Systolic blood pressure >90mmHg with reduced peripheral perfusion ('wet and cold')

These patients, although not meeting the criteria for cardiogenic shock, have a worse outcome than their well-perfused counterparts. Their cardiac output is low, their tissue perfusion compromised, and their blood pressure is only being maintained with peripheral vasoconstriction. Initial therapy should be closely monitored (with invasive monitoring if necessary) and unless there is a striking response they should be thought of and managed as cardiogenic shock.

Shocked (systolic blood pressure <90mmHg)

Initial contact with ICU staff may be in the ED or cardiac catheterization laboratory. The mainstay of therapy is to improve cardiac and respiratory function and end organ perfusion whilst addressing the underlying cause. Primary PCI is the treatment of choice for all shocked STEMI patients.

- Urgent echocardiography is essential.
- High flow oxygen +/– CPAP/invasive ventilation as required for coexistent respiratory failure.
- Treat cause/precipitant, e.g. coronary revascularization, surgical repair of papillary muscle rupture/ventricular septal rupture.
- Inotropic therapy (see above).
- Diuretic therapy.
- IABP.
- Consider LVAD.

Vasodilating agents such as ACE inhibitors or GTN should be avoided as they may exacerbate hypotension. Patients with LV systolic dysfunction who stabilize with the above therapy should ideally be commenced on a low dose ACE inhibitor and β-blocker once euvolaemic and prior to hospital discharge if tolerated.

Right ventricular infarction

This is usually a complication of inferior myocardial infarction and can also result in cardiogenic shock. If suspected, a right-sided ECG should be performed with ST-elevation in leads $V_{3-5}R$ (same positions as V_{3-5} but on the right side of the chest), indicating RV infarction. Isolated RV infarction is uncommon but should be suspected in a patient with hypotension, raised JVP, and a clear chest. The initial management is based around cautious fluid resuscitation guided by invasive monitoring in order to maintain LV filling pressures. Diuretics/vasodilators should be avoided. Inotropic therapy should be introduced if these measures are insufficient.

RV infarction may present with pulmonary oedema if:
- Complicated by sino-atrial or atrio-ventricular node dysfunction and extreme bradycardia (sinus or heart block)
- There is extensive coexistent infarction of the LV inferior wall.

CHF and ICU referral

The prognosis of CHF has improved greatly over the past 30 years with the advent of many pharmacological and device-based disease-modifying therapies that both improve symptoms and prolong life. CHF patients are a heterogenous group and prognosis can vary widely between patients.

Myocardial stunning (reversible myocardial dysfunction following ischaemia) can commonly complicate large myocardial infarctions, therefore LV systolic dysfunction seen on echocardiography may be reversible. This should be borne in mind when selecting patients for further management in ICU.

The appropriateness of ICU involvement in decompensated patients needs to be decided individually following consideration of:

- Comorbidities
- Previous level of function
- Life expectancy
- Reversibility of the precipitant
- Patient wishes.

Further reading

Birks E (2010) Left ventricular assist devices. *Heart* **96**, 63–71.

Stevenson LW (2003) Clinical use of inotropic therapy for heart failure: looking backward or forward? Inotropic infusions during hospitalization. *Circulation* **108**, 367–372.

Dickstein K, Cohen-Solal A, Filippatos G et al. (2008) ESC Guidelines for the diagnosis and treatment of acute and chronic heart failure 2008: the Task Force for the Diagnosis and Treatment of Acute and Chronic Heart Failure 2008 of the European Society of Cardiology. Developed in collaboration with the Heart Failure Association of the ESC (HFA) and endorsed by the European Society of Intensive Care Medicine (ESICM). *Eur Heart J* **19**, 2388–2442.

Nicol E, Fittall B, Roughton M, Cleland J, Dargie H, and Cowie M (2008) NHS heart failure survey: a survey of acute heart failure admissions in England, Wales and Northern Ireland. *Heart* **94**(2), 172–177.

6.5 Conventional immune modifiers and biologic therapies

Introduction

This chapter concentrates on immunomodulatory agents with properties that increase the risk of infection. The risk is often dose dependent, and the use of more than one immunosuppressive agent compounds this risk. The underlying disease process and certain co-morbidities (e.g. diabetes mellitus) confer additional risk. Agents may increase the risk of infection through specific inhibition of leucocyte function, direct toxic effects on the bone marrow, and/or alteration of the usual host defence mechanisms. In some cases, specific prophylactic measures are recommended during routine therapy.

Immunosuppressed patients are at risk of common infections, opportunistic infections, or atypical infections at unusual sites. They may not display typical features of an infective illness nor an acute inflammatory response, therefore a high index of suspicion is essential to identify an unusual or subacute presentation, especially if there has already been a poor response to conventional broad-spectrum antibiotic therapy.

Immunosuppressant agents

Azathioprine and 6-mercaptopurine

Azathioprine is as a steroid-sparing agent during long-term immunosuppression and a disease-modifying antirheumatic drug (DMARD) in inflammatory arthritidies.

Mechanism of action

Azathioprine is the pro-drug of 6-mercaptopurine, a purine analogue that impairs DNA replication in dividing cells by inhibiting nucleotide synthesis. Both agents suppress lymphocyte proliferation and interfere with antigen recognition, lymphocyte adhesion, and cell-mediated cytotoxicity. Immunosuppressant activity is prolonged by intracellular accumulation of active metabolites. The half-life is prolonged in renal impairment.

Adverse effects

Bone marrow suppression

- Dose-related leucopenia can occur in up to 27% of patients.
- Patients with low thiopurine methyltransferase (TPMT) activity are at a significantly increased risk of bone marrow suppression. This defect is genetically determined, with partial deficiency being present in up to 10% of the general population. It is considered prudent to test for TPMT activity before commencing therapy.
- Allopurinol impairs renal excretion of 6-mercaptopurine and will increase the risk of bone marrow suppression.

Infection risk

- Infectious complications are reported in up to 9% of patients and can relate to either common pathogens or opportunistic infections.
- Bacterial infections are usually associated with leucopenia.

- Viral infections can affect up to 6% of patients. There is an association with disseminated herpes zoster infection.

Corticosteroids

Corticosteroids have dose-dependent anti-inflammatory and immunosuppressive properties.

Mechanism of action

Corticosteroids are transported into the nucleus of cells and interact with specific DNA sequences, resulting in the altered transcription of genes that are associated with inflammation and immunity. Effects include:

- Decreased production of pro-inflammatory cytokines
- Reduction in circulating leucocyte levels, except neutrophils
- Impaired bactericidal ability of neutrophils and monocytes.

Adverse effects

Corticosteroids are not associated with significant bone marrow suppression. They have well-documented systemic side-effects, including cushingoid appearance, weight gain, hypertension, osteoporosis, diabetes mellitus, and myopathy.

Demargination

The apparent neutrophilia associated with steroid therapy is caused by reduced adherence of neutrophils to the endothelium of blood vessels. Circulating neutrophils are less able to migrate to sites of infection, further impairing the usual host immune responses.

Infection risk

Corticosteroids increase the risk of common, atypical, and opportunistic infection. There is an increased frequency of infection with common bacterial, viral (herpes virus), and fungal (Candida) pathogens.

Risk is dose dependent and increased in hospitalized patients, the elderly, those with severe underlying disease, and in patients receiving additional immunosuppressant agents. Inhibition of the usual inflammatory and febrile responses can cause 'masking' of many of the typical presenting features of infectious illness. Specific considerations include:

- Tuberculosis—corticosteroid therapy is associated with a five-fold increase in tuberculosis (especially doses >15mg/day for 1 month)
- Pneumonia caused by *Pneumocystis jirovecii* (PCP, pneumocystis pneumonia) is unusual with corticosteroid therapy alone and PCP prophylaxis is not recommended.

Ciclosporin

Ciclosporin is central to several antirejection regimens in solid organ transplant recipients. It is often considered in active inflammatory arthritis and psoriasis if more usual agents are contraindicated.

Mechanism of action

Ciclosporin acts primarily on T lymphocytes by binding to intracellular cyclophilin proteins to interrupt calcineurin-mediated signalling pathways. It prevents the transcription of several genes associated with cytokine synthesis (including IL-2, IL-3, IL-6, IL-8, TNF, and IFNγ). Ciclosporin is predominantly metabolized in the liver by the cytochrome P450 enzyme system, raising the possibility of multiple drug interactions.

Adverse effects

Ciclosporin is not associated with significant bone marrow suppression, leucopenia, or lymphopenia. It has dose-dependent systemic side-effects, including:
- Nephrotoxicity
- Hypertension
- Seizures.

Infection risk
- In transplant recipients, who require high doses, the infection rate is approximately 38%.
- Ciclosporin increases the risk of viral pneumonias (predominantly cytomegalovirus), bacterial infections, and fungal sepsis.

Cyclophosphamide

Cyclophosphamide, an alkylating agent, is a highly effective treatment for autoimmune and inflammatory disease. It is reserved for disease with significant organ involvement (e.g. lupus nephritis, systemic vasculitis) and cancer chemotherapy regimens.

Monthly pulsed intravenous cyclophosphamide is generally preferred for inflammatory diseases since, compared to oral preparations, it has a lower rate of toxicity and is less likely to cause haemorrhagic cystitis.

Mechanism of action

Cyclophosphamide alkylates DNA cross-strands, causing errors in replication and transcription. Cell division is impaired, causing bone marrow suppression and inhibition of lymphocyte proliferation. T and B lymphocyte lines are affected equally, with counts being suppressed by up to 80%.

Adverse effects

There is a cumulative risk of toxicity related to dose and duration of therapy. Acute effects include haemorrhagic cystitis and haematological derangement. Long-term risks include gonadal suppression and ovarian failure, increased risk of malignancy (especially bladder, skin, and haematological), and pulmonary fibrosis.

Bone marrow suppression
- Leucopenias can affect both neutrophil and lymphocyte counts.
- The typical cell count nadir occurs approximately 9–14 days after treatment and bone marrow recovery is usually evident by 21 days.
- Thrombocytopenia and anaemia are longer-term complications.

Infection risk

Cyclophosphamide is associated with an increased risk of infection even if the blood counts are normal. The development of neutropenia (<3000/μl) or the co-administration of high dose corticosteroids is associated with a significantly increased risk.
- Bacterial infection—increased risk (up to 21%). Reported cases include pneumonia, sinusitis, urinary tract infection, abscesses, and septicaemia.

- PCP—particularly in patients with leucopenia or in patients also on corticosteroids. These at-risk groups should have PCP prophylaxis (usually co-trimoxazole).
- Other opportunistic infection—increased risk of fungi and nocardia.
- Reactivation of latent infection, including Varicella zoster, human papilloma virus, and tuberculosis. Reactivation of Varicella zoster may be a direct effect of cyclophosphamide and may present once therapy has finished (i.e. an immune reconstitution syndrome, which presents with deterioration due to inflammation or unmasked infection after initial improvement).

Leflunomide

Leflunomide is predominantly used to treat the inflammatory arthritides and psoriasis. There is increasing evidence that it could be used to maintain remission in other systemic inflammatory conditions if alternative immunosuppressive therapy is contraindicated.

Mechanism of action

Leflunomide inhibits pyrimidine biosynthesis to produce a variety of different biologic effects, including disruption of antigen presentation by dendritic cells, inhibition of leucocyte adhesion and neutrophil migration, inhibition of inflammatory cytokine production, and impaired reactivation of memory T lymphocytes.

Adverse effects

Adverse effects (particularly hypertension and liver function test disturbances) and intolerances are seen in up to 60% of patients.

- Leucopenia (including neutropenia) and eosinophilia are both most common when additional immunosuppressants are prescribed.
- Increase in common infections (particularly respiratory tract infections).
- Charcoal or colestyramine resin can help reverse adverse effects.

Methotrexate

Methotrexate is a popular immunomodulatory agent. Low doses are used for inflammatory arthritides and psoriasis. High-dose methotrexate ($>50mg/m^2$) is cytotoxic and is used as chemotherapy in the treatment of solid organ and haematological malignancies.

Mechanism of action

Proposed mechanisms include:
- Inhibition of folate-dependent enzymes (especially dihydrofolate reductase), causing decreased nucleic acid and protein synthesis
- Promotion of adenosine release, leading to inhibition of neutrophil function and reduced synthesis of proinflammatory cytokines.

Adverse effects

- Serious adverse effects are rare and most are related to methotrexate's antifolate properties (folate is usually prescribed with methotrexate). Risk factors for adverse effects include older age, folate deficiency, drug interactions (e.g. trimethoprim/sulfamethoxazole, phenytoin, NSAIDs, probenecid) and renal dysfunction (methotrexate is predominantly renally excreted; the risk of toxicity increases with falling GFR).

Bone marrow suppression
- Usually presents as either leucopenia or pancytopenia (mortality 17%) and is the major factor limiting dose escalation.
- Severe cases may respond to oral or intravenous folinic acid 'rescue'. Unlike folic acid, folinic acid does not require dihydrofolate reductase in order to function as a vitamin (initial dose = methotrexate dose).

Infection risk
- Intercurrent infections are predominantly upper respiratory tract and/ or urinary tract infections. However, whether or not methotrexate increases the overall risk of infection has not yet been well established.
- There are case reports of pneumonia related to PCP, cryptococcus, cytomegalovirus, and disseminated herpes zoster infection.

Methotrexate pneumonitis
The incidence of methotrexate-associated lung injury is 2–8%. Cases can present at any stage of treatment, although most occur within 1 year of starting therapy. Pneumonitis is more likely to develop in those with:
- High-dose therapy
- Daily rather than weekly administration
- Pre-existing lung disease
- Abnormal PFTs prior to therapy
- Methotrexate pneumonitis is discussed in ▯ Drug-induced lung disease, p 438.

Mycophenolate mofetil
Mycophenolate mofetil (MMF) is commonly used to prevent graft rejection in organ transplant recipients. It is increasingly used as a steroid-sparing agent in systemic lupus erythematosus (particularly lupus nephritis) and systemic vasculitidies, where ongoing studies are addressing its ability to induce and maintain sufficient immunosuppression to achieve disease remission.

Mechanism of action
MMF inhibits synthesis of purine nucleotides, causing decreased lymphocyte proliferation and antibody production. Additional immunosuppressive properties include inducing T-cell apoptosis, reduced adhesion molecule expression, and inhibition of lymphocyte recruitment.

Adverse effects
The risk of adverse effects has been most extensively investigated in organ transplant recipients, but it is likely that these risks will extend to patients with inflammatory conditions. Patients with inflammatory disease may have additional bone marrow suppression and immunoparesis as a result of their underlying disease.

Bone marrow suppression
- Bone marrow suppression is common. It is dose dependent and usually reversible with dose reduction or temporary withdrawal of therapy.

Infection risk
- There is an increased risk of infection by common and opportunistic pathogens.

- Viral infections—Varicella zoster (VZV). Renal transplant recipients more susceptible to CMV infection.
- MMF may have a protective effect against PCP.

Sulfasalazine

Sulfasalazine (covalently-bound sulfapyridine and 5-aminosalicylic acid) is used to treat inflammatory arthritidies and inflammatory bowel disease.

Mechanism of action

This is not fully understood. Colonic bacteria cleave sulfasalazine to sulfapyridine (largely absorbed) and 5-aminosalicylic acid (excreted in faeces). Sulfapyridine may inhibit lymphocyte function and synthesis of inflammatory cytokines. Sulfasalazine also has antifolate properties.

Adverse effects

Dose-dependent adverse effects (e.g. gastrointestinal intolerance, neurological disturbances, haemolysis) usually respond to dose reduction.

Hypersensitivity reactions (e.g. skin reaction, pneumonitis, hepatitis, agranulocytosis, aplastic anaemia) are idiosyncratic and require immediate drug withdrawal.

Bone marrow suppression

- Leucopenia occurs in 1–2% of patients. It is usually mild, dose dependent, and responds to either dose adjustments or withdrawal of treatment.
- Severe agranulocytosis, related to idiosyncratic hypersensitivity mechanisms can also occur and requires immediate, permanent discontinuation of therapy. It is most common within 3 months of starting sulfasalazine and there is usually evidence of bone marrow recovery within 1–2 weeks of drug discontinuation.

Infection risk

To date, sulfasalazine has not been associated with an increased risk of either common or opportunistic infections. Those patients who develop leucopenia, and particularly significant neutropenia, are assumed to be at increased risk.

Tacrolimus

Tacrolimus is a fungal-derived macrolide antibiotic. It is used to prevent graft rejection in organ transplant recipients and in many inflammatory conditions, including rheumatoid arthritis, systemic sclerosis, and Crohn's disease.

Mechanism of action

Tacrolimus binds to the FK binding proteins in cytoplasm. This inhibits calcineurin, causing reduced transcription of proinflammatory cytokines. It also inhibits of prolactin gene transcription (a potent immune activator) and prevents lymphocyte activation (predominantly T-helper cells).

Adverse effects

Important adverse effects include nephrotoxicity, hyperkalaemia, hypertension, impaired glucose tolerance, and neurotoxicity (headache, tremor, seizure).

Tacrolimus is not associated with significant bone marrow suppression.

Infection risk
- There is an increased risk of viral infection, bacterial infection, and fungal sepsis.
- Tacrolimus may be associated with a higher risk of fungal sepsis than ciclosporin (an alternative calcineurin inhibitor).

Biologics

The recent introduction of biologic therapy has greatly improved the efficacy of treatments for many inflammatory conditions. Biologic therapies are specifically engineered to target, and usually inactivate, specific molecules or cell surface receptors integral to the inflammatory process. These agents are usually highly effective, producing profound decreases in the systemic inflammatory burden. However, they also suppress host immune responses, which increases the risk of common, atypical, and opportunistic infections, and may lead to reactivation of latent infections. In the presence of a confirmed or suspected infectious processes, biologic therapy should be discontinued immediately and should not be reconsidered until the infection has completely resolved.

Abatacept

Abatacept is indicated for the treatment of refractory rheumatoid arthritis that is not responding to traditional DMARD therapy (North America) or anti-TNF-α therapy (Europe).

Mechanism of action

Abatacept is a co-stimulatory inhibitor that modulates T-lymphocyte activation. It blocks the interaction between surface membrane receptors on antigen-presenting cells (CD80 and CD86) and T lymphocytes (CD28), removing the second antigenic signal essential for T-cell activation.

Adverse effects

Abatacept is a relatively new agent therefore the complete adverse effect profile has not been fully described.

Infection risk
- Bacterial infections—increased risk of serious bacterial infections which persists after withdrawal of therapy. Upper and lower respiratory tract infections are the most commonly reported.
- Tuberculosis—patients with evidence of previous tuberculosis exposure were excluded in the original clinical trials therefore the risk of risk of tuberculosis reactivation remains unclear.
- There is currently no evidence to suggest increased rates of atypical and/or opportunistic infections.

Alemtuzumab

Alemtuzumab is used as single agent treatment for B-cell chronic lymphocytic leukaemia and may also have a role in the treatment of relapsing–remitting multiple sclerosis and pre-transplant (i.e. perioperative) induction of immunosuppression.

Mechanism of action

Alemtuzumab is a humanized monoclonal antibody which targets CD52 receptors on the surface of lymphocytes and monocytes to produce prolonged T-lymphocyte depletion.

Adverse effects

Infusion-related reactions

These are common and can include pyrexia, hypotension, urticaria, and dyspnoea.

Bone marrow suppression

Lymphopenia and neutropenia are expected and can be prolonged (CD4+ and CD8+ may take up to 12 months to return to pretreatment levels). Autoimmune thrombocytopenia has also been described.

Infection risk

- Alemtuzumab increases the risk of bacterial, viral, fungal, and protozoal infections, and has been associated with increased rates of serious infection.
- Prolonged lymphopenia and neutropenia is associated with an increased risk of opportunistic infections, therefore during these episodes prophylaxis against PCP and viral infections is recommended.
- Viral infections—alemtuzumab is particularly associated with an increased risk of cytomegalovirus infection and viraemia. Patients should be monitored for evidence of cytomegalovirus throughout, and for 2 months after, the course of treatment.

Anakinra

Anakinra (an IL-1 receptor antagonist) is considered less potent than other biologic therapies and is not yet widely used in the treatment of inflammatory arthritides. It may be useful in systemic onset juvenile idiopathic arthritis and other inflammatory conditions.

Mechanism of action

Anakinra inhibits the activity of IL-1, a potent pro-inflammatory cytokine.

Adverse effects

Bone marrow suppression

Cases of neutropenia and thrombocytopenia are rare.

Infection risk

Infection risk is increased, particularly if the patient is also receiving corticosteroids or anti-TNF therapies.

- Bacterial infections, particularly pneumonia and cellulitis.
- There is no evidence to suggest an increased risk of tuberculosis or other opportunistic infections.

Gemtuzumab

Gemtuzumab is reserved for the treatment of patients aged over 60 who experience their first relapse of CD33 positive acute myeloid leukaemia and are not considered candidates for alternative cytotoxic chemotherapy.

Mechanism of action

Gemtuzumab is a humanized monoclonal antibody that is conjugated to the cytotoxic antibiotic calicheamicin. It binds to the CD33 surface antigens expressed by myeloid blast cells and, following internalization of the antibody–antigen complex, releases calicheamicin to induce blast cell apoptosis.

Adverse effects

Infusion-related reactions

- Varying degrees of hypersensitivity reactions have been described. These can vary from transient fever, chills, and hypotension to frank anaphylaxis, pulmonary involvement, and/or ARDS.

Bone marrow suppression

- CD33 is expressed by all non-progenitor myeloid cells, therefore significant myelosuppression is to be expected if the dosing is correct. Most patients will develop prolonged neutropenia and often thrombocytopenia as well, with recovery evident after approximately 40 days.

Infection risk

- During treatment up to 30% of patients will experience at least one infective episode. The risk of opportunistic infections is increased during any neutropenic phase. No specific infectious associations have been identified, but cases of pneumonia, systemic sepsis, and herpes simplex have been reported.

Hepatotoxicity

- Gemtuzumab is associated with an increased risk of hepatotoxicity (hyperbilirubinaemia, transaminitis), which is often transient. Patients who have previously undergone haemopoietic stem cell transplants appear to be at an increased risk of veno-occlusive disease of the liver.

Rituximab

Rituximab was originally used in the treatment of B-cell non-Hodgkin's lymphoma. It is increasingly used in rheumatoid arthritis and systemic lupus erythematosis with vital organ involvement.

Mechanism of action

Rituximab is a chimeric monoclonal antibody targeted at CD20 cell surface receptors. Treatment almost entirely depletes B lymphocytes, causing reduced inflammatory cytokines and immune complexes. Stem cells and existing plasma cells are preserved. Multiple treatment courses can be associated with falling immunoglobulin levels and an attenuated vaccine response. There is a prolonged elimination process, and rituximab can be detected in serum several months after treatment.

Adverse effects

Bone marrow suppression

Following treatment, there is prolonged, almost total, B-lymphocyte depletion, with evidence of recovery developing approximately 6 months after treatment. CD19 expression may be used as marker for B-cell recovery. Severe pan-leucopenia is rare.

Infection risk

- Bacterial infection—small additional risk of serious infection.
- Viral infection—there are reports of severe CMV infection and reactivation of latent hepatitis B and refractory/relapsing babesiosis.
- Progressive multifocal leukoencephalopathy—caused by reactivation of polyomavirus JC (the JC virus). The risk is not fully quantified.

- Tuberculosis—the risk remains unclear. Most patients receiving rituximab will already have received anti-TNF therapy and will have been screened for tuberculosis.
- Opportunistic infection—there is no evidence of increased risk.

TNF-α blocking therapy

The TNF-α blocking therapy group comprises three established agents (adalumimab, etanercept, and infliximab) and two new agents (certoluzimab and golimumab). They are often highly effective. They are usually reserved for severe disease that has been refractory to traditional therapy, although earlier use is increasingly emerging in practice. Current indications include inflammatory arthritides and spondyloarthropathies, uveitis, inflammatory bowel disease, and psoriasis.

Mechanism of action

All agents block the activity of TNF-α, a cytokine associated with endothelial cell activation, T-cell stimulation, regulation of inflammatory cytokine release, and angiogenesis. Etanercept is a TNF receptor-p75/Fc fusion protein, adalumimab a fully human monoclonal antibody, and infliximab is a humanized monoclonal antibody (part mouse/part human) that binds TNF in soluble and membrane-bound phases.

Adverse effects

A large number of adverse effects have been described, many of which are idiosyncratic. Between-drug variations have not been fully established.

Established acute adverse effects include autoantibody formation (particularly anti-nuclear antibody), central and peripheral demyelination, psoriaform skin rashes, paradoxical exacerbation of existing psoriasis, worsening of cardiac failure, and development of acute, rapidly progressive interstitial lung disease.

Bone marrow suppression

Cases of leucopenia, pancytopenia, and aplastic anaemia are rare.

Infection risk

TNF-α is an integral component of the immune response, therefore infection by common and opportunistic organisms is a significant concern. This risk is compounded by co-prescription with corticosteroids, is highest in the first year of therapy, and persists for the duration of treatment.

Specific considerations include:

- Bacterial infection—the risk is increased. Common sites of infection include respiratory tract, skin, soft tissues, bone, and joints (native and prosthetic). Mycobacterial infection is a particular concern (see box).
- Viral infection—herpes simplex virus (HSV), CMV, VZV, and molluscum contagiosum have been reported. Stable hepatitis B infection may be reactivated.
- Fungal infection—TNF-α blocking therapy increases the risk of new invasive and disseminated fungal infections. Latent infections can be reactivated (histoplasmosis, coccidioidomycosis). Invasive fungal infections may present with malaise, fevers, weight loss, cough, increasing breathlessness, pulmonary infiltrates on CXR, and/or fungaemia with severe systemic illness and septic shock.
- There is an increased risk of perioperative infection. TNF-α blocking therapy should be discontinued before any elective surgery.

- Particular vigilance is required for granulomatous infections such as listeriosis, histoplasmosis, coccidiomycosis, and mycobacterial infection.

TNF-α blocking therapies and tuberculosis

TNF-α is essential for the maintenance of granulomas, so TNF-α blocking therapies increase the risk of tuberculosis (including reactivation of latent infection). Reactivation of latent infection usually presents shortly after commencing therapy; the risk of new infection persists throughout treatment.

- The clinical manifestations of active infection are often atypical. There is a higher risk of miliary tuberculosis and disseminated, extrapulmonary disease. Patients with disseminated disease may not display pulmonary involvement.
- Non-specific, constitutional presentations can include malaise, fever, anorexia, and weight loss, therefore a high index of suspicion may be required in all patients and especially those from areas with a high endemic risk of tuberculosis.
- Before commencing TNF-α blocking therapy all patients should be screened (including clinical risk assessment, tuberculin skin test, and CXR). Those with significant risk factors or evidence of previous tuberculosis exposure receive prophylactic isoniazid.
- In the presence of proven, or strongly suspected, active tuberculosis infection TNF-α blocking therapy should be discontinued and antituberculous therapy commenced. Discontinuation of TNF-α blocking therapy during active tuberculosis infection can cause a paradoxical worsening of infection.
- TNF-α blocking therapies increase the risk of non-tuberculous mycobacterial infections (e.g. *Mycobacterium avium intracellulare*).

Tocilizumab
Tocilizumab is a new therapy for moderate to severe rheumatoid arthritis and severe systemic juvenile idiopathic arthritis that has failed to respond to conventional therapy.

Mechanism of action
Tocilizumab is a humanized antibody that blocks the IL-6 receptor. IL-6 is a pro-inflammatory cytokine that mediates inflammatory disease processes and host immune responses to infection.

Adverse effects
Long-term experience is lacking.

Bone marrow suppression
- Transient leucopenia (particularly neutropenia).

Infection risk
This has not been fully determined. Clinical trials suggest that tocilizumab is associated with a small increase in the risk of serious infection, especially when co-prescribed with methotrexate.

- Slight increased risk of diverticular complications (particularly diverticulitis and perforation).

- Opportunistic infections have been reported, but there are insufficient data available to fully assess the risk.

Ustekinumab

Ustekinumab is a biologic therapy recently licensed for use in moderate to severe psoriasis and under development for use in psoriatic arthritis and inflammatory bowel disease.

Mechanism of action

Ustekinumab is a human monoclonal antibody that binds to the shared p40 chain that is present in IL-12 and IL-23, blocking receptor activity. Downstream effects include reduced production of proinflammatory cytokines and reduced activation of T lymphocytes (especially Th17 cells), natural killer (NK) cells, and antigen-presenting cells.

Adverse effects

Clinical trial evidence, based on a relatively small number of patients, has not suggested an increased risk of serious or opportunistic infections or tuberculosis.

Diagnosis and management of infections secondary to immunomodulatory and biologic therapy

Only those infections that are unusual or have particular problems associated with respiratory intensive care are considered here.

Appropriate antimicrobial therapy may not be sufficient to resolve life-threatening infection in an immunocompromised patient. Serious consideration must always be given to reducing or stopping the immunosuppressive drug. In such circumstances stopping immunosuppressive therapy may be the only way to keep a patient alive, although resulting in flare of disease or loss of a transplanted organ.

Viral infections

Varicella zoster

VZV commonly reactivates to produce shingles in the immunocompromised. It can spread rapidly to involve many dermatomes and produce hemorrhagic pneumonia, hepatitis, and other systemic involvement. Disease progression can be very rapid.
- Diagnosis usually evident clinically but PCR of vesicle fluid definitive.
- Reactivation of VZV can produce encephalitis in the absence of skin lesions; PCR on CSF is diagnostic.
- Initial treatment—intravenous aciclovir 10mg/kg 8 hourly. Step down to oral famciclovir/valaciclovir for 7–10 days.
- The skin lesions are highly infectious, although most adults are immune. Pregnant healthcare workers should avoid contact with VZV unless they know they are immune.

Cytomegalovirus

Reactivation is very common in immunocompromised patients. There are variable clinical effects, ranging from mild fever to fulminant pneumonia, hepatitis, and other systemic effects.
- Diagnosis best by PCR in blood/BAL, with quantification of viral load.

- Treatment may not be indicated if low viral load, as reactivation can occur without clinical disease. Standard therapy is intravenous ganciclovir.
- Intravenous immunoglobulin (IVIG) has been used for severe pneumonia.

Respiratory syncytial virus

Respiratory syncytial virus (RSV) is a common respiratory virus, especially in infants and young children. It can produce a severe pneumonitis in the immunocompromised with prolonged viral shedding.

- Diagnosis from PCR from throat swab/respiratory secretions.
- Treatment is with ribavirin intravenously, as administration by aerosol is impracticable on ITU. The intravenous formulation may not be generally available.
- RSV is highly infectious and can spread to other immunocompromised patients or cause severe disease in pre-term infants or children <2 years with cyanotic heart disease/chronic lung disease. Prophylaxis of such patients with palivizumab, a humanized monoclonal antibody to RSV, is highly effective.

Influenza/parainfluenza

These are common infections with potential life-threatening pneumonia in the immunocompromised. Secondary bacterial pneumonia is common.

- Diagnosis by PCR from throat/nasal swab is highly sensitive and will determine viral species and sub-type.
- Parainfluenza treatment is ribavirin. Aerosolized steroids may be beneficial but trial data are lacking.
- Influenza A treatment is oseltamivir (no intravenous preparation). Zanamivir 2 puffs twice daily effective, but resistance is common.

Hepatitis B

Reactivation of chronic hepatitis B can occur with immunosuppressant therapy, typically in chronic carriers but it can also occur in those who have apparently cleared the virus. Rises in viral load can be associated with acute hepatitis.

- Diagnosis is by combined viral antigen detection, viral DNA load, and antibodies to viral proteins. Given that blood products are screened for hepatitis B, infection will generally be a reactivation if it presents while in ITU.
- Entecavir or lamivudine give good initial control of viral replication, although longer-term resistance can arise. Intravenous formulations may be difficult to source. Chronic carriers should have been identified at screening and started on prophylactic lamivudine prior to immunosuppressant therapy.
- Active hepatitis B is highly infective by blood transmission. Heathcare workers should be immunized.

Bacterial infection

Clostridium difficile

C. difficile infections are significantly associated with immunosuppressive therapy, even in the absence of broad-spectrum antibiotic treatment.

- Toxin detection in stool is diagnostic but sensitivity significantly increased by two separate tests.

- Luminal delivery of antibiotics is preferable—vancomycin 500mg four times daily nasogastrically. If ng delivery unsuccessful or impractical use intravenous metronidazole or consider retention enema (vancomycin 500mg diluted to 1L with 0.9%NaCl delivered via rectal tube and clamped for 1h). The use if IVIG has been described.
- As far as possible, source isolation of *C. difficile* infected patients should be practised. Spores of the organisms are not killed by alcohol wipes; hand washing with soap is required.

Mycobacterium tuberculosis

M. tuberculosis is frequently reactivated in patients who are immunosuppressed. Onset can be insidious; it can affect many extrapulmonary targets and a high degree of suspicion must be kept for this infection.

- Ziehl–Nielsen staining of biological fluids is very helpful, although it has low sensitivity other than for sputum. Culture may take 6 weeks.
- γ-interferon release assays (e.g. T spot test) can be very helpful, as they indicate active immune response to tuberculosis and are useful even in the immunosuppressed. In white Caucasians this will generally indicate active infection; patients from regions where tuberculosis is endemic may have positive tests resulting from childhood infection. When immunosuppressed they are very likely to reactivate, so most would advocate chemoprophylaxis with isoniazid (plus pyridoxine) for 9 months if there is no evidence of active disease.
- Active disease requires initial treatment with four drugs: isoniazid, rifampicin, pyrazinamide and ethambutol for 2 months, plus isoniazid with rifampicin for another 4 months, but be guided by sensitivities.
- Smear-positive tuberculosis is reasonably infectious, emphasizing the importance of universal precautions and use of face-masks with respiratory care.

Atypical mycobacteria

Immunosuppression can be associated with a variety of atypical mycobacterial infections. Unlike tuberculosis, some of these species grow very rapidly. They can present as pulmonary disease, skin infections, and abscesses. Therapy can be difficult and *in vitro* sensitivities do not necessarily predict *in vivo* effects.

Nocardia

Nocardia are Gram-positive branching rod-shaped organisms usually only causing infection in the immunocompromised.

- They typically produce abscesses in diverse sites, e.g. lung, brain, bone, heart, skin.
- Diagnosis suspected on Gram staining. Definitive diagnosis on culture.
- Treatment needs to be prolonged (6–12 months):
  - Co-trimoxazole
  - Add amikacin in severe infection
  - Carbapenems are a useful alternative to co-trimoxazole
  - Abscesses should be drained.

Fungi

Aspergillus spp.

This is a common environmental fungus that most often causes pneumonia in the immunosuppressed, but can produce abscesses in the brain and elsewhere.

- Diagnosis on histology/culture but can colonize respiratory tract so not diagnostic from upper airway secretions.
- Serum galactomannan, a fungal cell wall component, may be useful in invasive disease.
- Invasive disease best treated by voriconazole. Amphotericin is also effective.

Pneumocystis jirovecii

P. jiroveci (formerly *carini*., still referred to as PCP). This is a cause of pneumonia in the immunosuppressed. Although it looks like a protozoan, its genome indicates that it is a fungus.

- In non-HIV positive patients, onset of illness is more abrupt and microbial load much lower.
- Interstitial lung infiltrates with relative sparing of apices and bases is typical, with absence of pleural fluid, but other patterns are possible.
- BAL specimens showing organisms on silver stain or by immunofluorescence are diagnostic 'gold standard' but of low sensitivity.
- PCR much more sensitive, with excellent negative predictive value, but in the non-HIV population only about 50% positive predictive value. However, positive result in the presence of immunosuppression is highly suggestive of active infection.
- Treatment is with co-trimoxazole. In severe disease with PO_2 <8.0kPa, prednisolone improves outcome. The alternative is clindamycin plus primaquine.

Cryptococcus neoformans

C. neoformans is a widespread yeast-like microbe. It causes meningitis, but can also result in pulmonary and cutaneous disease.

- Serum and cerebrospinal fluid (CSF) cryptococcal antigen is very sensitive and specific for this organism. Additionally, the yeast forms may be seen on direct microscopy of samples stained with India ink. It typically produces a lymphocytic infiltrate in the CSF with a low sugar.
- Treatment is with amphotericin B together with flucytosine, usually for 2 weeks, followed by maintenance with fluconazole life-long or until immune state normal.
- Elevated CSF pressure is very common and usually symptomatic. Daily lumbar puncture with removal of CSF until pressure is <20cmH$_2$O may be required. The alternative is insertion of a CSF reservoir or shunt.

Multicellular parasites

Strongyloides stercoralis

S. stercoralis is a common intestinal nematode human parasite endemic in the tropics/subtropics that can auto-infect the host via the lower gut. Chronic infection can last for decades. In immunosuppressed individuals, parasite burden can become intense, resulting in a 'hyperinfection' syndrome, with parasites invading the lung and other tissues. It carries a high mortality and is frequently associated with Gram-negative sepsis.

• Serology confirms infection, but can be falsely negative in immunosuppressed patients.
• In hyperinfection, larvae can be found in many sites.
• Although eosinophilia is typical of chronic infection, it is usually absent in hyperinfection.
• The treatment of choice is ivermectin for at least 7 days in hyperinfection. Although unlicensed in the UK, ivermectin is generally available via hospital pharmacies for this indication.

6.6 Chronic obstructive pulmonary disease

COPD is one of the most frequent causes of hospital admission and the most common cause of chronic and acute respiratory failure, both type 1 and type 2. Despite this, the importance of COPD is often underestimated by clinicians and the complex multidimensional nature of COPD is poorly understood. Although the management of patients admitted to hospital with exacerbations of COPD has improved in the last decade, principally as a result of the greater use of NIV, many patients receive sub-optimal care and there is often a reluctance to admit patients to ITUs because of mistaken pessimism about the likely outcome.

Patients with COPD experience poor physical functioning, live with distressing symptoms, become socially isolated, often have a poor quality of life, and commonly experience clinical depression. As their disease progresses they require frequent hospital admissions. COPD also takes its toll on patient's spouses, carers, and their families, who may have to assist patients with basic activities such as washing or dressing. Partners may also suffer the frustration of not being able to enjoy recreational activities with their spouses.

Definition

COPD is a chronic, progressive, usually fatal disease characterized by poorly reversible obstruction of the airways that leads to breathlessness, cough, sputum production, wheeze, and frequent exacerbations. It affects the airways, the alveoli, and the pulmonary vasculature, and also has effects on skeletal muscle and other organs. It is a preventable and treatable condition.

Airflow obstruction is generally defined as meaning a post-bronchodilator FEV_1 less than 80% of the predicted value and an FEV_1/FVC ratio less than 70%.

Terminology

Chronic obstructive pulmonary disease

COPD is now the recommended name for a group of conditions previously known as chronic airflow limitation (CAL), chronic obstructive airways disease (COAD), chronic obstructive lung disease (COLD), chronic bronchitis, and emphysema.

- COPD is the preferred term because it includes the airways, the lung parenchyma, and the pulmonary circulation.

Emphysema

Emphysema is defined as 'abnormal, permanent enlargement of airspaces distal to the terminal bronchiole, accompanied by destruction of their walls and without obvious fibrosis'.

- It can be classified into panacinar, centriacinar, or paraseptal.
- The pattern of emphysema has no effect on the clinical symptoms it produces, but the two forms of emphysema have distinct mechanical properties: lung compliance is greater in panacinar emphysema, leading to a greater contribution to airflow limitation from loss of elastic recoil.

- Bullae are areas of emphysema larger than 1cm in diameter that are locally over-distended.

Chronic bronchitis

Chronic bronchitis is a state of chronic mucus hypersecretion.

- It was defined for the purposes of epidemiology by the British Medical Research Council as a cough productive of sputum for more at least 3 months in each year for not less than 2 successive years.
- Epidemiological studies have shown that there is no relationship between the rate of decline in the FEV_1 or mortality and the symptoms of chronic bronchitis.

Historical terminology

The terms 'blue bloater' and 'pink puffer' have been used to characterize different physiological phenotypes of COPD. Despite their linguistic appeal, they are rarely used now as they represent an oversimplification and are seen less commonly as a result of modern management.

- 'Blue bloaters' were defined as patients with chronic bronchitis who developed alveolar hypoventilation with cyanosis, CO_2 retention, and oedema as a result of recurrent exacerbations. These patients were thought to have relatively little emphysema.
- 'Pink puffers' were rarer. They were defined as patients who developed progressive dyspnoea on exertion, without a preceding history of chronic bronchitis. They were hyperinflated and worked hard to maintain a supra-normal minute volume to keep the $PaCO_2$ normal. They generally had severe emphysema.

The use of these terms should now be abandoned.

Aetiology of COPD

Smoking

- Smoking accounts for approximately 80% of the attributable risk of COPD in the UK.
- There is a clear dose–response relationship between total tobacco consumption and the risk of developing COPD and the severity of the disease.
- Approximately 50% of smokers will develop COPD if they live long enough.

Environment

Environmental factors and occupational dust exposures are also important causes of COPD. The best characterized are coal dust, cotton dust, grain dust cement dust, oil fumes, and cadmium fumes.

Genetic susceptibility

The development of COPD is thought to be related to genetic susceptibility factors. Currently the only characterized genetic risk factor is alpha-1 antitrypsin (α-1 AT) deficiency.

Alpha-1 antitrypsin deficiency

α-1 AT (or α-1 antiprotease) is the major protease inhibitor in serum and the lung, which it protects from potential damage from enzymes released by activated neutrophils, including neutrophil elastase.

- α-1 AT deficiency is a rare cause of COPD, accounting for ~2% of cases.

- There is considerable variability in the clinical manifestations of patients with α-1 AT deficiency: some patients having minimal or no symptoms and others develop severe emphysema at an early age.
- Smoking is still the major factor influencing the development of emphysema, but some non-smokers develop airflow limitation in later life, possibly related to a history of asthma or pneumonia.
- The risk of developing COPD is affected by the α-1 AT genotype.

Socio-economic status
The incidence of COPD has always had a strong socio-economic bias and this persisted even in the years when cigarette smoking was relatively evenly distributed across socio-economic groups. This may be partly explained by an increased risk of COPD in people with:
- Low birthweight
- Frequent childhood infection
- Damp housing
- A diet low in fish, fruit, and vegetables.

Other factors
Two other risk factors have been proposed: recurrent bronchopulmonary infections (the 'British hypothesis') and pre-existing atopy and airway hyper-responsiveness (the 'Dutch hypothesis').

Prevalence and mortality
- The prevalence of spirometrically confirmed COPD in adults aged over 40 years is 9–10%.
- Up to 65% of patients with COPD are not diagnosed as many accept breathlessness and limited exercise tolerance as features of ageing and regard their smoker's cough as normal.
- There has been a marked increase in the prevalence of COPD in women over the last decade.
- Overall 5-year survival from diagnosis is 78% in men and 72% in women, and 30% and 24%, respectively, in severe disease.
- Approximately one-third of deaths are due to respiratory causes, one-third to cardiac causes, and a quarter to cancer.
- As well as the effects of smoking, there is increasing evidence that systemic inflammation in COPD may have a direct effect on the heart.

Pathophysiology
Pathological changes
The pathological changes of COPD are complex and correlate poorly with the physiological abnormalities.
  Within the lungs COPD is associated with:
- Increased volume and number of submucosal glands
- Increased number of goblet cells in the mucosa
- Mucosal inflammation
- Emphysema
- Inflammatory exudate within airway lumens.

The airflow obstruction that characterizes COPD is located primarily in the small peripheral airways. Pathologically, the changes in these airways are subtle but include:
- Loss of alveolar attachments that act like guy ropes to hold open the airway

- Increased surface tension as a result of replacement of surfactant by inflammatory exudates
- Occlusion of the lumen by exudates
- Oedema and inflammation of the mucosa
- Bronchoconstriction.

In hypoxaemic patients with COPD, characteristic changes occur in peripheral pulmonary arteries: the intima of small arteries develops accumulations of smooth muscle, and muscular arteries develop medial hypertrophy.

Physiological changes

Decreased maximal expiratory flow, hyperinflation, and impaired gas exchange are fundamental to the pathophysiology of COPD.

- The relationship between exercise capacity and FEV_1 is poor and there is a better correlation with measures of hyperinflation such as inspiratory capacity.
- Expiratory flow limitation contributes to hyperinflation by preventing the exhalation of sufficient volume in the time available to allow the EELV to fall to the relaxation volume determined by elastic recoil.
- Loss of lung recoil due to emphysema also leads to increased EELV as there is less force to balance the recoil of the chest wall.
- Dynamic hyperinflation refers to the acute and variable increase in EELV above its baseline value that occurs in flow-limited patients as a consequence of the lack of sufficient time for the lungs to deflate fully prior to the next inspiration.
- In COPD the inspiratory load is increased as a result of airway obstruction. In addition, the force of contraction is reduced as a consequence of:
  - Hyperinflation altering the mechanical advantage of the muscles (both intercostal and diaphragmatic)
  - Malnutrition
  - Respiratory muscle fatigue (in some cases).

Inspiratory muscle dysfunction is central to the development of hypercapnia.

- Pulmonary gas exchange abnormalites may arise as a result of:
  - Alveolar hypoventilation
  - Impaired alveolar–capillary diffusion
  - Ventilation–perfusion mismatching
  - Increased physiological dead space.
- When patients with COPD exercise they are frequently limited by leg discomfort rather than breathlessness, reflecting the skeletal muscle dysfunction that is a systemic feature of COPD. The causes of skeletal muscle dysfunction probably vary from patient to patient and include deconditioning, malnutrition, hypoxia, hypercapnia, and increased oxidative stress.

Clinical features

Symptoms

Patients with mild airflow obstruction are often asymptomatic, but as COPD develops symptoms progress.

- The cardinal symptoms are cough, wheeze, and breathlessness.
- When patients first develop symptoms they are usually mild and intermittent.

- Patients with moderate COPD invariably have some symptoms, but the severity varies considerably.
- Patients with severe COPD are almost always breathless on minimal exertion and have reduced exercise capacity. They generally cough, especially in the mornings, and frequently wheeze. They may have symptoms of complications such as peripheral oedema, and their sleep may be disturbed (but not by acute breathlessness, as in asthma).
- Breathlessness:
  - Usually develops insidiously and may be regarded as a normal part of ageing
  - Correlates poorly with the degree of airflow obstruction
  - May be worse in the morning, but does not vary markedly from day to day or within a day
  - May vary according to environmental conditions and is sensitive to changes in the weather, particularly temperature and humidity.
- Weight loss is a common symptom in advanced COPD. It is due to a combination of the effects of the increased WOB, reduced calorie intake because of increased breathlessness, and the metabolic effects of COPD.

Signs

The findings on clinical examination in patients with COPD are as variable as the symptoms.
- There is a very poor correlation between the clinical signs and the severity of airflow obstruction.
- Examination is often normal in patients with asymptomatic or mild disease.
- There may be signs of hyperinflation (depressed liver, loss of cardiac dullness, reduced crico-sternal distance, increased AP diameter of chest).
- Polyphonic wheezes or abnormally quiet breath sounds may be heard.
- If there is a component of chronic bronchitis coarse crackles may be heard.
- Expiration is prolonged.
- There may be signs of complications, particularly cor pulmonale (peripheral oedema and elevated venous pressure, RV heave, loud pulmonary second sound, tricuspid regurgitation) and weight loss or cachexia.

Diagnosing COPD

Spirometry is fundamental to diagnosing COPD and a confident diagnosis can only be made if spirometry confirms the presence of airflow obstruction. Most guidelines now advocate post-bronchodilator values as they may show less variability. A lack of bronchodilator response is not recommended as part of the diagnosis of COPD.
- Repeated FEV_1 measurements can show small spontaneous fluctuations.
- The results of a bronchodilator challenge performed on different occasions may vary considerably.
- The definition of the magnitude of a significant change is purely arbitrary and many patients with COPD have a significant bronchodilator response.

Differential diagnosis

The differential diagnosis of patients presenting with symptoms suggestive of COPD includes:

- Asthma
- Bronchiectasis
- LV dysfunction
- Carcinoma of the bronchus
- Obliterative bronchiolitis.

Severity assessment

Because COPD is heterogeneous no single measure can give an adequate assessment of the true severity of the disease in an individual patient. Severity assessment is nevertheless important because it has implications for therapy and relates to prognosis.

- FEV_1 correlates poorly with symptoms but is predictive of 5-year mortality and is still widely used in guidelines to classify patients (Table 6.4).

Table 6.4 Classification of severity of airflow obstruction

Severity	Post-bronchodilator FEV_1/FVC	Post-bronchodilator FEV_1 (% predicted)
Stage 1 – mild	<0.7	≥80%
Stage 2 – moderate	<0.7	50–79%
Stage 3 – severe	<0.7	30–49%
Stage 4 – very severe	<0.7	<30%

- Multicomponent severity indices such as the BODE index give a better indication of prognosis over 12 months. It includes the body-mass index (B), the degree of airflow obstruction (O), dyspneoa (D), and exercise capacity (E), measured by a 6-min walk test.
- Acute Physiology and Chronic Health Evaluation (APACHE) II and III and the physiological components of Simplified Acute Physiology Score (SAPS) II can be used to predict mortality in patients admitted to ICU but organ-specific scoring systems such as the COPD and Asthma Physiology Score (CAPS) appear more accurate.

Even the best severity assessment will overlook aspects of the disease in individual patients and they should not be used in isolation to make critical decisions such as whether to aggressively treat a patient.

Oxygen therapy

Home oxygen therapy is indicated in patients with PaO_2 <7.3kPa when stable or PaO_2 <8kPa when stable and one of secondary polycythaemia, nocturnal hypoxaemia (SaO_2 less than 90% for more than 30% of the time), peripheral oedema, or pulmonary hypertension.

The use of home oxygen therapy is therefore an indicator of severe underlying disease, but it is unhelpful as a prognostic indicator during exacerbations.

Exacerbations

Exacerbations are common at all levels of lung function and are not just a feature of patients with severe disease.

- They occur, sometimes frequently, in patients with FEV_1 >50% and are often unreported.
- They cause disruptive and frightening symptoms and are a direct cause of worsening health status.
- Recovery from exacerbations is slow and often incomplete and they lead to step-wise decline in lung function and physical status.

A number of factors are known to cause exacerbations of COPD, including bacterial and viral infections as well as environmental factors such as air pollution.

Definition of an exacerbation of COPD

A sustained worsening of the patient's symptoms from his or her usual stable state that is beyond normal day-to-day variations and is acute in onset. Commonly reported symptoms are worsening breathlessness, cough, increased sputum production, and change in sputum colour. The change in these symptoms often necessitates a change in medication.

The clinical features of an exacerbation of COPD can be quite different in different patients, but changes in breathlessness, cough, and sputum production are common.

- The diagnosis is made clinically and does not depend on the results of investigations, but in hospitalized patients investigations may assist in ensuring appropriate treatment is given.
- Perform CXR, ECG, arterial blood gases (record FiO_2), FBC, urea and electrolytes (U+Es), sputum, and blood cultures, and, if necessary, a theophylline level.
- The differential diagnosis of an exacerbation includes pneumonia, pneumothorax, heart failure, and pulmonary emboli.

Management of exacerbations

Bronchodilators

- Increased breathlessness is usually managed with more frequent short-acting bronchodilators administered via both nebulizers and hand-held inhalers.
- If a nebulizer is used and the patient is hypercapnic or acidotic the nebulizer should be driven by compressed air, not oxygen (to avoid worsening hypercapnia).
- Patients should be changed to hand-held inhalers as soon as their condition has stabilized because this facilitates earlier discharge.

Steroids

- Oral steroids lead to faster improvement in lung function, earlier discharge, and a prolonged time to the next exacerbation.
- In ICU, variable absorption from the gastrointestinal tract means intravenous steroids are preferred.

- The National Institute for Health and Clinical Excellence (NICE) guideline recommends that in the absence of significant contraindications oral corticosteroids should be used, in conjunction with other therapies, in all patients admitted to hospital with an exacerbation of COPD.

Antibiotic therapy
- The bacteria that have been isolated during exacerbations are generally sensitive to most broad-spectrum antibiotics.
- Antibiotics should only be used to treat exacerbations of COPD associated with a history of more purulent sputum.

Oxygen
- Patients are often hypoxic during exacerbations and oxygen is commonly used to relieve symptoms and raise arterial oxygen saturations.
- The aim of supplemental oxygen therapy is to maintain adequate levels of oxygenation (SaO_2 >90%), without precipitating respiratory acidosis or worsening hypercapnia.
- In patients with a chronic respiratory acidosis (and therefore a high bicarbonate in blood gases), uncontrolled oxygen therapy can result in carbon dioxide narcosis and ultimately respiratory arrest.

Oxygen therapy is discussed in greater detail in 📖 Oxygen therapy, p 74.

The role of ICU
The indications for ventilation are no different in COPD to other causes of respiratory failure.

NIV is now considered the treatment of choice for persistent hypercapnic respiratory failure during exacerbations, despite optimal medical therapy.
- It is associated with fewer complications than intubation.
- It reduces mortality.
- It shortens the length of hospital stay.
- It can be provided in specialized ward, HDU, or ITU setting.
  Some patients may require intubation and ventilation:
- Those who do not respond adequately to NIV
- Those with multiple-organ system impairment
- Those unable to maintain or protect their airway.

Prognosis
There is often inappropriate pessimism about the outcome of IPPV in COPD. If a patient has a reasonable functional status, has suffered an acute exacerbation (as opposed to a chronic decline), and especially if there is only single-organ failure, outcomes are generally good.

The decision on whether to intubate a patient may be difficult and involves balancing health status with an estimate of expectation of survival.
- The mortality rate of patients requiring IPPV for acute respiratory failure due to COPD is significantly lower than mortality in patients with ARF due to other respiratory causes.
- In general ICU stays are short. In a UK study of nearly 4000 admissions the median ICU stay was 4 days and in a US study the mean duration of mechanical ventilation was 2.3 days.
- Overall, survival is good, but differences in admission criteria around the world result in widely differing ICU mortality rates being reported.

In the UK study the mortality rates was 23% whereas in other international studies it has ranged from 7 to 10%. Overall, median survival is between 1 and 2 years, with 30–40% of patients surviving for 3 years.

- Increased risk of hospital mortality is associated with:
  - Older age
  - Worse breathlessness/poor exercise capacity
  - Length of stay in hospital before ICU admission
  - Need for intubation in first 24h in ICU
  - Need for >72h mechanical ventilation
  - pH
  - PaO_2/F_iO_2 gradient
  - Low albumin
  - Multiple-organ failure.

Reversible features

- The key to reversibility is to identify an acute deterioration in symptoms.
- A clear CXR during an exacerbation should not be interpreted as a lack of reversible pathology precipitating admission. Outcome in these cases is in general better than when a 'reversible' cause (such as pneumonia or LVF) is identified on CXR.

Ventilatory management

The approach to mechanical ventilation will depend on the underlying pathophysiological abnormalities (e.g. bronchospasm, dynamic hyperinflation, emphysema) and the reason for the exacerbation (e.g. pneumonia, LVF). The approach to ventilation should be tailored to the individual.

- Hypoxaemia is not usually difficult to correct unless there is coexisting consolidation.
- Expiratory airflow limitation, loss of elastic recoil, small airway collapse during tidal ventilation, and dynamic airway collapse all lead to dynamic hyperinflation—inspiration starting before the lungs reach their resting volume.

Full mechanical ventilation

The ventilatory principles are similar to those used in asthma, although the airflow limitation is rarely as severe. Compliance in COPD is often increased.

- Aim for the patient's normal saturation or, if this is unknown, 88–92%.
- Aim for normal H^+, not normal CO_2.
- Adjust settings to allow the lungs to empty as fully as possible.
- Increase inspiratory flow rates to 80–100L/min or decrease pressure ramp time to 25ms.
- Aim for approximately 8mL/kg tidal volume.
- I:E ratio at least 1:3, possibly 1:4 or 1:5.
- Inspect the expiratory flow trace and make sure that it reaches close to zero. Always re-examine this trace after ventilatory adjustments.
- Consider calculation of the expiratory time constant (R × C). End inspiratory and end expiratory holds will allow accurate calculation of compliance and resistance respectively (see p 231, Monitoring on a ventilator). Expiration should be at least three times the expiratory time constant to allow 95% of this exponential process to complete.

- Aim to minimize $PEEP_i$. $PEEP_i$ can be estimated by slowly adding extrinsic PEEP. When extrinsic PEEP approaches $PEEP_i$, compliance reduces and the inspiratory pressure will rise (if using VCV) or the tidal volume will fall (if using PCV). PEEPi can be measured in passive patients with an expiratory occlusion.

Partial ventilatory support
- Use a flow trigger.
- Synchrony is a significant problem—see 📖 Pressure support ventilation, p 144. Over-supported breaths and $PEEP_i$ lead to frequent wasted inspiratory efforts. A balance must be found between reducing WOB (requires increased support) and reducing wasted efforts (requires decreased support).
- Aim for a respiratory rate of 25–30 per minute.
- Extrinsic PEEP is essential to reduce the WOB imposed by $PEEP_i$ (see 📖 Positive end expiratory pressure, p 119). Changes in WOB with PEEP can be assessed by observing the $P_{0.1}$. If the addition of PEEP reduces WOB, the $P_{0.1}$ will usually reduce.
- If the expiratory trigger is adjustable on the ventilator, increase it to around 50%.
- Concerns about difficulties weaning are misplaced. Newer modes of ventilation and improved ventilators mean that 'being stuck on a ventilator' is an unlikely clinical scenario. NIV can be successfully used to shorten duration of IPPV and facilitate weaning. Refer to 📖 Weaning from mechanical ventilation, p 333, for further details.

Recovery and discharge planning
- The patient's recovery from an exacerbation should be monitored by regular clinical assessment of their symptoms and observation of their functional capacity.
- Patients should be established on optimal maintenance bronchodilator therapy prior to discharge and patients who have had an episode of respiratory failure should have satisfactory oximetry or arterial blood gas results prior to discharge.
- Patients may need temporary or even permanent domiciliary support on discharge.
- Follow-up and home care arrangements, e.g. visiting nurse, oxygen therapy, should be agreed before discharge.
- Over the last few years there has been considerable interest in hospital-based rapid assessment units and early discharge schemes for patients with exacerbations of COPD. They are effective ways of shortening the duration of hospital stay or preventing admission and provide safe and cost-effective alternatives that many patients prefer.

Excessive dynamic airway collapse and tracheobronchomalacia

The significance of these conditions is uncertain. They may be present without symptoms.
- Excessive expiratory airway collapse has been reported to occur in patients with COPD, but there is controversy about its significance.

- The posterior tracheal wall collapses normally on expiration. Excessive dynamic airway collapse has been defined as narrowing by prolapse of the posterior wall by >50% (but this can be seen in normal individuals).
- Acquired tracheobronchomalacia may be caused by weakness of the anterior or lateral walls of the trachea, or both.
- In ICU, excessive dynamic airway collapse presents with (usually rapid) failure of extubation because of respiratory distress, wheezing, and stridor.
- It may also present with expiratory airflow obstruction resistant to steroid and bronchodilator therapy.
- The airway collapse can be visualized by bronchoscopy or rapid CT scanning.
- Treatment is to manage the underlying condition and to electively use CPAP or NIV. In rare cases stenting or surgery may be considered.

Further reading

1 Barbera JA, Roca J, Ferrer A, et al. (1997) Mechanisms of worsening gas exchange during acute exacerbations of chronic obstructive pulmonary disease. Eur Respir J **10**(6), 1285–1291.
2 Gibson GJ (1996) Pulmonary hyperinflation a clinical overview. Eur Respir J **9**(12), 2640–2649.
3 Management of chronic obstructive pulmonary disease in adults in primary and secondary care (partial update). NICE clinical guideline 101 (2010). Available at http://guidance.nice.org.uk/CG101.
4 O'Donnell DE and Parker CM (2006) COPD exacerbations. 3: Pathophysiology. Thorax **61**(4), 354–361.
5 Rabe KF, Hurd S, Anzueto A, et al. (2007) Global strategy for the diagnosis, management, and prevention of chronic obstructive pulmonary disease: GOLD executive summary. Am J Respir Crit Care Med **176**(6), 532–555.
6 Wildman MJ, Harrison DA, Brady AR, and Rowan K (2005) Case mix and outcomes for admissions to UK adult, general critical care units with chronic obstructive pulmonary disease: a secondary analysis of the ICNARC Case Mix Programme Database. Crit Care **9**, S38–S48.

6.7 Drug-induced lung disease

Drug-induced lung disease (DILD) is a relatively uncommon, although potentially serious, cause of iatrogenic morbidity or mortality. As the number of drugs available increases so does the potential for these to cause harm. A review in 1972 identified only 19 drugs responsible for DILD. This number has now increased to almost 400.[1] The clinical syndromes resulting from DILD are widespread and include:

- Asthma
- SLE
- Bronchiolitis organizing pneumonia obliterans
- Hypersensitivity pneumonitis
- Interstitial pneumonia or fibrosis
- Non-cardiogenic pulmonary oedema
- Parenchymal haemorrhage
- Pleural effusion
- Eosinophilic pneumonia
- Pulmonary vascular disease.

DILD should be considered when alternative causes of respiratory disease have been largely excluded, or when the response to treatment of another suspected respiratory disorder is poor. A high index of suspicion is required. Early diagnosis of DILD allows the suspect drug to be withdrawn, and prevents disease progression.

Pathophysiology

- Direct lung toxicity—some drugs, such as chemotherapy agents, can have a direct toxic effect on the lungs.
- Direct pharmacological effect—for example β-adrenergic antagonists in asthmatics.
- Indirect pharmacological effect—drugs may be biotransformed in the lung. This phase 1 oxidative reaction converts lipid-soluble compounds to more water-soluble forms to aid excretion. It is catalysed by enzymes such as cytochrome P450 and may produce reactive metabolites, e.g. oxygen free radicals, hydrogen peroxide, and hydroxyl radicals. These all cause cell damage and cell wall lipid peroxidation, triggering an inflammatory response with release of leukocytes and cytokines and resultant lung injury. Fibrosis may occur during the healing process. Examples include paraquat, oxygen toxicity, nitrofurantoin, and bleomycin.

Epidemiology

DILD can occur in any age group and some reactions are more common in women (aspirin-induced bronchospasm and ACE-I induced cough) or men (amiodarone pneumonitis). There are age-related, genetic, and racial differences in the frequency of certain reactions.

Co-morbidities may predispose to DILD. This may be related to:

- The disease being treated—rheumatoid arthritis and methotrexate
- Radiation therapy
- Renal failure—reduced drug clearance.

The incidence of DILD is unknown. 'Pneumotox online'[2] grades the frequency of DILD reported in the world literature using a star system, with * representing <5 cases, up to **** allocated to drugs with >100 cases of pulmonary toxicity in the literature (Table 6.5).

Table 6.5 Drugs associated with a high number of case reports of lung injury

Drugs with >100 case reports of lung injury	Drugs commonly used in ICU with reports of DILD
Amiodarone	Aspirin***
Angiotensin-converting enzyme inhibitors	Anticoagulants (oral)***
β-blockers	Adrenaline*
Bleomycin	Angiotensin-converting enzyme inhibitors
Blood transfusions	Antidepressants***
Captopril	β-blockers
Ergot compounds	Carbamazepine***
Heroin	Cyclophosphamide***
Iodine radiographic contrast media	Heparin**
l-tryptophan	Insulin**
Methotrexate	Lisinopril**
Nitrofurantoin	Morphine***
Paraffin oil	Sulfamides/sulfonamides***
Phenytoin	Sulfasalazine***
Salbutamol	
Steroids	

*Isolated case report; **~10 case reports; ***20–100 case reports; ****>100 case reports.

Source: Pneumotox.com (accessed 4 May 2010).

Diagnosis
With a few exceptions, because of its relative rarity DILD is usually a diagnosis of exclusion and should not be made until alternative diagnoses have been excluded. There are no specific clinical, radiological, and pathological findings. Many drugs responsible for DILD can cause several different disease processes. The only sure way to confirm DILD is for the signs and symptoms to resolve on stopping the precipitating agent and for them to recur when the drug is restarted. Understandably, restarting the drug is rarely done.

Clinical presentation

Symptoms

These are largely non-specific and reflect the type of lung disease presenting: dyspnoea, cough, wheeze, haemoptysis. Weight loss and clubbing may occur with chronic disease.

Signs

Physical signs are similarly non-specific: tachypnoea, fever, hypoxaemia, crepitations.

Investigation

Chest X-ray

- May be normal.
- Diffuse infiltrates, ground glass opacification, consolidation, or ARDS are common patterns, but none are pathognomonic of DILD.

Bronchoalveolar lavage

Usually not specific and reflects the type of lung injury.

- Hypersensitivity pneumonitis—lymphocytes 40–80%.
- Eosinophilic pneumonitis—eosinophils present in lavage fluid.
- Non-cardiogenic pulmonary oedema—non-specific watery lavage fluid.
- Alveolar haemorrhage—haemorrhagic BAL fluid.
- Foamy alveolar macrophages in amiodarone-induced pulmonary toxicity.

High-resolution CT scan

HRCT provides superior imaging of the diseased lung and is more able to demonstrate parenchymal abnormalities such as ground glass opacities and fibrosis. Again, however, the changes seen are not specific to DILD. In one series of 13 cases of DILD investigated by HRCT the differential diagnoses was wide and all required lung biopsy for confirmation.

Lung biopsy

Lung biopsy may be performed by either an open surgical technique or, more commonly, the transbronchial route. Open-lung biopsy is the more useful because a larger, more representative sample can be acquired. Although there are few pathognomonic histopathological changes for DILD, lung biopsy does help exclude other causes of lung disease, such as infection, haemorrhage, and tumour. Underlying lung disease may complicate the picture.

Management

Withdraw suspect drug

If at all possible stop the suspected drug.

Steroid therapy

Steroid therapy is recommended to suppress the inflammatory reaction in DILD. Evidence that steroids actually improve or accelerate the resolution of DILD is lacking.

Alternative treatment for underlying disease

In many cases the underlying disease will still require treatment. Avoid using alternatives agents from the same pharmacological group as the suspect drug.

Drugs commonly associated with DILD

Amiodarone

Amiodarone-induced pulmonary toxicity usually presents months or years after starting therapy. Risk factors are cumulative dose and age. Patients typically present insidiously with cough, fatigue, dyspnoea, and low-grade fever. There are usually bilateral infiltrates on CXR and reduced diffusing capacity for carbon monoxide.

An acute form has been reported only a few days after starting therapy and may be associated with high FiO_2. If lung function deteriorates after 3 or more days of therapy with amiodarone, consider a bronchoalveolar lavage—it helps to rule out infection and the presence of foamy alveolar macrophages, with fibrosis and hyperplasia of type II alveolar cells, supports the diagnosis. The mechanism of pulmonary toxicity is not certain but may be either an immunological response or due to free radical production.

Treatment

Drug withdrawal has a delayed effect because of the long half-life of amiodarone. Treatment is supportive. Steroids are sometimes added.

Bleomycin

The most common pulmonary side-effect is pneumonitis. Approximately 3% of patients treated with bleomycin will die from pulmonary toxicity.

Patients present with dry cough, dyspnoea, and fever. Bilateral bibasal infiltrates are often found on CXR, and CT usually reveals small linear and subpleural nodules in the lung bases. Infection, pulmonary metastases, and lymphangitis carcinomatosis must be excluded. Risk factors are:
- Cumulative dose of bleomycin
- Age
- Smoking
- Inspired oxygen concentration (animal work suggests a powerful relationship; human studies are less clear)
- Other cytotoxic drug use.

Treatment

Stop bleomycin. High-dose steroid therapy is normally used, although there is little evidence of its efficacy. Most clinicians keep supplemental oxygen to a minimum for anyone who has received bleomycin at any time in the past.

Carbamazepine

Carbamazepine can cause a spectrum of drug-related side-effects, including acute diffuse interstitial pneumonitis, organizing pneumonia, pulmonary eosinophilia syndrome, pulmonary oedema, pulmonary haemorrhage, and pleural effusions. It may be accompanied by signs of a systemic drug eruption (skin rash, Stevens–Johnson syndrome, deranged liver function, eosinophilia).

BAL may show a lymphocytosis and transbronchial biopsy may show changes consistent with an organizing pneumonia.

Treatment

Drug withdrawal and steroids have been reported to resolve symptoms in >60% of patients within 2 weeks.

Cyclophosphamide

Cyclophosphamide is an alkylating agent used in many chemotherapeutic regimes for haematological and solid malignancies. It is also used in vasculitidies and, paradoxically, sometimes for idiopathic pulmonary fibrosis.

In addition to its immunosuppressive effects, rendering the patient susceptible to traditional and opportunistic pulmonary infections, cyclophosphamide therapy is associated with direct pulmonary damage, which can result in ARDS, organizing pneumonia, diffuse alveolar damage, and irreversible pulmonary fibrosis. The incidence of pulmonary side-effects is low.

The diagnosis is based on history and exclusion of other aetiologies to explain the respiratory disease (for example, infection or tumour infiltration). HRCT typically shows ground glass opacities.

Treatment

Treatment is supportive in conjunction with drug withdrawal and steroid therapy. Response is variable. Once alveolar and interstitial damage is established, progression to fibrosis is the norm, and prognosis is poor.

Methotrexate

Methotrexate can cause a variety of lung toxicity, but is classically associated with interstitial pneumonitis (incidence 2–8%).

Patients present with progressive dyspnoea, cough, and fever. Hypoxaemia and tachypnoea are always present. Diagnosis is often difficult but there should be a history of exposure to methotrexate, pulmonary infiltrates on CXR, and the exclusion of other diseases (particularly infection, including opportunistic infection).

Methotrexate pneumonitis is most likely within 1 year of starting therapy. Risk factors include high-dose therapy, daily administration, and pre-existing lung disease.

Treatment

Stop methotrexate. High-dose steroid therapy. Most patients respond well, but mortality is 13%.

Nitrofurantoin

Nitrofurantoin is still used to treat urinary tract infections and is the most common antimicrobial associated with DILD. It may be missed in the history if it is intermittently prescribed.

There is an acute form that develops hours to days after initiation of therapy, and a chronic form that presents after weeks to years of continuous prophylactic therapy.

Typical symptoms include cough, dyspnoea, chest pain, arthralgia, and a rash. Patients may be hypoxaemic and have abnormal transaminases and an eosinophilia. Bibasal reticular shadowing is present on CXR and CT shows ground glass shadowing or consolidation, and subpleural linear opacities.

Treatment
Resolution is usually rapid after drug withdrawal, and mortality is low.

Sulfasalazine

Sulfasalazine is used as a disease-modifying drug in rheumatoid arthritis and in the treatment of inflammatory bowel disease. Although systemic side-effects are well described, pulmonary side-effects are relatively rare.

The typical presentation is of cough and fever. Sputum production, rash, and chest pain have been described, but are inconsistent features.

CXR may show diffuse interstitial infiltration, and bloods typically show an eosinophilia. The most common histological appearances are of eosinophilic pneumonia, but fibrosis is possible.

Treatment
The majority of patients improve within weeks of drug withdrawal. Steroid use has been described.

1 Camus P and Rosenow EC (2004) Iatrogenic lung disease. *Clin Chest Med* **25**(1), XIII–XIX. The entire volume reviews all forms of DILD.
2 Pneumotox online. The Drug Induced Lung Diseases. Available at: http://www.pneumotox. com (accessed 4 May 2010). An online service run by the Groupe d'Etudes de la Pathologie Pulmonaire Iatrogen (GEPPI), which records and grades the level of evidence for drugs causing DILD.

6.8 Extrapulmonary causes of respiratory failure

Respiratory failure can occur in patients with normal pulmonary parenchyma. In these patients the problem is usually ventilatory failure (i.e. type 2 respiratory failure) with hypercapnia. Oxygenation is often relatively preserved and any hypoxia easily reversed with supplemental oxygen. However, oxygen therapy may exacerbate hypercapnia in patients with chronic hypercapnia.

They may also have underlying respiratory disease (e.g. 'overlap syndrome' of COPD and sleep apnoea) that may aggravate their non-pulmonary conditions and lead to respiratory failure out of proportion to the primary diagnosis. These patients frequently present to secondary care with unrelated problems and are identified on the basis of abnormal investigations.

This section will focus on patients who often present with an acute episode on the background of often unrecognized chronic respiratory failure. These patients may therefore be seen by intensive care, respiratory, or emergency/acute medicine physicians. Many patients with respiratory failure of extrapulmonary origin require long-term home ventilation (see 📖 Long-term (home) ventilation, p 354).

Control of respiration

Normal respiratory function is controlled by a neural network located in the lower brainstem (pontine, dorsal, and ventral respiratory groups). Motor neurones project down the spinal cord to the diaphragm, intercostal, and abdominal muscles. Disease anywhere along this path may lead to respiratory failure.

During sleep arterial PCO_2 rises by 0.2–0.4kPa in normal individuals as a result of hypoventilation caused by:
- Decreased response to ventilatory stimuli
- Supine-related reduction in FRC
- Altered V/Q matching
- Reduced respiratory and upper airway muscle tone.

In patients with abnormal respiratory function, clinically significant hypoventilation often first occurs during sleep. This is usually most pronounced during REM sleep, when there is paralysis of the skeletal muscles.

Causes

Neuromuscular disease
Brainstem lesions
- Cerebrovascular accident (CVA).
- Multiple sclerosis.

- Syringobulbia.
- Chiari malformation.
- Polio.
- Space-occupying lesions.
- Multiple system atrophy.
- Congenital central hypoventilation syndrome.
- Central depression by opioid and other sedative drugs.

Spinal cord lesion
- Cervical spine injury.
- Multiple sclerosis.
- Syringomyelia.

Peripheral neuropathy
- Guillain–Barré syndrome.
- Critical illness polyneuropathy.
- Drugs and alcohol.
- Metabolic (diabetes and porphyria).
- Vasculitis.
- Congenital neuropathies.
- Motor neurone disease.

Neuromuscular transmission disease
- Myasthenia gravis.
- Eaton–Lambert syndrome.
- Botulism.

Muscle disease
- Muscular dystrophies.
- Myotonic dystrophy.
- Periodic paralysis (hypo and hyperkalaemic).
- Acid maltase deficiency (Pompe's disease).
- Congenital myopathies.

Chest wall disorders
- Obesity hypoventilation syndrome.
- Congenital kyphoscoliosis.
- Thoracoplasty (for TB in pre-chemotherapy era).
- Ankylosing spondylitis.

Upper airway disease
- Trauma (including post-surgery, e.g. thyroidectomy).
- Foreign body.
- Tracheal stenosis following prolonged intubation.
- Infection, including epiglottitis, laryngotracheobronchitis, peritonsillar abscess.
- Allergy—swelling of lips, tongue, pharynx, larynx (including vocal cords).

Approach to patient with type 2 failure

There is a huge range of presentations of patients with type 2 respiratory failure, from acute blockage of the airway to long-term sleep-related hypoventilation that presents with apparently unrelated symptoms.

In general patients present in one of three ways:

- As an emergency with acute decompensation, often on the background of unrecognized chronic respiratory failure.
  Precipitating factors include:
  - Respiratory tract infection
  - Pulmonary aspiration, as many of these patients have co-existing bulbar dysfunction
  - Upper airway obstruction
  - Other intercurrent illness or medical intervention (e.g. surgical disease requiring operative intervention under general anaesthesia, or use of opioid analgesia)
- As a consequence of disease progression, perhaps with sleep-disordered breathing characterized by:
  - Disrupted sleep pattern
  - Daytime somnolence
  - Headaches (due to hypercapnia) on awakening
  They may also suffer from:
  - Dyspnoea on exertion (impaired mobility may mask this)
  - Orthopnoea (due to diaphragmatic weakness)
- As a consequence of failure to wean from acute ICU ventilation in a patient with chronic respiratory insufficiency (perhaps unrecognized at the time of ICU admission), or who has developed critical illness polymyoneuropathy.

Symptoms

Enquire specifically about speed of onset of symptoms.

- Dyspnoea (patients with chronic respiratory failure are often undistressed by extreme hypoxia).
- Orthopnoea (reflecting diaphragmatic weakness).
- Features of nocturnal hypoventilation:
  - Unrefreshing sleep (due to recurrent arousals caused by hypoxia and hypercapnia).
  - Daytime somnolence (Epworth sleepiness scale >11 abnormal; see box).
  - Morning headache ('hangover'-like, due to hypercapnia).
  - Enuresis.
  - Nocturnal choking.
  - Witnessed apnoeas by bed partner.
- Other:
  - Loss of appetite and weight.
  - Decreased intellectual performance.
  - Recurrent respiratory infections.
  - Inability to clear secretions.
  - Clinical signs of cor pulmonale.
  - Other organ involvement giving a clue to primary diagnosis.

Epworth Sleepiness Scale
0 = would never doze; 1 = slight chance of dozing; 2 = moderate chance of dozing; 3 = high chance of dozing
  Situations
- Sitting and reading.
- Watching TV.
- Sitting, inactive in public (e.g. theatre, cinema).
- As a car passenger for 1 hour without a break.
- Lying down to rest in the afternoon.
- Sitting talking to someone.
- Sitting quietly after lunch without alcohol.
- In a car, while stopped at traffic for a few minutes.

Total possible = 24

Signs
- Look for features of primary disease (e.g. frontal balding in myotonic dystrophy, ptosis in myasthenia).
- Stridor.
- Respiratory rate changes.
- Features of cor pulmonale.
  - Raised JVP.
  - Parasternal heave.
  - Loud P2.
  - Peripheral oedema.
- Heart rate.
- Blood pressure.

Note: It is easy to miss the usual signs of respiratory distress in muscle-wasted patients, but tachycardia and hypertension are often seen.
- Evidence of cardiorespiratory instability in acute onset disease (e.g. autonomic dysfunction in Guillain–Barré syndrome).
- Formal neurological examination often necessary; particularly look for evidence of bulbar dysfunction, specifically the ability to cough and clear secretions.
- Reduced level of consciousness/somnolence.
- Body mass index (may need heavy range scales).
  - Ask about shirt collar size.

Investigations
The investigations required will be determined to some degree by the speed of onset of illness and the time available before instituting therapy.

Minimum
- SpO_2 on air. 88% approximates to PaO_2 of 8kPa.
- Arterial blood gas to confirm the presence of respiratory failure.
  - Hypercapnia $PaCO_2$ >6kPa (45mmHg) +/– hypoxia (remember to document FiO_2 clearly).

- H$^+$ (or pH): is the patient acidotic or is this compensated (i.e. chronic respiratory failure)?
- ECG showing evidence of right heart strain.
- If ECG abnormal an echocardiogram can be helpful in looking for evidence of pulmonary hypertension.
- Chest radiograph excluding any cardiorespiratory cause of respiratory failure.
- Full blood count: erythrocytosis in chronic hypoxaemia (Hb >16g/dL).

More advanced

- Vital capacity (VC): ideally erect and supine. VC is linked to the likelihood of sleep disordered breathing (SDB):
  - Normally less than 20% drop in VC on recumbency
  - VC > 60%: predicted SDB unlikely
  - VC 40–60%: onset of SDB with REM hypopnoeas
  - VC 25–40%: REM and non-REM hypoventilation
  - VC < 25%: diurnal respiratory failure.
- In acute decompensation, an FVC <15mL/kg is often considered an indication for intubation and ventilation.
- Overnight pulse oximetry with patient breathing air. OxyHb saturation <88% for 5 min is considered evidence of significant desaturation.
- Overnight transcutaneous CO_2 measurement >6.5kPa to confirm hypoventilation.
- Full pulmonary function tests: spirometry, lung volumes, gas transfer if coexistent pulmonary disease suspected (e.g. COPD in a smoker).
- Maximal inspiratory pressure <60cmH$_2$O.
- Sniff nasal inspiratory pressure (SNIP). A value of –70cmH$_2$O in males and –60cmH$_2$O in females is unlikely to be associated with respiratory muscle weakness. <40cmH$_2$O is significant, suggesting muscular weakness. Values in between are equivocal.

Still more advanced

- Limited (home) sleep study: measures of airflow, thoraco-abdominal movement, oximetry, heart rate.

Specialized

- Full polysomnography: in cases of diagnostic uncertainty (do they have coexistent sleep apnoea syndrome?).

Treatment: general principles

Acute upper airways obstruction

This requires urgent definitive control of the airway. Options include:
- Deep inhalational anaesthesia with sevoflurane to facilitate intubation, avoiding muscle relaxant use

- Awake fibreoptic-assisted intubation
- Tracheostomy under local anaesthesia, usually performed by ENT surgeons
- In extreme emergency, cricothyroidotomy puncture (e.g. minitrach).

Ventilation

In hypercapnic respiratory failure both the hypercapnia and hypoxia can be corrected by ventilatory support (assuming no coexisting lung disease).

The speed of onset of respiratory failure often governs the speed with which this must be instituted. In acute decompensation immediate ventilatory support may be appropriate. It may then be converted to NIV for long-term support.

In many patients a planned approach can be undertaken as the insidious onset of respiratory failure does not necessitate rapid correction.

Early in the process the patient's views should be ascertained and ventilatory support only instituted if this is in accordance with the patient's wishes.

The first decision is usually to choose between invasive and non-invasive support.

The indications for intubation are:
- Airway protection
- Failure of clearance of secretions
- Major haemodynamic instability
- Agitation or significant reduction in level of consciousness (GCS <8).
- Significant bulbar involvement.

In patients with acute muscle denervation, suxamethonium should be avoided as it may precipitate fatal hyperkalaemia.

In most patients, NIV is preferred. A range of patient–ventilator interfaces exists:
- Nasal mask
- Nasal pillows
- Full facemask.

In the acute setting a full facemask is generally favoured, but is a matter of physician preference. Once hypercapnia is controlled the interface can be changed to nasal mask/pillows, depending on patient predilection.

For long-term use, NIV is preferred for patients who require ventilatory support for less than 16–20h per day. 24-h NIV is now feasible, but may well not be socially acceptable to the patient.

There is more detailed discussion of long-term ventilatory support in 📖 Long-term (home) ventilation, p 354.

Specific conditions
Obesity hypoventilation
- Increasingly common indication for NIV.
- Definition: obesity (BMI >30kg/m^2) and diurnal hypercapnia (PaCO$_2$ >6kPa).
- Exact incidence/prevalence uncertain but increasing as obesity increases.
- About 1 in 3 obese individuals has obesity hypoventilation syndrome (OHS).
- Distinct condition to obstructive sleep apnoea (OSA), which is characterized by multiple episodes of apnoea/hypopnoea during sleep with daytime somnolence but normal diurnal blood gases. Many patients with OHS have coexisting OSA.

Treatment
- NIV improves hypercapnia and symptoms.
- Weight loss: dietary advice, pharmacological approaches (e.g. orlistat), bariatric surgery.
- Failure to recognize/treat OHS is associated with increased hospitalization and reduced survival compared to weight-matched controls.
- Treatment improves survival (18-month mortality 23% in untreated patients reduces to 3% with treatment) and quality of life.
- If hypoxia persists despite adequate ventilation, additional oxygen can be used to overcome it.

Acute inflammatory postinfectious polyneuropathy (Guillain–Barré syndrome)
- Most common cause of neuromuscular respiratory failure, with an incidence of 1–4/100000/year.
- Occurs 1–3 weeks after bacterial/viral infection or immunization.
- Initially sensory symptoms proceed to muscular weakness due to demyelinating motor neuropathy.
- Ventilation required in 20% of patients.
- Treat with intravenous immunoglobulin (5 days, total dose 2g/kg).
- Generally muscle strength recovers over weeks or months, allowing weaning from ventilation.

Chronic neuromuscular diseases
- There is increasing use of NIV in this group of patients.
- Cochrane Collaboration review has found some evidence that nocturnal mechanical ventilation improves symptoms. In three small studies survival was improved in patients with motor neurone disease (MND) (without prominent bulbar involvement).

- Duchenne muscular dystrophy (DMD) is the best investigated group and there is definite improvement in survival with nocturnal NIV. However, pre-emptive institution of NIV in DMD does not improve survival and is poorly tolerated.
- Myotonic dystrophy is a more complicated patient group as daytime somnolence and sleep disorder is multi-factorial. They may have:
  - Some degree of central drive failure
  - OSA
  - Respiratory muscle weakness
  - Obesity hypoventilation
  - CNS involvement with central drowsiness and personality change.

The response to treatment in myotonic dystrophy is often less satisfactory as a result of the complexities of the issues involved.

Patients with respiratory failure of non-pulmonary cause present an on-going problem because of their acute presentation, chronic hypercapnia requiring long-term respiratory support, and the need to negotiate other medical problems, e.g. anaesthesia. It is prudent for the care of such patients to be brought under the aegis of a single consultant with a specific commitment to, and expertise in, the care of these challenging groups, ideally supported by a specialist team of nursing and paramedical staff.

Further reading

Annane D, Orlikowski D, Chevret S, Chevrolet JC, and Raphaël JC (2007) Nocturnal mechanical ventilation for chronic hypoventilation in patients with neuromuscular and chest wall disorders. *Cochrane Database of Systematic Reviews* **4**. Art No:CD001941.DOI10.1002/14651858. CD001941.pub2.

Consensus Conference (1999) Clinical indications for non-invasive positive pressure ventilation in chronic respiratory failure due to restrictive lung disease, COPD and nocturnal hypoventilation—A consensus conference report. *Chest* **116**, 521–534.

Crummy F, Piper AJ, and Naughton MT (2008) Obesity and the lung. 2. Obesity and sleep disordered breathing. *Thorax* **63**, 738–746.

Nogues MA and Benarroch E (2008) Abnormalities of respiratory control and the respiratory motor unit. *The Neurologist* **14**(5), 273–288.

6.9 Haematological malignancy in ICU

1 in 50 adults will at some time suffer a serious haematological disorder. The range and complexity of available therapies is steadily increasing and there is a move away from limiting treatment on the basis of chronological age (median age at presentation is 60–70). Consequently, a growing number of ICU admissions are related to a haematological disorder or its treatment.

General principles of treating haematological malignancy

Chemotherapy

Chemotherapy works by being more toxic to malignant cells than healthy cells. Usually given in pulses or cycles, which are timed so that, hopefully, the patient's bone marrow and other susceptible healthy tissues have regenerated between cycles, but the malignancy has not. This gradually reduces tumour burden without progressive deterioration in healthy tissue.

Chronic myeloid leukaemia
- Long-term disease control generally possible with continuous daily administration of well-tolerated oral agents.

Low-grade lymphoma and chronic lymphocytic leukaemia
- May be aggressive but generally indolent.
- Sometimes do not require therapy.
- Limited disease is potentially curable with three cycles of intravenous chemotherapy followed by radiotherapy.
- Widespread disease is not curable, but durable remissions possible with six to eight cycles of intravenous chemotherapy.
- Usually outpatient therapy.

High-grade lymphoma
- Aggressive and rapidly fatal if untreated.
- Both limited (three cycles of intravenous chemotherapy plus local radiotherapy) and widespread (six to eight cycles of intravenous chemotherapy) disease are potentially curable.
- Usually outpatient therapy.

Acute leukaemia
- Aggressive and rapidly fatal if untreated.
- May be curable with three to four cycles of aggressive intravenous chemotherapy.
- Usually prolonged (weeks to months) inpatient stays.

Autologous SCT

Marrow toxicity is often a dose limiting factor in chemotherapy administration. Autologous stem cell transplant (SCT) is used as a way of avoiding this by physically sheltering some marrow stem cells from chemotherapy by removing them from the body. These cells are re-infused after chemotherapy has been completed and eliminated from the body. This technique is used to give very large doses of chemotherapy in myeloma and relapsed high-grade lymphoma.

Allogeneic SCT

This may also be used as a way to give high doses of chemotherapy. Donor marrow is infused after the chemotherapy is completed and eliminated from the patient's system. Unlike autologous SCT there may also be direct attack on malignant cells by the transplanted (i.e. donor) immune system (graft versus leukaemia effect).

However, allogenic SCT requires thorough eradication of the recipient immune system, magnifying the infection risk. The donor marrow may attack healthy host tissues and organs in addition to attacking malignant cells (graft versus host disease).

This is high mortality rate therapy and is used most commonly as the final phase of curative intent treatment for the worst prognosis diseases.

Serious complications of therapy

Following allogeneic SCT

See Fig. 6.4 for complications in the first 30 days following allogeneic transplant.

Acute graft versus host disease

Acute graft versus host disease (aGvHD) occurs within the first 100 days following allogeneic SCT. It classically affects the liver, gut, and skin, and may range from minor dysfunction to fulminant liver failure, catastrophic gut fluid and blood loss, and eythroderma with widespread epidermal sloughing. Treatment is with high doses of methylprednisone and other potent immunosuppressants if methylprednisolone is unsuccessful. Very high mortality if steroids ineffective. Infection is the most common cause of death.

Chronic graft versus host disease

Chronic graft versus host disease (cGvHD) occurs more than 100 days following allogeneic SCT. It classically causes progressive pulmonary fibrosis, a scleroderma-like skin disease, dry eyes and mouth, gut mucosal atrophy and strictures, fasciitis, and joint contractures. It may range from minor changes to marked cosmetic change, organ failure, malnutrition, and crippling joint dysfunction. Infection is the most common cause of death.

Following chemotherapy

Neutropenic sepsis

For many haematological disorders, chemotherapy sufficient to kill enough malignant cells to permit cure or lengthy remission requires drug doses high enough to produce temporary bone marrow failure with each cycle. Neutropenia (and thus neutropenic sepsis) is therefore a consequence of adequate cancer therapy.

However, multiply relapsed patients have often had enough chemotherapy to cause permanent bone marrow failure. Advanced haematological malignancy may also infiltrate the bone marrow and produce marrow failure. Haematology patients with neutropenic sepsis can, therefore, be split into two groups:

• Advanced, untreatable disease/multiply relapsed patients. Marrow function is irreversibly impaired and there may be multiple additional co-morbidities from disease or previous therapy. These patients are rarely appropriate for ICU admission.

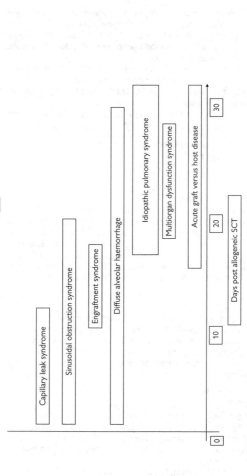

Fig. 6.4 Timing of serious early complications of allogeneic SCT. Capillary leak syndrome = unexplained weight gain, widespread tissue oedema, diuretic non-responsiveness. Sinusoidal obstruction syndrome = small hepatic vessel thrombosis producing a triad of painful hepatomegaly, hyperbilirubinemia, and unexplained fluid retention occurring within 21 days of the transplant. Engraftment syndrome = fever, erythrodermatous skin rash, and non-cardiogenic pulmonary oedema occurring with neutrophil recovery. Idiopathic pneumonia syndrome = multilobar infiltrates, progressive hypoxia, and no identifiable pulmonary infection.

• Active, neutropenia-inducing therapy. These patients are usually deemed to have a chance of cure or long-term remission if fit enough for the necessary therapy. They are often appropriate for ICU admission.

The neutropenic patient

Immunocompetence is generally maintained when the neutrophil count is >0.5 × 10^9/L. Neutropaenia as a result of chemotherapy can be expected to be transient, usually beginning 7–10 days post chemotherapy and lasting:
• Up to 1 week for most outpatient chemotherapy regimens
• ≥3 weeks with more aggressive inpatient regimens, such as those used in acute leukaemia or bone marrow transplantation.

Neutropenia increases the likelihood and severity of infection and masks the usual evidence of an infective process. It is often contemporaneous with loss of gastrointestinal mucosal integrity, which further increases infection risk and impairs adequate nutrition and drug absorption, as well as increasing fluid loss and causing significant pain.

Likelihood of infection
This can be reduced by isolating patients, as much as possible, from sources of infection.
• Positive pressure rooms, minimizing sharing of equipment between patients—patient-unique stethoscopes, disposable tourniquets, barrier nursing, use of apron and disposable gloves by anyone directly touching the patient.
• No flowers unless in self-contained, sealed bag.
• Bottled water should be fizzy and consumed within 24h of opening (risk of pseudomonas contamination).
• No visitors who are unwell with any symptom suggesting infection.

It can also be reduced by minimizing the duration of neutropenia. Daily granulocyte macrophage colony-stimulating factor (GCSF) may achieve this.

There is no convincing evidence that 'neutropenic diets', which ban many fresh foods for fear of contamination with living organisms, have any impact on the infection rate and they may deprive the patient of useful nutritional options.

Severity of infection
Infection must be treated promptly with broad-spectrum antibiotics. All hospitals treating patients with haematological malignancies in the UK are now required to have an agreed neutropenic infection antibiotic policy. This should be available within the ICU. Most policies will require an HRCT to exclude fungal infection after 48–72h if patients are not responding to initial therapy.

Altered or reduced evidence of infection
The use of regular paracetamol and other antipyretics should be discouraged as fever is often the only initial sign of infection in severely immunocompromised patients. Regular screening of neutropenic patients for virulent organisms should be undertaken. In the event the patient becomes febrile the choice of antibiotics may be modified if a resistant or unusual

colonizing organism has been identified (e.g. MRSA, vancomycin-resistant enterococci (VRE), extended spectral β-lactamases (ESBL)). Screening should include weekly nose and throat and line swabs, stool and urine for microscopy culture and sensitivity.

Patients who are heavily immunocompromised, such as those who have received allogeneic SCTs or are receiving drugs such as fludarabine or the monoclonal antibody campath-1H, should have regular (usually twice weekly) CMV PCR performed.

Specialised blood products

Irradiation

The purpose of irradiation is to destroy leukocytes in the transfusion. This is necessary in those patients so immunocompromised that trans-fused leukocytes might be able to proliferate and mount an attack on the recipient. If this occurs it is invariably fatal. Currently, recipients of alloge-neic SCT, those within 6 months of autologous SCT, patients who have had Hodgkin's lymphoma, and those within 6 months of campath-1H or fludarabine are considered at risk. FFP does not need to be irradiated (it contains no viable white cells).

CMV negative blood

The purpose of this is to minimize the risk of transfusing CMV-infected leukocytes into an immunocompromised patient. Since all UK blood prod-ucts are now universally leukodepleted (leukocytes are filtered out with high, but not total, efficiency) there is some argument that this is suffi-cient, but some transplant centres still require blood products for patients receiving allogeneic SCT who are CMV negative to be screened for CMV. FFP does not need to be CMV negative (it contains no viable white cells).

HLA and human platelet antigen matched platelets

Just as red cells may be separated into different blood groups depending on the surface antigens they express, the same is true of platelets. In general these platelet antigens can be ignored but some heavily transfused patients will develop antibodies to them which can produce refractoriness to platelet transfusion. This is circumvented by switching to:

- Single-donor (also called 'apheresis') platelets (standard platelet units are pooled from multiple donors and contain a range of platelet antigens), then to
- HLA-matched platelets, then to
- human platelet antigen matched platelets.

Guidelines on platelet transfusion thresholds

Although in most laboratories the normal range for the platelet count is $150–450 \times 10^9$/L this is far more than is required for normal haemostasis. Depending on the severity of haemostatic challenge and the consequence of haemorrhage, platelet counts significantly lower will provide adequate haemostasis (see Table 6.6).

Table 6.6 Thresholds for platelet transfusion

Platelet count	Provides adequate haemostasis for
>100	No increased risk of haemorrhage with any intervention
>80	Any intervention except ocular or neurosurgery
>50	Most minor surgery, insertion of intravenous lines, lumbar puncture (guidelines differ on this, with some recommending >80)
>30	Multiple dental extraction
>20	Septic or febrile patients not requiring invasive procedures, intubated patients with respiratory failure (coughing on the ETT increases intracranial pressure; hypercapnia and fever both increase intracranial blood flow, therefore ICU patients on average will probably require a higher platelet count than normal patients)
>5–10	Patients not acutely unwell who do not require invasive procedures

Common supportive medications

Patients receiving chemotherapy for haematological malignancy are often on a variety of supportive medications. The more common ones are listed below.

- Allopurinol—a xanthine oxidase inhibitor used to prevent urate nephropathy, most effective in the first 10 days post chemotherapy.
- Rasburicase—a recombinant urate oxidase that is more effective than allopurinol, most effective in the first 10 days post chemotherapy.
- Aciclovir—herpes virus prophylaxis, commonly used in SCT recipients and patients on fludarabine, high-dose methylprenisone, or campath.
- Co-trimoxazole—PCP prophylaxis, commonly used in SCT recipients and patients on fludarabine, high-dose methylprenisone, or campath.
- Nystatin or amphotericin lozenges—topical antifungals to prevent oral/oesophageal candida, commonly used in SCT recipients and patients on intensive inpatient chemotherapy.
- Posoconazole or other systemic antifungal—to prevent systemic, especially pulmonary, fungal infection, commonly used in patients receiving chemotherapy who have a previous systemic fungal infection or patients at high risk, particularly those receiving allogeneic SCT.
- Levofloxacin or other 4-quinolone antibiotic—to reduce the risk of Gram-negative sepsis, commonly used in patients receiving SCT or intensive inpatient chemotherapy.
- G-CSF—daily subcutaneously or every 7–10 days pegylated subcutaneously. To reduce the duration and severity of neutropenia. Not proven to reduce mortality but shown to reduce length of hospital stay. Commonly used in patients receiving intensive chemotherapy, especially if serious infection or co-morbidities.
- Mouthcare—analgesic and antiseptic mouthwashes, used to minimize discomfort of oral mucositis.
- Anti-emetics, e.g. ondansetron, metoclopramide, cyclizine.

- Opiate analgesia—reduces the pain of oral and oesophageal mucositis, especially with intensive chemotherapy regimens and SCT.

Haematology patients and ICU admission

Some 40–50% patients with haematologic malignancy (HM) admitted to ICU survive to hospital discharge, although only 6% patients with HM receiving CPR survive to discharge. Survival figures have improved considerably in the last decade. The use of critical care outreach teams is responsible for some of that progress.

Despite improved survival, fewer than half of patients referred to ICU with HM are admitted. Of those not admitted because they are considered too sick to benefit, 25% are still alive 1 month later. Of those considered too well to benefit, one in three is later admitted and only 80% are still alive a month later.

Patients who have received an allogeneic SCT represent a particularly difficult to treat group. Of these, 20% require ICU admission, most commonly with:

- Respiratory failure (40%).
- Neutropenic sepsis (25%).
- Almost all require mechanical ventilation and only one-third survive to ICU discharge. Median survival after ICU discharge is less than a year. Patients with two organ failure following allogenic SCT have a near 100% mortality.

In HM patients who have not received an allogenic SCT, mechanical ventilation has better outcome, with >50% surviving to ICU discharge.

This probably reflects, in large part, how medically unwell such patients become with the haematological therapy rather than the haematological disorder *per se*. Most studies show survival is not influenced by:

- Type of hematological malignancy
- Neutropenia or other cytopenia
- Bacteremia
- Age.

Survival is chiefly influenced by haemodynamic and ventilatory status on admission to ICU.

The role of scoring systems in estimating survival is not well defined but some data suggest that scores such as SOFA and APACHE II may be useful. In one study of the latter:

- 100% mortality only predicted with a score >45
- Score <35 significantly underestimates survival.

A patient in whom it is considered worthwhile to treat the underlying HM aggressively (i.e. relatively fit, significant chance of response and durable remission) should be considered for ICU if they are ill enough to require it. The haematological disorder itself should not be grounds for denial of ICU admission or of ventilatory support. The longer-term prognosis of a number of haematological diseases is illustrated in Fig. 6.5.

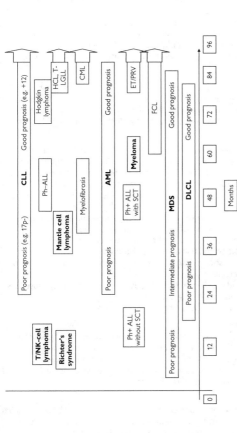

Fig. 6.5 Median survival from initiation of treatment in common haematological disorders. HCL, hairy cell leukaemia; FCL, follicular lymphoma low-grade lymphoma); CLL, chronic lymphocytic leukaemia; CML, chronic myeloid leukaemia; ALL, acute lymphoblastic leukaemia; Ph+/-, presence/absence of the Philadelphia chromosome t(9;22); T-LGLL, T-large granular lymphocyte leukaemia (a very indolent leukaemia); ET/PRV, essential thrombocythaemia/ primary polycythaemia; DLCL, diffuse large-cell lymphoma (a common high-grade lymphoma); 17p, 17p deletion; T/NK, T cell/natural killer cell; AML, acute myeloblastic leukaemia; MDS, myelodysplasia syndrome.

6.10 Inhalational injury

Inhalational injury has direct pulmonary and indirect systemic effects. These effects depend on the concentration, length of exposure, and nature of the substances inhaled. There are some similarities in the pattern of lung damage produced irrespective of the substance inhaled, including the development of ARDS, chemical pneumonitis, and increased airway reactivity. Common causes of inhalation injury include smoke inhalation, thermal injury, drowning, chemicals, and aspiration of gastric contents.

Smoke inhalation

Smoke inhalation is usually the consequence of exposure to products of incomplete combustion of carbon containing materials in an enclosed space, such as a house or aeroplane. Rarely, significant smoke inhalation can occur during medical procedures (e.g. diathermy of airway lesions).

Epidemiology

In the UK the frequency of house fires is falling, with a corresponding reduction in the number of injuries and deaths (>1000 deaths in 1979, 443 in 2007). This significant reduction is probably due to the increased use of smoke detectors, the improved design of new homes, and legislation that has led to the use of materials that are less flammable in furniture manufacture.

- 44% of deaths are due to smoke inhalation alone and a further 20% are due to the combination of inhalational injury and burns.
- In the UK deaths are more common in males and the elderly.
- Smoke inhalation and burns are associated with:
  - Poverty—associated with hazards in the home and reduced use of smoke detectors
  - Co-morbid conditions, such as epilepsy or diabetes, may cause loss of consciousness during cooking or smoking
  - Risky behaviour, e.g. alcohol and drug abuse.

Content of smoke

Smoke contains a wide variety of products of combustion. These products vary over the course of an individual fire and vary considerably between fires depending on the temperature and the materials involved.

Smoke also impedes escape, exacerbating the inhalational injury and increasing the chances of thermal burns.

Oxygen

A fire is a hypoxic environment and the FiO_2 can fall to between 0.05% and 0.15%. This leads to confusion and loss of consciousness, especially if associated with other factors contributing to tissue hypoxia.

Carbon monoxide

Carbon monoxide is produced when combustion occurs in a hypoxic environment. It has a high affinity for Hb, displacing oxygen and impairing oxygen delivery. Carbon monoxide also impairs tissue oxygen utilization by combining with the mitochondrial oxygen transport system.

Non-smokers typically have carboxyhaemoglobin (COHb) levels of around 2% and even heavy smokers have COHb levels <10%. It is always abnormal to see a COHb level >10% and this is the simplest and most reliable method of diagnosing smoke inhalation. The level rises in proportion to the exposure.

COHb has a half-life of 4h, but this reduces to 40min if 100% oxygen is administered. As COHb has predictable elimination kinetics it is possible to extrapolate the measured level to the peak level at the time of rescue (exposure carboxyhaemoglobin, eCOHb). Mortality and morbidity correlate with the eCOHB level.

The reduction in oxygen-carrying capacity is not thought to be the full explanation for most of the consequences of smoke inhalation. Carbon monoxide does have direct cellular toxic effects, but it is likely that many of the sequelae are due to the other contents of smoke, such as particulate matter.

Carbon dioxide

Variable amounts of carbon dioxide are produced in a fire environment. In combination with variable respiratory drive, this makes if difficult to predict the effect on $PaCO_2$. Carbon dioxide initially acts as a respiratory stimulant, but then reduces conscious level, ultimately depressing respiratory drive. Arterial blood gases should be performed as soon as possible in a smoke inhalation victim. A raised $PaCO_2$ should not deter the administration of high FiO_2.

Cyanide

Cyanide is a product of the combustion of nitrogen-containing polymers. It inhibits cytochrome c oxidase in the mitochondrial electron transport chain, impairing cellular respiration. Cyanide poisoning as a result of smoke inhalation is now very uncommon due to the use of safer materials in manufacturing. Cyanide analysis is not practicable in an emergency. A persistent metabolic acidosis may suggest the diagnosis, but caution should be used in interpreting this finding as there are many other potential explanations in a fire victim.

Particulate matter

Much of the damage due to smoke inhalation can be attributed to the particulate matter that is deposited in the airways. This causes an inflammatory response and a release of cytokines from activated macrophages and neutrophils, producing not only local but also systemic inflammation.

Other chemicals

Aldehydes, acrolein hydrochloric acid, and numerous other chemicals are found in smoke. Individually most of these cause lung injury and contribute to the induced inflammatory response.

Heat

As gases have a relatively low specific heat capacity, smoke does not induce thermal burns. However, smoke inhalation and thermal burns often coexist and smoke inhalation may be associated with facial and upper airway burns. Smoke inhalation can occur in the absence of any thermal burns and the converse is also true. It is important to recognize that thermal injury and smoke inhalation have significantly different mechanisms and consequences, and require different management. Thermal injury to the airway is discussed below.

Diagnosis

Features in the history suggesting smoke inhalation are:

- Fire in an enclosed space
- Loss of consciousness
- The need to be rescued
- Coughing, wheeze, or dyspnoea
- The presence of soot in expectorated sputum or in the airways on bronchoscopy.

Clinical signs are often absent on initial examination. An elevated COHb confirms the diagnosis.

Initial management

- From the time of rescue, 100% oxygen should be administered. This helps to correct hypoxaemia and to hasten the elimination of carbon monoxide.
- Subsequent management includes CPAP or intubation and ventilation if hypoxia persists.
- Over subsequent days sputum production may increase dramatically (bronchorrhoea) and physiotherapy will be required. Increased airway reactivity and bronchospasm are common after smoke inhalation. Bronchodilators should be prescribed prophylactically.
- Fluids should be initially prescribed according to estimated requirements using a standard calculation such as the Parkland formula. Smoke inhalation will increase the fluid requirement over and above any such calculation because of the additional inflammation induced.

Specific interventions

- Heparin and N-acetylcysteine are possibly beneficial in children but evidence is sparse for their benefits in adults. These beneficial effects are limited to animal studies and single-centre trials. As heparin has not been shown to be of benefit in larger multicentre studies routine use cannot yet be recommended.
- Steroids and bronchial lavage have been used but there is no trial evidence to support routine use.
- All other experimental interventions that have been shown to be efficacious in animals have not been shown to work in human trials.

Ventilatory strategy

Protective ventilation strategies should be employed. A number of animal and clinical studies have reported the successful use of a variety of ventilatory strategies.

- High-frequency percussive ventilation and high-frequency oscillation have been reported to be of benefit (in particular when used in combination with heparin).
- Many of these studies are old, and it is difficult to be certain whether these techniques are uniquely beneficial in smoke inhalation. They may merely reflect the known benefits of limited tidal volume and airway pressure.

- It would therefore seem sensible to use techniques that are familiar to the clinicians managing these patients, but to rigorously apply lung protection strategies.

Long-term outcome

The outcome of patients with isolated smoke inhalation is good. Features resulting in a poor outcome are:
- Coexisting burns
- Co-morbidity
- Significant ischaemic injury at the scene.

Some patients develop asthma-like symptoms due to increased airway reactivity. If burns are also present, smoke inhalation increases the occurrence of respiratory failure, multiple organ failure, and death expected for that size of burn without smoke inhalation.

Thermal injury to the airway

Inhalation of high-temperature gases or vapours can damage the airway, leading to swelling and airway occlusion. The upper airway will dissipate most of the thermal energy of a hot gas and so injury is usually confined to that area.
- Patients with facial burns, particularly in the perioral and nasal regions, may have an upper airway burn.
- In the absence of a burn around the mouth or nose an upper airway burn is highly unlikely. Rare exceptions include the impaction of hot food in the larynx, the direct application of hot liquids from the neck of a kettle or tea pot, or the direct application of a current from an electric cable onto the mucosa. In each of these cases a highly unusual clinical history will also be present.
- Occasionally an inhalation injury is much more extensive and also damages the lower airway. This can occur if the thermal load is high, such as in a steam burn, which has a much higher thermal capacity than air. Superheated steam has 200 times the heat capacity of hot air.

History and examination

A patient with upper airway burns may present initially with no or few symptoms. The key to the diagnosis is the recognition that in addition to perioral or perinasal burns the patient has symptoms suggesting upper airway burns:
- Minor voice changes
- Hoarseness
- Stridor.

On examination facial burns may not be obvious due to initial lack of swelling and because the burn is obscured by the presence of soot.
- Cleaning or wiping the soot away may reveal a burn.
- Close examination of the lips, nares, and oropharynx is necessary.

In the presence of symptoms and signs of upper airway burns urgent measures to secure the airway are mandatory.

Securing the airway

Airway swelling may progress rapidly and may become so severe that it completely obstructs the airway. In the absence of other complications the oedema may reach its maximum at between 24 and 48h, but the airway narrowing may become critical within a few hours of the injury. As a consequence the presence of any symptomatic airway swelling should be managed as an emergency.

Swelling will be made worse by fluid therapy and supine positioning.

Technique

There is no clear evidence base to demonstrate that any one approach is superior to the others. The priority is the rapid placement of an ETT that is sufficiently long ('uncut') to prevent its accidental migration from the trachea as the facial swelling increases.

- A rapid sequence induction or modified rapid sequence without muscle relaxants is the standard approach.
- Suxamethonium does not cause hyperkalaemia in the very early period following a burn (when this problem is encountered). However, a concern remains regarding the use of muscle relaxants if the airway is severely oedematous. Being unable to intubate or ventilate is a real possibility in these circumstances.
- Inhalational induction avoids apnoea, but has a higher risk of aspiration.
- Fibreoptic intubation or even a tracheostomy under local anaesthesia should be considered if there is likely to be significant airway difficulty.

These dilemmas may be avoided if the decision to intubate is taken promptly.

Whichever technique is used, it is advisable in this challenging situation that the clinician is skilled and experienced in the chosen technique and the ETT is both sufficiently long and adequately secured.

Near-drowning

Near-drowning is survival after an immersion injury. Drowning is death as a result of immersion.

Epidemiology

- According to the World Health Organization an estimated 376,000 people drowned in 2002.
- In the USA approximately 6000 people drown per year.
- In the UK 435 people drowned in 2005. UK data suggest that the rate of drowning is 0.5–3.26 per 100,000 population per year.
- Near-drowning and other injuries related to water result in up to 10 hospital admissions per 100,000 population annually.
- Men are three times more likely than women to be affected.
- Children are at proportionally higher risk of drowning than any other age group.
- Conditions causing reduced or loss of consciousness will increase the risk of drowning, including:
  - Hypoglycaemia
  - Diabetes
  - Cardiac disease, including arrhythmias (e.g. long QT syndrome)
  - Epilepsy

- Sedative medication
- Intoxication.

Pathogenesis

The amount of water aspirated in drowning can be relatively small. Animal experiments show that significant hypoxaemia occurs with aspiration of <2.2mL/kg water and that volumes up to 22mL/kg can cause persistent hypoxaemia.

A small proportion of patients appear at post mortem to have no evidence of water in the lungs, so-called 'dry drowning'. Plausible mechanisms for this include breath holding, laryngeal spasm, and loss of consciousness, leading to death from other causes. Alternatively, only a small amount of water may have been aspirated, and this would have been absorbed into the circulation by the time of post mortem.

Hypothermia is both a potential cause and a consequence of drowning. As a treatment, mild hypothermia may be of some benefit, but if it occurs after near-drowning in warm water it is a poor prognostic sign.

Freshwater vs salt water

Salt water drowning tends to result in:

- Hypernatraemia
- Hypermagnesaemia
- Pulmonary oedema (due to the osmotic gradient)
- Less frequent microbiological contamination.

Freshwater drowning is associated with:

- Hyponatraemia
- Haemolysis from fresh water aspiration
- Pulmonary oedema—possible mechanisms include increased capillary permeability, neurogenic pulmonary oedema, and reduced surfactant
- More frequent microbiological contamination.

Investigations

- CXR—the majority of near-drowning victims have radiological evidence of pulmonary oedema. Further deterioration in the CXR findings are expected in the following 24h.
- ECG—in addition to ventricular arrhythmias, the ECG should be reviewed for evidence of long QT syndrome.
- Arterial blood gases—hypoxia is common. Persistent severe metabolic acidosis is a poor prognostic sign.
- Electrolyte disturbances are common (sodium and magnesium).
- If Hb is low, check for haemolysis.

Management

At scene

- Extraction of the patient from the water should be considered carefully (where practically possible) to reduce the chance of further insult.
  - Vertical removal may lead to hypotension and cardiac arrest.
  - Cervical spine trauma may be present (particularly with a history of diving, water slide use, trauma, or alcohol).
- Immediate resuscitation improves the chances of survival.
- Gravitational drainage of fluid from the lungs may be beneficial.
- Oxygen should be administered and the patient rapidly transferred to hospital.

- If obtunded, the airway compromised, or if hypoxic despite supplemental oxygen, then intubation and ventilation may be needed. Lesser degrees of hypoxaemia can be treated with CPAP.

Hospital
- Steroids are not beneficial.
- Mild hypothermia has been recommended as a treatment for encephalopathy after near-drowning.
- Invasive monitoring of ICP can be used to guide therapy in raised ICP but has not been shown to improve outcome.
- Should ARDS develop management should be according to current protocols to reduce VILI.

Microbiology
Bacterial and fungal infections are recognized complications and should be treated as guided by cultures. The pathogens vary according to whether it is salt or freshwater. *Aeromonas* spp, *Burkholderia pseudomallei*, and *Chromobacterium violaceum* are more common following fresh water near-drowning. In salt water near-drowning the overall incidence of secondary infection is lower but more unusual organisms such as *Francisella philomiragia* are isolated more frequently.

The type of microorganism retrieved from the lungs can be used as a test to determine whether the cause of death of a body found in water was drowning.

Aspiration of gastric contents

Gastric contents may be aspirated during coma, in the presence of neurological disorders, or during anaesthesia (particularly emergency and obstetric anaesthesia). Other risk factors include pain, alcohol ingestion, hiatus hernia, gastro-oesophageal reflux, prolonged vomiting, and head injury.

The sequelae are related to the volume, the acidity, and the presence of microorganisms. Aspiration of gastric contents may result in:
- Airway obstruction
- Chemical pneumonitis
- Bacterial infection.

This subject is also discussed in 📖 Pneumonia, p 493.

Prevention
- Patients with reduced conscious level—consider airway protection (intubation) if GCS <8, or suspicion of loss of glottic function.
- Neurological disorders—in progressive disorders, the decision to protect the airway needs a full and frank discussion about the consequences of tracheal intubation and tracheostomy. In the interim, techniques such as thickened feed or PEG feeding may reduce the aspiration risk.
- Perioperative technique:
  - Awareness of risk factors.
  - Preoperative fluid and food restrictions.
  - Use of rapid sequence induction of anaesthesia.
  - Use of regional anaesthetic techniques.

- Preoperative gastric acid suppression and antacids such as sodium citrate will reduce the consequences of aspiration should it occur.

Treatment
Treatment is supportive and arterial blood gases, CXR, and continued monitoring of vital signs, including pulse oximetry, are useful in guiding therapy.
- Aspiration of solid food particles should be managed by fibreoptic or rigid bronchoscopy and suction.
- The routine use of antibiotics or steroids has no evidence base.
- Despite this antibiotics are frequently prescribed if there is evidence of a developing respiratory tract infection.

Other forms of aspiration
Pulmonary damage from aspiration of other substances is relatively uncommon, as chemicals that are ingested tend to injure the upper airway and oesophagus rather than the lower respiratory tract.
- Chemical pneumonitis has been reported with barium compounds and with antacids such a magnesium trisilicate. This led to the introduction of non-particulate antacids and non-ionic contrast media.
- Acute inhalation of particles and chemicals can occur if there is a massive amount of dust or debris in the atmosphere. The immediate and long-term consequences of this may be severe.
  - Victims of the 9/11 terrorist attacks in New York had a significant fall in FEV_1 at 6 months and 1 year, and this did not recover in the subsequent 7 years.
  - It was previously assumed the consequences of acute dust and particulate matter inhalation were mild and self-limiting. These observations reinforce the need for preventative measures in rescue workers and also the need for long-term follow up of people with prolonged or severe exposure to dust and chemical inhalation.

Further reading
1 Aldrich TK. Gustave J. and Hall CB (2010) Lung function in rescue workers at the World Trade Center after 7 years. *New Engl J Med* **362**(14), 1263–1272.
2 Enkhbaatar P, Herndon DN, and Traber DL (2009) Use of nebulized heparin in the treatment of smoke inhalation injury. *J Burn Care Res* **30**(1), 159–162.
3 Henderson H and Wilson RC (2006) Water incident related hospital activity across England between 1997/8 and 2003/4: a retrospective descriptive study. *BMC Public Health* **6**, 210.
4 Ibsen LM and Koch T (2002) Submersion and asphyxial injury. *Crit Care Med* **30**(11 Suppl), S402–S408.
5 Layon AJ and Modell JK (2009) Drowning Update 2009. *Anesthesiology* **110**, 1390–1401.

6.11 Interstitial lung disease

Definitions and nomenclature

The interstitial lung diseases (ILDs), also known as diffuse parenchymal lung diseases, represent some 200 entities. The terminology and classification used to describe this body of disorders is potentially confusing. Recent guidelines and consensus statements from international societies have helped in this regard.[1,2] Fig. 6.6 is an overview of ILD classification.

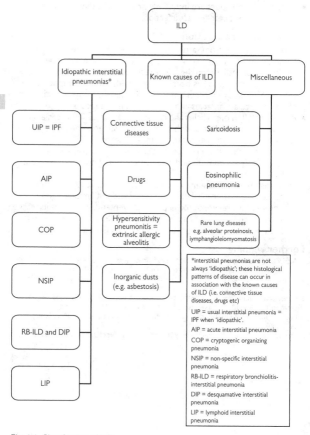

Fig. 6.6 Classification of ILDs.

Abbreviations

CFA	Cryptogenic fibrosing alveolitis
UIP	Usual interstitial pneumonitis
IPF	Idiopathic pulmonary fibrosis
COP	Cryptogenic organizing pneumonia
BOOP	Bronchiolitis obliterans organizing pneumonia
AIP	Acute interstitial pneumonitis

Cryptogenic fibrosing alveolitis

Cryptogenic fibrosing alveolitis (CFA) should be reserved to describe a syndrome characterized by breathlessness, bibasal inspiratory crepitations, and diffuse CXR infiltrates without an identifiable cause. The idiopathic interstitial pneumonias are the most common disorders to present with CFA syndrome, and idiopathic pulmonary fibrosis is the most common idiopathic interstitial pneumonia.

Nomenclature

CFA = Syndrome of breathlessness, bibasal inspiratory crepitations, and diffuse chest x-ray infiltrates, without an identifiable cause
UIP (if idiopathic) = IPF
AIP = Hamman Rich = idiopathic ARDS
COP = BOOP

Idiopathic interstitial pneumonias

These are a group of disorders originally recognized to be separate conditions based on distinctive patterns of lung injury and fibrosis in lung pathology specimens. With the increasing use of HRCT scanning, it is now recognized that some interstitial pneumonias may have distinctive corresponding patterns of disease on imaging. The interstitial pneumonias are not always 'idiopathic' and can be a consequence of underlying connective tissue diseases or adverse drug reaction.

- Usual interstitial pneumonia (UIP) in its idiopathic form is synonymous with idiopathic pulmonary fibrosis (IPF).
- AIP is synonymous with the Hamman–Rich syndrome.

- COP is synonymous with bronchiolitis obliterans organizing pneumonia (BOOP). Severe fulminant COP can present with acute respiratory failure.
- NSIP is probably a spectrum of disorders, our understanding of which is still evolving. In addition to the idiopathic form, NSIP commonly occurs in association with connective tissue diseases. NSIP rarely manifests with acute respiratory failure and the prognosis is generally better than for IPF.
- Respiratory bronchiolitis-ILD (RB-ILD) and desquamative interstitial pneumonia (DIP) are not strictly 'idiopathic' since they occur almost exclusively in smokers and often resolve on smoking cessation. DIP is rare and occasionally presents with acute respiratory failure.
- Lymphoid interstitial pneumonia is a rare disease that may be associated with autoimmune disorders and HIV infection. It does not present with acute respiratory failure.

General principles of diagnosing and managing ILD on the ICU

Acute respiratory failure with bilateral diffuse radiographic infiltrates is a common presentation to the ICU. Bilateral infective pneumonia, pulmonary oedema, and ARDS all occur more frequently in an ICU setting than acute- or acute-on-chronic ILD. In general, the key principles are:
- Establish quickly if the patient has a background ILD. In addition to case notes and chest radiology, previous abdominal CT scans often include a few cuts at the lung bases that may indicate underlying ILD.
- Investigate for treatable/reversible disease.
- If there is a known ILD, establish if this has been confidently diagnosed as IPF. This has important implications for management and prognosis.

Clinical clues that raise the suspicion of ILD
- Failure of clinical response to pneumonia or heart failure treatment is a common scenario that leads to investigations for ILD.
- Exposure to birds or moulds (causing hypersensitivity pneumonitis).
- Drug exposure (Drug-induced lung disease, p 438).
- Finger clubbing—usually denotes chronic ILD with fibrosis but may develop over a few months in evolving inflammation and fibrosis. Lymphangitis carcinomatosis may present with clubbing, diffuse CXR infiltrates, and respiratory failure.
- Most ILDs have no fever or a low-grade fever. High fevers suggest infection or vasculitis.
- Peripheral blood eosinophilia may indicate a drug-induced ILD, vasculitis (Alveolar haemorrhage and pulmonary vasculitis, p 388) or eosinophilic pneumonia. Note, however, that eosinophilic pneumonia can occur with a normal blood eosinophil count.

The CXR in ILD
- There are no characteristic CXR changes that reliably distinguish ILDs from other causes of pulmonary infiltrates and respiratory failure.
- Acute inflammatory change cannot always be distinguished from established fibrosis on CXR.
- Pleural effusions rarely occur with ILDs.

- 'Migratory' CXR changes, i.e. infiltrates that appear and disappear over a few days, are suggestive of organizing pneumonia or pulmonary vasculitis/hemorrhage, but may occur in pulmonary oedema.

HRCT in ILD
- HRCT should be performed early in suspected ILD. Interpretation can be more difficult in the presence of secondary complications such as hospital-acquired pneumonia or ARDS.
- HRCT images are best interpreted jointly by a clinician and a radiologist experienced in ILD.
- The following conditions may (but not always) present with highly characteristic CT findings, allowing a confident diagnosis to be made in the correct clinical context:
  - IPF
  - Subacute hypersensitivity pneumonitis
  - Lymphangitis carcinomatosis
  - Sarcoidosis.

BAL in ILD
The principal role of BAL is to exclude infection.

General principles of BAL
- BAL should be considered early in the course of admission in suspected ILD.
- Liaise with colleagues in microbiology and pathology prior to sending the sample.
- In a mechanically ventilated patient BAL is generally a safe procedure with a low complication rate (<5%) and very low mortality (<0.5%).
- In self-ventilating patients requiring high-flow oxygen, BAL is liable to precipitate destabilization and the requirement for invasive ventilation. BAL may be performed with non-invasive ventilatory support.
- The cellular content of normal BAL is >95% macrophages, with <5% neutrophils. BAL differential cell count is not usually useful for diagnosing, or distinguishing between, interstitial pneumonias presenting with respiratory failure, ARDS, or infection since all are typified by excess neutrophils (5–60% or higher) in lavage fluid. Occasionally BAL cytology will yield an alternative diagnosis, such as carcinomatosis.

Diagnoses that may be confirmed on BAL results
- Infective pneumonia, including tuberculosis, and opportunistic infection (particularly *Pneumocystis jirovecii*, CMV pneumonitis).
- Carcinomatosis.

Diagnoses that may be supported by BAL results
- Excess eosinophils support a diagnosis of drug-induced pneumotoxicity or pulmonary eosinophilia.
- 'Foamy alveolar macrophages' are a feature of amiodarone lung.
- Haemosiderin-laden macrophages are seen in pulmonary haemorrhage.
- Lymphocyte predominance raises the possibility of hypersensitivity pneumonitis.

Technical notes on BAL
- The site of BAL should be determined based on radiological appearances. In diffuse disease, the default site is usually the right middle lobe.
- Pre-oxygenate the patient with 100% oxygen for 5min.
- 'Wedge' the bronchoscope into the bronchial orifice.
- Instill 40–50mL aliquots of sterile saline, waiting 10s before gently aspirating.
- The first aspirate is strictly a 'bronchial wash', not a BAL. This might be sufficient to diagnose bacterial pneumonia but is unreliable and is not sufficient for opportunistic infections or useful cytology.
- Repeat instillation/aspiration up to a maximum instilled volume of 240mL. In ventilated patients the yield may be quite low; expect a return of approximately 20–30% of instilled fluid.
- In addition to cytology, standard microscopy, and culture, specifically request stains/immunofluorescence for acid-fast bacilli, *Pneumocystis jirovecii*, fungi, and viruses.

Transbronchial lung biopsy in ILD
- In general transbronchial lung biopsy (TBLB) is of limited value in diagnosing and managing ILD in an ICU setting.
- Although apparently safe, based on the experience of centres familiar with TBLB in ventilated patients, there is a 10% chance of pneumothorax, which may lead to persistent air leak.
- The tissue sample size from TBLB is usually insufficient to make a definitive histological diagnosis.
- TBLB may be diagnostic in infections and carcinomatosis, and yield tissue that might support other diagnoses.
- TBLB cannot reliably diagnose or distinguish between interstitial pneumonias.

Surgical lung biopsy in ILD
A surgical lung biopsy (SLB) should be considered in patients with sus-pected ILD in whom BAL has both excluded infection and failed to yield a confident diagnosis. In such cases SLB leads to a change in management (including withdrawal of therapy) in 60–80% of cases.

General principles of SLB
- SLB is most useful (and may be safer) earlier in the course of disease. However, a lung biopsy even after prolonged ventilation may change management.
- When liaising with thoracic surgical colleagues, make it clear that as well as histology, a fresh (unfixed) sample of lung should be sent to microbiology.
- High-dose corticosteroid therapy will often influence the histological pattern of disease, but does not necessarily prevent a histological (or microbiological) diagnosis from being made.
- Short-term complications are common, especially air leak, which may occur in around 30–40% of cases.

- Major morbidity and death attributable to SLB is hard to quantify, but is probably uncommon (<5%).

Diagnoses that may only be confirmed by SLB
- DAD—this is the histological pattern of disease seen in ARDS or AIP.
- End-stage fibrosis (prognostically if not diagnostically useful).
- Cryptogenic organizing pneumonia.
- Vasculitis.
- CMV pneumonitis and other opportunistic infections.
- Aspiration pneumonitis.
- Carcinomatosis.
- Lymphoma.

Idiopathic pulmonary fibrosis

Epidemiology
- The most commonest of the idiopathic interstitial pneumonias, 4000–5000 new cases in the UK per year.
- Median age of presentation 65–70 years; uncommon <50 years.
- Male:female 2:1.
- A weak association with smoking.

Pathophysiology
- The underlying histological pattern of disease is UIP, speculated to a be consequence of repeated subclinical type 1 alveolar epithelial cell injury, patchy aberrant wound healing, hyper-proliferation of type II alveolar cells, and excess collagen deposition at sites of 'fibroblastic foci'.
- Acute exacerbation of IPF (see below) is usually characterized histologically by DAD on a background of UIP.

Clinical features
- Onset of breathlessness typically 1 year prior to presentation.
- Dry cough.
- Finger clubbing is present in around two-thirds of cases.
- Fine bibasal, mid, and late inspiratory crepitations.
- Some patients have 'benign' stable disease for many years.
- Most patients experience periods of relative stability interspersed with acute declines, some of which may be severe (acute exacerbations).

Acute exacerbation of IPF
- Defined as an acute clinically significant deterioration of unidentifiable cause in a patient with underlying IPF.
- Over a 1-year period, approximately 10% of patients with IPF will experience an acute exacerbation.
- The cause of acute exacerbations is unknown. A viral aetiology has been implicated.

Diagnostic criteria for acute exacerbation in IPF (adapted from reference 3)
- Previous or concurrent diagnosis of IPF.
- Unexplained worsening or development of shortness of breath <30 days.
- HRCT—new infiltrates (ground glass or consolidation) on background consistent with UIP.
- No evidence of infection based on endotracheal aspirate or BAL.
- Exclusion of left heart failure, PE, or known cause of ALI.

Diagnosis of IPF
IPF can be confidently diagnosed based on typical clinical findings and HRCT but may require a BAL or lung biopsy to exclude other conditions.

HRCT in IPF
- Bibasal, subpleural cystic change ('honeycomb fibrosis') is virtually diagnostic of IPF in the correct clinical setting.
- There is comparatively little ground-glass attenuation in stable disease.
- In acute exacerbation of IPF, there is newly evolved extensive diffuse ground glass change or patchy/peripheral changes with focal consolidation. These changes are not reliably distinguishable from infection.

Medical management of IPF
There is no proven effective therapy for IPF. There are promising emerging data for the use of N-acetylcysteine (combined with corticosteroids and azathioprine), endothelin antagonists, and pirfenidone (an antifibrotic drug) in IPF but definitive trial outcomes are awaited. High-dose corticosteroids are not effective in stable IPF. Young patients with IPF should be considered for lung transplantation. International guidelines recommend best supportive care with palliation of symptoms for all patients with IPF.

Medical management of acute exacerbation of IPF
It is first necessary to distinguish acute exacerbation of IPF from other, potentially treatable, coexisting diseases, principally infective pneumonia, LV failure or thrombo-embolic disease (Fig. 6.7). If the diagnosis is acute exacerbation the following should be noted:
- There are no controlled trials in exacerbation of IPF and therefore no good evidence that therapy is effective.
- High-dose corticosteroid therapy (e.g. intravenous methylprednisolone 500mg to 1g over three consecutive days, followed by prednisolone 60mg daily, with slow dose reduction after 2–4 weeks) is the most commonly used treatment.
- There is anecdotal evidence for the use of immunomodulation therapy in addition to corticosteroids, e.g. with cyclophosphamide or ciclosporin A.
- Microthromboembolic disease has been postulated to play a pathogenic role in acute exacerbation in IPF but there is no good evidence that anticoagulation is effective.

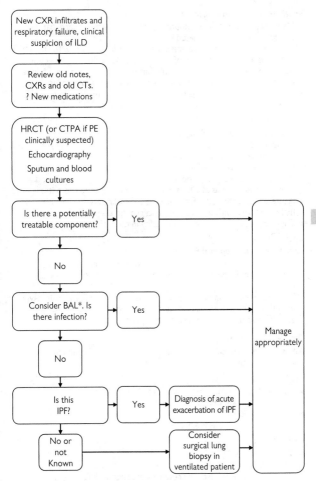

Fig. 6.7 ILD algorithm for the ICU. *In the self-ventilating/non-invasively ventilated patient BAL may precipitate the need for invasive ventilation.

Ventilatory management in IPF
- Mechanical ventilation is seldom appropriate in acute exacerbation of IPF due to the high associated mortality.
- Invasive ventilation may be appropriate in some patients with stable IPF if there is a reversible cause of acute decompensation, e.g. infection.
- Ventilatory management is difficult, but fibrotic disease generally does not respond well to high inspiratory or expiratory airway pressures.
- Ventilatory management is to allow medical treatment time to work. The main therapeutic aim of ventilation is to avoid VILI.

Prognosis in IPF
- The overall median survival from diagnosis is 3–4 years.
- A subgroup of patients have 'benign' stable disease for many years. This may represent around 10–20% of cases and this group is not reliably identifiable at presentation.
- Most patients experience periods of relative stability interspersed with acute declines, some of which may be severe (acute exacerbations).
- Acute exacerbation of IPF has around 60% mortality at 3 months, and higher in those with more severe background disease.
- The short- and medium-term mortality in mechanically ventilated patients with acute exacerbation of IPF is over 90%.

Lung transplantation in IPF
- Lung transplantation is appropriate for young (generally <65 years) patients with IPF who are otherwise physically and psychologically robust.
- In appropriate patients with acute exacerbation of IPF, liaise closely with the regional transplant centre; mechanical ventilation should not generally be used as a 'bridge' to transplantation.

Acute interstitial pneumonia

AIP is a catastrophic acute ILD (i.e. absence of pre-existing lung disease), also known as the Hamman–Rich syndrome.

Epidemiology
- The incidence of AIP is unknown, but it is uncommon.
- Most cases present in patients aged 50–70 years.
- Males:females 1:1.
- There are no obvious risk factors.

Pathophysiology
- The cause of AIP is unknown.
- The pathological pattern of disease is DAD, identical to that seen in ARDS and in most cases of acute exacerbation of IPF.

Clinical features
- Typically rapidly worsening breathlessness over a few days or weeks.
- Sometimes preceded by a viral pro-dromal illness and dry cough.
- A low-grade fever may be present.
- Finger clubbing has been described but is unusual; it raises the possibility of underlying IPF.
- Bibasal lung crepitations are usually present, but breath sounds may be normal.

Diagnosis of AIP

A presumptive diagnosis of AIP can be made based on integration of clinical features, radiology, and exclusion of infection, but a confident diagnosis requires a surgical lung biopsy. The HRCT pattern of disease is as seen in acute exacerbation of IPF, but without significant honeycomb change.

Medical management of AIP

- There are no controlled studies of treatment of AIP.
- Treatment is typically intravenous methylprednisolone 500mg to 1g daily for at least three consecutive days, followed by prednisolone 60mg daily and subsequent dose reduction after 2–4 weeks.

Ventilatory management for AIP

Because of its rapid onset in the absence of previous lung disease, the majority of individuals with AIP will be mechanically ventilated, often within a few hours or days of admission.

- Ventilatory management is difficult, but fibrotic disease generally does not respond well to high inspiratory or expiratory airway pressures.
- Ventilatory management is to allow medical treatment time to work. The main therapeutic aim of ventilation is to avoid VILI.

Prognosis in AIP

- The overall mortality is probably 70–80%.
- There is some evidence that early diagnosis and treatment lead to a lower mortality.
- In those that respond, improvement in gas exchange is usually observed within the first 3–4 days of starting corticosteroid treatment.
- The median time on a ventilator in survivors is probably 10–15 days, with a large range.
- Long-term survivors usually make a full recovery with little physiological defect.

Cryptogenic organizing pneumonia

COP is usually a comparatively benign interstitial lung disease, sensitive to corticosteroid therapy and associated with a very low mortality. Occasionally COP can be fulminant and present with acute respiratory failure.

Epidemiology

- The incidence COP is unknown but it is uncommon.
- May present at any age, mean age 55–60 years.
- Males:females 1:1.
- There are no known risk factors.

Pathophysiology

- Histologically organizing pneumonia is characterized by 'plugs' of organizing granulation tissue within alveolar ducts and airsacs, with a bronchocentric pattern.
- Organizing pneumonia is not always 'cryptogenic'; it can be associated with viral pneumonia, drugs, radiotherapy, and other causes.

Clinical features

Most patients with COP present with clinical features largely indistinguishable from infective pneumonia. The diagnosis usually becomes apparent when treatment for pneumonia fails.

- Dry cough, fever, and fatigue are common.
- Haemoptysis is uncommon.
- Finger clubbing is unusual.
- Chest crepitations are common, bronchial breathing is heard infrequently.
- Rapidly progressing breathlessness and respiratory failure are features of fulminant COP.

Diagnosis of COP

A presumptive diagnosis of COP can be made based on clinical features, imaging, and exclusion of infection or pulmonary oedema, but a definitive diagnosis requires a lung biopsy. COP is a cause of migratory CXR infiltrates.

Medical management of COP

- Typical mild COP responds very well to corticosteroid therapy. It is rare for COP to progress to fibrotic lung disease.
- There is little data on the treatment of severe fulminant COP, but overall it probably responds better to treatment than other ILDs.
- Treatment is usually with pulse methylprednisolone 500mg to 1g daily for at least three consecutive days, followed by prednisolone 60mg daily for 2–4 weeks followed by dose reduction and a total treatment period of 3–6 months.

Ventilatory management of COP

Because of its rapid onset, and likely favourable outome in comparison to other ILDs, individuals with fulminant COP should be considered for mechanical ventilation.

Natural history and prognosis

- COP generally has an excellent prognosis.
- There is very little data on fulminant COP. Fatalities have been described, but a response to treatment would be expected.
- In those that do respond to treatment, gas exchange and radiographic infiltrates improve rapidly.
- Relapse in COP is not uncommon.

Sarcoidosis

Sarcoidosis is a multisystem granulomatous disease of unknown aetiology. Although the disease affects the lungs in over 90% of patients, sarcoidosis very rarely presents with acute respiratory failure and only occasionally progresses to chronic respiratory failure.

Epidemiology

- There are around 3000 new cases of sarcoidosis a year in the UK.
- Most cases present between the ages of 20 and 50 years, with another smaller peak after 60 years.
- Males: females 1:1.
- The disease is more common and runs a more aggressive course in Afro-Caribbean patients.

Pathophysiology
- Characterized by non-caseating granulomata, with variable associated inflammation and scarring.

Clinical features

Sarcoidosis has been described in virtually all organs, but the most common clinical manifestations are skin, pulmonary, and ocular sarcoidosis. Neurological and cardiac disease is uncommon but potentially life-threatening. The clinical presentation is therefore variable. Pulmonary sarcoidosis presents as one of four 'stages' based on the CXR appearances:

- Stage 1 disease—bilateral hilar lymphadenopathy (BHL), normal lung parenchyma, and usually minimal chest symptoms. Co-presentation with erythema nodosum and arthralgia (Löfgren's syndrome).
- Stage 2 disease—BHL with interstitial lung infiltrate, usually nodular and mainly mid and upper zone dominant. Patients may be breathless and have a dry cough.
- Stage 3 disease—interstitial infiltrate without BHL. Symptoms as for stage 2 disease.
- Stage 4 disease—established lung fibrosis without BHL. Breathlessness, productive cough if secondary bronchiectasis has developed, and occasionally chronic respiratory failure.

Rarely, stage 2 or 3 disease presents with acute respiratory failure and extensive radiographic disease.

Diagnosis of sarcoidosis

The clinical presentation is often highly suggestive of sarcoidosis, especially when presenting with Löfgren's syndrome or with skin or eye manifestations, but a definitive diagnosis requires histological confirmation from an accessible site of disease.

- The plain CXR may be very suggestive of sarcoidosis in the correct clinical setting. The abnormalities are as described above. Pleural effusion is very rare in sarcoidosis.
- Sarcoidosis can present with a very wide variety of HRCT abnormalities, but the presence of lymphadenopathy and micronodular changes along bronchovascular bundles, subpleurally, and in the upper and mid zones is typical.
- Bronchial and transbronchial biopsies have a high diagnostic yield in pulmonary sarcoidosis.
- Blood tests are not often helpful in diagnosis. Sarcoidosis can cause hypercalcaemia. The serum ACE is often raised in active disease but is not specific to sarcoidosis.

Medical management of sarcoidosis

Sarcoidosis is usually a benign disease. Spontaneous remission is a feature of the natural history of pulmonary sarcoidosis and occurs in 60–80% of patients with stage 1 disease, 40–60% of patients with stage 2 disease, 10–20% of patients with stage 3 disease, and never in stage 4 disease. Progression or resolution of disease is usually evident in the first 2–3 years after presentation.

Treatment with corticosteroids is warranted in the following situations:
- Pulmonary sarcoidosis associated with declining lung function and radiographic progression

- Hypercalcaemia
- Ocular, cardiac, and neuro-sarcoidosis.

Pulmonary sarcoidosis is usually responsive to corticosteroids at initial doses of 20–40mg daily. Therapy is usually required for 18–24 months to minimize the risk of relapse.

Finally, a couple of tips....
- Think of TB in diffuse infiltrative lung disease and respiratory failure; it is a great mimicker.
- Always consider drug reactions (📖 Drug-induced lung disease, p 438); pneumotox.com is a valuable resource for checking previously reported drug reactions.

1 American Thoracic Society/European Respiratory Society (2002) International multidisciplinary consensus classification of the idiopathic interstitial pneumonias. *Am J Respir Crit Care Med* **165**, 277–304.
2 British Thoracic Society in collaboration with the Thoracic Society of Australia and New Zealand and the Irish Thoracic Society (2008) Interstitial lung disease guideline. *Thorax* **63** (Suppl 5), 1–58.
3 Collard HR, Moore BB, Flaherty KR, *et al.* (2007) Acute exacerbations of idiopathic pulmonary fibrosis. *Am J Respir Crit Care Med* **176**, 636–43.

6.12 Pleural disease

Pneumothorax

Pneumothorax is the presence of air in the pleural cavity and may be classified as:

- Primary (spontaneous), which occurs in otherwise healthy individuals
- Secondary, which occurs in the presence of underlying lung disease.

The majority of pneumothoraces in the ICU setting are secondary.

Primary pneumothorax may be managed with either observation, if small and minimal symptoms, or by fine needle aspiration of air in the first instance.

Risk factors for pneumothorax in ICU setting

Traumatic

- Trauma.
- Barotrauma from mechanical ventilation.
- Iatrogenic.
  - Central venous line placement.
  - Thoracocentesis.
  - Cardiopulmonary resuscitation (CPR).

Underlying lung disease

- ARDS.
- COPD.
- Asthma.
- CF.
- Sarcoidosis.
- Malignancy.
- IPF.
- Lymphangioleimyomatosis (rare).

Infection

- PCP.
- Tuberculosis.
- Severe adult respiratory syndrome.

Pleural disease

Diagnosis

In a mechanically ventilated patient diagnosis may be difficult.

- Clinical deterioration may be noted with increasing peak airway pressures or falling tidal volumes due to decreasing compliance.
- The usual signs of resonant percussion note and reduced breath sounds may be difficult to detect.
- There may be worsening hypoxaemia and, if there is progression to tension pneumothorax, cardiorespiratory collapse.

Chest X-ray

An erect CXR is rarely possible and even significant pneumothoraces may be difficult to detect in a supine ventilated patient (see box).

- In patients with very stiff lungs the lungs may not collapse readily.

- Loculation of pleural air may occur as a result of pleural inflammation and the lung may be tethered at many points.
- The supine position results in an atypical distribution of air; anteromedial, basal and subpulmonary collections are common. They may not produce an obvious lung edge and therefore the classically described radiological features may be absent.

Signs of pneumothorax on a supine CXR include:
- Hyperlucent hemithorax
- Increased lucency towards bases
- Deep sulcus sign (the costophrenic angle is abnormally deepened, causing a deep 'V')
- 'Double hemi-diaphragm' sign (one above and one below on affected side)
- Increased definition of the mediastinal border (including increased cardiophrenic lucency; there is normally an opaque diaphragmatic border at the midline)
- Unusually clear or sharp heart border.

Pneumomediastinum, pneumopericardium, or surgical emphysema should raise suspicion of a coexisting pneumothorax.

> **Traps for the unwary on CXR**
> - Bilateral pneumothoraces.
> - COPD with bulla.
> - Skin folds.

Ultrasound
Ultrasound may be useful to exclude pneumothorax by visualizing the lung–chest wall interface. Aerated lung does not transmit ultrasound well and neither does a pneumothorax, therefore it requires an experienced operator and is less useful in the presence of surgical emphysema or pre-existing lung disease, especially bullous lung disease.
- In a normal subject, the lung–chest wall interface is seen to slide to and fro with respiration. This 'lung sliding' or 'gliding' indicates that the visceral and parietal pleura are apposed.
- The comet tail (or B line) can be used to identify the visceral pleura. The comet tail is a band that extends vertically through the scanning field. It originates in the visceral pleura.
- The presence of lung sliding and comet tails excludes pneumothorax.

In the supine patient the use of a linear array probe to check every intercostal space anteriorly is recommended.

Computerized tomography
CT is helpful for diagnosis in the presence of bullae or surgical emphysema, as well as picking up small or loculated pneumothoraces. It does require patient transfer, and the risk/benefit ratio may be finely balanced.

Management
Not all pneumothoraces in spontaneously ventilating patients require drainage.

- Administration of high-flow oxygen increases the pleural gas reabsorption rate.
- The insertion of a small bore chest drain in the 'safe triangle' (see below) is the recommended treatment of secondary pneumothoraces. The drain is then connected to an underwater seal bottle and should be left on free drainage.
- The use of clamps is not recommended. A bubbling drain should never be clamped since this may lead to tension pneumothorax.
- Suction is generally not advised because of the risk of re-expansion pulmonary oedema. It may be considered if there is persistent bubbling after 48h, although it remains controversial.

Management of large or persistent (>48h) air leak (see 📖 Complications of ventilation, p 244)
- Check the drainage system for air leaks, especially around connectors.
- Involve respiratory physicians.
- Replacement with a large bore chest drain may be effective.
- Early thoracic referral is advised for consideration of open pleurectomy or video-assisted thoracic surgery (VATS) pleurodesis.
- High-volume, low-pressure suction may be considered but evidence of benefit is unclear.
- In patients with persistent air leak who are too unwell to consider general anaesthetic, such as in ARDS, pleurodesis may be considered.

Following initial management, divers and pilots should be referred to thoracic surgery for bilateral pleurodesis.

Tension pneumothorax
Approximately 50% of mechanically ventilated patients with pneumothorax develop a tension pneumothorax. The risk is increased by delay in diagnosis and it is potentially life-threatening.

Signs of tension pneumothorax
- Cardiorespiratory collapse.
- Mediastinal shift and tracheal deviation (depending on underlying lung disease and unilateral lung collapse).
- Worsening hypoxaemia.

In a mechanically ventilated patient:
- Worsening hypoxaemia.
- Increased peak airway pressures (volume control modes).
- Inadequate tidal volumes (pressure control modes).

Note: These signs are non-specific but should raise the possibility of pneumothorax.

Management of tension pneumothorax
If tension pneumothorax is suspected clinically, do not wait for radiological confirmation.
- Give 100% oxygen; insert a large bore cannula in the second intercostal space anteriorly to allow the release of the air under pressure.
- A chest drain should then be inserted promptly in the 'safe triangle' and connected to an underwater seal bottle.

Surgical emphysema

This may develop as sign of pneumothorax or as a complication of management. Whilst uncomfortable, it is usually not of significant clinical importance and will resolve as the pneumothorax resolves. Rarely, airway compromise may occur.

- Chest drains should be placed on suction to encourage air to escape via the drainage bottle rather than into the subcutaneous tissues.
- In severe cases involving the face and neck, consider subcutaneous drains, including cannulae, or subcutaneous incisions and then 'milking' the skin.

Pleural effusion

Pleural effusions are common in critically ill patients and the differential diagnosis is wide. Although clinical history and examination may point to the diagnosis, pleural aspiration and evaluation of the fluid is often required. Radiology, including ultrasound, may give important diagnostic information as well as aid investigation.

Pleural effusions may be classified as transudates or exudates, defined by a pleural protein less then or greater than 30g/L, respectively. In borderline cases Light's criteria should be used (see box).

Light's criteria

The following suggest an exudate:
- Pleural fluid protein:serum protein ratio >0.5
- Pleural fluid lactate dehydrogenase (LDH): serum LDH ratio >0.6
- Pleural fluid LDH more than two-thirds the upper limits of normal serum LDH.

The causes of each of pleural effusions are listed in Table 6.7.

Table 6.7 Causes of pleural effusion

Causes of transudates	Causes of exudates
Cardiac failure (common)	Malignancy (common)
Liver failure (common)	Parapneumonic (common)
Hypoalbuminaemia (common)	Empyema (common)
Peritoneal dialysis (common)	Post cardiac surgery (common)
Nephrotic syndrome	Post MI
Hypothyroidism	PE
Mitral stenosis (rare)	Tuberculosis
	Pancreatitis
	Oesophageal rupture
	Subphrenic or hepatic abscess
	Benign asbestos effusion
	Rheumatoid arthritis (rare)
	Autoimmune (rare)
	Amyloid (rare)
	Yellow nail syndrome (rare)

Imaging

- CXR may simply show diffusely increased shadowing on the affected side. Even in an upright patient, as much as 300mL may be present before the costophrenic angle is obliterated on CXR.
- Ultrasound is far superior to CXR in detecting fluid and is strongly recommended in all cases to mark a suitable spot for diagnostic aspiration or chest drain insertion.
- Ultrasound may differentiate between a transudate and an exudate: a transudate is always anechoic, whereas an exudate may be anechoic or highly echogenic. The presence of septations suggests a complex effusion that warrants drainage.
- CT scanning may provide further diagnostic information, for example in PE or malignancy, and can distinguish between benign and malignant pleural thickening.

Diagnostic aspiration

- Send protein, glucose, LDH, cytology. Establish pH.
- As well as sending a sample to microbiology for microscopy and culture, the yield is further increased if pleural fluid is also sent in blood culture bottles.
- A 50mL sample is adequate, sending at least 30mL for cytology.

Protein

- A transudate is defined by pleural protein <30g/L, an exudate has >30g/L. If the pleural protein is between 25 and 35g/L then Light's criteria (see box) can be used to assist diagnosis.

pH

pH <7.2 in the presence of infection indicates an empyema and requires prompt drainage.

- Measure the pH of all non-purulent samples using a blood gas syringe and analyser. Do not put pus through the blood gas analyser.
- pH <7.2 may also be seen in effusions due advanced malignancy, oesophageal rupture, and rheumatoid arthritis.

Glucose

- Low pleural glucose (<3mmol/L) is commonly seen in pleural infection and rheumatoid arthritis. It may also be low in malignancy, oesophageal rupture, and lupus.
- Although less sensitive, low pleural glucose may be a surrogate marker for pH as indicator of an empyema.

Haematocrit

- Pleural haemotocrit may be used to distinguish between a blood-stained effusion, commonly seen in malignancy, and a haemothorax.
- Pleural fluid haematocrit >50% of the peripheral blood haematocrit indicates a haemothorax.

Cell count

- Lymphocytosis suggests the effusion is chronic in nature and is seen in TB, malignancy, post-coronary artery bypass graft (CABG), and congestive cardiac failure (CCF).
- Neutrophilia is usually due to an acute inflammatory process, including bacterial or viral infection, and PE with infarction.

- Eosinophilia suggests a drug-induced cause or the previous presence of air in the pleural space. It may also occur in malignancy.

Cytology
- The most common malignancies causing effusions are lung, mesothelioma, breast, and lymphoma. However, pleural cytology alone is often insufficient to make a diagnosis.
- The mean diagnostic rate from pleural aspiration in malignancy is approximately 60%.
- If the initial sample is negative, repeat aspiration should be considered.
- Massive (majority of hemithorax) unilateral effusions are most commonly due to malignancy; if cytology is negative then further investigation is warranted.

Acid fast bacilli
- In effusions due to TB there may be no or little associated lung field changes.
- The diagnostic yield from AFB smears and culture is low (around 25%). However, a positive culture confirms the diagnosis and gives antibiotic sensitivities.
- The diagnostic rate increases to over 95% with pleural biopsy culture. This may be performed by ultrasound/CT guided biopsy or at thoracoscopy. Biopsy samples must be sent for culture as well as histology.

Management
In the critically ill patient initial management of the effusion may take priority over the need for investigation of the cause, if not already known. In the majority of cases the management consists of addressing the underlying cause. Symptomatic effusions should be considered for drainage.

Empyema and parapneumonic effusions
See pleural infection below.

Bilateral effusions
- Bilateral effusions in the critically ill patient are common. They are usually transudates due to cardiac failure or low protein states, although these can present as unilateral effusions.
- If history and clinical findings support the diagnosis of a transudate then diagnostic aspiration need only be performed if there is poor response to treatment or if there are atypical features.
- Chest drains should be avoided in a transudate. If required for acute symptom relief, a therapeutic pleural aspiration (500–1000mL) may be considered.

Post-coronary artery bypass graft effusions
Post-CABG effusions are usually small and left sided but can present as large, bilateral effusions.

They are typically classified as early (within 1 month) and late, with differing pathogenesis. Early effusions appear to be due to an immune response to the cardiac injury and are frequently haemoserous.

With both types, the majority will resolve with conservative management only. Therapeutic aspiration is sometimes required.

Late effusions may be associated with trapped lung, and intervention may be required.

Pleural tips

- *Pulmonary embolus.* The effusion is often small, with disproportionate dyspnoea.
- *Pancreatitis.* Effusions have a raised pleural amylase. This can also be found in oesophageal rupture, ruptured ectopic pregnancy, and malignancy. Check isoenzyme: a raised salivary isoenzyme suggests oesophageal rupture or malignancy; pancreatic isoenzyme suggests a pancreatic cause.
- *Chylothorax and pseudochylothorax* are suggested by the milky appearance on sampling. Request pleural cholesterol and triglycerides: chylothorax has raised trigycerides, usually >1.24mmol/L. The most common causes of chylothorax are lymphoma and trauma post surgery. Pseudochylothorax is indicated by pleural cholesterol >5.18mmol/L and is most commonly due to chronic pleural effusion (e.g. chronic rheumatoid effusion).

Haemothorax

Haemothorax is the presence of blood in the pleural space. It is defined as a pleural haematocrit of >50% of the peripheral blood haematocrit.

The signs are those of a pleural effusion and there may be associated haemodynamic instability.

Causes

Trauma

By far the most common cause of haemothorax is trauma.

- Blunt—the presentation may be delayed by several hours to days.
- Penetrating.
- Iatrogenic, including cardio-thoracic surgery, subclavian cannulation, and chest drain placement.

Non-traumatic causes

- Malignancy.
- Coagulopathies (including anticoagulation therapy).
- PE with infarction.
- Associated with primary pneumothorax (vessel rupture within a pleural adhesion).
- Spontaneous aortic dissection.
- Pulmonary arterio-venous malformations.
- Catamenial (menstrual).

Management tips.

- In major haemothorax (usually related to trauma) the initial priority is resuscitation, using blood products as appropriate.
- A wide bore (>32Fr gauge) chest drain should be inserted by blunt dissection and the output monitored carefully.
- Massive haemothorax (>1000mL initial drainage) can cause cardiovascular collapse and is an indication for early surgical intervention (see box).

- Prompt drainage of all but the smallest of haemothoraces is recommended to prevent complications. However, if pleural adhesions have already formed primary surgical intervention is advised, as tube drainage is unlikely to be effective and may cause further bleeding.
- Coagulopathies should be corrected prior to chest drain insertion whenever possible.
- If drainage is ineffective, multiple chest drains are not recommended as they are a further potential source of infection with little evidence of additional benefit. Surgical intervention is required to prevent long-term complications and impairment of lung volumes.

Indications for surgical intervention
- Massive or significant initial bleed.
- Persistent bleeding (>200mL/h) or haemodynamic instability.
- Clot retention despite tube drainage.
- Secondary infection (empyema).
- Significant adhesions.

Complications
Complications of haemothorax usually relate to incomplete drainage and include:
- Clot retention
- Secondary infection (empyema)
- Trapped lung (failure of lung to re-expand after drainage due to fibrin formation).

Pleural infection
Pleural effusions affect up to 40% of patients with pneumonia. They may be classified as:
- Simple parapneumonic (gram stain negative or pH >7.2)
- Complicated parapneumonic (gram stain positive, pH <7.2, loculations)
- Empyema (frank pus).

Pleural infection confers a high morbidity and mortality, and early intervention is vital.

Causes
- Hospital-acquired pneumonia (HAP).
- Community-acquired pneumonia (CAP).
- Iatrogenic (including post operative, chest drain insertion).
- Primary empyema.
- Thoracic trauma.
- Mediastinal infections (e.g. mediastinitis, oesophageal rupture).
- Abdominal infections.

Bacteriology
This depends on the source of infection. In HAP, empirical antibiotics should cover MRSA (the most commonly cultured organism in this presentation) as well as Gram negatives and anaerobes. In CAP the most common pathogens cultured are the *Strep. Milleri* Group, *Strep.*

Pneumoniae, Staphylococci and mixed anaerobes. In around 40% no organism is cultured, often due to prior antibiotic use.

Clinical features

Clinical features are that of the underlying infection with additional features of a pleural effusion. An empyema or complicated parapneumonic effusion should be suspected in effusions that are slow to resolve, or have ongoing fever or raised CRP. An empyema exacerbates catabolism in the critically ill patient and may cause further weight loss and low albumin.

Imaging
Chest X-ray

In a simple parapneumonic effusion a fluid meniscus may be seen. There is often underlying consolidation. If the fluid is loculated a rounded, pleural-based opacity may be present which may mimic the appearance of a tumour.

Ultrasound

Ultrasound is ideal for locating fluid and is superior to CT for detecting loculations, allowing identification of the optimal site for drain placement. It also has the significant advantage of being available at the bedside.

Computerized tomography

Contract-enhanced CT scanning is essential when surgical intervention is being considered.

It may help to distinguish between a lung abscess and an empyema; a lung abscess is seen as a thick-walled cavity without lung compression whereas an empyema is thin and smooth-walled with associated lung compression.

Management

Frank pus or pH <7.2 at diagnostic aspiration indicates the need for prompt chest drainage.

- Simple parapneumonic effusions will usually resolve without drainage by treatment of the underlying infection. Large effusions may require therapeutic aspiration for symptom relief.
- Complicated parapneumonic effusions and empyema require early drainage and appropriate antibiotics. The initial use of small bore chest drains is as effective as wide bore drains, and is associated with fewer complications and less patient discomfort. Small bore chest drains require regular saline flushes to prevent tube blockage. In a slowly resolving effusion or with thick pus, replacement with wide bore drain is sometimes necessary.
- Thoracic surgical referral is indicated if there is slow or incomplete initial drainage. Patients unfit for general anaesthetic may be considered for rib resection and drainage under local anaesthetic.
- The benefit of fibrinolytics in poorly draining empyema is controversial. The largest RCT of streptokinase in the management of empyema found no benefit. Routine use of fibrinolytics is not recommended.
- Maintenance of good nutrition is vital; an empyema is a further cause of significant catabolism in the critically ill patient and contributes to mortality.

Author's tips
- Bilateral empyema is rare. The main cause is bacterial mediastinitis secondary to mediastinal disruption (e.g. acute oesophageal rupture).
- Consider Lemierre's syndrome (acute oropharyngeal infection with *Fusobacterium* species, leading to septic thrombophlebitis of the internal jugular vein and empyema).

Chest drains

Chest drains are widely used in thoracic, respiratory, and emergency departments. They are used relatively frequently in ICU. Their insertion and management carries a small but definite risk to the patient. Inserting a chest drain just because you can see fluid is not good practice and each individual drain should be considered on the risks vs benefits presented to the patient (see also 📖 Complications of ventilation, p 244).

Indications
- Pneumothorax.
  - All ventilated patients.
  - Spontaneous pneumothorax after failed aspiration.
  - Large or symptomatic secondary pneumothorax.
- Empyema and complicated parapneumonic effusions.
- Haemothorax.
- Large post-operative effusions.
- Malignant pleural effusions.

Chest drains should generally be avoided in a transudate. If required for acute symptom relief, a therapeutic pleural aspiration (500–1000mL) may be considered.

Drain size
- Small-bore, Seldinger insertion chest drains (typically 10–14F) are recommended for the initial management of pneumothorax and pleural effusions, including empyema.
- Wide-bore (>24F), blunt dissection drains should be considered first line for traumatic haemothorax. Insertion of a wide-bore drain is also appropriate in persistent empyema or pneumothorax despite initial small bore drain insertion.
- A blunt dissection technique may be considered in ventilated patients with a high PEEP to avoid the risk of lung penetration during drain insertion.
- Regardless of technique, adequate training and supervision must be ensured.

Management tips
- Drain placement should be in the 'safe triangle' (Fig. 6.8) where possible.
- Check clotting. Avoid drain insertion until INR <1.5.
- Ultrasound is strongly recommended to confirm the presence and position of fluid and identify loculations.
- Secure drain with a strong suture (e.g. 1.0 Silk) and a clear dressing. Do not use 'purse string' sutures as they cause pain and a poor cosmetic result.

- Perform CXR to check position.
- If there is no 'swing' (movement of the fluid in the tubing with respiration) then either the tube is blocked or the drain is not in the pleural space. Flushing the drain with sterile saline, via a three-way tap, may restore tube patency. If patency cannot be restored then the drain should be removed and re-sited.
- Ensure adequate analgesia whilst the drain is *in situ*; simple paracetamol-based analgesia is usually sufficient for smallbore drains.

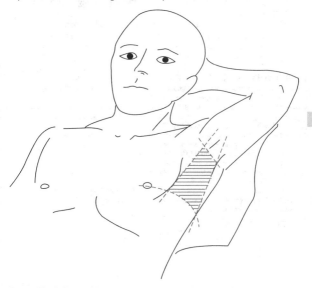

Fig. 6.8 The 'safe triangle'.

Use of clamps

- Pneumothorax—do not clamp a bubbling chest drain or if there is subcutaneous emphysema. A clamp may be considered for detection of small air leaks, under close nursing and medical supervision. This is not advised for ventilated patients.
- Pleural effusion—clamping of the drain may be required to control evacuation of fluid to prevent re-expansion pulmonary oedema.
- No more than 1.5L should be drained at one time, clamping the drain for 1h before releasing.

The routine use of clamps for patient transfers is not advised: care should be taken to keep the drain below the level of insertion.

Suction

Suction is not routinely advised.

- High volume/low pressure ($-20cmH_2O$) may be considered for management of persistent pneumothorax.
- Thoracic surgical referral should be considered at this point.

Chest drain removal

- Unless chemical pleurodesis is planned, removal is indicated when there is no further fluid drainage or bubbling and imaging shows full re-expansion of the lung.
- After chemical pleurodesis the drain is kept in for 24–48h.
- The drain should be removed in expiration and a suture placed as necessary. For small-bore drains, an occlusive dressing is often sufficient.

Further reading

American College of Surgeons (2008) *Advanced Trauma Life Support Manual*, 8th edn. American College of Surgeons Committee on Trauma.

Davies H, Davies R, Davies C, on behalf of the British Thoracic Society Pleural Disease Group (2010) Management of pleural infection in adults: British Thoracic Society Pleural Disease Guideline 2010. *Thorax*, **65** (suppl 2), ii41–53.

Havelock T, Teoh R, Laws D, *et al.*, on behalf of the British Thoracic Society Pleural Disease Group (2010) Pleural procedures and thoracic ultrasound: British Thoracic Society Pleural Disease Guideline 2010. *Thorax*, **65** (suppl 2), ii61–76.

Hooper C, Lee G, Maskell N, on behalf of the British Thoracic Society Pleural Disease Group (2010) Investigation of a unilateral pleural effusion in adults: British Thoracic Society Pleural Disease Guideline 2010. *Thorax*, **65** (suppl 2), ii4–7.

MacDuff A, Arnold A, Harvey J, on behalf of the British Thoracic Society Pleural Disease Group (2010) Management of spontaneous pneumothorax: British Thoracic Society Pleural Disease Guideline 2010. *Thorax*, **65** (suppl 2), ii18–31.

6.13 Pneumonia

Introduction

Pneumonia is a syndrome of inflammation and consolidation of the lung parenchyma. It is most commonly due to infection (usually bacterial) but may be due to non-infectious causes such as eosinophilic pneumonia and organizing pneumonia. This chapter will concentrate predominantly on pneumonia due to infectious causes, but it will also discuss briefly the diagnosis, clinical features, and management of non-infectious pneumonia. The diagnosis of pneumonia is usually made on the basis of a history suggestive of infection, focal signs within the lung, and the presence of new changes on chest radiograph.

- *CAP* begins outside the hospital or is diagnosed within 48h of admission to hospital.
- *HAP* occurs more than 48h after hospital admission.
- *Health-care associated pneumonia* occurs in patients who have had recent contact with the healthcare system (e.g. nursing home residents or those in extended care facilities).

Pneumonia may be an expected terminal event in frail elderly patients or in patients with progressive chronic disease/malignancy. In these situations palliative care is usually more appropriate than active investigation, antibiotic therapy, and respiratory support. It is particularly important to try to determine if the patient has made an advanced directive detailing their wishes regarding treatment.

Pathogenesis

Despite the constant presence of microbes in the upper airways, the lungs usually remain sterile. Pneumonia develops when the defense mechanisms that enable the lungs to remain sterile are overwhelmed. This can occur because of:
- Reduced host defence
- Particularly virulent pathogens
- An overwhelming inoculum.

Reduced host defence
- Age—the incidence of CAP in the over 65s is four times that in the general population.
- Alcohol excess—impairs cough reflexes, swallowing, mucociliary transport, and leucocyte function.
- Malnutrition—impairs immune function and respiratory muscle strength, resulting in inadequate cough.
- Smoking—impairs the mucociliary transport system, and humoral and cellular defences. It also affects bacterial adherence to epithelial cells, resulting in increased adherence of bacteria such as *S. pneumoniae* and *H. influenzae* in the oropharynx.
- Aspiration—micro-aspiration is a normal occurrence with no clinical sequelae as small volumes are easily dealt with by host defenses.

Bulbar dysfunction, impaired consciousness, or gastric disorders can lead to much larger volume aspiration, causing both chemical pneumonitis and infection.
* Mucocilliary dysfunction—immotile cilia syndrome, Kartagener's syndrome, Young's syndrome, and CF all predispose to infection.
* Immune defects—both inherited or acquired. Patients with haematological disorders, and those receiving immunosuppressive drugs or chemotherapy, are at increased risk of developing pneumonia. Clinical signs and radiological appearances may be atypical.
* Underlying lung disease—there is an increased incidence of pneumonia in patients with underlying structural lung diseases such as COPD and bronchiectasis.
* Chronic non-respiratory diseases such as diabetes mellitus or cardiac disease carry increased risk.

Bacterial virulence factors
Bacteria have developed techniques for overcoming host defenses.
* Secretion of exoproducts resulting in:
  * Reduced immune effector cell function—S. aureus can contain the PVL virulence factor, a pore-forming toxin that targets various immune cells, including neutrophils, and has potent cytotoxic and inflammatory actions. The presence of this factor is associated with the development of a severe pneumonia in young people that is often fatal.
  * Enzymatic break down of local immunoglobulin
  * Impaired mucociliary clearance
* Avoidance of immune surveillance.
  * Growth in biofilms.
  * Microcolonies of bacteria such as *Pseudomonas aeruginosa* surround themselves with a polysaccharide gel that prevents macrophages from engulfing them.
  * Endocytosis means that bacteria can 'hide' within epithelial cells. Pneumococci traverse eukaryotic cells within vacuoles without intracytoplasmic multiplication, partly via platelet-activating factor receptor-mediated endocytosis.

Overwhelming inoculums
The lungs' defences, even if functioning appropriately, can be overwhelmed if they encounter very large numbers of bacteria. This most frequently occurs with aspiration of gastrointestinal contents, where large numbers of anaerobic and Gram-negative enteric bacteria of relatively low pathogenicity can cause pneumonia. It may also occur in near-drowning when infection with a range of pathogens may occur. Some of these, e.g. *Aeromonas* spp. are not among the normal causes of CAP. The pathogens vary according to whether it is salt- or freshwater near-drowning. *Aeromonas* spp., *Burkoholderia pseudomallet*, and *Chromobacterium violaceum* are reported with relative higher frequency following freshwater near-drowning but less commonly in saltwater near-drowning, where the overall incidence of secondary infection maybe lower and *Francisella philomiragia* is more common.

Community-acquired pneumonia

Epidemiology

- CAP is common. The annual incidence in the non-institutionalized is 4.7–11.6 per 1000 population, rising to 25–44 per 1000 in the >65 age group.
- There is seasonal variation, with CAP occurring more frequently in winter.
- CAP is the sixth leading cause of death in the UK and USA.
- The mortality rate in patients admitted to hospital with CAP in the UK is reported to be between 6% and 14%.
- In the UK 5–10% of hospitalized patients require ICU admission and of these up to 50% will die.

Microbiology

A wide variety of pathogens can cause CAP. It is not always possible to identify the agent. In research studies an agent is identified in about 60% of cases but this can drop to as low as 20% in clinical practice.

The causative agent identified differs in studies of patients treated as outpatients, inpatients, and those requiring ITU admission (Table 6.8).

Table 6.8 Most common aetiologies of CAP (from American Thoracic Society/Infectious Diseases Society of America)

Place of care	Organisms
Outpatient	*Streptococcus pneumoniae*
	Mycoplasma pneumoniae
	Haemophilus influenzae
	Chlamydophila pneumoniae
	Respiratory viruses
Inpatient (non-ICU)	*Streptococcus pneumoniae*
	Mycoplasma pneumoniae
	Haemophilus influenzae
	Chlamydophila pneumoniae
	Legionella species
	Aspiration
	Respiratory viruses
Inpatient (ICU)	*Streptococcus pneumoniae*
	Staphylococcus aureus
	Legionella species
	Gram-negative bacilli
	Haemophilus influenzae

There are some epidemiological associations with specific causes of infection that may be helpful in planning empiric treatment in selected cases (Table 6.9).

Table 6.9 Risk factors related to specific pathogens in CAP

Risk factors	Organisms
Alcohol excess	S. pneumoniae, oral anaerobes, Klebsiella pneumoniae, Acinetobacter species, Mycobacterium tuberculosis
COPD	H. influenzae, Pseudomonas aeruginosa, Gram-negative enterobacteria
Bronchiectasis	P. aeruginosa, Burkholderia cepacia, S. Aureus
Aspiration	Gram-negative enteric pathogens, oral anaerobes
Intravenous drug abuse	S. aureus MSSA or MRSA
Exposure to bat or bird droppings	Histoplasma capsulatum
Exposure to birds	Chlamydophila psittaci (if poultry, avian influenza)
Exposure to rabbits	Francisella tularensis
Exposure to farm animals or parturient cats	Coxiella burnetti (Q fever)
HIV infection (early)	S. pneumoniae, H. influenzae, M. tuberculosis
HIV infection (late)	As for HIV early infection plus Pneumocystis jirovecii, Cryptococcus, Histoplasma, Aspergillus, atypical mycobacteria (especially Mycobacterium kansasii), P. aeruginosa, H. influenzae
Hotel or cruise ship in previous 2 weeks	Legionella species
Travel to the Mediterranean	
Travel to or residence in south-western USA	Coccidioides species, Hantavirus
Travel to or residence in south-east and east Asia	Burkholderia pseudomallei, avian influenza, SARS
Influenza active in community	Influenza, S. pneumoniae, Staphylococcus aureus, H. influenzae
Injection drug use	S. aureus, anaerobes, M. tuberculosis, S. pneumoniae
Endobronchial obstruction	Anaerobes, S. pneumoniae, H. influenzae, S. aureus
In context of bioterrorism	Bacillus anthracis (anthrax), Yersinia pestis (plague), Francisella tularensis (tularemia)

Diagnosis

Pneumonia may present as a subacute illness, an acute illness, or a respiratory emergency. History and examination can sometimes be misleadingly normal. The presence of an infiltrate on chest radiograph in conjunction with evidence of infection is central to the accurate diagnosis of pneumonia.

History

Pneumonia may be suggested by one or more of the following features in the history:
- Cough
- Fever
- Pleuritic chest pain
- Dyspnoea
- Sputum production.

Some patients may have gastrointestinal symptoms and confusion.

Examination
- Most patients are febrile and have a raised respiratory rate.
- Crackles and signs of consolidation may be present.
- Localized chest signs are the most reliable clinical feature.

Investigation

Radiography

Clinical signs and symptoms may not be typical and their sensitivity is limited when compared to the chest radiograph in predicting pneumonia.

Occasionally chest radiographs give a false negative result. This may be because the radiograph was taken very early in the course of the disease or the patient may have been significantly volume depleted.

In these circumstances it is reasonable to treat as pneumonia if there is high clinical suspicion and repeat the chest radiograph at 24–48h. See Figs 6.9 and 6.10 for examples of CXR abnormalities caused by pneumonia.

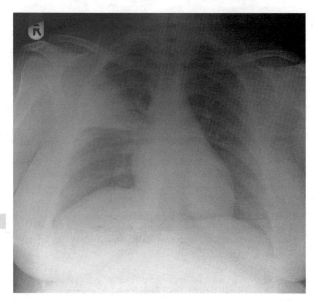

Fig. 6.9 Community-acquired pneumonia. Opacification in the right upper and mid zones is sharply demarcated inferiorly by the horizontal fissure, allowing confident localization to the right upper lobe (anterior segment).

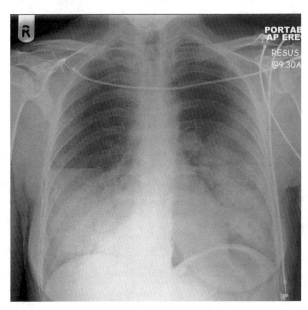

Fig. 6.10 Bilateral community-acquired pneumonia. Opacification in the right lower zone and left mid and lower zones. The right-sided opacity is sharply demarcated superiorly by the horizontal fissure and the adjacent right heart border is obscured, allowing confident localization to the right middle lobe. On the left the heart border is preserved, indicating that this is lower lobe consolidation.

Microbiological testing
Sputum samples and blood cultures should be sent for microbiological testing in all cases of CAP admitted to hospital. Routine testing has limitations, including:
- Time delay in obtaining results
- Relatively low yield of some tests
- Little evidence that microbiological-guided treatment offers significant benefit over empirical treatment in terms of mortality
- Previous antibiotic treatment for many patients presenting to hospital
- The danger of contaminant results (up to 10% in some studies of blood cultures) adversely altering treatment regimes.

Positive microbiological tests remain important as they may significantly alter the care of an individual patient. They also help to provide the epidemiological data that empirical treatment guidelines are based upon.

The severity of pneumonia, healthcare setting, other co-morbidities, and previous antibiotic therapy should guide the use of additional tests.

Table 6.10 Clinical indications for more extensive diagnostic testing (from ATS/IDAS)

Indication	Blood culture	Sputum culture	*Legionella* UAT	Pneumococcal UAT	Other
ICU admission	X	X	X	X	Xa
Failure of outpatient antibiotic therapy		X	X	X	
Cavitating lesion	X	X			Xb
Leucopoenia	X			X	
Active alcohol abuse	X	X	X	X	
Chronic severe liver disease	X			X	
Severe obstructive/ structural lung disease		X			
Asplenia (anatomic or functional)	X			X	
Recent travel (within past 2 weeks)			X		Xc
Positive *Legionella* UAT result		Xd	NA		
Positive pneumococcal UAT result	X	X		NA	
Pleural effusion	X	X	X	X	Xe

NA, not applicable; UAT, urinary antigen test.

aEndotracheal aspirate if intubated, possibly bronchoscopy or non-bronchoscopic BAL.

bFungal and tuberculosis cultures.

cSee above.

dSpecial media for *Legionella*.

eThoracentesis and pleural fluid cultures.

Specific microbiological tests

- Blood cultures—have a relatively low yield, revealing a causative organism in 7–16% of hospitalized patients. They are more likely to be positive in patients with severe disease. There is a significant incidence of false positive blood cultures from contaminants, particularly *S. aureus* (up to 10% in some studies) and this may lead to inappropriate antibiotic prescribing. The low sensitivity, (<20%) and specificity (<30% in some studies) have led to some authorities questioning their utility in routine practice. They continue to be recommended because in the sickest patients sensitivity may be increased, as bacteremia is more common, and the value of a positive result remains significant.
- Sputum culture and Gram stain—have a low yield in many patients with CAP. This often reflects technical problems with collection

and processing. As a result quoted sensitivity and specificity both vary from around 10% in some studies to over 90% in others. If sputum is collected a good quality sputum sample and careful processing are vital.

- Urine antigen tests—are available for streptococcus and legionella. They are more sensitive than blood cultures, provide a rapid result, and remain positive after antibiotics. They do not give any information about potential drug resistance.
  - The BINAX NOW urine pneumococcal antigen test has a sensitivity of 70–90% and a specificity of 80–100%.
  - The legionella urine antigen test only detects *Legionella pneumophilia* group 1 infection (accounting for ~80% of community legionella infections). It has a sensitivity of around 40% and a specificity of 100%. There is some evidence it is more sensitive (up to 86%) in cases of severe disease.
- BAL—Segments of the lung may be lavaged bronchoscopically with 100–150mL of normal saline to recover organisms. This provides a relatively uncontaminated sample of lower respiratory tract flora. This invasive test may be appropriate in a minority of patients if there is suspicion of an unusual organism, particularly in the context of immune-compromise. It is also useful in the management of patients with HAP or VAP. The sensitivity and specificity of this test is difficult to calculate as choosing an appropriate reference standard is problematic and patient populations are heterogeneous. A review of 23 studies of BAL in patients with VAP showed a mean sensitivity of 73% and specificity of 81%.For patients who have not yet commenced treatment the presence or absence of a particular bacteria at culture is felt to be reliable and ATS/IDAS guidelines suggest results should be used to refine empirical antibiotic prescribing. Bronchoscopic sampling does not reduce mortality or ICU length of stay in VAP.
- Protected catheter specimen—provides a sample of lower respiratory tract flora, similar to BAL. It is not possible to direct sampling to a specific lobe which may be involved on chest radiograph as can be done with BAL. It is easier to perform than bronchoscopy. There is a limited amount of data on its utility, but it is felt to have a similar or slightly lower sensitivity and specificity to BAL.
- Thoracentesis—patients with significant pleural effusions should have thoracentesis to obtain samples for culture and Gram stain, pH, protein, LDH, and glucose. The aspiration of fluid with a pH below 7.2 or frank pus suggests an empyema and should prompt chest tube drainage. Culture may not always be positive in empyema because of pretreatment with antibiotics and the difficulty of culturing some anaerobic organisms.
- Transthoracic needle sampling of lung tissue has a limited role in non-responding or immunocompromised patients. It may be useful when other diagnoses, particularly malignancy, are suspected. In one small study in stable haematology patients the sensitivity for detecting malignancy in appropriate patients was 50%. There is, however, a significant (around 10%) risk of pneumothorax, which is likely to be higher in critically ill ventilated patients.

Assessment of severity

CAP encompasses a wide spectrum of illness from the mild and easily treatable in the community to the severe and life-threatening. An assessment of the severity of the disease is crucial in guiding appropriate investigations, antibiotics, and other treatment, and on deciding on the most appropriate place of care for the patient. There are a number of severity assessment tools that are well recognized and evidence based. The two most commonly used are the British Thoracic Society CURB 65 scoring system and the Pneumonia Severity Index (PSI).

Curb 65

The CURB 65 tool allocates one point for each of the following features:

- **C**onfusion (mini-mental test score less than 8 or new onset disorientation to time place and person)
- **U**rea > 7mmol/L
- **R**espiratory rate ≥30/min
- **B**lood pressure (SBP < 90mmHg or DBP ≤ 60mmHg)
- **65**—age ≥ 65 years

Patients with a score of 3 or more should be treated as severe pneumonia, and those with a score of 4 or 5 should be considered for ICU admission. This tool has been validated as a predictor of mortality in ward patients

Score	Mortality (%)
0	0.7
1	3.2
2	13
3	17
4	41.5
5	57

The PSI stratifies patients into five bands based on history, examination, and selected laboratory and radiographical findings. It is more complex to use than the CURB 65 as it requires multiple pathological and physiological variables, and so is only really suitable for use with computerized support.

Both the PSI and the CURB 65 score have a limited ability to predict the likelihood of needing intensive care admission and the prognosis of those patients admitted to ITU. Studies have found that 27–30% of patients admitted to ITU have low PSI scores, and that a significant number of patients with high CURB 65 and PSI scores never require ITU.

APACHE scoring

The APACHE (acute physiology and chronic health evaluation) scoring system has better prognostic accuracy in ITU patients with pneumonia than CURB 65 or PSI scoring. The APACHE II score was found to be an accurate predictor of mortality in 95% of ITU patients, with an APACHE score of 25 or above being associated with a very high risk of death.

Severity assessment tools are useful in supporting clinical decision making and identifying the sickest patients but they cannot include all relevant parameters and they should not replace clinical decision making. In addition, being population statistics, they do not have the ability to predict the outcome in an individual patient.

Which patients need admission to ITU?

It is important to be able to identify cases of severe pneumonia and stratify which patients will benefit from ITU care. The decision comprises an assessment of:

- The severity of physiological derangement, which will affect the need for advanced organ support and high-level monitoring
- Previous level of function and co-morbidities
- The patient's wishes (e.g. have they made an advanced directive).

Up to 45% of patients who end up on ITU are initially admitted to general medical wards. Delayed treatment of shock and respiratory failure are associated with increased mortality and it is therefore important to try and recognize those patients who might benefit from ITU as early as possible.

The ATS/IDAS guidelines suggest that patients be admitted to ITU if they have either *one major* criterion:

- Septic shock requiring vasopressors
- Severe hypoxia requiring mechanical ventilation

or *three minor* criteria:

- Respiratory rate >30 breaths/min
- $PaO_2:FiO_2$ ratio <250mmHg
- Multilobar infiltrates
- Confusion/disorientation
- Uremia (urea >7.3mmol/L)
- Leucopoenia (white blood cell count <4000cells/mm^3)
- Thrombocytopenia (platelet count <100,000cells/mm^3)
- Hypothermia (core temperature <36°C)
- Hypotension requiring aggressive fluid resuscitation.

Treatment

Initial treatment of CAP is often empirical because microbiological results are not usually available and in many cases a causative organism is never identified. In addition, clinical features and radiological diagnosis are not sufficiently specific to differentiate between causative organisms. Antibiotic regimes are aimed at covering the likely causative organism and should be determined with reference to:

- General patterns of expected pathogens according to pneumonia severity and additional risk factors.
- Regional and local patterns of microbial resistance.
- Considerations of tolerability and toxicity of antimicrobial agents in the individual patient.
- Antibiotic therapy should be started as soon as possible once the diagnosis has been made. The British Thoracic society and the ATA/IDSA antibiotic guidelines are shown in Table 6.11 and the box, respectively.

Obviously, if a specific pathogen is identified antibiotics should then be reviewed and tailored to its treatment.

Table 6.11 The British Thoracic society antibiotic guidelines

Place of care	Preferred antibiotic	Alternative antibiotic
Community	Amoxicillin	Erythromycin/ clarithromycin
Hospital treated, not severe	Oral amoxicillin plus clarithromycin or erythromycin If intravenous therapy required: ampicillin or benzylpenicillin plus clarithromycin or erythromycin	Respiratory floroquinolone; moxifloxacin or levofloxacin
Hospital treated, severe	Co-amoxiclav or cefuroxime or cefotaxime or ceftriaxone plus erythromycin or clarithromycin (with or without rifampicin)	Fluoroquinolone with enhanced pneumococcal activity Levofloxacin plus benzylpenicillin

ATS/IDSA recommendations for antibiotic use in patients with pneumonia on ICU

A β-lactam (cefotaxime, ceftriaxone, or ampicillin-sulbactam)
plus
  either azithromycin or a respiratory fluoroquinolone

  If Pseudomonas is a consideration
Antipneumococcal, antipseudomonal β-lactam
  (piperacillin/tazobactam, cefepime, imipenem, or meropenem)
plus
  either ciprofloxacin or levofloxacin
or
the above β-lactam
  plus
  an aminoglycoside and azithromycin
or
the above β-lactam
plus
  an aminoglycoside and an antipneumococcal fluoroquinolone
(for penicillin-allergic patients, substitute aztreonam for above β-lactam)
  If community-acquired MRSA (CA-MRSA) is a consideration, add vancomycin or linezolid.

Drug resistance

Current levels of *in vitro* resistance to β-lactams among streptococcal species are normally not clinically significant when appropriate doses of drugs such as amoxicillin, ceftriaxone, and cefotaxime are used, but there may be clinically significant cefuroxime resistance.

Macrolide resistance seems to be a more significant clinical problem and the ATS/IDAS guidelines recommend that macrolides are not used as sole agent therapy in areas where resistance exceeds 25%.

Resistance to fluoroquinolones has been reported but appears less significant.

Risk factors for drug resistance are:
• Age over 65
• Previous antibiotic treatment within 3 months
• Alcoholism
• Medical co-morbidities
• Immunosuppression
• Exposure to a child in a daycare centre.

Community-acquired MRSA and PVL S. aureus

CA-MRSA causing pneumonia is an emerging problem. It is not typically as resistant to antibiotics as hospital-acquired MRSA, but it is often more virulent. Risk factors for CA-MRSA include:
• Participation in contact sports
• Living in densely packed accommodation, e.g. military barracks, prisons
• Intravenous drug use
• Male homosexuality.

CA-MRSA frequently carries the PVL virulence factor, which can cause rapid-onset necrotizing pneumonia and multiorgan failure. Patients often deteriorate rapidly, and should be considered for ITU support at an early stage.
• Treatment is normally with linezolid or vancomycin (aiming for trough concentrations between 15 and 20mcg/mL).
• Linezolid is thought to be more effective as it decreases toxin production and has better lung penetration.
• Critically ill patients with PVL *S. aureus* infections may also benefit from intravenous immunoglobulin, which appears to neutralize the endotoxins.

Drotrecogin alfa (activated protein C)

Drotrecogin alfa has been shown to offer a survival benefit in selected septic patients at high risk of death (APACHE II score ≥25).
• In patients with severe pneumonia, drotecogin alfa was associated with a reduction in mortality of 9.8%.
• The greatest benefit was in patients with streptococcal pneumonia treated early.
• Drotrecogin alfa is recommended (in ATS/IDAS guidelines) for use in the treatment of patients with persistent septic shock despite adequate fluid resuscitation within 24h of admission.
• It may be beneficial in other selected patients with severe pneumonia.

Corticosteroids

Steroids are not recommended in the routine treatment of CAP.

The role of corticosteroids in patients with septic shock remains controversial. The Corticus trial (randomized double-blind trial of 499 patients with septic shock) found no improvement in outcome at 28 days overall, or in the subgroup of patients with inadequate adrenal reserve. A recent meta-analysis suggests, however, that there may be a role for corticosteroid therapy in patients with severe septic shock not responsive to fluid and vasopressor therapy.

Some patients with pneumonia (e.g. those with underlying lung diseases) may also have a degree of adrenal suppression from recent oral steroid therapy and they should receive additional hydrocortisone.

Trial of NIV

The role of NIV in patients with pneumonia is evolving. The role of BiPAP is well established in patients with infective exacerbations of COPD and hypercapnic respiratory failure. There is conflicting evidence for the use of CPAP in patients with hypoxaemic respiratory failure:

- A meta-analysis suggested that CPAP reduced the risk of intubation, length of ITU stay, and ITU mortality in a heterogeneous group of patients.
- A trial looking at a large cohort of ICU patients with acute hypoxaemic respiratory failure, where 54% had pneumonia, found that despite an early improvement in physiology there was no reduction in the need for intubation or improvement in outcomes.
- Other studies have shown that delayed intubation leads to excess mortality in pneumonia.

We recommend the following:

- A trial of NIV may be appropriate in patients with CAP who are in respiratory failure but who do not need circulatory support and do not need immediate intubation to correct hypoxia or manage secretions.
- If such a trial is performed it is important to stay alert for early signs of non-invasive failure and avoid delayed intubation. Trials therefore should be performed on the ITU, by teams experienced in the use of NIV.

Ventilatory management

The ventilatory management of patients with pneumonia is similar to any other cause of hypoxaemic respiratory failure, with no particular mode of ventilation having been shown to be superior. Ventilatory principles that have demonstrated improved outcome in ARDS should be employed and the ventilatory strategy should be aimed at minimizing VILI.

- Tidal volume 6mL/kg.
- Plateau inspiratory pressure <30cmH$_2$O.
- Permissive hypercapnoea.
- Permissive hypoxia.

The response to PEEP and increased mean airway pressures in patients with pneumonia, particularly those with lobar or unilateral disease, is unpredictable. In addition to its cardiovascular effects, rising levels of PEEP may worsen gas exchange in patients with pneumonia as the pulmonary blood flow is preferentially diverted to the less compliant (consolidated) lung and the shunt fraction increased.

H1N1 influenza

In 2009 a new H1N1 strain of influenza A virus emerged, causing a global pandemic. This strain represents a genetic reassortment of swine, human, and avian influenza.

It is transmitted via large droplets, either aerosolized or via contaminated surfaces. It appears to have a higher attack rate than seasonal flu with secondary infection rates of around 30% in household contacts.

Most patients present with fever, cough, sore throat, malaise, and headache, although vomiting and diarrhoea are also common. A small minority of patients develops a progressive illness characterized by respiratory or cardiopulmonary insufficiency, confusion, severe dehydration, or exacerbations of chronic conditions.

In the USA it is estimated that about 0.3% of cases required hospital admission. Early results from Mexico and the western states of the USA suggested a relatively high mortality rate. As more was discovered about the high community prevalence, it became clear that the case fatality rate was lower than for other forms of seasonal influenza.

Risk factors for more severe illness and ITU admission include chronic lung disease, pregnancy, and BMI > 35. H1N1 was common between 1918 and 1957, which may explain why those over 60 were less severely affected.

The antiviral neuraminidase inhibitor drugs *Oseltamivir* and *Zanamivir* have been recommended for the treatment of patients with suspected influenza during a flu pandemic. This is based on evidence that these drugs shorten the duration of illness (by around a day) and reduce transmission and the likelihood of secondary complications. A recent Cochrane review has raised concerns about the quality of this evidence and as a result their use in healthy adults has been questioned. There remains, however, a consensus that these agents should be used in patients with more severe illness and patients at higher risk of complications. They should ideally be started within 48h of the illness for maximum benefit, but in critically ill patients starting them after this period may still confer some benefit. The intravenous antiviral peramivir may be used in patients where the oral or inhaled route is not practicable.

Primary viral pneumonia is a common finding in severe cases of H1N1 influenza and a relatively frequent cause of death. In hospitalized patients who have developed viral pneumonia the most common finding is patchy change on chest radiograph. Ground glass shadowing is also seen in some patients.

During the initial viral pneumonia, single-organ failure is the most common disorder. Compliance is relatively preserved. Case series suggest that BIPAP and HFOV were the most useful ventilatory modes. Aggressive diuresis is also reported to have beneficial effects.

Secondary bacterial infection occurred in 20% of patients with H1N1 admitted to ITU in Australia and New Zealand. *S. pneumoniae* and *S. aureus* were the most common organisms but the usual causes of HAP should also be considered. Clues to the fact that a patient with H1N1 influenza is developing a secondary bacterial pneumonia include:

- Late (4–7 day) deterioration in respiratory function
- Recurrent fever after a period of being afebrile
- Development of late multiple-organ failure
- Positive sputum culture

- Lobar consolidation on chest radiograph
- Leucocytosis.

Follow-up

Most patients with a good clinical response to treatment do not need routine follow-up, particularly non-smokers and age <50years.

If patients are smokers or age >50 years, they should have a follow-up CXR at 2–3 months to ensure complete radiographic resolution as there is a low incidence of underlying malignancy in this group.

Failure to respond to treatment

Incomplete response to treatment is a relatively common problem in CAP and some patients, particularly those on ITU, may deteriorate after initial stabilization. Age, severity of pneumonia, co-morbidities, and the nature of the infectious agent can all affect the rate of resolution.

CXR changes may progress even as the patient is clinically improving, but some evidence of response is usually seen within 72h.

Overall, 6–15% of hospitalized patients do not respond to initial antibiotic treatment. It is important to recognize non-responders so they can be reassessed and appropriate therapeutic changes made. Patients may fail to respond to treatment for a number of reasons:

- Resistant bacterial pathogen—rates vary from area to area and close liaison with a local microbiologist is important. Patients may be infected with bacteria such as *Pseudomonas aeuriginosa*, with innate resistance to some first-line antibiotics.
- Misdiagnosis of non-bacterial aetiological agent—not all pneumonia is bacterial in origin and some causes will have innate resistance to antibiotic treatment:
  - Fungi: aspergillus, coccidiomysis
  - Mycobacteria
  - Viruses
  - Parasites: *Pneumocystis carinii*.
- Defective host immune response—undiagnosed immunocompromised state. HIV testing should be considered routinely in CAP in areas of high prevalence.
- Complications of infection:
  - Lung abscess
  - Empyema
  - Metastatic infection
  - ARDS
- Non-infectious aetiology:
  - Malignancy
  - Hypersensitivity pneumonitis
  - Eosinophilic pneumonitis
  - Drug-induced pneumonitis
  - COP
  - AIP
  - Pulmonary vasculitis
  - Sarcoidosis
  - Pulmonary alveolar proteinosis
  - Pulmonary oedema
  - PE.

Non-infectious diseases mimicking pneumonia

A number of non-infectious aetiologies can coexist with pneumonia or resemble it.

Neoplasms

Neoplasms may be mistaken for pneumonic change (most typically broncho-alveolar cell lung cancers) and may also coexist with it if they cause endobronchial obstruction leading to pneumonia.

- The incidence of underlying endobronchial carcinoma in non-resolving pneumonia is up to 8% in case series.
- Smokers and those >50 years are at greatest risk of having an underlying malignancy.

Inflammatory disorders

Inflammatory disorders can cause symptoms similar to pneumonia.

- Systemic vasculitidies such as Wegner's granulomatosis can cause systemic symptoms, fever, and pulmonary infiltrates, and should be considered. Most patients with Wegner's are antineutrophilic cytoplasmic antibody (c-ANCA) positive.
- COP (also known as BOOP) often presents with a subacute history of fever and malaise, with dyspnoea and dry cough. Patchy infiltrates are seen on chest radiograph .These characteristically move between different zones. It is normally steroid responsive.

Eosinophilic lung disease

There is a spectrum of eosinophilic lung disease, including eosinophilic pneumonia, where the lung infiltrate is due to eosinophils. Globally, parasites are the major aetiological factor and these diseases are rare in the developed world. Eosinophilic pneumonia can also occur due to drug hypersensitivity and inhaled antigens.

Pulmonary infiltrates are also seen in Churg Strauss syndrome, which may occur in the context of an established diagnosis of asthma and is characterized by peripheral blood eosinophilia and systemic vasculitis. About 50% of patients are perinuclear ANCA (p-ANCA) positive.

Acute eosinophilic pneumonia has an onset of 1–5 days. Symptoms include myalgia, pleuritic chest pain, and dyspnoea. Fever is present and crackles occur on chest auscultation. Chest radiograph shows diffuse infiltrates with peripheral sparing.

Diagnosis rests on a combination of the clinical picture, chest radiograph findings, laboratory tests, and, in some cases, bronchiolar lavage and lung biopsy. The diagnostic criteria for acute eosinophilic pneumonia are:

- Acute onset
- Fever
- Bilateral infiltrates on chest film
- Severe hypoxemia
- Lung eosinophilia (BAL >25% eosinophils or a predominance of eosinophils at open lung biopsy)
- The exclusion of other known causes of eosinophilia such as drug hypersensitivity and parasitic infection.

Most eosinophilic lung disease responds to steroids, but it is important to look for and treat specific parasitic infections and drug reactions.

Drug-induced hypersensitivity

Drug-induced hypersensitivity pneumonitis can also mimic pneumonia, with fevers, an inflammatory response, and diffuse alveolar changes.

It is a recognized complication of a large number of agents, including amiodarone, disease-modifying agents used in rheumatoid arthritis such as leflunomide, and biological agents such as rituximab.

A careful drug history is important, although symptoms may lag behind the start of a new drug regime.

The website pneumotox.com is an invaluable resource on the respiratory complications of drugs.

Acute interstitial pneumonia (Hamman–Rich syndrome)

AIP is a rare and devastating disease of unknown aetiology that generally presents in previously healthy individuals. It has a rapid onset with fever, cough, and shortness of breath being the most common symptoms. There is an equal gender distribution with most patients being over the age of 40. Typically the chest radiograph shows bilateral, diffuse airspace opacification, and CT scanning shows patchy, bilateral areas of ground glass attenuation, often accompanied by airspace consolidation. Features are similar to those of ARDS. The pathological appearance is of organizing diffuse alveolar damage. Diagnosis is based on the clinical syndrome of idiopathic ARDS and a lung biopsy showing typical changes. Treatment is supportive. Despite no controlled trials, high-dose steroid therapy is often used. Mortality is over 60%, with only a minority of patients surviving more than 6 months.

An approach to the non-responding patient

Review history

In patients failing to respond history and presentation should be reviewed. Risk factors for immunocompromise or unusual infections should be considered.

Review microbiology

Initial microbiological studies should be pursued, if they were collected. Further evaluation is aimed at detecting complications and obtaining microbiological information.

Ensure the patient is receiving appropriate treatment at the appropriate doses for organisms identified or suspected.

Review radiology

CT imaging of the chest can reveal lung abscesses, effusions, or empyemas, as well as pulmonary emboli and underlying lung disease such as emphysema, fibrosis, and malignancy. It may be useful in directing bronchoscopy and lung biopsy if those are required.

Consider bronchoscopy and BAL

Bronchoscopy is useful for obtaining specimens for further investigation of infectious and non-infectious aetiologies. It has a very good pick-up rate for many infections. The absence of certain easily grown organisms in BAL samples, such as pseudomonas or MRSA at bronchoscopy (excepting prior treatment), is good evidence that these organisms are not present. Bronchoscopy may reveal evidence of non-infectious aetiologies such as diffuse alveolar haemorrhage, acute eosinophilic pneumonia, or neoplasm.

Transbronchial biopsies can give evidence of interstitial lung disease and can improve the pick-up of organisms such as PCP in immunocompromised patients. They are associated with an increased risk in critically unwell patients.

Aspirate pleural fluid if present

Empyema is a significant cause of non-response. Significant fluid collections should be sampled and drained. Fluid should be cultured for AFBs as well as standard culture. Low pH or turbid appearance of pleural fluid are immediately suggestive of an empyema. All empyemas need draining as well as prolonged antibiotic treatment, including cover for anaerobes. Complex, organized collections may require surgical intervention.

Consider lung biopsy

Occasionally, patients in whom the diagnosis remains unclear may need to proceed to open or VATS lung biopsy. The quoted mortality of surgical lung biopsy is around 6%, and a careful risk–benefit analysis needs to be made.

Aspiration pneumonia

Microaspiration is a phenomenon that occurs in many healthy individuals, often without clinical sequelae. Aspiration refers to the aspiration of large volumes of exogenous or endogenous substances into the lower airway.

Predisposing factors include:

- Reduced conscious level
- Neurological disease, particularly with dysphagia
- Gastrointestinal conditions, reflux, motility disorders
- Medical procedures—endotracheal intubation, occasionally bronchoscopy, upper gastrointestinal endoscopy
- Protracted vomiting, large volume nasogastric feeding
- Prolonged periods in the recumbent position.

Aspiration can cause airway obstruction, chemical pneumonitis, and bacterial infection.

Airway obstruction

Fluids or solids can cause mechanical obstruction. Solid particles can lodge at various levels. There may be unilateral wheeze and atelectisis on chest radiograph. If they remain *in situ* bacterial infection may occur. It is essential to remove the obstruction using suction for fluids and a rigid or fibre optic bronchoscope for particles.

Chemical pneumonitis

Chemical pneumonitis occurs following the aspiration or inhalation of substances toxic to the lungs, normally acid stomach contents.

- A significant inoculum (over 25mL) produces an initial flash chemical burn to the airways.
- This is followed by respiratory distress and hypoxia (caused by oedema, reduced surfactant activity, and alveolar haemorrhage) within 24h, sometimes progressing to ARDS.
- Treatment is supportive. Steroid treatment has been shown not to be of value and may increase the incidence of Gram-negative infection. Prophylactic antibiotics have not been shown to be beneficial.

- Patients who survive normally recover completely within 7 days. Some may develop secondary fibrosis.

Bacterial infection

Bacterial pneumonia following aspiration may be a secondary infection following airway obstruction or chemical pneumonitis, or it may be a primary event following aspiration of fluid-containing bacteria (especially anaerobes) that are resident in the stomach and upper airways.

- These infections can present indolently as the bacteria are not normally virulent.
- Microbiological samples may be negative as the organisms are hard to culture.
- Most patients have a mixed infection containing anaerobic and aerobic bacteria.
- First-line treatment should be with clindamycin or co-amoxiclav. Metronidazole should not be used alone as it is associated with a significant rate of treatment failure as a sole agent.

Pneumonia in the immunocompromised host

The immunocompromised host presents a number of challenges. It may present atypically and can have a much wider variety of infections. These considerations dictate a more aggressive investigative strategy. Organisms causing pulmonary infection in this group include:

- Bacteria
- Fungi
- Viruses
- PCP
- Nocardia
- Mycobacterium tuberculosis.

Particularly in patients who have undergone chemotherapy or radiation treatment for malignancy, a number of non-infectious disease processes may also occur:

- Radiation-induced pneumonitis
- Drug reactions
- Progression of the primary disease.

The spectrum of disease affecting patients with HIV has changed significantly with the widespread use of highly active antiretroviral therapy (HAART). PCP remains a common cause of respiratory infection in the UK, but its incidence has decreased. TB co-infection remains very common, particularly in the Third World, and may present atypically. These patients are also at increased risk of non-infectious disease, including Kaposi's, lung cancer, lymphoma, and emphysema. Outcomes have improved; in the early 1990s the mortality for patients ventilated with PCP pneumonia approached 100%, now it is around 50%. These improvements owe much to improved supportive care and better ventilatory strategies in ITUs, as well as the advent of HAART.

In immunocompromised patients chest radiograph changes may be subtle or even non-existent due to immune suppression. HRCT scanning can help further delineate subtle changes. Serological samples are not helpful. Microbiological samples and sometimes biopsies for histopathological staining are needed. Bronchoscopy should be performed early, and a wide variety of organisms, including fungi, PCP, and viruses, need to be sought. Some of these require special laboratory procedures and liaison is important. Transbronchial and lung biopsy improve the diagnostic yield further but carry a risk of morbidity and mortality (see above).

Hospital-acquired pneumonia

Healthcare-associated pneumonia patients tend to a spectrum of pathogens similar to those found in HAP.

VAP is a subgroup of HAP that develops in ventilated patients. It is reported to affect 7–9% of all intubated patients and is discussed in 📖 Complications of ventilation, p 244, and 📖 The microbiology laboratory, p 49.

HAP accounts for around 15% of nosocomial infections and carries a significant mortality. However, although the crude mortality rate for HAP is often quoted as 30–70%, many critically ill patients die of their underlying disease. Most episodes of HAP occur outside the ITU, but the patients at highest risk are those patients being mechanically ventilated.

HAP is caused by a different spectrum of pathogens than those in the community. This is particularly true of patients who develop late-onset (after 5 days) HAP. Multidrug-resistant pathogens are a concern and are seen more frequently with:

• Antimicrobial therapy in the preceding 90 days
• Current hospitalization of 5 days or more
• High frequency of antibiotic resistance in the community or in the specific hospital unit
• Significant previous healthcare contact
• Nursing home residents
• Immunosuppression.

The diagnosis of HAP should be suspected in the context of new radiographic infiltrates on chest radiograph in combination with clinical signs of infection. The clinical pulmonary infection score (CPIS, see 📖 Complications of mechanical ventilation, p 244) has been proposed to aid diagnosis of VAP.

• Routine tracheal aspirates in ventilated patients can be misleading.
• Treatment should normally be started on clinical grounds because delays in initiating therapy are associated with excessive mortality.
• Empirical treatment can lead to overtreatment and should be reviewed promptly in light of microbiological sample results, which should be collected prior to changes in treatment.
• In ventilated patients BAL or protected brush specimens should be obtained.
• Quantative or semi-quantative culture may improve the relevancy of the clinical information obtained from these samples.
• When starting empirical therapy the key question is whether the patient has risk factors for multidrug-resistant disease (as detailed above). This significantly alters the choice of initial antibiotics.
• If the patient is likely to have multi-drug resistant (MDR) organisms a combination of agents should be used.
• For many patients short antibiotic courses of 7 days are adequate, but patients with proven pseudomonas infection require longer treatment periods.

The American Thoracic Society has made recommendations about antibiotics for use in patients with HAP depending on the likely organism, but clinicians should always refer to local antibiotic policies as well such international guidelines.

Table 6.12 American Thoracic Society recommendations for treatment of HAP according to likely organisms

Early onset/no risk factors for MDR disease	Late onset/risk factors for MDR organisms
S. pneumoniae	Pseudomonas aeruginosa
H. influenzae	Klebsiella pneumoniae extended spectrum beta-lactamase
Meticillin-sensitive S. aureus	Acinetobacter species
	MRSA
Antibiotic-sensitive enteric Gram-negative bacilli	
Suggested antibiotics	**Suggested antibiotics**
Ceftriaxone or	Antipseudomonal cephalosporin (ceftazidime) or antipseudomonal carbepenem(imipenem or meropenem)
Levofloxacin, moxifloxacin or	or Lactam/lactamase inhibitor
Ampicillin/sulbactam or	(piperacillin–tazobactam)
Ertapenem	*plus*
	antipseudomonal fluoroquinolone
	(ciprofloxacin or levofloxacin) or
	aminoglycoside
	(amikacin, gentamicin, or tobramycin)
	plus
	linezolid or vancomycin

Further reading

Davidson C and Treacher D (2002) *Respiratory Critical Care*. Arnold, London.
Macfarlane J, Boswel T, Douglas G, et al (2004) BTS Guidelines for the Management of Community Acquired Pneumonia in Adults. Available at: www.Brit-thoracic.org/guideline.
Mandell LA, Wunderink RG, Anzueto A, et al (2007) Infectious Diseases Society of America/American Thoracic Society consensus guidelines on the management of community-acquired pneumonia in adults. *Clin Infect Dis* **44**(Suppl 2), S27–S72.
Niederman MS, Craven DE, Bonten MJ, et al (2005) Guidelines for the management of adults with hospital-acquired, ventilator-associated, and healthcare-associated pneumonia. *Am J Respir Crit Care Med* **171**(4), 388–416.
Woodhead M, Blasi F, Ewig S, et al (2005) ERS Guidelines for the management of adult lower respiratory tract infections. *Eur Respir J* **26**, 1138–1180.

6.14 **Respiratory disease in pregnancy**

Between 1997 and 2005 there were 24 maternal deaths directly related to underlying respiratory disease in the UK reported to the Confidential Enquiry into Maternal and Child Health (CEMACH).[1] Worldwide, opportunistic respiratory infections in HIV-infected mothers have had a significant impact on maternal morbidity and mortality.

Diseases related to pregnancy can present as, or be complicated by, respiratory failure, and previously unknown underlying respiratory or cardiac disease can manifest for the first time during pregnancy.

In 2005 the Intensive Care National Audit and Research Centre (ICNARC) reported that 7 per 1000 critical care unit admissions were obstetric patients, many of whom had respiratory failure. These women have a low mortality and 96% will survive.[2]

Physiological changes in pregnancy

Pregnancy results in significant physiological changes affecting the cardiovascular, respiratory, renal, and gastrointestinal systems. These changes reduce maternal respiratory reserve and will exacerbate any pre-existing respiratory disease.

Respiratory changes

Physiological changes in the respiratory system start in the first trimester of pregnancy and are hormonally mediated. These changes are necessary to accommodate the growing uterus upwards into the abdomen, meet increased maternal oxygen requirements (↑15–20%), and facilitate foetal gas exchange.

Anatomical changes
- Diaphragm is displaced upwards.
- Ligament laxity increases.
- Anteroposterior and transverse diameters of the chest increase as a result of lower rib flaring and subcostal angle elevation.
- Chest wall compliance decreases.
- Prostaglandin reduces bronchial smooth muscle tone.

Alterations in lung volumes in pregnancy
- Tidal volumes ↑40% from 500 to 700mL.
- Minute ventilation ↑50%.
- Inspiratory reserve capacity ↑10%.
- Total lung capacity is ↓5%.
- Expiratory reserve capacity, FRC, and residual volume ↓20% (more in supine position).

Alterations in respiratory rate and arterial blood gases
From the first trimester progesterone stimulates the respiratory centre, resulting in hyperventilation (see Table 6.13).
- Respiratory rate increases from 16 to 20 breaths/minute.
- The carbon dioxide response curve is shifted to the left, dropping maternal baseline $PaCO_2$ to 3.6–4.1kPa. This benefits maternal haemoglobin oxygen-carrying capacity by shifting the oxygen dissociation curve to the left.

- Respiratory alkalosis is compensated by metabolic renal adaption.
- ↑maternal oxygen consumption.

Table 6.13 Arterial blood gas values in pregnancy

	PaO₂ (kPa)	PaCO₂ (kPa)	H⁺ (nmol/L)	HCO₃ (mmol/L)
Non-pregnant	13.3	4.5–5.3	35–45	22–26
Pregnant	13.5–14.0	3.6–4.1	40–45	18–21

Immunological changes

The maternal immune system becomes suppressed during pregnancy to prevent foetal rejection. This is partly hormonally mediated. As a consequence the mother may be more prone to infection, particularly viral and fungal infections.

- ↓lymphocyte proliferation.
- ↓natural killer cell activity.
- ↓number of T helper cells.
- ↓lymphocyte cytotoxic activity.

Respiratory failure in pregnancy

The underlying causes of respiratory failure during pregnancy fall into three main categories:

- Causes specific to pregnancy (see box)
- Causes not specific to pregnancy (e.g. pneumonia)
- Exacerbation of underlying pulmonary disease.

Investigations

The basic investigations for respiratory disease in pregnant women are similar to those for non-pregnant women.

Radiology

Radiological investigations can be performed without exposing the foetus to any specific risks.[3] The foetal radiation exposures for commonly performed investigations are given in Table 6.14. All doses are substantially below the mean dose required to cause foetal death or gross malformation, although there is a very low theoretical risk of inducing childhood malignancy.

Table 6.14 Radiation exposures for common radiological procedure

Investigation	Fetal radiation exposure (mGy)
CXR	<0.01
CTPA	0.01–0.06
Radionuclide lung scintigraphy	0.11–0.22

Foetal monitoring

The foetus is viable after 24 weeks' gestation and foetal outcome is generally better after 32–34 weeks' gestation. Delivery decisions in critically unwell patients are often difficult, and foetal assessment is a vital component in the overall evaluation. Foetal delivery may not guarantee improvement in maternal respiratory function.

Delivery plans should be made after multidisciplinary consultation considering foetal wellbeing, gestation, maternal status, and aetiology of maternal compromise.

Preterm labour may be triggered by the illness.

Causes specific to pregnancy

Causes of respiratory failure specific to pregnancy:
- Pre-eclapmsia
- HELLP syndrome
- Acute fatty liver of pregnancy
- Amniotic fluid embolism
- Peripartum cardiomyopathy
- Tocolytic-induced pulmonary oedema
- Chorioamnionitis
- Endometritis
- Ovarian hyperstimulation syndrome.

Pre-eclampsia and eclampsia

The incidence of severe pre-eclampsia in the UK is 5 per 1000 pregnancies and the incidence of eclampsia is 5 per 10000 pregnancies. In the CEMACH report, triennium 2003–2005, the mortality rate was 0.85 per 100000 maternities. It is a multisystem disorder with diffuse maternal endothelial cell dysfunction. The only cure is delivery.

Definition of pre-eclampsia and eclampsia

- Pre-eclampsia is defined as pregnancy-induced hypertension (systolic blood pressure ≥170mmHg or diastolic blood pressure ≥ 110mmHg, on two occasions) with proteinuria (>0.3g in 24h) with or without peripheral oedema.
- Eclampsia is pre-eclampsia with one or more superimposed grand mal convulsions.
- Women may have only moderate hypertension (diastolic blood pressure ≤100mmHg) but other sinister clinical features of severe disease, for example
  - Headache
  - Visual disturbance
  - Papilloedema
  - Epigastric pain
  - Liver tenderness
  - Abnormal liver enzymes
  - Clonus
  - Falling platelet count.

Respiratory complications

The respiratory complications associated with pre-eclampsia/eclampsia are primarily pulmonary oedema and ARDS related to:
- Lung parenchymal endothelial dysfunction
- ↓colloid osmotic pressure
- LV dysfunction
- Iatrogenic fluid overload.

Initial management
- Maternal and foetal monitoring.
- Intravenous access, FBC, coagulation, U+E, liver function tests (LFTs), serum urate.
- Urinalysis.
- Blood pressure control.
- Seizure control (or prophylaxis in patients at risk of developing seizures).
- Consider timing of delivery.

Blood pressure control
- Aim to lower blood pressure to 130–140/90–100mmHg.
- Avoid rapid reduction.
- May require cautious fluid bolus with associated vasodilation.
- May require combination drug therapy.
- Consider invasive blood pressure monitoring.
- Monitor foetus with continuous CTG recording.

Labetalol
- Oral: If tolerated, administer 200mg. Repeat if necessary after 1h.
- Intravenous: If no response to oral dose, or not tolerated, administer slow 50mg intravenous bolus. Repeat if necessary after 20min. Start intravenous maintenance infusion initially at 20mg/h (max. 160mg/h).

Hydralazine
- Slow 10mg intravenous bolus. If necessary give further 5mg intravenous boluses every 20min. Start maintenance infusion initially at 2mg/h (max. 20mg/h).

Nifedipine
- 10mg orally (not sublingually). Repeat 6 hourly.

Seizure control (or prophylaxis)
- 4g loading dose of magnesium sulphate over 5–10min.
- Further infusion of 1g/h, maintained for 24h after last seizure.
- Magnesium is more effective than phenytoin or diazepam for seizure control, with better maternal and neonatal outcome. Phenytoin or diazepam should not be used as first-line agents.
- If recurrent seizures consider:
  - Further bolus of 2g magnesium sulphate
  - Increase infusion rate to 1.5g or 2.0g/h
  - Single dose of diazepam (further doses may increase maternal mortality)
  - Intubation with thiopental.

- Assess clinically for magnesium sulphate toxicity by monitoring deep tendon reflexes and respiratory rate or measure plasma levels (therapeutic level 5–7mg/dl).

Fluid balance
- Fluid restriction.
- Catheterise, hourly urine volumes.
- Oliguria is common with severe pre-eclampsia.
- Total fluids should be limited to 80mL/h.
- Aim for urine output of 30mL/h, but may be less.
- CVP trends are more helpful than actual values. There is poor correlation with PAOP in pre-eclampsia.

Renal failure is rare in women with pre-eclampsia and renal function usually improves within 24–48h of delivery. In contrast, the risk of developing pulmonary oedema is high.

Delivery
Delivery depends on:
- Foetal gestation
- Foetal development *in utero*
- Severity of maternal disease.

HELLP
HELLP syndrome is a complication of severe pre-eclampsia and eclampsia. It may also develop in the postnatal period and is associated with increased maternal and perinatal mortality.

Signs and symptoms
- Epigastic or right upper quadrant pain.
- Mucosal bleeding and bruising.
- Malaise.
- Nausea and vomiting.
- Headache.

Diagnosis
HELLP is characterized by microangiopathic haemolytic anaemia (confirm with blood film), raised LDH (>600U/L), elevated liver enzymes (aspartamine transaminase (AST) >70U/L), hyperbilirubinaemia and thrombocytopaenia (platelet count <100 × 10^9/L). Hypertension and proteinuria are also present in the majority of patients, although they not essential for diagnosis; when absent, diagnosis may be difficult.

Differential diagnosis includes viral hepatits, cholestasis, acute fatty liver of pregnancy, thrombotic thrombocytopaenia, haemolytic uraemic syndrome, disseminated intravascular coagulation (DIC), antiphospholipid syndrome and autoimmune haemolytic anaemia.

In HELLP syndrome, coagulopathy is not typically a predominant feature.

Management
Management of HELLP depends on maternal stability, gestation, and foetal condition.
- Acute: treat hypertension and administer magnesium sulphate for seizure prophylaxis (as above).

- Administer platelets if actively bleeding or platelet count <20 × 10⁶/mL.
- Consider corticosteroids.
  - Improve foetal lung maturity (if <34 weeks' gestation).
  - Increase rate in resolution of maternal biochemical and haematological abnormalities, although does not improve outcome.
- Delivery may be delayed for 24–48h to allow foetal lung maturity in stable patients. Mode of delivery (caesarean section or vaginal) dependant on maternal and foetal status.

Complications
- Acute hepatic failure.
- Hepatic rupture/haemorrhage.
- Placenta abruption.
- Acute renal failure.
- ARDS.
- DIC.
- Intracranial haemorrhage.
- Sepsis—increased incidence.

Amniotic fluid embolism

The incidence of amniotic fluid embolism (AFE) has been reported as 1 in 8000–80,000 pregnancies. In the 2003–2005 CEMACH report the mortality rate was 0.8 per 100,000 pregnancies, the third leading cause of maternal death. It has a poor maternal outcome with the individual risk of death between 25% and 86%. Most events occur during labour or in the immediate postpartum period.

Factors increasing incidence of AFE
- Advanced maternal age.
- Multiparity.
- Uterine hyperstimulation.
- Intrauterine death.
- Polyhydramnios.
- Placental abruption.
- Maternal history of atopy.

Pathogenesis of AFE

Amniotic fluid in the maternal circulation causes the release of a cascade of systemic inflammatory mediators (similar to that occurring in sepsis), precipitating pulmonary vascular spasm, pulmonary hypertension, acute right heart failure, V/Q mismatch, hypoxia, and systemic hypotension. Death may occur at this stage.

A second phase follows with left heart failure, myocardial suppression, pulmonary oedema, DIC and multiorgan failure.

Bleeding from DIC is often a predominant feature.

Signs and symptoms

These may be subtle or profound and include:
- Respiratory symptoms—dyspnoea, chest pain, bronchospasm, hypoxia
- Cardiovascular collapse, arrhythmias
- Neurological symptoms—confusion/agitation, dizziness, parasthesia, nausea

- Coagulopathy
- Foetal distress.

Management
- Immediate delivery of foetus if not already performed.
- Cardiovascular resuscitation and support.
- Correction of coagulopathy.

Treatment options also described in literature
- Plasma exchange.
- Continuous haemofiltration to remove inflammatory mediators.
- Inhaled nitric oxide and prostaglandins for pulmonary hypertension.
- Serum protease inhibitors.
- High-dose steroids.

These treatments are usually carried out as a last resort. There is little evidence regarding their efficacy.

Peripartum cardiomyopathy

The incidence of peripartum cardiomyopathy ranges from 1 in 3000 to 1 in 4000 pregnancies and varies between different countries. It is a disorder of LV systolic function that occurs in previously healthy women in late pregnancy and early postpartum period. The aetiology is unknown but possibilities include an autoimmune disorder, myocarditis, myocyte apoptosis, or a viral trigger.

Risk factors
- Multiparity.
- Increased maternal age.
- Pre-eclampsia and gestational hypertension.
- Chronic hypertension.
- African origin.
- Twin pregnancies.
- Use of tocolytic agents.

Presentation
- Dyspnoea, orthopnoea, paroxysmal nocturnal dyspnoea.
- Peripheral oedema.
- Cough.
- Abdominal discomfort secondary to hepatic congestion.
- Pulmonary or systemic embolization from thrombus formation in the dilated cardiac chambers.
- May be misdiagnosed as asthma, or the normal pregnancy related respiratory changes described above.

Diagnosis
- Based on history and timing of symptoms.
- Pulmonary oedema and cardiomegaly on CXR.
- Echocardiographic evidence.
- ECG—may show sinus tachycardia, dysrythmias, LV hypertrophy, inverted T waves, Q waves and non-specific ST segment changes.
- Viral PCR.
- Endomyocardial biopsy.

Diagnostic criteria for peripartum cardiomyopathy
- Development of heart failure in the last month of pregnancy or first 5 months post partum.
- Absence of identifiable cause for cardiac failure.
- Absence of recognizable heart disease prior to the last month of pregnancy.
- LV systolic dysfunction demonstrated by echocardiography.

Specific echocardiographic criteria
- Ejection fraction <45%, fractional shortening <30% or both.
- End-diastolic dimension >2.7 cm/m^2 body surface area.

Treatment of peripartum cardiomyopathy
The first-line treatments for peripartum cardiomyopathy are outlined in Table 6.15.

Table 6.15 Treatment of peripartum cardiomyopathy

Treatment	Antenatal	Postnatal
Diuretics	Furosemide	Furosemide
Vasodilators	Hydralazine, nitrates, amlodipine	ACE inhibitors
Beta blockade	Metoprolol	Carvedilol
Anticoagulation (ejection fraction <30%)	LMWH or unfractionated heparin	Warfarin
Inotropic support	Dobutamine, dopamine and milrinone	Dobutamine, dopamine and milrinone

In severe cases, the use of intra-aortic balloon counterpulsation may be life-saving.

Suggested future therapies have directed treatment against a proposed inflammatory or auto-immune mechanism:
- Immunosuppression, e.g. azathioprine or steroids.
- Immunoglobulins.
- Antiretroviral therapy if viral trigger proven (PCR testing, endomyocardial biopsy).

Prognosis
- ~50% of women recover completely within 6 months.
- ~20% of women require cardiac transplantation.
- The remainder may gradually improve over a few years or have persistent cardiac dysfunction.

Tocolysis
Tocolytic agents are used to inhibit preterm labour. Common agents used are β-agonists, prostaglandin synthetase inhibitors, oxytocic antagonists, calcium channel blockers, indometacin and magnesium sulphate. Combination therapy can be used.

Tocolytic therapy has been associated with pulmonary oedema. Primarily this is due to β-agonists used alone or in combination, with an incidence of 5%.

β-agonists lead to fluid overload and cardiovascular decompensation by a number of mechanisms:
- Activation of renin angiotensin system
- Stimulation of cardiac output by 40–60% above normal pregnancy values.
- Co-administration with intravenous fluid leading to iatrogenic fluid overload.

Prevention
- Limit tocolysis to one single agent. β-agonists are no longer recommended as first-choice agents.
- Limit co-administered intravenous fluid.
- Avoid β-agonists in patients with underlying cardiac disease.
- Limit duration of maintenance therapy.

Pulmonary oedema
Reduced colloid oncotic pressure, increased blood volume and cardiac output are normal physiological changes associated with pregnancy but also predispose the pregnant patient to pulmonary oedema.

Common causes of pulmonary oedema in pregnancy
- Iatrogenic fluid overload.
- Tocolysis.
- Excessive syntocinon administration.
- Pre-eclampsia.
- Infection.
- Cardiogenic.

Treatment
- Treat underlying cause.
- Caution with intravenous fluid administration.
- Careful fluid balance—catheterize, consider CVP monitoring.
- Echocardiography to exclude underlying cardiac pathology if cause uncertain and no response to treatment.

Causes not specific to pregnancy
Some causes of respiratory failure are not specific to pregnancy, but occur with greater frequency in pregnant patients or have higher rates of complications in pregnancy.

Pulmonary embolism
The incidence of venous thromboembolism in pregnancy is 0.5–3 per 1000 pregnancies and is the leading cause of *direct* maternal mortality in the UK (1.56 per 100000 maternities) and USA. Women are at increased risk from the first trimester through to the postpartum period. A parturient with an untreated DVT has a 24% chance of developing a PE, with a mortality rate of 15%.[4]
- If a pregnant woman presents with chest pain and increasing breathlessness the diagnosis of VTE must be considered. If the diagnosis is likely (see 📖 Pulmonary embolism, p 529), consider commencing treatment before the diagnosis is confirmed.

Blood coagulability during pregnancy

Pregnancy is a state of hypercoagulability, a protective physiological change which is aimed at reducing haemorrhage at delivery. Pregnancy results in:

* ↑Fibrinogren levels.
* ↑Clotting factors VII, VIII, IX, X, XII.
* ↑von Willebrand factor levels.
* ↓Protein S, factor XI, and XIII levels.
* Inferior vena cava and pelvic veins being compressed by the gravid uterus, leading to venous stasis.

Approximately 50% of pregnant women who develop a VTE have a coexistent thrombophilia.

The presentation, investigation, and management of PE are discussed in detail in 📖, Pulmonary embolism, p 529. Points specific to pregnancy are:

* PE is most common in postpartum period but can occur any time during pregnancy.
* D-dimers normally rise throughout pregnancy and are therefore of limited diagnostic value.
* Anticoagulation:
  * Antenatal—use LMWH. Consider unfractionated heparin in patients at high risk of haemorrhage.
  * Stop anticoagulation 12h before induction of labour and 24h before scheduled caesarean section.
  * Postnatal—recommence LMWH or unfractionated heparin (if high risk of postpartum haemorrhage). Timing of re-introduction variable depends on mode of delivery, regional anaesthesia, and bleeding status.
  * Warfarin may be used postnatally but not until 72h post partum. Target INR 2–3.
  * Duration of treatment—anticoagulation should continue throughout remaining pregnancy and at least 6 weeks post partum. Overall treatment should be for at least 3 months.

Bacterial pneumonia

The incidence of pneumonia in pregnancy is reported as 0.04–1%. Although this is similar to non-pregnant patients, the complication rate is increased. Maternal mortality has been quoted at 3%. The average gestational age is 32 weeks at the time of infection. The risks of intrauterine infection, preterm birth, and neonatal mortality are increased and average birth weight at delivery is reduced.

Risk factors for developing pneumonia in pregnancy

* Anaemia.
* Asthma.
* Corticosteroids.
* HIV infection.
* Alcohol abuse.

The most common bacterial pathogens identified are:

* *Streptoccocus pneumoniae*
* *Haemophilus influenzae*
* *Mycoplasma pneumoniae*
* Legionella (accounts for 5% of antepartum pneumonias with a mortality rate of 20%).

Management

Same as for non-pregnant patients. Antibiotic treatment as recommended by the BTS guidelines and liaison with local microbiologist. Discuss antibiotic choice with pharmacy for safety profile during pregnancy.
- Safe antibiotic profile—penicillins, cephalosporins, and macrolides.
- Cautionary use—gentamicin, metronidazole.
- Antibiotics to avoid during pregnancy—tetracyclines, flouroquinolones, streptomycin, fluconazole, and sulphonamides (in the third trimester).

Viral pneumonitis

Viral pathogens are responsible for 5% of identified causes of pneumonia in pregnancy.
- VZV is the most common pathogen. Primary infection complicates 3 in 1000 pregnancies. It results in marked hypoxia in pregnancy. Mechanical ventilation is required in 7–11%.
- Influenza A carries a high morbidity rate in pregnancy.

Treatment of non-immune pregnant women with VZV exposure (RCOG guidelines[5])
- Administer VZV immunoglobulins (up to 10 days post exposure).
- If rash develops administer oral acyclovir 800mg five times a day if >20 weeks' gestation. If <20 weeks' gestation consider aciclovir (unknown safety profile).
- If patient >36 weeks' gestation or symptoms are deteriorating despite oral acyclovir commence intravenous acyclovir (10mg/kg three times a day for 5 days).

Influenza infection

Although pregnant women are not at greater risk of contracting influenza (the most recent pandemic was caused by H1N1, 'swine'flu'), they are at a greater risk of developing complications, particularly in the second and third trimesters.[6] If the diagnosis seems likely it is recommended that they receive antiviral agents within 48h and, if necessary, before laboratory confirmation is received. Antibiotics should be considered if there is little response to antivirals, persistent pyrexia, or lower respiratory tract infection, and particularly if there is underlying co-morbidity; however, remember to exclude other possible pregnancy-related conditions (e.g. chorioamniitis). If early delivery is considered, the usual guidelines on maternal steroid administration to promote foetal lung maturity should be followed. ECMO has been used successfully in severe disease.

HIV infection

HIV infection has lead to rising maternal mortality secondary to opportunistic infections, especially in developing countries. PCP and TB are common pathogens.

Antiretroviral therapy

Antiretroviral therapy in pregnancy has two main goals:
- Prevention of vertical (mother-to-child) transmission
- Prevention of maternal disease progression.

During pregnancy antiretrovirals should be continued if required for maternal disease stage preconception. If antiretrovirals are not required for maternal disease (CD4 lymphocyte count >350 × 10^6/L and low viral load), therapy should be commenced at 28–32 weeks' gestation to prevent vertical transmission at the time of delivery. Women requiring antiretroviral therapy (CD4 count falling and/or high viral load) but not on treatment at the time of conception should commence therapy (but defer until the start of the second trimester).

Pneumocystis jirovecii (carinii)

Active treatment with trimethoprim-sulfamethoxazole plus folic acid supplementation. There is potential foetal teratogenicity but administer if maternal benefit outweighs risk. Add steroid therapy if significantly hypoxaemic.

Tuberculosis

Treatment of tuberculosis is similar for non-pregnant patients: isoniazid (first-line agent), rifampicin (administer vitamin K in the third trimester to avoid neonatal coagulopathy), and ethambutol.
- Streptomycin is contraindicated.

Acute respiratory distress syndrome

The aetiology of ARDS in pregnancy includes all the causes affecting non-pregnant patients plus causes related to pregnancy:
- Uterine sepsis
- Placental abruption
- Chorioamnionitis
- Endometritis
- Pre-eclampsia/eclampsia
- HELLP syndrome
- Acute fatty liver of pregnancy
- Amniotic fluid embolus
- Obstetric haemorrhage
- Aspiration pneumonitis (although not unique to pregnancy, occurs more frequently)
- Tocolytic therapy
- Trophoblastic embolization.

The incidence of ARDS during pregnancy is estimated at 16–70 per 100,000 pregnancies. The mortality rate is high, quoted at 23% antenatally and 50% postnatally in one series of 83 obstetric patients. Neonatal outcome is poor, with high rates of foetal death, spontaneous preterm labour, and perinatal asphyxia. The cause of ARDS is not predictive of maternal outcome.

The principles of treating pregnant patients with ARDS are similar to those for non-pregnant patients. Maternal survival is the most important treatment goal, but permissive hypoxia and hypercapnia may disrupt foetal gas transfer across the placenta.

Management
- Foetal monitoring.
- Place patient in left lateral position.
- Aim for maternal blood gas targets: PaO_2 >9.3, SpO_2 95%, $PaCO_2$ <6.0, H^+ <50nmol/L.

- The use of nitric oxide (NO) in pregnant patients with ARDS has not been evaluated and does not have FDA approval in this setting. Successful NO use in maternal pulmonary hypertension has been reported.
- Prone positioning has unknown foetal consequences.

Exacerbation of underlying disease

All pre-existing diseases which compromise respiratory function will be exacerbated by the physiological changes of pregnancy. The following is not an exclusive list.

Asthma

Asthma complicates 4–8% of pregnancies. Adequate asthma control is important for improving maternal and foetal outcome.

- Severe or poorly controlled asthma may be associated with prematurity, caesarean section, pre-eclampsia, and growth restriction as a result of acute or chronic foetal hypoxia.
- Studies suggest that 11–18% of pregnant women with asthma will have at least one ED visit for acute asthma and of these 62% will require hospitalization.
- The normal physiological changes in pregnancy may obscure early recognition of an acute severe asthma attack.

Management of acute asthma exacerbation

Management is essentially the same as in the non-pregnant patient, described in detail in 📖 Asthma, p 395.

- Aim to maintain SpO_2 >95%, PaO_2 >9.3kPa.
- Foetal wellbeing must be assessed.
- Methylxanthines are safe in pregnancy but care needed with drug-level monitoring.

Cystic fibrosis

As management for CF has improved, nearly 80% of patients now reach adulthood and are capable of childbearing. There was one maternal death secondary to CF in the 2003–2005 CEMACH report.

- Every year 30–40 women with CF in the UK (140 in the USA) become pregnant.
- The long-term outcome of CF women is not worsened by pregnancy, but mortality rate is increased during pregnancy.
- Hospital admissions, respiratory tract infections, diabetes, and nutritional deficiency all increase during pregnancy.

Lung function

Lung function is the most significant predictor of pregnancy outcome in CF patients. Maternal survival is positively correlated with pre-pregnancy FEV_1 values. An FEV_1 <50% predicted is associated with poor maternal and foetal outcome. It is considered a contraindication to pregnancy, although successful pregnancies have been reported in stable patients with lower FEV_1 values.

- Burkholderia cepacia colonization can cause unpredictable rapid decline in respiratory function.
- Cor pulmonale and pulmonary hypertension are absolute contraindications to pregnancy.

Management
- Aggressive treatment of chest infections.
- Effective chest physiotherapy.
- Nutritional support to maintain weight gain both ante and postnatally. Consider total parenteral nutrition.
- Antibiotic choice must consider foetal teratogenicity.
- Diabetic control.

Myasthenia gravis

Pregnancy may exacerbate, improve, or have no effect on maternal myasthenia gravis. Exacerbations can occur in any trimester or the post-partum period.
- Maternal mortality is inversely proportional to the duration of disease prior to pregnancy.
- Pregnancy has no long-term effect on the course of myasthenia gravis.

Myasthenia crisis

Precipitation of a crisis can be caused by pregnancy, pyrexia, surgical or emotional stress, and certain drugs. Infection during pregnancy or the postnatal period should be treated aggressively.

Management
- Monitoring of muscle weakness during pregnancy can be performed by regular checks of PFTs.
- During labour replace oral acetycholinesterase inhibitors with parenteral administration because of poor absorption in this period.
- Treatment with magnesium sulphate in pre-eclampsia and eclampsia should be avoided as severe muscle weakness can ensue.

1 CEMACH (2007) Confidential Enquiry into Maternal and Child Health. Saving Mothers' Lives. Reviewing Maternal Deaths to make Motherhood safer. 7th report. 2003–2005. CEMACH, London, pp. 131–44.

2 Harrison DA, Penny JA, Yentis SM, et al (2005) Case mix, outcome and activity for obstetric admissions to adult, general Critical Care units: a secondary analysis of the ICNARC Case Mix Programme Database. *Crit Care* **9**(suppl. 3), S25–S37.

3 Scarsbrook AF and Gleeson FV (2007) Rational imaging. Investigating suspected pulmonary embolism in pregnancy. *BMJ* **334**, 418–19.

4 Ie S, Rubio ER, Alper B, and Szerlip H (2001) Respiratory complications of pregnancy. *Obstet Gynaecolog Survey*, **57**(1), 39–46.

5 Byrne BMP, Crowley PA, Carrington D. Chicken Pox in pregnancy. Royal College of Obstetrics and Gynaecology. Guideline No.13 2007. Setting Standards To Improve Women's Health. Available at: http://www.rcog.org.uk/files/rcog-corp/uploaded-files/GT13Chickenpoxinpregnancy2007.pdf (accessed 23 June 2009).

6 Department of Health and Royal College of Obstetricians and Gynaecologists (2009) Pandemic H1N1 2009 Influenza: Clinical Management Guidelines for Pregnancy. Available at: www.rcog.org.uk/news/swine-flu.

6.15 Pulmonary embolism

Pulmonary embolism (PE) is the most common preventable cause of death in surgical patients and may be responsible for up to 15% of in-hospital mortality. The non-specific nature of symptoms and signs make diagnosis difficult, and PE is often undetected pre mortem.

Pathophysiology

Over 75% of pulmonary emboli result from clot formation and fragmentation within the deep venous system of the legs and the major vessels of the pelvis. Less common causes include:

- Amniotic fluid emboli (see 📖 Respiratory disease in pregnancy, p 515).
- 'Fat' emboli (actually bone marrow micro-emboli) resulting from fracture of a long bone or major orthopaedic surgery
- Air emboli caused by central venous cannulation, pulmonary barotrauma, or, rarely, pneumothorax
- Septic emboli, most commonly due to right-sided endocarditis. They may result in multi-focal pulmonary consolidation and systemic sepsis.

Contrary to popular belief, pulmonary infarction is uncommon in PE. This is because the bronchial circulation usually remains intact. Unless there is a concomitant impairment to gas diffusion (e.g. pulmonary oedema), the lung tissues can also continue to obtain oxygen directly from alveolar air.

Large or diffuse PE result in a sudden increase in RV afterload, which may lead to acute RV dilatation, RV ischaemia, and a fall in cardiac output. Most patients who die from PE do so from cardiogenic shock.

While obstruction of the pulmonary circulation is the principal cause of abnormal physiology in PE, the release of vasoactive and bronchoactive mediators from platelets (e.g. serotonin) can also cause widespread V/Q abnormalities.

Epidemiology

The reported annual incidence of PE is 23–69 per 100,000 population with an attributed mortality of around 200,000 per year in the USA. Hospital mortality is reported at 6–15%.

Classification

The classification of acute PE has recently been revised by the European Society of Cardiology to encourage early risk stratification and improve clinical decision making.

- High-risk PE (previously massive)—associated with a systolic arterial blood pressure <90mmHg and RV dilatation or dysfunction (based on imaging tests or biomarker evidence of acute myocardial injury).
- Intermediate risk PE (previously sub-massive)—associated with RV dilatation or dysfunction (based on imaging or biomarkers) but a normal systolic arterial blood pressure (≥90mmHg).
- Low-risk PE (previously non-massive)—not associated with any haemodynamic compromise or RV embarrassment.

Diagnosis

The presentation of PE is non-specific. Neither the symptoms nor signs listed below have a high sensitivity or specificity for PE. A high index of suspicion is required, but the use of clinical prediction scores improves diagnostic accuracy.

Clinical presentation

Symptoms

- PE may present as syncope, collapse, or cardiac arrest.
- Acute breathlessness and/or chest pain (central or pleuritic) are common.
- Haemoptysis is reported in ~10 %.
- In ventilated patients PE may present as unexplained episodes of hypoxaemia, hypotension, dysrhythmia, or weaning difficulties.

Signs

Physical signs are often absent but may include:

- Tachycardia, tachypnoea, and a low-grade fever (<38°C)
- Central cyanosis, suggesting a large PE
- Elevation of the JVP, a parasternal heave, prominent splitting of the second heart sound with a loud P_2, which all suggest elevated right heart pressures.

Predisposing factors

Look for evidence of a DVT and other risk factors.

Major risk factors

- Recent surgery, particularly major abdominal, pelvic, or orthopaedic surgery (especially lower limb).
- Late pregnancy, recent caesarean section, pre-eclampsia.
- Malignancy, particularly abdominal, pelvic, or metastatic disease.
- Lower limb abnormalities, e.g. trauma or varicose veins.
- Reduced mobility, e.g. hospitalization or institutional care.
- Previous proven PE.

Minor risk factors

- Cardiovascular co-morbidity, e.g. congenital heart disease, heart failure, hypertension, central venous line *in situ*.
- Oestrogens, e.g. oral contraceptive pill, hormone replacement therapy (HRT).
- Thrombophilias, e.g. anti-thrombin, protein C or S deficiencies.
- Miscellaneous—occult malignancy (present in approx 10%), obesity, neurological disability, inflammatory bowel disease, dialysis.

Major risk factors increase relative risk by a factor of 5–20. Minor risk factors increase relative risk by a factor of 2–4.

Pre-test clinical probability scoring systems

The non-specific presentation of PE makes it challenging, even for experienced clinicians, to identify. Early (pre-test) clinical probability scoring has been shown to improve clinical decision making and diagnostic accuracy. In these schemes points are awarded for suggestive clinical features or risk factors. Patients can then be stratified into low, intermediate, or high probability groups and appropriate tests can be arranged, if indicated. Various scoring systems have been tested but the Wells and Geneva scores are the most extensively validated.

Wells score
- DVT symptoms and signs: 3 points
- PE as likely or more likely than alternative diagnoses: 3 points
- Tachycardia (HR >100bpm): 1.5 points
- Immobilization or surgery in last 4 weeks: 1.5 points
- Previous DVT or PE: 1.5 point
- Haemoptysis: 1 point
- Cancer: 1 point

Interpretation: <2 low; 2–6 intermediate; >6 high pre-test probability

Geneva score
- Age
  - 60–79 years: 1 point
  - ≥80 years: 2 points
- Previous DVT or PE: 2 points
- Recent surgery: 3 points
- Tachycardia (>100bpm): 1 point
- $PaCO_2$
  - <4.8kPa: 2 points
  - 4.8–5.19kPa: 1 point
- PaO_2
  - <6.5kPa: 4 points
  - 6.5–7.99kPa: 3 points
  - 8.0–9.49kPa: 2 points
  - 9.5–10.99kPa: 1 point
- Chest radiograph
  - Plate atelectasis or elevation of hemidiaphragm: 1 point each

Interpretation: ≤4 low; 5–8 intermediate; ≥9 high pre-test probability

British Thoracic Society
The British Thoracic Society has simplified these scores, mindful of the fact that most patients are seen by relatively junior physicians in busy EDs. Their simplified score requires the clinician to answer two questions:
- Does the patient have clinical features compatible with acute PE?
- If yes, look for:
  (1) A major risk factor (see above)
  (2) The absence of another reasonable explanation, e.g. pneumonia.

A clinical probability score can then be assigned:
- High when both (1) and (2) are present
- Intermediate when either (1) or (2) are present
- Low when neither (1) or (2) are present.

Investigation

Electrocardiogram
- May be normal, but sinus tachycardia is common.
- Signs of right heart strain may be present, e.g. right-axis deviation, anterior T-wave inversion, right bundle branch block.
- The classic triad of $S_1Q_3T_3$ is fairly uncommon.

Chest X-ray
- May be normal (Fig. 6.11).
- Non-specific abnormalities include an elevated hemidiaphragm, linear atelactasis, opacification, or a pleural effusion (Fig. 6.12).
- Wedge-shaped pulmonary shadowing, due to infarction, and localized pulmonary oligaemia (Westermark's sign) are less common.

Arterial blood gases
- May be normal.
- Low $PaCO_2$ and H^+ concentration (hyperventilation).
- Low PaO_2.
- Increased A–a gradient.

D-dimers
D-dimers are fibrin degradation products. They are sensitive (87–99% sensitivity) markers of acute venous thromboembolism but lack specificity. Any condition that results in fibrinolysis (e.g. malignancy, infection, pregnancy, inflammatory disease) may cause a false positive. As such, they have limited use in ICU.

D-dimers in non-ICU patients
- In patients with low or intermediate clinical probability, a negative enzyme-linked immunosorbent assay (ELISA) D-dimer reliably excludes PE and further imaging is not necessary.
- If a less sensitive assay is used, e.g. the qualitative red cell agglutination test (SimpliRED), PE can only be excluded in patients with low pre-test clinical probability and a negative result.
- D-dimer testing should not be performed in patients with high pre-test clinical probability, in whom it does not improve diagnostic accuracy; appropriate imaging should be ordered instead.

Biomarkers
Acute RV strain leads to a rise in serum troponin and BNP (and N-terminal pro B type natriuretic peptide (NT-proBNP)) in intermediate and high-risk PE. Both assays are of proven prognostic value and they have a high negative predictive value for subsequent complications. Whichever test is available locally should be requested and used for early risk stratification.

Diagnostic imaging tests
Multi-detector CTPA and V/Q lung scanning are highly sensitive imaging tests for acute PE. However, they necessitate transfer of the patient to another department and, in the case of CTPA, involve administration of intravenous contrast, neither of which may be desirable or possible in an unstable, critically ill patient.

CT pulmonary angiography
CTPA can demonstrate filling defects in segmental and subsegmental pulmonary arteries (Figs 6.12 and 6.14). Multidetector-row CT allows for shorter image acquisition times, reducing the patient movement artefact. It has now largely replaced conventional pulmonary angiography.
- Investigation of choice.
- Rapid.

- Accurate (reported accuracy up to 98%).
- Widely available.
- Allows detection of RV enlargement.
- May reveal alternative diagnosis.
- In pregnancy, foetal radiation dose is about one-third that of V/Q scanning.

But
- CTPA is dependent on experienced radiological input
- CTPA cannot completely exclude small subsegmental clots.

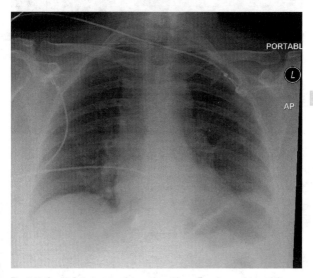

Fig. 6.11 Case 1. Patient post pelvis surgery with acute cardiovascular instability. Normal chest radiograph.

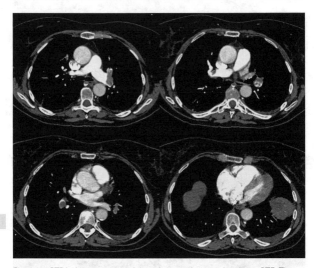

Fig. 6.12 CTPA shows extensive, bilateral non-occlusive and occlusive PTE. The right heart is dilated with RV:LV >1 and LV is under-filled, indicating imminent cardiovascular collapse. CXR is usually normal in PE. Although PE may cause subtle radiological signs (such as basal atelectasis or localized pulmonary oligaemia) these signs are so non specific that other investigations are always required.

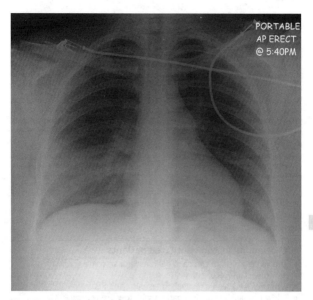

Fig. 6.13 Case 2. Patient with right-sided chest pain and tachycardia. Abnormal chest radiograph with right lower zone opacification.

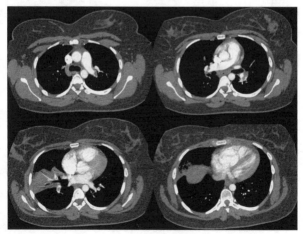

Fig. 6.14 CTPA shows extensive, bilateral non-occlusive and occlusive PTE. Right lower zone consolidation where the right lower PA is largely occluded is a developing pulmonary infarction. The right heart is dilated with RV:LV >1, indicating severe PTE. There was rapid improvement with peripherally administered thrombolysis.

V/Q scanning

Ventilation and perfusion should be well matched throughout healthy lungs. A focal perfusion defect in an area of normally ventilated lung suggests a PE and V/Q scanning is an alternative when intravenous contrast should be avoided, e.g. renal impairment.

The distribution of ventilation is assessed by inhaled xenon or aerosolized technetium diethylenetriaminepentaacetic acid (DTPA). The perfusion phase involves intravenous administration of technetium-labelled macro-aggregated albumin. A gamma camera acquires the images for both phases of the study. Each phase lasts about 10min, but with washout times the whole investigation takes about 1h.

- The test is technically difficult to perform in ventilated patients.
- IPPV can interfere with V/Q relationships, making the interpretation more difficult.
- The results are often inconclusive in acute and chronic lung disease, the elderly, those with CXR changes, and patients with coexisting cardiorespiratory insufficiency.

For these reasons, V/Q scanning is of limited value in ICU patients and is rarely used.

V/Q scanning in non-ventilated patients

- The investigation of choice in patients with a normal CXR and no previous cardiorespiratory disease.
- A normal V/Q scan effectively rules out acute PE.
- A low probability scan in a patient with low pre-test clinical probability makes the odds of PE very low and further tests are not required.
- In patients with other pre-test clinical probability scores, low and intermediate probability scans are essentially non-diagnostic and further investigation should be considered, especially if the clinical story is convincing.
- A high probability scan should be considered diagnostic of acute PE, unless the pre-test clinical probability is low or the patient has had a previous event.

Echocardiography

- Trans-thoracic echocardiography (TTE) can be performed at the bedside by many suitably trained ICU physicians.
- TTE findings described in PE include acute RV dilatation, paradoxical septal motion, moderately elevated pulmonary artery pressures with tricuspid regurgitation, a hyperdynamic empty LV, and McConnell's sign (RV free wall hypokinesia with apical sparing; this sign has a high specificity and positive predictive value but a low sensitivity).
- TTE may be diagnostic in a minority, revealing a clot travelling through the right heart or lodged in the proximal pulmonary artery. However, TTE is not sufficiently sensitive to be used as a single-imaging modality and it should certainly not be used to rule out PE.
- Its primary role is as a means of identifying acute, prognostically significant RV distress in patients with confirmed PE.

- It may identify other explanations for the presentation such as pericardial tamponade, myocardial infarction, LV failure, and aortic dissection.

Compression ultrasound scanning of the leg veins
- DVT and PTE are both presentations of the same disease.
- Compression ultrasonography (CUS) is portable, non-invasive, and simple to perform.
- In non-ICU populations, CUS has been shown to be a sensitive means of detecting proximal DVT (sensitivity 97%). However, the sensitivity decreases in patients with distal DVT (73%) or those without symptoms (53%).
- The diagnostic performance of CUS has not been rigorously tested in ICU populations.
- A positive CUS only establishes a diagnosis of venous thromboembolism. It does not provide direct evidence of PE.

Portable imaging tests

TTE and CUS are less sensitive tests for PE (and DVT) than CTPA and V:Q scanning. However, they may secure a diagnosis in unstable patients who cannot be safely transferred to other departments, or those in whom intravenous contrast media are contraindicated. Although not supported by an evidence base and liable to false negatives, this pragmatic approach may be all that is possible in some ICU patients.

Medical management
High-risk PE
These patients are at risk of rapid death unless patency of the pulmonary circulation can be restored, RV afterload reduced, and RV coronary blood flow maintained.
- Give oxygen.
- Fluid resuscitation is initial therapy for hypotension.
- If shock persists or circulatory collapse is imminent, consider thrombolysis followed by an intravenous infusion of unfractionated heparin. Alteplase (10mg bolus then 90mg over 2h) is preferable to streptokinase as the latter can exacerbate hypotension.
- Cardiac output monitoring may be useful in optimizing any further cardiovascular support.
- Consider inotropic and vasopressor support. There is no evidence for any particular agents. Use of an inodilator without vasopressor may result in a reduction in systemic blood pressure and further impair right coronary perfusion, which will exacerbate RV ischaemia. A combination of an inodilator and vasopressor achieves the best balance of inotropy and coronary perfusion without excessive elevation in PVR.

Low-risk PE
The main priority is to prevent a second, more severe event in those patients without haemodynamic upset or RV embarrassment.
- Oxygen if hypoxaemic.
- Low molecular weight heparin (LMWH) until the patient has been established on oral anticoagulation (INR 2.0–3.0 for 2 days).

LMWH can be given for the full treatment period if warfarin is contraindicated (e.g. pregnancy).
- Oral anticoagulation with warfarin (target INR range of 2.0–3.0) for 3 months is adequate treatment for patients with a transient risk factor (e.g. post-op or related to a fracture); indefinite treatment should be considered if a risk factor cannot be identified or the risk of PE is persistent, e.g. malignancy.
- Recurrent PE should be treated with life-long anticoagulation.

Intermediate-risk PE

These patients have prognostically significant abnormalities of RV structure and function, and close haemodynamic monitoring is mandatory.
- Based on the current evidence base, initial treatment should be as for low-risk PE.
- Late thrombolysis should only be considered if there is evidence of persistent haemodynamic deterioration.

Inferior vena cava filters

Inferior vena cava (IVC) filters reduce the incidence of subsequent PE, but have not been shown to improve long-term survival. Filters are indicated in patients with confirmed PE who cannot be treated conventionally or in whom conventional treatment has failed, for example:
- Patients with contraindications to thrombolysis
- Those who develop major bleeding complications during anticoagulation
- Those with recurrent PE despite therapeutic anticoagulation.

Traditional, non-retrievable filters lead to an increased incidence of subsequent DVT and other thrombotic complications and life-long anticoagulation is often necessary.

Modern retrievable filters do not present the same thrombotic risk and may be particularly useful in critically ill patients with temporary risk factors (e.g. lower limb trauma, post op) in whom a further PE might prove fatal.

The use of IVC filters without anticoagulation does not address the underlying disorder. These patients are at risk of extension of the lower limb venous thrombosis and resultant venous insufficiency.

Pulmonary embolectomy

- Mechanical embolectomy and fragmentation at right heart catheterization may be life-saving in haemodynamically unstable patients in whom thrombolysis has failed or is contraindicated. However, local expertise is essential and mortality rates have been high (6–17%) in the small series which have been reported.

Ventilatory management

Intubation and mechanical ventilation should be considered in patients presenting with acute PE and refractory hypoxaemia. It may be life-saving, but carries considerable risk.

Potential advantages
- Relieves exhaustion.
- Reduces oxygen consumption by reducing the work of breathing.
- Improves oxygenation due to high delivered FiO_2 or alveolar recruitment of atelectatic areas.
- Improves oxygenation by reversing abnormal pathophysiology occurring as a result of other diseases.

Potential disadvantages
- Since associated RV dysfunction is likely, and mechanical ventilation is likely to lead to a further increase in PVR, there is a significant risk of haemodynamic instability or cardiovascular collapse both on induction of anaesthesia and during ventilation.
- Arterial oxygenation may not improve despite adequate ventilation because of profound V/Q mismatch.

Ventilatory strategy
- Conventional ventilatory strategy should focus on providing adequate oxygenation while avoiding measures which increase PVR (pulmonary over-distension, excessive PEEP, lobar or alveolar collapse, patient–ventilator dysynchrony, increased sympathetic tone, acidosis, hypercapnia, sympathomimetics).
- Measures to support the circulation (fluid loading and inotropes) will be necessary.
- There is limited animal evidence that high-frequency jet ventilation may produce greater improvements in alveolar ventilation, PaO_2 and cardiac index than conventional ventilation strategies.
- A positive outcome will clearly depend far more on effective antithrombotic treatment and appropriate short-term cardiovascular support than any specific ventilatory intervention.

Prevention

Thromboprophylaxis is an attractive strategy given the high mortality rate of what is a potentially preventable event. Graded compression stockings should be considered in all patients without specific contraindications and anticoagulant prophylaxis should be provided to patients at increased risk of venous thromboembolism (VTE) (see below). Mechanical thromboprophylaxis (e.g. IVC filters) should be reserved for patients with major risk factors for both VTE and bleeding.

The evidence for anticoagulant thromboprophylaxis
Surgical patients
- Thromboprophylaxis with LMWH, fondaparinux, or unfractionated heparin should be prescribed for all patients undergoing major surgical procedures (most open procedures under general anaesthetic) and patients with major trauma, spinal injuries, or burns as soon as local bleeding has been controlled.
- In general surgical patients this treatment has been shown to reduce the rate of symptomatic PE (from 2.0 to 1.3%; NNT 143), fatal PE (from 0.8 to 0.3%; NNT 182), and all-cause mortality (from 4.2 to 3.2%; NNT 97).
- Monoprophylaxis with aspirin is no longer recommended.

Medical patients
- Provision of 'routine' anticoagulant thromboprophylaxis to all patients cannot be justified based on the current evidence.
- RCTs have shown a low rate of symptomatic DVT or PE (0.5–1%).
- All RCTs to date have utilized asymptomatic DVT (detected by venography or CUS) as their principal end-point—this is 30 times more common than symptomatic DVT/PE and is of uncertain clinical importance.
- No study has proven a mortality benefit.
- In the one study[1] that included acute PE as part of a composite end-point, LMWH reduced the rate of PE from 0.34% to 0.28%. However, the low event rate precluded statistical analysis and mortality appeared higher in the treatment group.
- The NNT to prevent one symptomatic VTE event is therefore high (150–1600) and the risk of major bleeding with LMWH should be considered (0.5–1.7% in the published studies).
- Certain groups are at significantly increased risk of VTE and a careful risk assessment is essential, e.g. previous VTE (relative risk (RR) 2.1–15.6), active malignancy (RR 1.6–6.5), pregnancy (RR 11.4).
- Careful consideration should be given to potential benefits and risks in other groups, e.g. COPD (RR 1.33), CCF (RR 1.36–1.72), age >75 in isolation (RR 1.03).

Further reading
Geerts WH, Bergqvist D, Pineo GF, Heit JA, Samama CM, Lassen MR, and Colwell CW, American College of Chest Physicians (2008) Prevention of venous thromboembolism, American College of Chest Physicians Evidence-based Clinical Practice Guidelines, 8th edn. *Chest* **133**(6), 381S–453S.

Samama MM, Cohen AT, Darmon JY, et al, Prophylaxis in Medical Patients with Enoxaparin Study Group (1999) A comparison of enoxaparin with placebo for the prevention of venous thromboembolism in acutely ill medical patients. *N Engl J Med* **341**, 793–800.

1 Leizorovicz A, Cohen AT, Turpie AG, Olsson CG, Vaitkus PT, and Goldhaber SZ, PREVENT Medical Thromboprophylaxis Study Group (2004) Randomized, placebo-controlled trial of dalteparin for the prevention of venous thromboembolism in acutely ill medical patients. *Circulation* **110**, 874–9.

6.16 Pulmonary vascular disease

Pulmonary hypertension (PH) is common in the ICU, most frequently secondary to ARDS, left heart disease (e.g. post cardiac surgery), acute pulmonary embolism, or parenchymal lung disease. Intercurrent illness in patients with pre-existing PAH is a rare cause of ICU admission.

PAH patients have limited haemodynamic reserve and a high mortality rate in surgical, obstetric, and ICU settings.

- Adults with PAH have a mortality rate of 7% associated with non-cardiac surgery.
- The maternal mortality of patients with PAH undergoing pregnancy has been estimated as 36%.
- CPR is rarely successful in the absence of a clearly identifiable and reversible cause for the arrest.

Pathophysiology

Pulmonary hypertension can arise from disease anywhere along the vascular pathway from the pulmonary arteries to the left side of the heart.

Classification

In the Dana Point 2008 classification, PH is classified according to the aetiology. It is based on clinical grounds, and is summarized below.

1 Pulmonary arterial hypertension
  - Idiopathic PAH (IPAH).
  - Heritable PAH.
  - Drugs and toxins induced.
  - Associated with connective tissue disease (CTDPH).
  - Associated with HIV infection.
  - Associated with portal hypertension.
  - Associated with congenital heart disease (ACHD-PH).
  - Associated with schistosomiasis.
  - Associated with chronic haemolytic anaemia.
2 Pulmonary veno occlusive disease (PVOD) and/or pulmonary capillary haemangiomatosis.
3 Pulmonary hypertension due to left heart disease.
4 Pulmonary hypertension due to lung disease and/or hypoxia.
5 Chronic thromboembolic pulmonary hypertension (CTEPH).
6 Pulmonary hypertension with unclear/multifactorial mechanisms, e.g. myeloproliferative disorders, splenectomy, sarcoidosis, histiocytosis, neurofibromatosis.

Class 1 Pulmonary arterial hypertension

PAH is thought to occur due to an imbalance of endothelial-derived mediators. There is a deficiency of prostacyclin (PGI2) and nitric oxide (NO), and an excess of endothelin-1 (ET-1).

This results in triad changes in precapillary arteries and arterioles, namely vasoconstriction, *in situ* thrombosis, and vascular remodelling, which act together to cause progressive luminal obliteration. Vascular remodelling describes the proliferation of fibroblasts, smooth muscle, and endothelial cells, causing thickening of the adventitia, media, and intima.

Other pathways have been implicated, including vasoactive intestinal peptide (VIP), serotonin, potassium channels, and hypoxia-inducible factor-1α.

Five to ten per cent of IPAH patients show a familial tendency, with the most common defect in one allele of the BMPR2 receptor (type 2 receptor for transforming growth factor-beta (TGFβ).

Physiological consequences

$$MPAP = CO \times PVR + PCWP$$

where MPAP is mean pulmonary artery pressure, CO is cardiac output, PVR is pulmonary vascular resistance, and PCWP is pulmonary capillary wedge pressure.

- Luminal obstruction → increased PVR → increased MPAP → RV pressure overload → RV dilatation and hypertrophy → RV systolic dysfunction.
- This leads to symptoms:
  - ↓stroke volume (SV)—shortness of breath and presyncope/syncope.
  - RV ischaemia—chest pain.
  - Tricuspid regurgitation (TR) and RV failure—peripheral oedema.
  - Right to left shunting through a patent foramen ovale—hypoxaemia.
  - Arrhythmias.
  - LV dysfunction due to interventricular dependence (RV pressure and volume overload produces leftwards late systolic septal shift, reducing LV filling during early diastole).

Class 2 Pulmonary venous hypertension
Pulmonary hypertension is secondary to LV diastolic dysfunction or valvular heart disease.

Class 3 Hypoxic lung disease
The major mechanism is increased PVR secondary to hypoxic pulmonary vasoconstriction (see 📖, Pathophysiology, p 2). The resulting pulmonary hypertension leads in the long term to pulmonary vascular remodelling. Parenchymal lung diseases such as ILD or COPD also cause vascular destruction. In ALI, a combination of alveolar hypoxia and intravascular fibrin and cellular debris cause an increased PVR.

Class 4 Chronic thromboembolic pulmonary hypertension
After an acute pulmonary embolism, the pulmonary artery fails to reca-nalize completely, perhaps due to a defective fibrinolytic system. This can cause subintimal fibrosis and in some cases lead to complete obliteration of the vessel lumen. The consequent pulmonary hypertension leads to vascular remodelling affecting all areas, including those spared from acute pulmonary embolism.

Epidemiology
The incidence of PH has doubled in 6 years. This may be due to greater awareness of the diagnosis, particularly in older patients (the mean age at diagnosis has increased from 36 in 1987 to 58 in 2008).

The prevalence doubled in 4 years, reflecting both the increased incidence and improved survival because of new agents directly targeting the pulmonary arteries.
- IPAH—incidence $2.6/10^6$/year, prevalence $14.5/10^6$, ♀:♂ 1.8:1.
- CTDPH—incidence $2.8/10^6$/year, prevalence $8.5/10^6$, ♀:♂ 5.4:1. Relative contributions of different connective tissue diseases: scleroderma 76%, mixed connective tissue disease 8%, SLE 8%, dermatomyositis/ polymyositis 4%, rheumatoid arthritis 3%, undifferentiated connective tissue disease 2%, Sjogrens's 1%.
- CTEPH—incidence $1.75/10^6$/year, ♂:♀ –1:1. A history of previous venous thromboembolism is present in 58% of cases and splenectomy in 7% of cases.
- ACHD-PH—5–10% of patients with CHD develop PAH.
- Portopulmonary hypertension—2–6% of patients with portal hypertension develop PAH.
- HIV-related pulmonary hypertension—0.5% of patients with HIV develop PAH.

Diagnosis of pulmonary arterial hypertension
Patients with PAH can deteriorate to a level requiring ICU support because of progression of right heart failure, sudden collapse, a com-plication of the pulmonary hypertension treatment, or a new unrelated problem.

Minor medical problems may have serious consequences because of the poor haemodynamic reserve seen in this condition, for example haemoptysis, infections, gastrointestinal bleeding, gastroenteritis, seizures, and arrhythmias.

An existing diagnosis of PAH is normally clear from the history. Symptoms are non specific: dyspnoea, fatigue, syncope or presyncope, chest pain, palpitations, and leg oedema. The following findings are typical.

Examination
- Low systemic blood pressure.
- Elevated JVP with prominent 'v' wave.
- RV heave.
- Loud pulmonary component of the second heart sound (P2) and split second heart sound.
- Pan-systolic murmur of TR at left sternal edge (louder on inspiration—Carvallo's sign).
- Early diastolic murmur of pulmonary regurgitation (Graham–Steell murmur).
- Normal lung auscultation.
- Tender, pulsatile hepatomegaly.
- Ascites.
- Peripheral oedema.
- Signs of the underlying aetiology (connective tissue disease, portal hypertension, adult congenital heart disease).

Investigations
Blood tests
- Elevated troponin.
- Raised N-terminal proB-type natriuretic peptide (NTproBNP).

ECG

Sensitivity 55%; specificity 70%; can be normal. Changes showing RV abnormalities predict decreased survival in IPAH.
- Right-axis deviation.
- R/S >1 in V1 with R >0.5mV.
- P pulmonale.
- ST depression in right-sided chest wall leads (V1–V4).
- Supraventricular arrhythmia (especially atrial flutter).

CXR

Abnormal in 94%.
- Hilar enlargement due to dilated pulmonary arteries (obscured aorto-pulmonary window).
- RA and RV enlargement.
- Reduced vascularity in lung peripheries.
- Signs of pulmonary venous hypertension (pulmonary venous congestion, pleural effusions) should be absent except in PVOD.

Transthoracic echocardiography
- Elevated pulmonary artery pressure from TR jet velocity.
- Elevated RA pressure (from inferior vena cava collapse during inspiration).
- RV and RA dilatation.
- RV hypertrophy and hypokinesis.
- Bowing of interventricular septum into LV during late systole/early diastole with D-shaped LV (indicates RV pressure and volume overload).

- Pericardial effusion.
- Increased RA pressure, pericardial effusion and septal bowing are poor prognostic indicators.
- Above changes are not specific for PAH and can be seen in acute decompensation of lung disease and severe LV diastolic dysfunction.
- Transoesophageal echocardiography/contrast TTE may give further information, particularly regarding the interatrial septum and mitral valve.

Pulmonary artery catheterisation

Swan Ganz catheter placement is essential in confirming the diagnosis and managing the complex haemodynamics in patients with PAH.

All three of the following haemodynamic conditions must be met:

- MPAP >25 mmHg.
- PCWP ≤15 mmHg.
- PVR ≥240 dynes/s/cm^5.

These conditions effectively exclude pulmonary venous hypertension and artefactual pulmonary hypertension secondary to high cardiac output, which can occur in type 2 respiratory failure, liver failure, and systemic arteriovenous fistulae (e.g. haemodialysis patients).

Other investigations

Other imaging is not immediately indicated (HRCT/CTPA) or is difficult/impossible in the ICU setting (V–Q scan, pulmonary angiogram, magnetic resonance angiogram of pulmonary arteries).

Treatment

The physiological objectives of treatment of patients with decompensated PAH are as follows:

- Optimize RV preload.
- Increase RV contractility (ideally without increasing heart rate).
- Reduce RV afterload (i.e. reduce PVR).
- Increase LV preload.
- Maintain systemic blood pressure and thereby coronary artery perfusion.

Optimize fluid balance with fluids/diuretics

In patients with PAH and RV dysfunction, both hyper and hypovolaemia can lead to a reduction in LV preload. The optimal filling pressure in patients with an RV infarct was found to be 10–14mmHg but in chronic PAH this depends on the individual patient. Close haemodynamic monitoring, usually via a Swan Ganz catheter or equivalent, allows measurement of RA pressure, PCWP, and cardiac output (CO). In addition to facilitating diagnosis, placement of such a device is helpful in monitoring the response to therapy.

Treat the cause of decompensation

- Any intercurrent illness should be appropriately treated.
- Treat arrhythmias. Loss of sinus rhythm is poorly tolerated by patients with PAH and may be the sole cause of decompensation. Either immediate or delayed DC cardioversion to sinus rhythm should be attempted despite unfavourable cardiac anatomy.

Mitigate aggravating factors

- Give oxygen—alveolar hypoxia causes hypoxic pulmonary vasoconstriction and increased PVR.
- Hypercapnia and acidosis also cause pulmonary vasoconstriction and should be reversed if possible.

Pulmonary vasodilator therapy

Evidence for the use of this therapy is extrapolated from chronic treatment of PAH and from treatment of secondary PH in conditions such as ARDS and post-cardiac surgery. These agents either increase levels of cAMP or cGMP (prostanoids and NO) or act as phosphodiesterase (PDE) inhibitors to reduce cAMP and cGMP breakdown (milrinone and sildenafil).

- Prostanoids
  - For example epoprostenol (PGI2, epoprostenol, treprostinil, iloprost).
  - Replace endogenous prostacyclin and enhance the level of cAMP in PA smooth muscle cells.
  - ↓PVR; ↓MPAP; ↑CO; ↓SVR.
  - Prostacyclin—$t_{1/2}$ 3–6min; given by continuous intravenous infusion; started at 1–2ng/kg/min, titrated upwards by 0.5–1ng/kg/min increases at intervals of 15–30min according to haemodynamic effect.
  - Treprostinil—usually given subcutaneously but can be given intravenously; $t_{1/2}$ 3–4h; starting dose 2ng/kg/min and titrate upwards.
  - Iloprost—usually given via nebulized route but can be given intravenously; nebulized dose 2.5–5mcg/dose six to nine times per day.
  - In awake patients, use of prostanoids is limited by systemic side-effects (hypotension, headache, diarrhoea, nausea and vomiting, jaw pain, flu-like symptoms).
  - Abrupt withdrawal may lead to rebound hypertension and decompensation.
- Nitric oxide
  - Replaces endogenous NO and enhances the level of cGMP in PA smooth muscle cells.
  - Given by inhaled route and therefore improves V/Q matching in well-ventilated lung only.
  - ↓PVR; ↓MPAP; →SVR; →CO; quickly inactivated by haemoglobin and therefore no systemic effect.
  - Continuous inhalation at dose of 10–20ppm is safe.
  - Side-effects—methaemoglobinaemia, forms NO_2 (an oxidant) with O_2; abrupt withdrawal may lead to rebound hypertension and haemodynamic collapse.
  - Requires specialist equipment for administration.
- Milrinone
  - PDE3 inhibitor which increases levels of cAMP in PA smooth muscle cells; acts as both an inotrope and vasodilator.
  - ↓PVR; ↓MPAP; ↑CO; ↓SVR.
  - Infusion 0.375–0.75mcg/kg/min. Avoid recommended bolus in critically ill patients.

- Side-effects—systemic hypotension; vasopressors (e.g. noradrenaline or vasopressin) have been used to counteract this.
- Probably inferior to PDE5 inhibitors, which produce more pulmonary vasodilatation and less systemic vasodilatation.
- Sildenafil
  - PDE5 inhibitor that increases levels of cGMP in PA smooth muscle cells.
  - ↓PVR; ↓MPAP; ↑CO; minimal ↓ in systemic blood pressure.
  - 20–80mg 8-hourly orally or via NGT; data emerging on administration via intravenous and nebulized route (10mg bolus).
  - Side-effects—synergistic effect with nitrates or nicorandil to produce a large drop in systemic blood pressure.
  - Little studied in ICU setting.
- Vasodilator combinations
  - Sildenafil has been used in combination with prostanoids, inhaled NO, and milrinone.
  - Intravenous milrinone and intravenous epoprostenol have both been used in combination with inhaled NO.
- Other agents
  - No longer used: nifedipine, nitroprusside, nitrates, hydralazine.
  - Not recommended: nesiritide (recombinant human BNP).
  - Possibly effective: zaprinast, dipyridamole.
  - Not studied in acute setting: endothelin receptor antagonists.

Inotropes/vasopressors
An ideal agent in this setting would:
- Maintain systemic blood pressure
- Not produce a tachycardia
- ↓PVR
- ↑CO.

Commonly used
- Dobutamine
  - Low dose: <5mcg/kg/min, ↓PVR, ↑CO.
  - High dose: 5–10mcg/kg/min, ↑heart rate, →PVR.
  - Main drawback is systemic hypotension due to peripheral β-agonist effect, which may necessitate the use of a peripheral vasoconstrictor such as noradrenaline.
- Noradrenaline
  - ↑PVR; ↑MPAP; →↑CO; ↑systemic blood pressure; ↓heart rate.
  - Initial dose 0.5–1mcg/min; titrate to desired response: 8–30mcg/min is usual range.
  - Needs to be used in combination with a vasodilator to mitigate vasoconstrictor effect on pulmonary circulation.
- Dopamine
  - ↑MPAP; ↑CO; ↑systemic blood pressure; ↑heart rate.
  - Low dose: 1–2mcg/kg/min, D1 action, vasodilatation, ↓systemic blood pressure.
  - Moderate dose: 5–10mcg/kg/min, β-agonist; ↑CO, ↑SV, →↑heart rate.
  - High dose: >10mcg/kg/min, α- and β-agonist; ↑heart rate, ↑SVR.

- Major problem is with tachycardia, which reduces RV filling time, increases the potential for ischaemia, and may induce tachyarrhythmias.

Rarely used
- Phenylephrine
  - Not recommended as noradrenaline has a superior haemodynamic effect in PAH.
- Isoprenaline
  - ↓PVR, ↑CO, no effect on PA pressure.
  - Infusion at 2–10mcg/min.
  - Main problems are tachyarrhythmias. In addition, it needs to be withdrawn gradually as PVR can rise rapidly. Despite these problems, isoprenaline has been used in heart transplantation patients with ↑PVR.
- Adrenaline
  - Not studied in PAH.
- Digoxin is not widely used. It may increase cardiac index but, when studied in PAH, PVR did not change and MPAP increased.

Promising novel agents
- Vasopressin
  - Acts via endothelial G-protein coupled with vasopressinergic (V1) receptors.
  - Causes systemic vasoconstriction and pulmonary vasodilatation (the latter via an NO-dependent mechanism).
  - Low dose (e.g. 0.06–0.1U/min) appears effective in treating refractory systemic hypotension in PAH patients.
  - High dose (e.g. >1U/min) has a harmful effect, with ↑PVR, ↑MPAP, ↓CO.
- Levosimendan
  - Acts via myocardial and vascular sensitization to calcium.
  - 'Inodilator'—pulmonary vasodilatation, positively inotropic, thereby improving right-sided ventriculo-vascular coupling.
  - Infusion at 0.2mcg/kg/min.
  - Also reduces SVR and is likely to require concomitant vasopressor therapy.

Combination of vasodilators/inotropes
- In most cases, a combination of pulmonary artery vasodilators and inotropes/vasopressors will be used.
- The precise choice of vasodilator agent will depend to a certain extent on availability and experience but is likely to be one of inhaled NO, intravenous prostanoid or oral sildenafil.
- The following table offers some guidance for the initial choice of the inotrope/vasopressor.

	Normotensive	Hypotensive
Normal HR	Dobutamine/milrinone	Dopamine/noradrenaline/vasopressin
Tachycardic	Milrinone	Noradrenaline/vasopressin/phenylephrine

Treatment of PAH resulting from critical illness, or chronic lung or heart disease, should address the underlying disorder, optimize RV and LV preload and afterload, and maintain coronary artery perfusion.

There is no current evidence to support the use of pulmonary arterial vasodilators in these circumstances.

Ventilatory management

There are two physiological consequences of positive pressure ventilation that dictate modern ventilation practice in patients with PAH, the effect of lung volume and the effect of ITP.

Effect of lung volume

There is a U-shaped relationship between lung volume and PVR. At low lung volumes, hypoxic pulmonary vasoconstriction causes increased tone in extra-alveolar vessels. At high lung volumes there is compression of alveolar vessels. PVR is minimized at a lung volume near FRC.

Effect of ITP

Increased ITP increases right atrial pressure and thereby decreases venous return and cardiac output. It uncouples pulmonary blood flow from alveolar ventilation.

The ideal strategy for ventilation of these patients therefore involves low tidal volumes and avoidance of either inadequate or excessive PEEP. Adoption of these strategies may be in some part responsible for the decline of cor pulmonale seen in ARDS from 61% to 25% over the last 15 to 30 years. In addition hypoxaemia, hypercapnia, and acidosis should also be avoided. In one study a mixture of hypercapnia and acidosis increased PVR by 54% and MPAP by 30%.

Further reading

Galie N, Hoeper MM, and Humbert M (2009) Guidelines for the diagnosis and treatment of pulmonary hypertension (ESC/ERS Guidelines). *Eur Respir J* **34**, 1219–1263.

Tsapenko MV, Tsapenko AV, Comfere TBO, *et al.* (2008) Arterial pulmonary hypertension in the intensive care unit. *Vasc Health Risk Manag* **4**(5), 1043–1060.

Zamanian RT, Haddah H, Doyle RL, *et al.* (2007) Management strategies for patients with pulmonary hypertension in the intensive care unit. *Crit Care Med* **35**(9), 2037–2050.

6.17 Thoracic surgical patients in ICU

Patient selection for thoracic surgery is not a science. It combines a mixture of objective measurement and the subjective assessment of the extremes of pulmonary dysfunction by the thoracic team. Co-morbidity can be extensive and neither a satisfactory scoring system nor an investigation exists that is reliably predictive of outcome. In general, a patient should survive a thoracotomy and lung resection if they are left with at least 35% of predicted normal lung function (usually an FEV_1 >1L), are pain free, have minimal secretions, and have sufficient nutrition and muscle bulk to breathe and cough.

The requirement for invasive ventilation following an elective thoracotomy usually indicates a failure of treatment.

Analgesia

Thoracic surgical techniques can be endoscopic, video-assisted, or open. Excellent pain relief is mandatory after thoracotomy. Most types of analgesia have been used for post-thoracotomy pain. No particular technique is consistently better than any other.

- Epidural analgesia (with or without opiates or clonidine) is usually regarded as the gold standard. However, even at T4, the failure rate (up to 17%) can be unacceptably high.
- Para-vertebral blocks sited surgically at the time of operation with one or two epidural catheters between parietal pleura and the chest wall have all the advantages of epidural analgesia but with unilateral motor, sensory and sympathetic blocks, good analgesia, and possibly a lower failure rate.
- Diaphragmatic or chest wall stimulation from chest drains can occur despite a good block, and so whatever regional technique is used it should include an opiate, either epidurally or intravenously by patient-controlled analgesia.
- Remifentanil target-controlled infusion has been used successfully in both ventilated and spontaneously breathing patients (effect site concentration 0.5–3ng/mL).
- Paracetamol (1g 6 hourly) can provide background pain relief.
- NSAIDs (diclofenac 75mg intravenously or 100mg per rectum) are excellent for short-term rescue analgesia but should be used sparingly in fluid-restricted patients. Avoid NSAIDs in pleurodesis (talc or pleural strip) as a good inflammatory response is required for pleural adhesion.

Beware the aquatic assassin (excess fluid)

Modern monitoring makes it easy to measure and optimize cardiovascular status post thoracotomy. However, fluid loading to normalize cardiac output and give pre-renal protection can compromise pulmonary function. The following features can disrupt the normal function of the alveolar–capillary junction, initiate inflammatory pathways, and predispose patients to pulmonary oedema:

- Handling of the lung at surgery.
- Lung collapse and re-expansion.
- One-lung ventilation.

This is exacerbated by any operative loss of lymphatic drainage and especially by fluid challenges.

Risk of pulmonary oedema:
pneumonectomy > lobectomy > wedge resection

Initial post-operative fluid replacement should be with a balanced salt solution (e.g. Hartmann's) given at a rate of 1mL/kg/h and should not exceed a total of 1500mL/24h for the first 2–3 days. In addition, the usually small blood loss should be replaced volume for volume with an appropriate colloid.
- Pre-operative use of a β-blocker and long-acting vasodilators may necessitate a low-dose infusion of vasopressor (noradrenaline 0.01–0.05mcg/kg/min) to maintain blood pressure and renal perfusion.
- A urine output of 0.5–1mL/kg/h should be sufficient to avoid renal failure but should not be pursued at the expense of lung function.
- These patients should be run very dry.

Post-thoracotomy respiratory failure

Post-thoracotomy respiratory failure rarely has a single aetiology and is often not recognized until late in the process. Symptoms may be exacerbated by alcohol or nicotine withdrawal. Once established, the clinical picture is unmistakable, depressing, and carries a high mortality.
Features include:
- Confusion or obtunded conscious level
- Retained secretions
- Hypoxia
- Hypercapnia (often >10kPa)
- Infection or sepsis
- Hypotension with or without cardiac failure
- Acidosis
- Renal failure.

Overt pulmonary oedema is rare. Oedema, infection, and inflammation can all contribute to the clinical picture but with no way of determining their individual contributions, therapy has to be widely based and address all of the possible pathologies. Management should address:
- Obvious causes
- Infection
- Cardiovascular support and fluid status
- Ventilatory support
- Weaning
- Sedation.

Obvious causes
Exclude or treat the most common causes of respiratory failure in this group.
- Pneumothorax (chest drain).
- Secretions with lobar/lung collapse (physio, suction bronchoscopy, mini-tracheostomy).
- Opiates (reduce or reverse).
- Muscle weakness from epidural motor block (reduce or stop infusion).

Infection

- In the absence of positive sputum or blood cultures treat initially as a community-acquired chest infection and exclude atypical pneumonia.
- Consider anaerobic cover for obstructed lung segments.

Cardiovascular support

By the time patients with post-thoracotomy respiratory failure come to the attention of ICU or the outreach team, it is common for them to be relatively fluid overloaded and/or hypotensive. Although there is little evidence, there is a strong argument for the early empirical use of inotropes (adrenaline or dobutamine) and diuretics (furosemide), even before the institution of full cardiovascular monitoring. In some patients, these measures, along with CPAP, may be enough to avoid full ventilation.

Should the patient require invasive ventilation, the continued use of inotropes must be supported by full cardiovascular monitoring. Although measurement of continuous cardiac output by thermodilution or pulse contour analysis is not mandatory, it greatly helps the therapy goals of optimizing the cardiac index whilst removing (or reducing the potential for) excess lung water.

In the early stages the distinctions between infection, pulmonary oedema, and ARDS are largely academic.

- Avoid fluid loading.
- There is no advantage to crystalloid or colloid.
- Start renal replacement therapy earlier rather than later.

Ventilatory support

There is no evidence that very early intubation and ventilation reduce morbidity. In the early phase of post-thoracotomy respiratory failure, nasal or full-face CPAP will improve oxygenation and may be sufficient. CPAP will not help with hypercapnia and interferes with the ability to cooperate with physiotherapy, cough, communicate, eat, and drink. Consider an early NGT.

BiPAP and its equivalents work well for cooperative patients with weak muscles and borderline lung function but are miserable for hypoxic, hypercapnic patients with secretions, stiff lungs, and a high respiratory drive. This group should be intubated and ventilated.

Pressure support and PEEP are the mainstays of a ventilation strategy that is aimed at maintaining low airway pressures, reducing lung water, clearing secretions, exercising ventilatory muscles, and early extubation. Unfortunately, high respiratory drives or airway pressures are common and may necessitate paralysis and PCV with permissive hypercapnia.

The further management of these patients should follow the normal principles of longer-term ventilation.

Weaning

Although some patients may be extubated after a few days of ventilation, weaning in this population is generally problematic. Most patients will have entered hospital with reduced respiratory function and been further compromised by surgery and the co-morbidities of prolonged ICU stay. By the time the weaning process is started they tend to have stiff lungs, poor lung volumes (restrictive defect), weak musculature, and high CO_2 levels with a compensatory metabolic alkalosis.

- The mode of weaning should be agreed by the team and applied *consistently* either by gradual reduction of pressure support or by intermittent, staged workouts on an RSBI protocol. Here the patient's 'normal' pressure support is reduced by 5cm. They are then allow to breathe for an hour (then two or three, etc.) or until the RSBI (respiratory rate divided by tidal volume in litres) >100–105. RSBI is also used to predict weaning success (see 📖 Weaning, p 333) but here is being used to exercise respiratory muscles to an 'objective' level of fatigue.
- It is difficult to wean a person reliant on hypoxic drive if they are not kept hypoxaemic.
- Ventilation post pneumonectomy carries quoted mortalities of 67–100%. Weaning may take weeks to months but will be achievable for a minority of patients.
- Be prepared to deal with the humanitarian and ethical issues surrounding the stable, alert patient with single-organ failure who may be neither well enough to leave the ICU breathing unsupported nor fit for home ventilation.

Chest drains

Thoracic surgeons understand chest drains. If in any doubt at all, ask for help.

> Remember **AAA** and **BBB** for drains inserted in theatre:
> The **A**nterior drain is draining **A**ir from the **A**pex.
> The drain at the **B**ack is draining **B**lood from the **B**ase.

Air leaks are common after any resection that leaves raw lung surfaces. They will usually settle within 2–3 days, especially if the residual lung tissue has expanded to fill the pleural space.

Chest drain insertion on ICU

Chest drain insertion is a common procedure, but may cause puncture of heart, lungs, liver, or spleen. Deaths and serious harm associated with chest drain insertion have been linked with common themes: inexperienced staff, incorrect insertion site, poor patient position, excessive insertion of dilator, anatomical anomalies, inadequate imaging, and lack of knowledge of existing guidelines. There is no evidence favouring one technique over another, and Seldinger insertion of small drains is associated with similar complications. Ultrasound guidance is strongly recommended when inserting a drain for fluid.

This topic is fully discussed in 📖 Pleural disease, p 481.

Indications for chest drain placement on ICU include:
- Pneumothorax:
  - In any ventilated patient
  - Tension pneumothorax (perform a needle decompression first)
  - Persistent or recurrent after needle aspiration
  - Large recurrent spontaneous Pneumothorax
- Large haemothorax (especially traumatic)
- Large pleural effusions (if compromising ventilation or weaning)
- Empyema (post-operative in cardiac and thoracic surgery).

You need to be certain that the 'pneumothorax' is not a large bulla, and that the lung is not adherent to the chest wall.

Clamping drains
Chest drains are usually only clamped after a pneumonectomy, with the drain unclamped for 5min in the hour.
- Only clamp on the advice of a thoracic surgeon or respiratory physician.
- Never clamp a bubbling chest drain.
- If the patient develops surgical emphysema or becomes breathless unclamp the drain.

Closed drainage systems
Each tube must be attached to its own drainage system, which should be below the level of the patient, appropriately filled with water, and kept upright at all times.
- Monitor air and fluid loss.
- Respiratory swing indicates patency of the system.
- Flutter valves allow early mobilization in pneumothorax.

Suction
Should a lung with an underwater seal chest drain not re-inflate with physiotherapy and coughing, high-volume low-pressure suction (15–25cmH$_2$O) can help.
- An effective cough in a pain-free patient will generate a higher pressure than suction, but ventilated patients often do not generate effective coughs so suction is advisable.
- Suction that is not working has similar effects to a clamped tube.

Re-expansion pulmonary oedema
When large pneumothoraces (with associated mediastinal shift and cardiovascular compromise) or sizeable pleural effusions are drained, the re-expanding lung can develop significant pulmonary oedema. It is most commonly seen after re-expanding chronically (72h or more) collapsed lung and usually presents dramatically and immediately after re-expansion. It can occur even in the absence of fluid loading and the quoted mortality is up to 11%.
- It may only require supportive therapy with oxygen and diuretics, but more severe cases may need inotropes or short-term ventilation with moderate to high levels of PEEP.

Double-lumen tubes in ICU
There are few absolute indications for the use of a double-lumen tube (DLT) in ICU. Relative elective indications for a DLT include:
- Prevention of soilage
- Facilitation of BAL.

Relative emergency indications include:
- Massive bronchopleural fistula
- Massive haemoptysis.

Differential ventilation for unilateral lung disease is very rare, used after the failure of conventional therapies, and requires a ventilator for each lung.

Red rubber Robertshaw DLTs are easier to insert, mostly self-lateralise correctly, and tend not to move from the correct position. The high-pressure, low-volume cuffs that anchor the tubes make them unsuitable, compared to plastic tubes, for long-term ventilation.

Broncho-pleural fistula

These usually occur 7–10 days post pneumonectomy as a result of an air leak through a poorly healing bronchial stump. They present with sudden breathlessness and expectoration of serosanguinous fluid (from the pleural cavity). Treatment is aimed at protecting the remaining lung from contamination and swamping by the leaking pleural fluid.

- Give high oxygen concentrations, insert a large chest drain, and lie the patient on the operated side.
- Send bacteriology samples but treat with broad-spectrum antibiotics that include anaerobic cover.
- Definitive treatment may require re-thoracotomy and over-sewing of the bronchial stump. The surgeon may wish to use an omentum or a muscle patch to reinforce the repair.

A massive air leak from a broncho-pleural fistula that interferes with ventilation should be treated with a DLT before being taken to theatre. Alternatively, an uncut 6–7mm diameter single-lumen tube can be slid into the normal bronchus aided by a fibre-optic bronchoscope.

Do not destroy a leaking bronchial stump with an endo-bronchial blocker. A persistent small-to-medium broncho-pleural fistula is better treated with two-lung ventilation through a single-lumen tube and with a large, functioning chest drain.

Massive haemoptysis

The treatment of choice for massive haemoptysis is selective embolisation of the relevant pulmonary artery. Although emergency isolation of one lung is of help whilst waiting for radiological intervention, the emergency changing of a single-lumen tube to a DLT should only be attempted by an expert. In less experienced hands it is probably safer to use an endo-bronchial blocker with a fibre-optic bronchoscope down the existing ETT and isolate the bleeding lung (do not use a fibre-optic laryngoscope as the suction lumen is too small to clear blood in the volumes needed). Failing either of the above, an uncut single-lumen tube can be passed into the bronchus on the protected side.

Emergency surgery may occasionally be required to control massive bleeding but only after stabilization and imaging.

Bullous lung disease

Laplace's law for spheres (tension ∝ radius × pressure) explains the preferential ventilation of bullae over normal alveolae. In health, patients with bullous lung disease achieve a dynamic equilibrium between pathological and normal lung. This is destroyed by IPPV or PEEP, causing two main problems:

- Compression of the remaining normal lung tissue
- Hyper-inflation of bullae with air-trapping, which can lead to total loss of cardiac output.

Both may be minimized by very low inflation pressures, little or no PEEP, and very long expiratory times.

In acutely over-inflated lungs with tamponade-induced loss of cardiac output and hypoxia, do not kill the patient by continued attempts at ventilation. Disconnect the ventilator and wait for the lungs to empty, restoring cardiac output.

6.18 Thoracic trauma

Chest trauma remains one of the most common causes of death in patients who suffer major trauma. UK practice has a predominance of blunt trauma, but penetrating trauma is increasing, especially in urban areas. In the USA, chest trauma is also predominantly due to blunt trauma (70%), but the proportion of penetrating trauma is greater (30%). The management of such injuries requires close attention to detail, but this is rewarded with good functional recovery.

The ED management of trauma is based on advanced trauma life support (ATLS) principles. These seek to identify and treat immediate life-threatening injuries, and has usually been implemented before the patient arrives in the ICU. A record of this will often be available on the trauma run-sheet that is commonly used in the ED for such patients. However, it is prudent to check the initial assessment has been completed, using the mnemonic:

- **A**irway obstruction
- **T**ension pneumothorax
- **O**pen pneumothorax
- **M**assive haemothorax
- **F**lail chest
- **C**ardiac tamponade.

Chest wall injuries

Rib fractures

The most common problem from blunt chest trauma is rib fractures, with potential underlying lung injury. These may be difficult to identify on plain CXR, but can often be palpated or presumed in the presence of crepitus. Multiple rib fractures, especially those involving two or more segments of a number of ribs, are associated with respiratory failure (type 1 or 2).

First rib fractures are associated with a tear in the thoracic aorta and indicate severe trauma, usually deceleration. The gold standard for the diagnosis of this injury is the aortogram, but it is not used as a screening tool. CT thorax with dynamic intravenous contrast may be used as part of the trauma series, and will usually detect mediastinal blood or aortic contrast leak.

Management involves analgesia, NIV, and regular physiotherapy to assist sputum clearance. Unilateral fractures can be managed with epidural analgesia and paravertebral or inter-pleural local anaesthetic infusion. The latter is particularly useful if there is already a chest drain *in situ*, as the local anaesthetic can be bolused into the drain, which is then clamped for 10–20min to allow the local to 'fix'. Do not clamp a bubbling chest drain. Bilateral fractures will usually require epidural analgesia, as the other two methods would require toxic volumes of local anaesthetic.

Multiple rib fractures alone rarely prevent weaning from mechanical ventilation: it is more likely that underlying lung contusion or ARDS prevents weaning. However, if gas exchange is good, yet the patient cannot sustain SBTs, the problem may be mechanical chest wall dysfunction. In these circumstances, discuss with thoracic surgery whether surgical fixation of multiple rib fractures may improve lung function.

Burns
- Circumferential burns to the chest wall can impair ventilation.
- Patients who are already on mechanical ventilation will demonstrate worsening compliance, while patients breathing spontaneously may develop type 2 respiratory failure.
- Escharotomy under general anaesthesia should be performed as an emergency by an experienced surgeon: blood loss can be considerable, as the incision must reach the deep chest wall layers.

Pleural injuries

Blood, air, and fluid can accumulate in the pleural space following traumatic injury. The management of this depends on the volume in the pleural space and also the need for mechanical ventilation.

Pneumothorax
- Tension pneumothorax is usually diagnosed clinically or radiologically in the ED and managed at this point. However, smaller pneumothoraces, especially bilateral ones, may sometimes only be picked up on CT thorax.
- If the pneumothoraces are less than 10% of chest cavity by volume, then they can be watched without immediate need for drainage. However, if patients require mechanical ventilation, either in ICU or in the operating theatre, a chest drain is indicated.
- The drain should be inserted in the 'safe triangle' (see 📖 Pleural disease, Fig. 6.8, p 481). The choice between Seldinger or blunt dissection is a personal one, as there is no clear benefit of either technique. There is a risk of trauma to underlying structures if the dilators required for the Seldinger technique are advanced significantly beyond the chest wall.
- A large-gauge drain should be inserted if fluid coexists or if a lung leak is suspected.
- Aseptic technique is vital. There is good evidence that empyema may follow drains inserted under less than ideal conditions.

Haemothorax

The drainage of a massive haemothorax may have been performed in the emergency room, or indeed in the pre-hospital setting via thoracostomy.
- Pleural collections that are less than 500mL on the CT scan may be observed: larger collections require drainage with a large-bore chest drain.
- Ultrasound to mark out the site of the effusion is beneficial unless the CT scan shows clear surface markings of maximal effusion thickness.
- On insertion of the chest drain, initial drainage >1000mL or ongoing losses of >200mL/h indicate a need for surgical involvement.

Intra-thoracic injuries

Pulmonary injuries

Pulmonary contusion is the most common parenchymal lung problem seen in the trauma patient. It may lead to the development of ARDS, and where extra-pulmonary causes of ARDS are present, direct and indirect lung injury may coexist. The ventilation strategy should follow the ARDSnet guidelines, including:
- Tidal volume 6mL/kg of ideal body weight
- Limitation of plateau airway pressure to 30cmH$_2$O

● Careful fluid management. In general, these patients should be managed with as limited an intravascular volume as other organ perfusion will allow.

The use of prone ventilation (see 📖 Adjuncts, p 188) is contentious, particularly in the trauma patient. The compounding factors in the trauma patient include the 'uncleared' cervical spine and application of external fixators to, for example, the pelvis or lower limbs. However, proning may have a place in the trauma patient with severe unresponsive hypoxia, where the above problems are relatively minor.

Tracheo-bronchial injuries

● Most tracheal injuries are in the cervical region and will have been diagnosed prior to arrival in the ICU.
● If the patient cannot be orally intubated across the tear, then tracheostomy is required.
● Bronchial injuries are very infrequent with blunt trauma, but may present with persistent pneumothorax and air leak (50%).
● Clinical suspicion is essential, especially where subcutaneous emphysema and air leak persists despite pleural drainage.
● Bronchoscopy will usually confirm the diagnosis, although up to half of these injuries take more than a month to diagnose. Open repair via thoracotomy should be performed as quickly as possible.

Heart and great vessel injuries

Myocardial contusion

● Myocardial contusion is the most common injury, and is usually diagnosed by ECG changes (ST-T wave changes in the anterior leads) and a rise in troponin.
● It may be difficult to differentiate from acute myocardial infarction, although myocardial contusion rarely produces persistent ST elevation and Q wave development.
● Inotropic support may be required.

Pericardial tamponade

● Pericardial tamponade should be suspected in patients with features of cardiac failure and high right-sided filling pressure. Tamponade is a clinical diagnosis, but suspicions may be raised on review of the thorax CT. Echocardiography may confirm the clinical diagnosis.
● Echocardiographic features of tamponade:
  • RV and right atrial diastolic collapse.
  • Interventricular septum deviation toward the LV cavity on inspiration.
  • Increase in transmitral inflow E wave velocity of >25% on inspiration and/or increase in tricuspid inflow E wave velocity by >40% on inspiration.
  • Inferior vena cava dilatation without collapse with inspiration.
● A haemopericardium that produces clinical signs requires discussion with a cardiothoracic surgeon, as drainage of the blood is rarely curative.
● Atrial and ventricular rupture from blunt trauma is usually fatal, but should be considered if a haemopericardium persists.

Aortic injury

A high index of suspicion is required in blunt trauma patients with marked acceleration/deceleration. The most common point of injury is at the ligamentum arteriosum, where the aorta becomes fixed to the posterior thoracic cage.

The clinical findings that should prompt specific investigation are:
• Widened mediastinum on semi-erect CXR
• Fracture to first rib, especially left side
• Pleural capping, again often on left
• Deviation of passage of NGT at level of arch of aorta
• Varying blood pressure between arms is not a common sign.

CT thorax with contrast will have already been performed in many patients with these signs, as part of the trauma series. Arch aortography is still the gold standard, although many cardiothoracic surgeons will delay this until they receive the patient if the CT scan is clearly diagnostic.

Diaphragm rupture
• Injury commonly occurs on the left side, and usually results in herniation of stomach into the thorax.
• NGT placement may confirm the diagnosis on CXR, and will also prevent gastric distension and rupture.
• Collapse of the left lower lobe and mediastinal shift to the right are common complications.
• Surgical repair is required urgently, and will involve an approach through either chest or abdomen.

Ballistic injuries

The nature of the wound produced by a missile depends on a number of factors and includes:
• Velocity and mass of missile(s)
• Anatomical site of entrance and path of missile
• Presence of restraining clothing, i.e. anti-ballistic jackets
• Behaviour of missile on entering tissue, e.g. Yaw (side-to-side movement), precession (tip rotation), tumble (end-over-end rotation)
• Contamination of wound by missile/fragments/clothing/human tissue
• Secondary injuries from, for example, blast, falling, fire.

The majority of these factors can be assessed by the history of the event. The anatomical course of the wounds will usually determine the radiological investigation, which will then guide surgical intervention. Initially, the patient should be examined closely front and back to search for and label all wounds. Photographs should be taken, and then a paperclip stuck next to each wound with sticky tape. This will allow plain X-ray to indicate the cutaneous markings of any wounds, and help determine the passage of a missile.

Classification of ballistic wounds

There are a variety of ways to classify such wounds, but the most common method studies the velocity of the missile(s) involved. This is not a classification of severity, as kinetic energy alone does not determine the nature of the wounds.

- Low velocity—includes most air weapons, stab wounds, some handguns, spears, darts, and other objects pushed by human hand into the body.
- Medium velocity—includes most handguns, high-powered air rifles, and shotguns.
- High velocity—includes most rifles, some handguns, and fragmentation munitions ('blast') injuries.

ICU management

The patient who has received a ballistic wound will usually present to the critical care unit after an initial process of stabilization and primary/secondary management has occurred. This will typically identify the most life-threatening injuries, but it is important to realize that injuries may be missed or develop over time: the latter is particularly true for fragmentation-type injuries, e.g. blast, bomb, or grenade injuries. Thus, the initial management on the critical care unit should include:

- Description of mechanism and time of injury
- Review of injuries detected, management, and investigation
- Effects of treatment already applied
- Plan for further treatment
- Antibiotic and tetanus regimes proposed
- Discussion with family.

Management of penetrating chest wounds

Penetrating wounds to the chest may cause a wide variety of wounds and injuries, and the above schema will help to determine initial investigation and treatment. The management of chest wounds is determined by the anatomical site of the wound and the nature of the wound. Any wound that crosses into the area of thorax bounded by a 'central rectangle' over the sternum is more likely to require surgical exploration. The 'central rectangle' does not have strict boundaries, but extends from the suprasternal notch to the xiphisternum and encloses the mediastinum and heart. Wounds that are exclusively outside this area are less likely to require surgical intervention, but may still be life-threatening. Thus, the sequence should be:

- Identify the number and site of entrance wounds.
- Identify the number and site of exit wounds.
- Attempt to plot, with radiological support, the course of each missile.
- Any missile that crosses the central rectangle will require some form of surgical exploration.
- If the passage of the missile(s) is completely outside the central rectangle, then usually tube thoracostomy and clinical observation will be adequate. If the tube thoracostomy drains >1000mL of blood or >200mL/h or food material/gastric contents, then surgical exploration

is required. The majority of low/medium-velocity wounds, and even some high-velocity injuries, outside the central rectangle will not require surgical exploration.

Surgical intervention

The type and timing of the surgical intervention is dependent on:
- Haemodynamic stability on arrival in hospital
- Central rectangle wound or not
- Provisional/actual diagnosis and anatomical location of injury
- Facilities/skills available.

Patients who arrive in cardiac arrest, or imminent cardiovascular collapse, are best treated by emergency room thoracotomy or sternotomy, with urgent descending thoracic aortic cross-clamp and identification of bleeding wounds. Injuries that are diagnosed after arrival in more stable patients will require careful consideration for surgical approach. Such injuries can include:
- Cardiac tamponade due to cardiac chamber rupture—must always be considered in wounds crossing the central rectangle
- Pulmonary bleeding
- Tracheo-bronchial rupture—often recognized because of massive surgical emphysema and failure to re-inflate the lungs despite tube thoracostomy
- Diaphragmatic rupture
- Hilar injuries—may present as intractable chest drain bleeding and/or persistent air leak despite tube thoracostomy
- Abdominal visceral injuries from chest wounds that have penetrated the diaphragm.

Late problems on the critical care unit following penetrating trauma

These problems are not unique to penetrating trauma, but cause most of the mortality/morbidity for patients who survive their initial penetrating wound:
- ARDS/ALI
- Sepsis from wound contamination
- Pleural empyema following contamination of stab/missile wounds to chest
- Mediastinitis following oesophageal perforation, often diagnosed late.
- Bleeding/fistulation from unremoved missiles.

Blast injuries

Although blast injuries (fragmentation injuries) fall into the category of high-velocity wounds, they are very different to a conventional high-velocity bullet wound. Typically, blast injuries are recognized to cause up to four different patterns of injury, which may all coexist:
- Primary injuries are caused by the pressure waves, both positive and negative, that emanate from a blast. They cause internal injuries such as blast lung, ruptured eardrums, and bowel perforation.
- Secondary injuries are due to fragments causing penetrating wounds and are managed as above.
- Tertiary injuries are caused by the victim being forced back against solid objects and sustaining blunt/penetrating trauma.

- Quaternary injuries are caused by secondary damage from the explosion, such as fire, falling objects, or falls from broken objects.

All four types of injuries may coexist, but the primary and secondary types are more common in patients close to the epicenter of the blast. Quaternary injuries are rare in open-space blasts, but common in urban explosions.

Management

The management consists of the standard ABCDE approach, with immediate management of life-threatening injuries. Particular problems include:

- Deafness from primary shock wave, which may make the patient very confused and may also apparently compound any neurological injury.
- Blast lung, which is similar to ARDS and is thought to be due to a combination of over- and under-pressure on the lung. It may lead to pneumothorax, shear injury to the lung, and tracheo-bronchial rupture. It is the most common cause of death in patients who survive the initial blast.
- Penetration of multiple missiles, often contaminated by other objects during bomb preparation. This should be managed as for conventional penetrating trauma. Gross contamination of these wounds is more common than in conventional high-velocity missile wounds.
- Blast injuries from shock waves that precede the fragment injuries.
- Burns from thermal energy.
- Rib fractures and underlying pulmonary contusion due to impact from tertiary/quaternary injuries.

A high index of suspicion for blast lung, as well as repeated clinical assessment, is essential to identify and treat the respiratory complications of blast injury.

6.19 Miscellaneous lung disease

Pulmonary arteriovenous malformations and hereditary haemorrhagic telangiectasia

Causes
- Hereditary haemorrhagic telangiectasia (HHT) accounts for at least 70% of all pulmonary arteriovenous malformations (PAVMs) (two genotypes, HHT1 and HHT2).
- Acquired PAVMs account for the other 30%, e.g. trauma, mitral stenosis, schistosomiasis, metastatic thyroid carcinoma.

Pathophysiology
- PAVMs are abnormal communications between pulmonary arteries and veins but may be fed by bronchial arteries (5% of cases).
- Precise pathogenesis is unclear.
- Gene mutations involving the TGF-β superfamily lead to abnormal vascular growth and development, e.g. endoglin (HHT1) and ALK-1 (HHT2), BMPR2 (pulmonary artery hypertension, PAH).

Epidemiology
- Female:male 2:1
- Uncommon in infancy and childhood.
- The size and number of lesions increase with age.

Clinical features
- HHT symptoms may develop before age 20, but acquired PAVMs typically develop later, between the fourth and sixth decades.
- Haemoptysis (may be massive) or haemothorax if PAVMs adjacent to the pleural surface rupture.
- Dyspnoea and arterial hypoxaemia at rest and/or on exercise.
- Platypnoea and orthodeoxia (dyspnoea and desaturation on adopting an upright position and relieved by recumbency, due to increased right-to-left intrapulmonary shunting).
- Migraines, strokes, and cerebral abscesses from paradoxical embolization.
- Pulmonary hypertension develops in ~10% of patients with PAVMs and HHT (type 2).
- Pregnancy
  - PAVMs will enlarge during pregnancy due to increased blood volume and cardiac output.
  - Beware of the possibility of spinal arteriovenous malformations (AVMs) in HHT patients if epidural anaesthesia is considered.

Investigations
CXR
- 1–5-cm nodules, but can be as large as 10cm, >50% in the lower lung fields and 80% involve the pleura.

Identify the presence of right-to-left intrapulmonary shunts
- Contrast echocardiography using agitated saline is most sensitive.
- Shunt fraction measurement (abnormal if >5%).

- Radionuclide lung perfusion scanning with imaging of the brain and kidneys.

Locate and assess anatomy of AVMs
- CTPA.
- Pulmonary angiography.

Assess pulmonary haemodynamics
- To exclude significant pulmonary hypertension prior to embolization of PAVMs.

Medical treatment
- Percutaneous coil embolization.

Hepatopulmonary syndrome
Hepatopulmonary syndrome (HPS) is characterized by the presence of intrapulmonary vascular dilatations in patients with established chronic liver disease of any aetiology leading to intrapulmonary shunting and significant arterial hypoxaemia. It can also develop in acute ischaemic hepatitis. The presence of orthodeoxia is strongly suggestive of HPS. The diagnosis is made by demonstrating an increased alveolar–arterial oxygen gradient and intrapulmonary shunting by contrast echocardiography. HPS independently worsens the prognosis of patients with cirrhosis. Liver transplantation confers a survival benefit and frequently leads to resolution of HPS, but the time course of resolution is variable.

Bronchiectasis
Causes
- Idiopathic ~50% of cases.
- Post-infectious (incidence is falling in developed countries with the widespread use of antimicrobial therapy).
  - Childhood infections, e.g. measles, pertussis.
  - Mycobacterial infections.
  - Pneumonia.
- Bronchial obstruction (tumour, foreign body, extrinsic compression).
- Allergic bronchopulmonary aspergillosis.
- α1-antitrypsin deficiency.
- Associated with inflammatory diseases, e.g. rheumatoid arthritis, Sjogren's syndrome, ulcerative colitis.
- Recurrent aspiration.
- Immunodeficiency, e.g. common variable immunodeficiency, selective IgA deficiency.
- Impaired mucocilliary clearance, e.g. cystic fibrosis, primary cilia dyskinesia (defective cilia), Young's syndrome (viscous mucus).
- Lymphatic obstruction.
  - Yellow nail syndrome (lymphoedema, pleural effusions, atrophic nails).

Pathophysiology
Bronchi are distorted and dilated due to a vicious cycle of defective host defenses and/or mucociliary clearance, microbial infections, and/or colonization and inflammation.

Clinical features
- Chronic cough productive of purulent sputum.
- Haemoptysis.
- Airflow limitation.

Investigations
Blood tests
- Autoantibodies, e.g. antinuclear antibody (ANA), rheumatoid factor (RhF), ANCA.
- Serum immunoglobulin levels (total and subclasses).
- Functional antibody levels after receiving vaccines for *Streptococcus pneumoniae*, tetanus and *Haemophilus influenzae*.
- Total IgA, IgE, and IgG levels for aspergillus.
- α1-antitrypsin level.

Sputum (and TB) cultures
HRCT of chest
- Dilated, thick-walled, non-tapering bronchi.
- Mucus plugs.
- Air trapping.

Bronchoscopy
- To exclude endobronchial obstruction.

Nasal biopsy if primary ciliary dyskinesia is suspected
Sweat test and genetics study if CF is suspected
Medical treatment of non-CF bronchiectasis
Evidence from RCTs is lacking.

Acute exacerbations
- For outpatients, a broad-spectrum oral antibiotic active against *H. influenzae* and *P. aeruginosa* for a minimum of 7–10 days, e.g. fluoroquinolones.
- For hospitalized patients, two intravenous anti-pseudomonal antibiotics with different mechanisms of action.
- The benefit of oral corticosteroids is unclear.

Maintenance therapy
- Inhaled corticosteroids.
- Prophylactic antibiotic use (various strategies).
  - Daily fluoroquinolone or daily clarithromycin/erythromycin or thrice-weekly azithromycin or nebulized anti-pseudomonal antibiotics, e.g. gentamicin, tobramycin.
- Sputum clearance techniques.
- Mucolytics—inhaled dry powder mannitol is being studied.

Haemoptysis
Bronchial artery embolization.

Bronchiolitis

Bronchiolitis and bronchiolitis obliterans are general terms describing inflammation in the small airways (measuring <2mm in diameter) leading to airflow obstruction and air trapping.

Cause
- Idiopathic.
- Inhalation of toxic agents/irritants.
- Drugs.
- Infections.
- Connective tissue disease, e.g. RA, SLE, Sjogren's syndrome, dermatomyositis.
- Post-organ transplantation, e.g. bone marrow, lung, heart–lung.

Constrictive, proliferative bronchiolitis and diffuse panbronchiolitis describe the underlying histopathological features. Treatment is directed at the underlying aetiology. Other therapies include oral and inhaled corticosteroids, inhaled bronchodilators, and macrolides. Diffuse panbronchiolitis mainly affects the Japanese and requires a prolonged course of macrolides (6–24 months).

Cystic fibrosis

Pathophysiology
- The most common inherited disease in Caucasian populations (autosomal recessive).
- Caused by mutations (~1200 identified) in a single gene on chromosome 7 (defective gene frequency ~4%) encoding for CFTR protein, functioning as a regulated chloride channel on cell surfaces.
- Abnormal chloride channel function causes the production of viscous secretions and impaired mucociliary clearance in the respiratory, gastrointestinal, and genitourinary tracts.
- Phenotypic expression is variable and depends on the underlying genetic patterns.
- High morbidity and mortality due to progressive lung disease and eventual respiratory failure.

Epidemiology
- In the UK, 96% of those affected are Caucasians.
- The live birth rate is 1 in 2500.

Clinical features
- Rhinosinusitis.
- Bronchiectasis.

Common pathogens causing chronic infection and acute exacerbations:
  - Pseudomonas aeruginosa.
  - Burkholderia cepacia complex (associated with more rapid decline of lung function and shortened survival).
  - Staph. aureus, H. influenzae.
  - Atypical mycobacteria, Aspergillus species.
- Haemoptysis (may be brisk).
- Spontaneous pneumothorax.

- Gastrointestinal complications: pancreatic insufficiency, distal intestinal obstructive syndrome, cholelithiasis.
- Diabetes.
- Osteoporosis.
- Infertility and subfertility.

Treatment of lung disease
Bronchodilators
Antibiotics
- Acute exacerbations.
  - Oral antibiotics for 14–21 days for mild exacerbations.
  - Intravenous antibiotics for 10–14 days, two agents directed by bacterial sensitivity.
- Maintenance therapy
  - Oral azithromycin three times weekly improves lung function.
  - Nebulized tobramycin for 1 month on alternate months improves lung function and reduces exacerbation rates in patients chronically infected with *P. aeruginosa*.

Corticosteroids
- Short courses of oral steroids for acute exacerbations in patients with reversible airflow obstruction or allergic bronchopulmonary aspergillosis.

DNase
- Nebulized DNase 2.5mg daily improves lung function.

Chest physiotherapy
Exercise
Others
- Pneumothorax is managed as for non-CF patients. Pleurodesis does not preclude subsequent lung transplantation.
- Bronchial artery embolization for massive haemoptysis.

Ventilation support
Nocturnal NIV is indicated for patients with daytime hypercapnia as a bridge to lung transplantation.

Lung transplantation
- The median age at transplantation is 26 years.
- Survival rates at 1 year, 5 years, and 10 years are 82%, 62%, and 51%, respectively, in a large UK cohort.

Lung transplantation
Epidemiology
~1700–2200 procedures performed for all conditions annually worldwide.

Cause of respiratory failure
Primary graft dysfunction
- Develops in the first 72h post transplantation.
- Manifests as ARDS.

- Caused by injury to the transplanted lung inflicted by retrieval/cold storage, reperfusion, mechanical ventilation, and post-transplant factors such as fluid overload, aspiration, and hypotension.
- Leading cause of death in the first year post transplantation.

Acute graft rejection

- Characterized by cough, fever, decline in lung function, infiltrates on CXR/HRCT.
- The risk is greatest in the first few months and declines with time.
- Recurrent episodes of acute rejection increase the risk of chronic rejection.

Chronic graft dysfunction

- Manifests as bronchiolitis obliterans syndrome (BOS)
  - Symptoms of respiratory tract infections or progressive dyspnoea.
  - Progressive airflow obstruction.
  - No effective treatment after onset.
  - CMV infection increases risk.
- Present in 50% of recipients at 5 years.
- Leading cause of death after the first year post transplantation.

Infections

- Bacterial bronchitis/pneumonia.
- PCP, viruses notably CMV, fungi.

Management

Differentiation between graft rejection and infection

- BAL may show a predominance of lymphocytes in rejection and polymorphonuclear cells +/– pathogens on special staining in infections (except for CMV infection, which causes a lymphocytic response).
- Transbronchial biopsy may show lymphocytic inflammation centred around the vessels +/– airways in rejection vs alveoli in infections.

Treatment

- Primary graft dysfunction.
  - Ventilatory support.
  - Nitric oxide.
  - ECMO in severe cases.
- Augmented immunosuppression for severe rejection.
- Antibiotics +/– antifungal +/– antiviral agents for infections.

Survival

- The overall median survival of lung transplantation is 5 years (data from the International Society for Heart and Lung Transplantation 2007).

Management of immunosuppression in severe illness

- Patients with lung transplants may present with severe sepsis, or indeed other coincidental illnesses. They will be receiving immunosuppressive therapy.
- Consider withdrawal of cyclosporine in profound sepsis or renal failure. Steroids should be continued and doses may need to be increased in severely unwell patients.

Unusual diffuse parenchymal lung diseases
Amyloidosis

Pathophysiology

Extracellular deposition of fibrils composed of a variety of precursor proteins that normally circulate in the plasma.

Amyloid light chain amyloid

Immunoglobulin light chain as precursor protein, associated with plasma cell dyscrasias, e.g. myeloma and Waldenstrom's macroglobulinaemia.

Amyloid A amyloid

Amyloid A (acute phase protein) as precursor protein, associated with chronic inflammatory or infective disorders.

Pulmonary manifestations

- Tracheobronchial infiltration may cause hoarseness, stridor, endobronchial obstruction.
- Pleural effusions.
- Lung nodules.

Extra-pulmonary manifestations

Heart

- Cardiomyopathy, dysrhythmias, myocardial ischaemia.

Skin

- Subcutaneous nodules/plaques, purpura.

Renal

- Proteinuria, nephrotic syndrome, chronic renal failure.

Gastrointestinal

- Hepatomegaly +/− splenomegaly, bleeding, dysmotility, malabsorption.

Bone

- Arthropathy, muscle enlargement.

Neurological

- Carpal tunnel syndrome, mixed sensory and motor peripheral neuropathy.

Treatment

- Bronchoscopic or surgical resection of pulmonary amyloid deposits.
- No specific treatment for organ damage.

Alveolar proteinosis

Pathophysiology

- Terminal bronchioles and alveolar sacs are filled with an amorphous, periodic acid-Schiff (PAS) positive lipoproteinaceous material.
- No associated lung inflammation or distortion.
- Idiopathic or associated with high-level dust exposures (e.g. silica), haematological malignancies, or following bone marrow transplant for myeloid malignancies.
- May be related to alveolar macrophage dysfunction and relative deficiency of GM-CSF.

Clinical features
- Asymptomatic or cough, dyspnoea, low-grade fever, malaise.
- CXR/HRCT—symmetrical ground-glass opacities.
- BAL fluid has a milky and opaque appearance.
- Alveolar macrophages are filled with a PAS-positive amorphous material.

Treatment
- Whole lung lavage with 10–15L of saline via a double-lumen ETT under general anaesthesia.
- GM-CSF.
- Lung transplantation.

Langerhans cell histiocytosis
Pathophysiology
- Precise pathogenesis is unknown.
- May be due to immune dysfunction involving the Langerhans cells (differentiated cells of the monocyte–macrophage lineage and function as antigen-presenting cells).
- May affect a single or multiple sites, e.g. the lung, brain, bones, skin, and lymph nodes.

Epidemiology
- Commonly affects adults aged 20–40 years.
- Strongly linked to cigarette smoking.

Pulmonary manifestations
- Dyspnoea, cough, chest pain, fever, malaise, and weight loss (asymptomatic in 20%).
- CXR/HRCT— nodules, cysts, or interstitial fibrosis affecting upper and mid zones.
- Complications—pneumothorax, pulmonary arterial hypertension, and veno-occlusive disease.

Extra-pulmonary manifestations
Skin
- Papular rash, oral and genital ulcers, gingival hypertrophy.

Pituitary gland
- Diabetes insipidus.

Bone
- Cysts and bone pain.

Treatment
- Smoking cessation—mandatory
- Corticosteroids may be beneficial in nodular disease.

Lymphangioleiomyomatosis
Pathophysiology
- Proliferation of atypical smooth muscle cells around and within the bronchovascular structures and lymphatics.

- Oestrogen is thought to play a role as women of child-bearing age are almost exclusively affected, either occurring sporadically or with tuberous sclerosis complex.

Pulmonary manifestations
- Progressive formation of diffuse thin-walled cysts measuring 0.1cm to several cm in diameter.
  - Recurrent pneumothoraces.
  - Airflow obstruction and hyperinflation resembling emphysema.
  - Progressive respiratory failure in most cases.
- Haemoptysis.
- Chylous pleural effusions.
- Pulmonary hypertension.

Extra-pulmonary manifestations
- Renal angiomyolipomas (benign tumours made up of adipose tissue, smooth muscle cells, and thickened blood vessels).
- Abdominal lymphangioleiomyomas (cystic lymphatic masses).
- Chylous ascites.
- Meningiomas.

Treatment
- Anti-oestrogens have been tried with no proven benefit.
- Studies of sirolimus are currently underway.
- Lung transplantation.

Neurofibromatosis
Pathophysiology
- Autosomal dominant.
- Arise from mutations in the NF1 (NF type 1) and NF2 (NF type 2) genes coding for tumour suppressor proteins.

Clinical features
NF type 1
- Café-au-lait spots.
- Axillary or inguinal freckling.
- Peripheral neurofibromas may cause skin nodules, nerve pain, spinal cord compression.
- Lisch nodules (pigmented hamartomas on the iris).
- CNS and soft tissue tumours.

NF type 2
- Few cutaneous manifestations.
- High incidence of CNS tumours, e.g. acoustic neuromas, meningiomas, spinal cord schwannomas, and gliomas.

Pulmonary manifestations of NF type 1
- Cystic and bullous changes with an upper lobe predominance, basal fibrosis, and ground-glass opacities have been reported in case series.
- Uncertain if lung disease is a primary manifestation of NF type 1.
- Others, e.g. rib deformity, lung neoplasms, kyphoscoliosis.
- No specific treatment.

Index